Handbook of Experimental Pharmacology

Continuation of Handbuch der experimentellen Pharmakologie

Vol. 55/III

Psychotropic Agents

Part III: Alcohol and Psychotomimetics, Psychotropic Effects of Central Acting Drugs

Contributors

L. G. Abood · G. K. Aghajanian · J. B. Appel · W. O. Boggan
D. A. Buxton · H. Coper · T. L. Chruściel · J. Ellingboe · C.-J. Estler
D. X. Freedman · H. J. Gärtner · S. R. Goldberg · D. T. Greenwood
H. Halbach · H. Heimann · L. E. Hollister · D. M. Kuhn · W. R. Martin
R. Mechoulam · N. K. Mello · J. H. Mendelson · D. N. Middlemiss
A. D. Poling · H. E. Shannon · A. T. Shulgin · R. D. Spealman

Editors

F. Hoffmeister · G. Stille

Springer-Verlag Berlin Heidelberg New York 1982

Professor Dr. F. Hoffmeister
Bayer AG, Institut für Pharmakologie, Aprather Weg 18a, D-5600 Wuppertal 1

Professor Dr. G. Stille
Institut für Arzneimittel des Bundesgesundheitsamtes,
Stauffenbergstraße 13, D-1000 Berlin 30

With 21 Figures

ISBN-13: 978-3-642-67772-4 e-ISBN-13: 978-3-642-67770-0
DOI: 10.1007/978-3-642-67770-0

Preface

The description of the pharmacology of psychotomimetics, cannabis, and alcohol in this third volume concludes the discussion on psychotropic agents.

As psychomotor stimulants these groups of psychotropic agents are of little or no therapeutic relevance, but since they are used in a nonmedical manner, or are even considered by some groups of the population as social commodities, their behavioral effects and psychopharmacological properties are not the concern of the pharmacologist alone. The same is true of psychotomimetics, as well as cannabis and its components. Psychotomimetics have a social history going back many hundreds of years and are among the most potent psychotropic agents known to man.

The closing description of psychopharmacology also deals with the psychotropic effects of a number of drugs not primarily considered to be psychotropic. Their psychotropic effects are either an inherent constituent of their therapeutic profile, as is the case with opiates, hypnotics, and caffeine, or they may occur indirectly as side effects or accompanying effects during therapy. This applies to β-adrenoreceptor antagonists and anticholinergics.

The editors are also aware that a description of psychotropic agents would not have been complete without discussing the medical, ethical, and legal aspects of the development, clinical testing, and use of such drugs.

Conscious of the fact that it is almost impossible to describe and discuss psychopharmacology completely, the editors express the hope that those topics of major importance have been included. It would not have been possible to compile the three volumes on psychotropic agents without the cooperation of numerous scientists from all over the world. Therfore, the editors would like to express their gratitude to all those who cooperated in making it possible to publish those three volumes.

Wuppertal/Berlin

F. Hoffmeister · G. Stille

List of Contributors

Professor Dr. L. G. Abood, University of Rochester, Center of Brain Research, Medical Center, Rochester, NY 14642/USA

Professor Dr. G. K. Aghajanian, Departments of Psychiatry and Pharmacology, Yale University School of Medicine and the Connecticut Mental Health Center, 3400 Park Street, New Haven, CT 06508/USA

Professor Dr. J. B. Appel, Behavioral Pharmacology Laboratory, Department of Psychology, University of South Carolina, Columbia, SC 29208/USA

Professor Dr. W. O. Boggan, Department of Psychiatry and Biochemistry, Medical University of South Carolina, Charleston, SC 29403/USA

Dr. D. A. Buxton, ICI Imperial Chemical Industries Ltd., Pharmaceuticals Division, Mereside Alderley Park, GB-Macclesfield, Ches. SK 10 4TG

Professor Dr. H. Coper, Institut für Neuropsychopharmakologie der Freien Universität, Ulmenallee 30, D-1000 Berlin 19

Professor Dr. T. L. Chruściel, Institute for Drug Research and Control, 30/34 Chałmska, P-00725 Warsaw

Dr. J. Ellingboe, Alcohol and Drug Abuse Research Center, Harvard Medical School, The McLean Hospital, 115 Mill Street, Belmont, MA 02178/USA

Professor Dr. C.-J. Estler, Institut für Pharmakologie und Toxikologie der Universität Erlangen-Nürnberg, Universitätsstraße 22, D-8520 Erlangen

Professor Dr. D. X. Freedman, University of Chicago, Department of Psychiatry, 950 East 59th Street, Chicago, IL 60637/USA

Dr. H. J. Gärtner, Psychiatrische Universitätsklinik, Osianderstraße 22, D-7400 Tübingen

Dr. S. R. Goldberg, National Institute on Drug Abuse, Addiction Research Center, P.O. Box 12390, Lexington, KY 40583/USA

Dr. D. T. Greenwood, ICI Imperial Chemical Industries Ltd., Pharmaceuticals Division, Mereside Alderley Park, GB-Macclesfield, Ches. SK 10 4TG

Professor Dr. H. Halbach, D-8210 Prien, Stetten

Professor Dr. H. Heimann, Psychiatrische Universitätsklinik, Osianderstraße 22, D-7400 Tübingen

Dr. L. E. HOLLISTER, Stanford University School, Veterans Administration Hospital, 3801 Miranda Avenue, Palo Alto, CA 94304/USA

Dr. D. M. KUHN, Behavioral Pharmacology Laboratory, Department of Psychology, University of South Carolina, Columbia, SC 29208/USA

Professor Dr. W. R. MARTIN, University of Kentucky, Albert B. Chandler Medical Center, College of Medicine, Department of Pharmacology, Lexington, KY 40536/USA

Professor Dr. R. MECHOULAM, The Hebrew University of Jerusalem, Department of Natural Products, IL-Jerusalem

Professor Dr. N. K. MELLO, Alcohol and Drug Abuse Research Center, Harvard Medical School, The McLean Hospital, 115 Mill Street, Belmont, MA 02178/USA

Dr. J. H. MENDELSON, Alcohol and Drug Abuse Research Center, Harvard Medical School, The McLean Hospital, 115 Mill Street, Belmont, MA 92178/USA

Dr. D. N. MIDDLEMISS, ICI Imperial Chemical Industries Ltd., Pharmaceuticals Division, Mereside Alderley Park, GB-Macclesfield, Ches. SK 10 4TG

Professor Dr. A. D. POLING, Western Michigan University, Department of Psychology, Kalamazoo, MI 49008/USA

Dr. H. E. SHANNON, National Institute on Drug Abuse, Addiction Research Center P.O. Box 12390, Lexington, KY 40583/USA

Dr. A. T. SHULGIN, 1483 Shulgin Road, Lafayette, CA 94549/USA

Dr. R. D. SPEALMAN, Harvard Medical School, New England Regional Primate Research Center, Southborough, MA/USA

Contents

Psychotomimetics

CHAPTER 1

Chemistry of Psychotomimetics. A. T. SHULGIN

CHAPTER 2

Pharmacology and Toxicology of Psychotomimetics. L. E. HOLLISTER. With 2 Figures

Cannabis

CHAPTER 7

Chemistry of Cannabis. R. MECHOULAM. With 6 Figures

CHAPTER 8

Pharmacology and Toxicology of Cannabis. H. COPER

Alcohol

CHAPTER 9

General Pharmacology and Toxicology of Alcohol. T. L. CHRUŚCIEL

CHAPTER 10

Behavioral Pharmacology of Alcohol. N. K. MELLO. With 4 Figures

CHAPTER 11

Biochemical Pharmacology of Alcohol. J. ELLINGBOE and J. H. MENDELSON

CHAPTER 12

Dependence-Producing Effects and Alcohol Dependence Syndrome
T. L. CHRUŚCIEL. With 1 Figure

Psychotropic Effects of Central Acting Drugs

CHAPTER 13

Psychotropic Effects of Opioids and Opioid Antagonists. S. R. GOLDBERG, R. D. SPEALMAN, and H. E. SHANNON

CHAPTER 14

Hypnotics. W. R. Martin. With 2 Figures

CHAPTER 15

Anticholinergics. L. G. ABOOD. With 3 Figures

Contents

Part I: Antipsychotics and Antidepressants

Contents

Part II: Anxiolytics, Gerontopsychopharmacological Agents, and Psychomotor Stimulants

Anxiolytics

Gerontopsychopharmacological Agents

Psychotomimetics

CHAPTER 1

Chemistry of Psychotomimetics

A. T. SHULGIN

A. Introduction

A presentation and discussion of the psychotomimetic drugs in a handbook concerned with psychotropic agents must, at the onset, emphasize the several properties that make this class of materials unique.

Most psychotropic drugs are intended to be either curative or cosmetic. They may be used to reverse a pathologic mental state, or they may be intended to alleviate a persistent symptom which, in turn, might then allow some normal repair process to take effect. In either case, treatment is provided a patient who shows some psychological inadequacy with the intent of normalization. The psychotomimetics, on the other hand, are generally studied in subjects who have good psychological balance. To the extent that the effects are considered disruptive, the rationale of research is the generation of an intoxication that bears some superficial resemblance to a psychosis. When such a transient and reversible "model psychosis" is produced, biochemical and psychological changes can both be observed. But to the extent that the effects are considered constructive, there are benefits to be found in the areas of insight, changes of motivation, self-analysis, entertainment, and even simply escape. These results may be effected through a process of disorganization and reorganization, by a sensory elaboration such as visual or auditory enhancement, or by intense reverie or fantasy. There has been only limited experimentation with these drugs in the treatment of pathologic states, and so there has been little recognition of any potential medical utility. This limitation, along with a generalized abuse potential inherent in such drugs, has led to severe legal classifications which have, paradoxically, further restricted human experimentation. This latter point is exacerbated by another unique property. The effects that are observed such as changes in interpretation, in insight, and in communicability, can be assayed only in man. At the present time, no assays or behavioral tests in animals exist that allow satisfactory prediction of the qualitative nature of a new and unexplored psychotomimetic drug.

Thus, this group of drugs stands apart from the remainder of the psychotropic drugs and must be discussed in terms other than those of neuropathy, pathology, and related clinical presentations. Rather, a generalized chemical subdivision will be made predicated upon structure and grouped with reference to the principal neurotransmitters. Functional relationships with these endogenous factors are still controversial.

I. Terminology

A number of names are currently in use to identify this group of drugs. "Psychotomimetic," the adjective used in this chapter, literally means psychosis-imitating. In the early work with these materials, it was believed that they led to an authentic psychotic state and might be of value in the search for endogenous psychotoxins or in biochemical unbalances that might he correlated with such mental states. To a clinician who interacts with mentally ill patients, these experiences might increase both understanding and compassion if he were to experience within himself the "psychotomimetic" syndrome. This concept fell into complete disrepute a decade ago, but today it has a balanced acceptability. The name remains neutral and medically unbiased and will be used in this chapter. The term "hallucinogen" is widely used, but it implies that the generation of hallucinations is a general property and, in fact, synthetic imagery of undocumentable origins is a rare property of these drugs. A third term, also widely used, is "psychedelic", which was coined in the mid-1960s to indicate mind-manifesting or mind-expanding properties. The term, however, has become associated with the broad and occasionally irresponsible popular use of these drugs. It is rarely seen in the medical and scientific literature due to the connotation of both condoning and encouraging paramedical use. The term "psychodysleptic" has been routinely employed in Europe for drugs of this classification to emphasize similarities to the psycholeptics (mood depressants) and psychoanaleptics (mood stimulators). A host of other terms proposed over the years (e.g., phantastica, delirients, schizogens, eidetikas, etc.) have historic interest but have never found wide acceptance.

II. Methods of Assay

Three broad areas of scientific discipline have been employed to rank and to attempt to explain the quantitative nature of the psychotomimetic drugs. The molecular structures of the active drugs themselves have been dissected and interpreted in completely physical terms; the materials have been titrated in animal models in a search for behavioral correlates that might relate to human activity; and most precisely, they have been studied in clinical experiments using humans.

The physical approach to explanations of biologic activity has been exclusively concerned with the geometry and measurable properties of the chemicals themselves. Intramolecular hydrogen bonding is a measurable property that can explain stabilization of unusual conformations (SMYTHIES et al., 1970), and it is widely felt that in the case of bifunctional molecules, the establishment of parameters, such as the separation of charged sites, might allow some definition of sites of action (KELLEY and ADAMSON, 1973). The natural molecular configuration of psychotomimetics can be determined using X-ray crystallography (BAKER et al., 1973), but these data are obtained from solid samples, whereas these drugs are, by definition, only active in solution. Computer calculations of orbital charge densities and charge distributions (SNYDER and MERRIL, 1965) have been correlated with potency, as have empirical measurements such as partition coefficients (BARFKNECHT et al., 1975) and strengths of charge transfer complexes (SUNG and PARKER, 1972). Such properties are, in general, simple to measure or calculate precisely, but successful generalizations have been restricted to studies of small classes of closely related drugs. There has been no successful extrapolation to new chemicals.

Biologic titration in animal models has given a wider correlation, but one which still lacks behavioral logic. In vitro experiments have concentrated largely on interactions of selected psychotomimetics with neurotransmitters. Their agonist or antagonist action on serotoninergic, dopaminergic, or cholinergic preparations often correlates closely with their relative potency in man, but a causal explanation for their action is not yet satisfactory. A number of in vivo tests have been developed, such as field behavior (BRIMBLECOMBE, 1963) and interference with conditioned responses in rats (SMYTHIES et al., 1969; TILSON and SPARBER, 1973), head twitching (CORNE and PICKERING, 1967) and interference with nest-building behavior of mice (SCHNEIDER and CHENOWETH, 1970), and the development of bizarre action patterns in cats (BENINGTON et al., 1958; JACOBS et al., 1977). None of these behavior patterns can be reasonably associated with the subtle effects of these drugs in man. An instructive example is the measure of psychotomimetic drugs on the body temperature of rabbits. In rectal hyperthermia measurements, a positive correlation between body temperature and psychotomimetic potency has been found to encompass drugs varying widely in chemical type, from the least potent (mescaline) to the most potent (LSD) (ALDOUS et al., 1974). Two recent critical analyses of these several behavioral systems (SILVA and CALIL, 1975; KUHN et al., 1977) have discussed their limited value.

A final weakness of many of these in vivo studies is that the level of drug used is often near a lethal dose for the species in question, and the responses observed may well be compounded by changes in the vital processes themselves.

The most reliable measure of the psychotomimetic character of a drug, but the most difficult to obtain, comes from clinical studies on human subjects. These are both ethically and legally difficult to perform. The ethical considerations involve the necessity of enlisting normal volunteers in good mental health, who must consent to a study wherein there will certainly be some disruption of this "normal" status. The classic requirements of a double-blind study, i.e., that the capsule with the active drug and the subject to whom it is given should be unknown to both the subject and the experimenter, are inapplicable. When the expected actions are those that embrace subtleties such as insight and interpretation of sensory integrity, it is obligatory to advise the subject of these possibilities, and the concept of "double-conscious" has gained acceptance (ALLES, 1959; SHULGIN et al., 1969). This implies a knowledge on the part of both the experimenter and the subject of the nature and the extent of psychological changes that might be expected. The legal complications result from the passage of statutes (at least in the United States) that effectively prohibit research with scheduled drugs (i.e., those with no recognized medical utility) in human subjects, without extensive approval and permission. New psychotomimetic drugs, those that are not legally recognized, can be studied with fewer restrictions, but the therapeutic potential of the better known materials will remain unexploited within the present structure.

III. Classification

The central action of the psychotomimetic drugs requires, by definition, that they express their effects by interference with the several neurotransmitters known to be of primary importance in the regulation and function of the central nervous system. There are a number of major neurotransmitters, directly or indirectly involved in the sensory, affective, and cognitive processes, any and all of which can be shown to be interfered with during the action of a psychotomimetic drug. The highest concentrations of serotonin are found in the brain stem and the hypothalamus. Destruction of the raphe system (rich in serotoninergic fibers) leads to sleeplessness in experimental animals, whereas the pharmacologic depletion of serotonin in the hypothalamus leads to sedation. This neurotransmitter, in these areas, appears to integrate the mechanisms that are associated with reactivity to external stimuli and that are reflected in the parasympathetic branch of the autonomic nervous system. The catecholamines, specifically dopamine and norepinephrine and to a lesser extent epinephrine, are also widely distributed in the brain, dopamine being most concentrated in the basic ganglia and norepinephrine, again largely in the hypothalamus. It is still unclear if any of these bases actually plays a primary role in neurotransmission in the brain, but certainly they act as regulators of synaptic transmission. The role of acetylcholine in the activation of cholinergic neurons is well established in brain neurochemistry, and it may well be these synaptic junctions that are modulated by the catecholamines and serotonin. GABA (γ-aminobutyric acid) has recently been accepted as a neurotransmitter playing an inhibitory role within the CNS. It, too, has agonists that will be discussed here.

It is convenient to arrange most of the known psychotomimetics into groups that appear to be chemically related to each of these neurotransmitters. It is appealing to think that each psychotomimetic drug might have some particular selectivity for the transmitter that it resembles (i.e., LSD for serotonin, both indoles; and mescaline for dopamine, both phenethylamines), but research has not allowed any such simple explanation of activity. Total brain biochemistry is an intricate interbalance of many neuronal amines working in concert, and it is this homeostasis that is disrupted by the administration of a psychotomimetic drug. In this chapter, the various psychotomimetics will be grouped on the basis of a resemblance of their structures to those of the neurotransmitters, but there should be no inference that these natural hormones are specifically or uniquely involved in the mechanism of action. These mechanisms, in the present state of pharmacology, are still largely unknown.

B. Psychotomimetics Structurally Related to Serotonin

Serotonin (1) contains an indole nucleus (2), which is substituted on the 3-position with a β-aminoethyl side chain, and on the 5-position with a hydroxyl group. The parent base of serotonin is tryptamine [(3-β-aminoethyl)indole] (3), and this structural moiety is found in a large number of psychotomimetic drugs. These will be presented

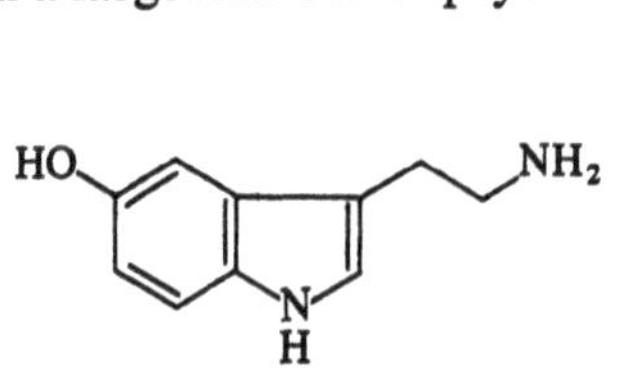

(1) Serotonin

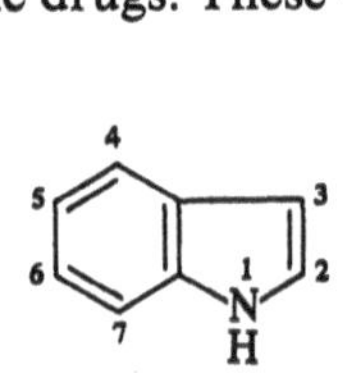

(2) Indole

in three subgroups: those that are indoles with chemical modifications on the chain nitrogen and/or on the aromatic ring; those that have the β-aminoethyl group brought into the form of a third ring system; and those that contain yet additional rings and structural complexity.

I. Indoles

All of the psychotomimetic indoles are substituted derivatives of tryptamine (3) with substituents located at one or more of the following locations: the aliphatic nitrogen, the aromatic ring, or the aliphatic chain α-position. These are indicated as areas (a), (b), and (c) in (3). Several drugs are known to be substituted in more than one location.

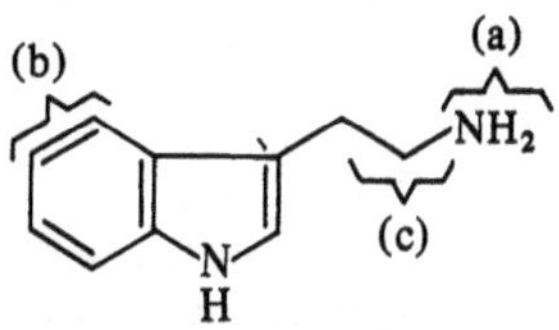

(3) Tryptamine

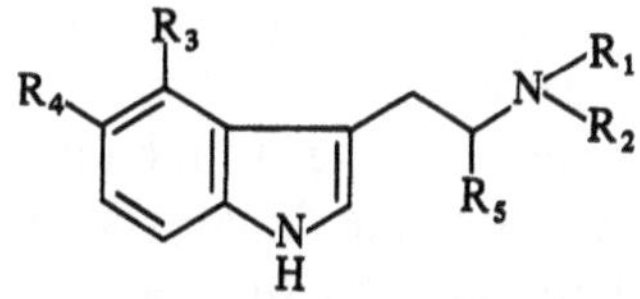

(4) Substituted tryptamine

1. Nitrogen-Substituted Tryptamine Derivatives

The *N*-substituted tryptamines that are known to be psychotomimetic are listed in Table 1. All are symmetrically disubstituted with aliphatic groups, and all are of approximately the same potency, active in man at between 60 and 100 mg. The simplest member, *N,N*-dimethyltryptamine (DMT, 4a) is known in nature, being a major alkaloid in a number of New World snuffs. It is rapidly deaminated in vivo following oral administration and so must be used parenterally or in admixture with an effective deaminase enzyme inhibitor. It has an unusually rapid onset of action (apparent within a minute or two following smoking or injection), and the effects are largely dissipated within an hour of administration. The diethyl homologue (DET, 4b) is slightly longer lived in action, and the higher homologues (4c, 4d, 4e) are separate in that they are active orally. DPT (4c) is of potential clinical use due to its rather abrupt termination of effect (GROF et al., 1973).

2. Ring-Substituted Tryptamine Derivatives

Psychotomimetic tryptamine derivatives are known in which there are oxygen substituents at either position 4 or position 5 of the indole nucleus, and in most cases the basic amine function is dialkylated.

The tryptamine analogues with an oxygen function in the 4-position of the indole ring (4f–4k) are all orally active and appreciably more potent than the parent refer-

Table 1. Nitrogen-substituted tryptamines (4) $R_3, R_4, R_5 = H$

Compound	R_1	R_2	Potency relative to DMT=1	Reference
4a DMT	$-CH_3$	$-CH_3$	1	SZARA (1956)
4b DET	$-CH_2CH_3$	$-CH_2CH_3$	1	SZARA (1957)
4c DPT	$n-C_3H_7$	$n-C_3H_7$	1	FAILLACE et al. (1967) SOSKIN et al. (1973)
4d DIPT	$i-C_3H_7$	$i-C_3H_7$	1.5	SHULGIN (1976)
4e	$-CH_2CH=CH_2$	$-CH_2CH=CH_2$	1	SZARA and HEARST (1962)

ence compound DMT (4a). The simplest of these, psilocin (4f) is a naturally occurring hallucinogenic component of the many "magic" mushrooms of the western hemisphere (HEIM and WASSON, 1962) where it is found to a large measure as the phosphate ester, psilocybin (4g). The two bases are approximately equivalent, both stoichiometrically and qualitatively in man, implying that dephosphorylation occurs metabolically. The demethylated homologues of psilocybin (*N*-monodemethyl, baeocystin; *N*-didemethyl, norbaeocystin) are reported congeners of psilocybin in several hallucinogenic species of mushroon (LEUNG and PAUL, 1967, 1968), but they are unexplored pharmacologically.

When the indolic oxygen function is located at the 5-position, the drugs become subject to the loss of the dimethylamino group by deamination (as with the simpler tryptamines) and thus are only active parenterally. 5-Methoxy-*N,N*-dimethyltryptamine (41) is found as a component of several snuff mixtures used by Indians in the New World. It has a remarkably rapid onset of action and a short duration (the entire intoxication cycle lasts perhaps 15 min). The analogue of 41 without the methyl group on the 5-position oxygen is a natural alkaloid known as bufotenine ($4,R_1,R_2=CH_3$; $R_3,R_5=H$; $R_4=OH$). This drug has been claimed to be psychotomimetic (FABING and HAWKINS, 1956), but it is now known to be a cardiovascular stimulant involving serotonin release (TURNER and MERLIS, 1959; ISBELL, 1967; FISCHER, 1968). The increase of bulk of the substituents on the terminal nitrogen seen in 4m again allows oral activity, as seen in the tryptamine counterparts in Table 2.

A second structural manipulation can be employed to protect the basic nitrogen from enzymatic deamination: the introduction of a methyl group alpha. This device is examined in more detail in Sect. C in the comparison of the phenethylamine and amphetamine structures. Within the tryptamines, α-methylation allows oral activity with the two psychotomimetics 4n and 4o.

II. Beta-Carbolines

The β-carboline ring system (5) has a great potential significance in brain biochemistry, as it can be synthesized in vitro under physiologic conditions from various natural tryptamines.

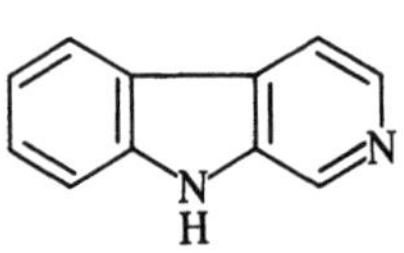

(5) β–Carboline

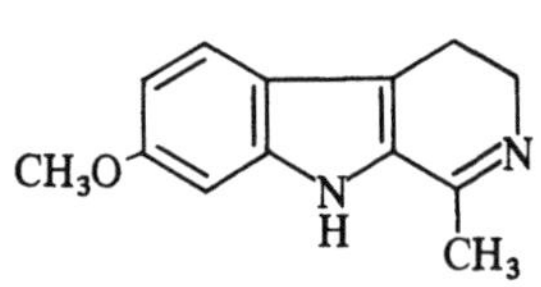

(6) Harmaline

Cyclization of biologic tryptamines can occur with formaldehyde or acetaldehyde to form tetrahydro-β-carbolines (called tryptalines), which are potent serotonin uptake inhibitors (KELLER et al., 1976) and monoamine oxidase inhibitors (MELLER et al., 1977). These products can be formed simply by the incubation of mammalian tissue (e.g., from the brain) with 5-methyl tetrahydrofolic acid as the source of formaldehyde (HSU and MANDELL, 1975; WYATT et al., 1975). Also, melatonin (5-methoxy-*N*-acetyltryptamine, a serotonin-derived natural hormone found in the pineal body) can be cyclized under physiologic conditions to form the biologically active carboline 6-methoxyharmalan (MCISAAC, 1961). A number of these "in vivo"-generated bases are

Table 2. Ring-substituted tryptamines (4)

Compound		R_1	R_2	R_3	R_4	R_5	Potency relative to DMT=1	Reference
4f	Psilocin	$—CH_3$	$—CH_3$	—OH	H	H	8	Wolbach et al. (1962)
4g	Psilocybin	$—CH_3$	$—CH_3$	$—OPO_3H_2$	H	H	6	Delay et al. (1959) Rinkel et al. (1960)
4h	CZ-74	$—C_2H_5$	$—C_2H_5$	—OH	H	H	8	Leuner and Baer (1965)
4i	CEY-19	$—C_2H_5$	$—C_2H_5$	$—OPO_3H_2$	H	H	6	Leuner and Baer (1965)
4j		$—CH_3$	$i—C_3H_7$	—OH	H	H	8	Repke and Shulgin (1979)
4k	4-OH-DIPT	$i—C_3H_7$	$i—C_3H_7$	—OH	H	H	4	Repke and Shulgin (1979)
4l	5-MeO-DMT	$—CH_3$	$—CH_3$	H	$—OCH_3$	H	10	Shulgin and Nichols (1978)
4m	5-OCH_3-DIPT	$i—C_3H_7$	$i—C_3H_7$	H	$—OCH_3$	H	10	Shulgin and Carter (1977)
4n	Monase-M	H	H	H	H	$—CH_3$	3	Hollister et al. (1960) Murphree et al. (1960)
4o	DMS	H	H	H	$—OCH_3$	$—CH_3$	20	Shulgin and Nichols (1978)

believed to be psychotomimetic agents, but efforts to document them as being endogenous factors in mental illness have failed.

The only β-carboline that has been extensively studies in man as a psychotomimetic agent is harmaline (6). It is the major active alkaloid found in the intoxicating South American drink *ayahuasca*, made from plants of the genus *Banisteriopsis*. As a pure chemical, harmaline is active in man at the 300–400 mg level, leading in many subjects to elaborate visual synthesis (NARANJO, 1973a), although in others there is little more than a generalized sedation. A second pharmacologic property of harmaline is that it is an effective inhibitor of the monoamine oxidase enzyme system (UDENFRIEND et al., 1968). Dimethyltryptamine (4a), which is normally inactive when given orally in man, is frequently found in *Banisteriopsis* extracts (POISSEN, 1965; AGURELL et al., 1968; DER MARDEROSIAN et al., 1968). Thus, the biologic activity of the native plant decoction may be due in large part to DMT that is protected from metabolic destruction by the presence of a relatively small amount of harmaline, itself without activity.

Several other substituted β-carbolines have been studied in man. Harmine [the completely aromatic counterpart of (6)] is inactive orally at levels of 1 g (PENNES and HOCH, 1957), but upon intravenous administration there are effects observed with doses of less than 50 mg (SLOTKIN et al., 1970). Limited studies (NARANJO, 1967) have been reported concerning the dihydroderivative of (6) (tetrahydroharmine) and the positional isomer of (6) in which the methoxyl is relocated into the position analogous to that found with serotonin (6-methoxy-harmalan); the former appears to be less active and the latter more active than harmaline itself.

III. Ergot-Related Drugs

All of the known psychotomimetic drugs that contain the alkaloid nucleus ergoline have a consistent structural feature of a carboxamide function at the 8-position and dehydration at the 9,10 position (see partial structure 7). The activity of this class of compounds is extremely sensitive to minor structural variations in this ring. Inversion of the hydrogen at the 5-position (to yield the isolysergic acid family), at the 8-position (to yield the L-lysergic acid family), and saturation of the 9,10-double bond (with hydrogen or solvent) all effectively eradicate the psychotomimetic properties of the product. Hydrogenation of the indolic double bond (to give 2,3-dihydro-LSD) reduces the potency by an order of magnitude (GORODETZKY and ISBELL, 1964). Although most of the better studied drugs are synthetic, they depend upon the use of lysergic acid as a starting material, and it must be obtained from natural sources.

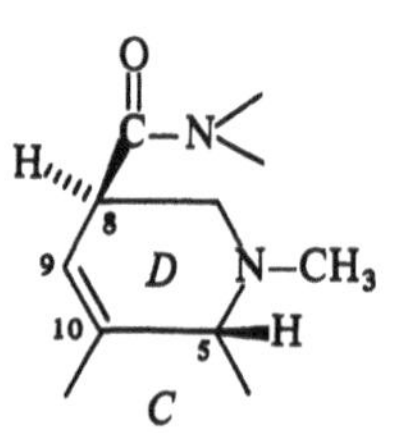

(7)
Ring D of the ergot alkaloids

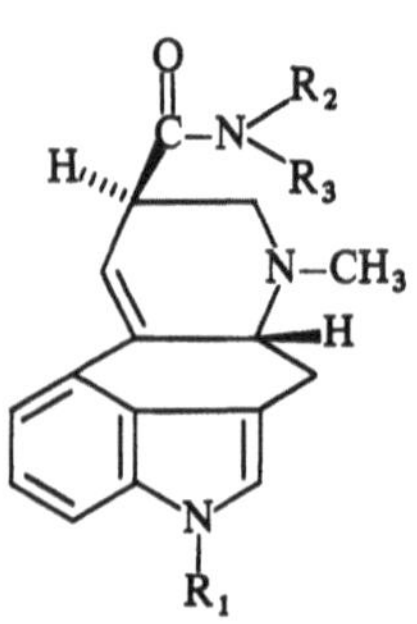

(8)

1. Synthetic Lysergic Acid Derivatives

The best studied of the synthetic ergot derivatives, and one of the most potent psychotomimetics yet reported, is the diethylamide, LSD (8, $R_1=H$; $R_2=R_3=C_2H_5$). It was originally prepared and studied in 1938 (STOLL and HOFMANN, 1943) as an ergot-related analogue of the medullary stimulant nikethamide (*N,N*-diethylnicotinamide). Its intense psychological effectiveness was discovered 5 years later. Its extremely high potency (50–250 µg, given orally) and the complexity and richness of the evoked response have prompted widespread experimentation. In the scientific community, its initial description as producing a model psychosis commanded the attention of researchers in the area of mental health. In the lay community, its fast-spreading reputation as a hallucinogenic drug quite literally ushered in the psychedelic era. There is a greater volume of literature – scientific, philosophic, and fictional – on this one material than on any other psychotomimetic drug.

The destructive effects of structural modification within the "D" ring mentioned above apply to LSD itself as well. However, substitution on the indolic nitrogen (1-position) or modifications of the identities of the amide nitrogen substituents can result in the maintenance of psychotomimetic activity albeit with some attenuation of potency. Table 3 lists these variations and their approximate potencies relative to LSD. Most of the homologues are less active than LSD, several are of similar potency, and none are of higher potency. Two of the listed compounds are pharmaceutical drugs: ergonovine (8 k, ergometrine) is used clinically as a uterine contractant, and methysergide (Sansert, 81) is popular as a prophylactic against migraine. The latter drug has shown side effects in clinical use similar to those seen with LSD, and the material has been employed as an LSD substitute in psychotherapeutic LSD therapy. The 2-bromo analogue of LSD (BOL-148) is of considerable pharmacologic interest, having served as a continuing challenge to proposed mechanisms of action in this family of drugs. It is even more potent than LSD as a serotonin antagonist (CERLETTI and ROTHLIN, 1955), but it is practically devoid of psychotomimetic activity (HOFMANN, 1959).

2. Natural Lysergic Acid Derivatives

A number of higher plants, largely of the family Convolvulaceae, are also sources of alkaloids of the lysergic acid family and have been employed as intoxicants. Three morning glory species are especially rich in centrally active bases and have proven active orally in man as psychotomimetics. The Aztec drug ololiuqui has been established botanically as *Rivea corymbosa* (SCHULTES, 1941). The Zapotecs employ, in addition to ololiuqui, a similar plant known as *badoh negro* which is the closely related morning glory *Ipomoea violacea* (MADDOUGALL, 1960); most of the many *Ipomoea* subspecies are, however, devoid of alkaloids (DER MARDEROSIAN and YOUNGKEN, 1966). The third plant of this group, and the richest yet known in alkaloid content, is the Hawaiian baby wood rose, *Argyeia nervosa*. Of the large number of alkaloids present in these species, the ones believed to account for the plants' activities are lysergamide (Ergine, 8 r) and the epimer with opposite configuration at the 8-position, isolysergamide. As a pure compound, isolysergamide produces a depressed and sedative effect at dosages of 2 mg (HOFMANN, 1963). The labile hydroxyethyl amides of these two bases are also present and might give rise by hydrolysis to the free amides. Ergonovine (8 k) is also present in small amounts and may contribute to the activity as well. The

Table 3. Lysergic acid amide derivatives (8)

Compound	R_1	R_2	R_3	Potency relative to LSD = + + + +[a]	Reference
8a LSD-25	H	$—CH_2CH_3$	$—CH_2CH_3$	+ + + +	
8b ALD-52	$—COCH_3$	$—CH_2CH_3$	$—CH_2CH_3$	+ + + +	ABRAMSON (1959)
8c OML-632	$—CH_2OH$	$—CH_2CH_3$	$—CH_2CH_3$	+ + +	ABRAMSON (1959) CERLETTI (1959)
8d MLD-41	$—CH_3$	$—CH_2CH_3$	$—CH_2CH_3$	+ + +	ABRAMSON (1959)
8e LAE-32	H	$—CH_2CH_3$	H	+ +	ROTHLIN (1957)
8f ALA-10	$—COCH_3$	$—CH_2CH_3$	H	+	USDIN and EFRON (1972a)
8g MLA-74	$—CH_3$	$—CH_2CH_3$	H	+	USDIN and EFRON (1972b)
8h LPD-824	H	$—CH_2CH_2CH_2CH_2—$		+ +	MURPHREE et al. (1958) CERLETTI (1959)
8i MPD-75	$—CH_3$	$—CH_2CH_2CH_2CH_2—$		+	USDIN and EFRON (1972c)
8j LSM-775	H	$—CH_2CH_2OCH_2CH_2—$		+ + +	GOGERTY and DILLE (1957)
8k	H	$—CH(CH_2OH)CH_3$	H	+	BIGWOOD et al. (1979)
8l UML-491	$—CH_3$	$—CH(CH_2OH)CH_2CH_3$	H	+	ABRAMSON and ROLO (1967)
8m	H	$n—C_3H_7$	$n—C_3H_7$	+ +	HOFMANN (1959)
8n LEP	H	$n—C_3H_7$	$—CH_2CH_3$	+ + +	ABRAMSON and ROLO (1967)
8o LMP	H	$n—C_3H_7$	$—CH_3$	+	ABRAMSON and ROLO (1967)
8p LME	H	$—CH_2CH_3$	$—CH_3$	+	ABRAMSON and ROLO (1967)
8q DAM-57	H	$—CH_3$	$—CH_3$	+ +	ABRAMSON (1959) CERLETTI (1959)
8r LA-111	H	H	H	+	HOFMANN (1963)

[a] Each loss of a + indicates the loss of a half order of magnitude of potency

Table 4. Components of the psychotomimetic convolvulaceae[a]

Compound	*Rivea corymbosa* %	*Ipomoea violacea* %	*Argyrea nervosa* %
Lysergamide (8r)	48 (a) 54 (b)	5–50 (a)[b] 58 (b) 10–16 (c)[b]	23 (d) 25 (c)
1-Hydroxyethyl lysergamide	c	c	6 (d)
Isolysergamide	17 (b) 35 (a)	9–17 (a) 18–26 (c) 8 (b)	18 (c) 31 (d)
1-Hydroxyethyl isolysergamide	c	c	4 (d)
Ergonovine (8k)	—	8 (b)	8 (d)
Total alkaloid content (wet weight)	0.012 (b)	0.06 (a, b)	0.3 (c)

[a] Reference: (a) GENEST (1965); (b) HOFMANN (1971); (c) HYLIN and WATSON (1965); (d) CHAO and DER MARDEROSIAN (1973)
[b] Range covering several varieties of *I. violacea*
[c] Possibly hydrolysed to lysergamide or isolysergamide during analysis. See HOFMANN (1971)

alkaloid composition of these three morning glories, insofar as these potentially contributing components are concerned, is given in Table 4. Most of the remaining alkaloids lack the 8-position carboxyl group, or even an intact piperidine ring, and have not been evaluated as psychotomimetic agents.

C. Psychotomimetics Structurally Related to Dopamine

I. Phenethylamines

Dopamine (9a) is the simplest of the catecholamine neurotransmitters and serves also as the metabolic precursor of the related compounds norepinephrine (noradrenalin, 9b) and epinephrine (adrenalin, 9c). These bases carry the carbon skeleton of phenethylamine (10) which is itself naturally present in human tissue (ASATOOR and DALGLEISH, 1959), including the brain (BORISON et al., 1977). The variability of its concentration in urine reflects clinical diagnosis (decreased in depression, FISCHER et al., 1973; increased in schizophrenics, POTKIN et al., 1979) and suggests that it may play a role as an endogenous stimulant. When administered exogenously, it is readily in-

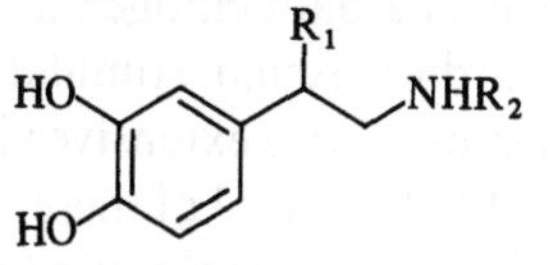

(9a) $R_1 = R_2 = H$
Dopamine
(9b) $R_1 = OH; R_2 = H$
Norepinephrine
(9c) $R_1 = OH; R_2 = CH_3$
Epinephrine

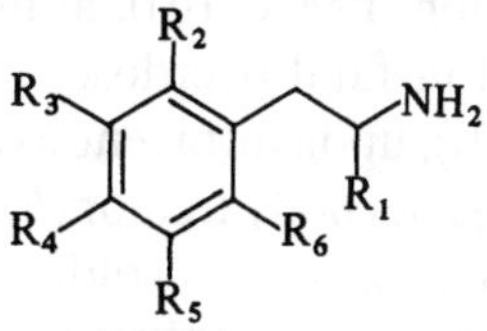

(10) $R_1, R_2, R_3, R_4, R_5, R_6 = H$
Phenethylamine

activated by the ubiquitous monoamine oxidase (MAO), and it is only with extensive ring substitution that the phenethylamines become centrally active. The best-studied phenethylamine psychotomimetic is mescaline (10a, $R_1=R_2=R_6=H$; $R_3=R_4=R_5=OCH_3$), which is itself immune to deamination by the MAO system. It and related phenthylamines are listed in Table 5, with comparisons of their relative potencies in man. Most of these materials have had their origin in the established activity of the phenylisopropylamine counterparts, which will be discussed in the next section.

It is apparent that no compounds with less than trisubstitution are centrally active, presumably due to rapid deamination in vivo. The mono-methoxy analogue 4-methoxyphenethylamine is inactive (BROWN et al., 1968), and the dimethoxy analogue similar to dopamine appears to be a mild stimulant but only at the rather high dosage of 1,500 mg (VOJTECHOVSKY and KRUS, 1967). This latter compound, because of its close resemblance to dopamine and its possible appearance in the urine of schizophrenic subjects (FRIEDHOFF and VAN WINKLE, 1962), has been thoroughly studied in its possible role in mental health. There is as yet no consensus as to its origins or its significance in the body. Two positional isomers of mescaline have been studied, but they appear to be of limited activity. The 2,3,4-isomer, "reciprocal" or "iso" mescaline, has been reported to be inactive in normal subjects, but highly potent in schizophrenic patients (SLOTTA and MÜLLER, 1936). The 2,4,5-isomer, which bears the substitution pattern of the potent neurotoxin 6-hydroxydopamine, has been reported as being similar to mescaline (JANSEN, 1931), but recent work suggests that its only indication of central availability is the potentiation of the action of mescaline (DITTRICH, 1971).

II. Phenylisopropylamines

As discussed above, an appropriate ring-substitution pattern can protect a phenethylamine derivative from desctructive metabolism by MAO deamination. A second structural modification has been frequently employed to this same end, i.e., the placement of a sterically hindering methyl group on the carbon alpha to the primary amine. Thus, amphetamine (10; $R_1=CH_3$, $R_2,R_3,R_5,R_6=H$) is a long lived and little metabolized stimulant, whereas phenethylamine, of intrinsically similar potency, is relatively inactive when administered orally. A large family of psychotomimetic drugs is known which are ring-substituted derivatives of amphetamine. These are presented in Table 6, with their potency relative to mescaline, and with appropriate leading references. There are some generalities that are not apparent from the table. The mono- and disubstituted isomers show, in addition to psychotomimetic action, considerable central stimulation. PMA (10i), although active as a hallucinogen at 60–80 mg, has been implicated in fatal overdoses involving cardiovascular stimulation (CIMBURA, 1974). DMA (10l), upon intravenous administration, elicits extensive visual distortion complicated by gross body tremor (FAIRCHILD, 1963). Several of these substituted amphetamine analogs have been studied as their *N*-methyl homologues (in analogy with the relationship between amphetamine and methamphetamine). Although most show a striking drop in potency, MDMA (the *N*-methyl homologue of MDA, 10m) retains full activity (SHULGIN and NICHOLS, 1978). Referring to Table 6, it is apparent by comparing compounds 10p, 10q, and from 10dd to 10nn, that the 2,4,5-trisubstitution pattern is needed for maximum potency, and that there is a great sensitivity to

Table 5. Substituted phenethylamines (10) (with R_1=H)

Compound	R_2	R_3	R_4	R_5	R_6	Potency relative to mescaline (10a=1)	Reference
10a Mescaline	H	OCH_3	OCH_3	OCH_3	H	1	BERINGER (1927)
10b Escaline	H	OCH_3	OCH_2CH_3	OCH_3	H	6	BRAUN et al. (1978)
10c Proscaline	H	OCH_3	$OCH_2CH_2CH_3$	OCH_3	H	6	BRAUN et al. (1978)
10d 2-CD	OCH_3	H	CH_3	OCH_3	H	20	SHULGIN and CARTER (1975)
10e 2-CB	OCH_3	H	Br	OCH_3	H	30	SHULGIN and CARTER (1975)
10f 2-CI	OCH_3	H	I	OCH_3	H	30	SHULGIN (1979)
10g 2-CE	OCH_3	H	—CH_2CH_3	OCH_3	H	20	SHULGIN (1979)
10h 4-Thiomescaline	H	OCH_3	SCH_3	OCH_3	H	10	BRAUN et al. (1978)

Table 6. Substituted phenylisopropylamines (10) (with R_1=CH_3)

Compound		R_2	R_3	R_4	R_5	R_6	Potency relative to mescaline (10a=1)	Reference
10i	PMA	H	H	OCH_3	H	H	6	SHULGIN et al. (1969)
10j	2,4-DMA	OCH_3	H	OCH_3	H	H	6	SHULGIN (1978)
10k	2,5-DMA	OCH_3	H	H	OCH_3	H	6	SHULGIN (1978)
10l	DMA	H	OCH_3	OCH_3	H	H	1	FAIRCHILD (1963)
10m	MDA	H	—OCH_2O—		H	H	3	NARANJO et al. (1967) TUREK et al. (1974) YENSEN et al. (1976)
10n	TMA	H	OCH_3	OCH_3	OCH_3	H	2	PERETZ et al. (1955) SHULGIN et al. (1961)
10o		H	OCH_3	$OCH_2\Phi$	OCH_3	H	2	SHULGIN (1978)
10p	TMA-2	OCH_3	H	OCH_3	OCH_3	H	20	SHULGIN (1964a)

Table 6 (continued)

Compound		R_2	R_3	R_4	R_5	R_6	Potency relative to mescaline (10a = 1)	Reference
10q	MEM	OCH_3	H	OCH_2CH_3	OCH_3	H	20	SHULGIN (1978)
10r	TMA-3	OCH_3	OCH_3	OCH_3	H	H	< 2	SHULGIN (1964a)
10s	TMA-4	OCH_3	OCH_3	H	OCH_3	H	4	SHULGIN et al. (1969)
10t	TMA-5	OCH_3	OCH_3	H	H	OCH_3	10	SHULGIN et al. (1969)
10u	TMA-6	OCH_3	H	OCH_3	H	OCH_3	10	SHULGIN et al. (1969)
10v	MMDA	H	OCH_3	$—OCH_2O—$		H	3	SHULGIN (1964b) SHULGIN et al. (1973)
10w	MMDA-2	OCH_3	H	$—OCH_2O—$		H	10	SHULGIN (1964a)
10x	MMDA-3a	OCH_3	$—OCH_2O—$		H	H	10	SHULGIN (1964a)
10y	MMDA-3b	$—OCH_2O—$		OCH_3	H	H	3	SHULGIN (1964a)
10z	MMDA-5	$—OCH_2O—$		H	H	OCH_3	10	SHULGIN (1978)
10aa		OCH_3	OCH_3	OCH_3	OCH_3	H	6	SHULGIN et al. (1969)
10bb	DMMDA	OCH_3	$—OCH_2O—$		OCH_3	H	12	SHULGIN and SARGENT (1967)
10cc	DMMDA-2	OCH_3	OCH_3	$—OCH_2O—$		H	5	SHULGIN and SARGENT (1967)
10dd	p-DOT (Aleph-1)	OCH_3	H	SCH_3	OCH_3	H	40	SHULGIN and NICHOLS (1978)
10ee	Aleph-2	OCH_3	H	SCH_2CH_3	OCH_3	H	80	SHULGIN (1978)
10ff	Aleph-4	OCH_3	H	SPr (*i*)	OCH_3	H	40	SHULGIN (1980)
10gg	Aleph-7	OCH_3	H	SPr (*n*)	OCH_3	H	60	SHULGIN (1980)
10hh	DOM(STP)	OCH_3	H	CH_3	OCH_3	H	80	SNYDER et al. (1967)
10ii	DOET	OCH_3	H	CH_2CH_3	OCH_3	H	100	SNYDER et al. (1968)
10jj	DOPR	OCH_3	H	Pr (*n*)	OCH_3	H	80	SHULGIN and DYER (1975)
10kk	DOBU	OCH_3	H	Bu (*n*)	OCH_3	H	40	SHULGIN and DYER (1975)
10ll	DOAM	OCH_3	H	Am (*n*)	OCH_3	H	10	SHULGIN and DYER (1975)
10mm	DOB	OCH_3	H	Br	OCH_3	H	400	SHULGIN et al. (1971)
10nn	DOI	OCH_3	H	I	OCH_3	H	400	SHULGIN (1978)

the identity of the substituent on the 4-position. This consistency has suggested a mechanism of action involving in vivo oxidation to a quinonoid intermediate to, in turn, some subsequent indole metabolite (ZWEIG and CASTAGNOLI, 1974, 1975).

Several of these racemic bases have been studied as separated optical isomers. The observation that the "R" isomer of DOM (10hh) can account for most of the psychotomimetic activity (SHULGIN, 1973) is consistent with this same absolute configuration being required for the 5-carbon of LSD, whereas the active isomer of amphetamine (a stimulant rather than a psychotomimetic) is the "S" isomer. This generality applies to the other primary amines studied as separated isomers (10m, 10ii, and 10mm) (COOK and FELLOWS, 1961; SNYDER et al., 1974; ANDERSON et al., 1978). The only known active *N*-methyl derivative (MDMA; see above) has a reversal of activity, the "S" isomer being the more active (ANDERSON, 1978).

D. Psychotomimetics Structurally Related to Acetylcholine: Atropine-Related Drugs

The third major neurotransmitter in the human nervous system is acetylcholine (11), and a number of psychotomimetics are known that are closely related to this compound structurally.

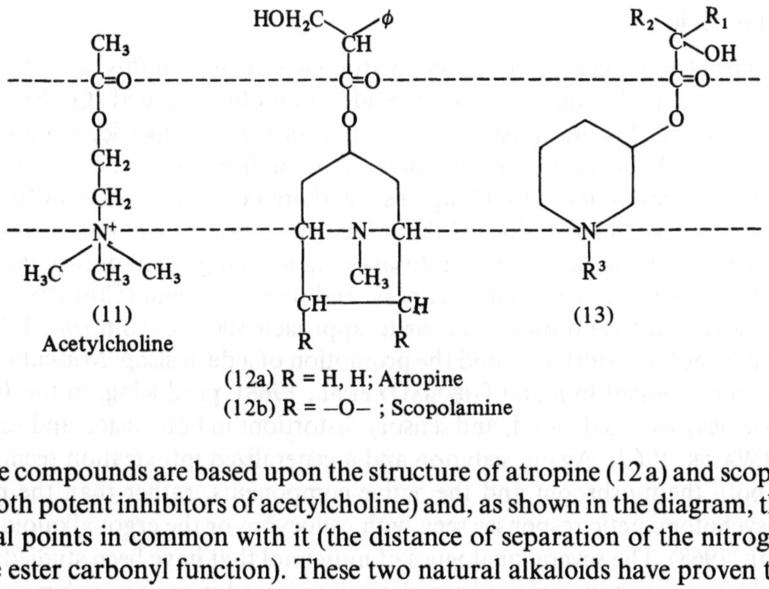

(11) Acetylcholine

(12a) R = H, H; Atropine
(12b) R = –O– ; Scopolamine

(13)

These compounds are based upon the structure of atropine (12a) and scopolamine (12b) (both potent inhibitors of acetylcholine) and, as shown in the diagram, they bear structural points in common with it (the distance of separation of the nitrogen atom from the ester carbonyl function). These two natural alkaloids have proven to be the active components of many plants from around the world renowned for centuries for their mystical powers. The belladonna plant, *Atropa belladonna*, was used in Europe in the Middle Ages as a witch's brew. Henbane, *Hyoscyamus niger*, was also widely cultivated in Europe (as was mandrake, *Mandragora officinarum*), and from this name come the alkaloidal names hyoscyamine and hyoscine (for 12a and 12b, respectively). Pituri, *Duboisia hopwoodii*, has been used broadly by the Australian aborigines, and many species of *Datura* have been used for centuries in the New World for religious purposes and as stupefacients.

The intoxication produced by these alkaloids, and the chemical relatives listed in Table 7, is distinctly different than that characteristic of the serotonin- and dopamine-related psychotomimetics already discussed. There are peripheral changes (dry mouth, nonreflexive pupillary dilation, urinary retention, tachycardia, muscular weakness) characteristic of parasympatholytic activity. Centrally, the hallucinations are usually clouded in amnesia, and there is intellectual impairment and confusion, often incoherence.

Table 1 lists several compounds that do not strictly follow the generalized formula (13). Atropine and scopolamine are with the structures drawn above. Benactyzine (13a) and Win-2299 (13j) are both open-chain compounds, esters of *N,N*-diethylaminoethanol with diphenylglycolic acid and thionyl cyclohexylglycolic acid, respectively. Ditran (JB-329, 13h) is actually a mixture of the listed piperidinyl compound and the ring-contracted pyrrolidinylmethyl analogue. And finally, the last-mentioned compound 13m, quinuclidinyl benzilate, has as the nitrogen substituent a two-carbon chain folded back to the 4-position of the piperidine to form the quinuclidine ring. This anticholinergic has been studied extensively in the chemical warfare research laboratories of several countries as an incapacitating agent. The potency given in the table is for a subcutaneous injection.

E. Miscellaneous Psychotomimetics

I. Ibotenic Acid

Another chemical implicated in normal neurologic function, in this case as an inhibitory transmitter, is the aliphatic amino acid γ-aminobutyric acid (GABA, 14) (see IVERSEN, 1978). The historic mushroom *Amanita muscaria* (fly agaric) contains a number of pharmacologically active alkaloids. Two of these, ibotenic acid (15a) and muscimol (15b), are potent GABA agonists and are believed to account for most of the psychopharmacologic action of the intact mushroom, including disorientation and deep sleep. Ibotenic acid, at lower dosages (up to 50 mg) leads only to facial flushing (WASER, 1967), a generalized weakness, and disequilibrium (CHILTON, 1975).

Moderately effective dosages appear to approach 100 mg (CHILTON, 1975), with considerable motor disturbance and the promotion of a deep sleep. Muscimol is some five times more potent in man (THEOBALD et al., 1968), producing, in the 10–15 mg range, dizziness, elevated mood, and sensory distortions in both vision and sound perception (WASER, 1967). Again, sedation and a generalized intoxication seem to characterize both the mushroom and the active components, rather than the more expected psychotomimetic responses seen with psilocybin or the ergot alkaloids (THEOBALD et al., 1968). The several analogues of muscimol that have been studied as effective GABA agonists have not yet been clinically assayed in man as either intoxicants or sedatives.

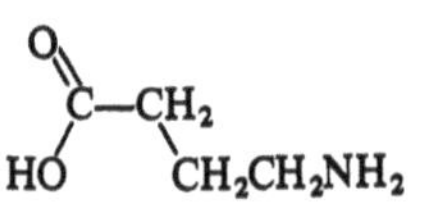

(14) GABA

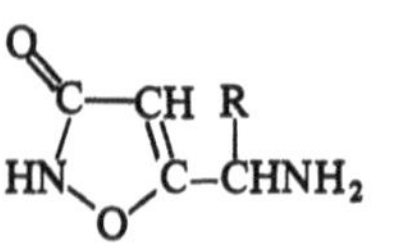

(15a) R = COOH Ibotenic acid
(15b) R = H Muscimol

Table 7. Anticholinergic psychotomimetics (13)

Compound		R_1	R_2	R_3	Effective dose range (mg)	Reference
12a	Atropine[a]				10– 15	KETCHUM et al. (1973)
12b	Scopolamine[a]				1– 4	KETCHUM et al. (1973)
13a	Benactyzine[a]	Phenyl	Phenyl	Ethyl	50–200	VOJTĚCHOVSKÝ et al. (1958)
13b	JB-841	Phenyl	Phenyl	H	> 20	ABOOD et al. (1959a)
					>100	ABOOD et al. (1959b)
13c	JB-18	Phenyl	Phenyl	Allyl	> 20	ABOOD et al. (1959a)
13d	JB-868	Phenyl	Phenyl	—$(CH_2)_2NHNMe_2$	> 20	ABOOD et al. (1959a)
13e	JB-344	Phenyl	Thionyl	CH_3	10– 20	ABOOD et al. (1959b)
13f	JB-318	Phenyl	Phenyl	Ethyl	10– 20	OSTFELD et al. (1958)
						ABOOD (1968)
13g	JB-851	Phenyl	Phenyl	—$(CH_2)_2NMe_2$	> 10	ABBOD et al. (1959b)
13h	JB-329[a] (Ditran)	Phenyl	Cyclopentyl	Ethyl	10	ABOOD et al. (1959b)
13i	JB-840	Phenyl	Cyclohexyl	CH_3	10	ABOOD et al. (1959b)
13j	Win-2299[a]	Thionyl	Cyclohexyl	Ethyl	5– 10	PENNES and HOCH (1957)
13k	JB-328	Phenyl	Cyclohexyl	Ethyl	5– 10	ABOOD et al. (1959b)
13l	JB-336	Phenyl	Phenyl	CH_3	5– 10	ABOOD (1968)
13m	QB, BZ[a]	Phenyl	Phenyl		0.2	SCHALLEK and SMITH (1952)

[a] Does not follow the generalized formula; see text

II. Dissociative Anesthetics

Two clinically useful anesthetics have recently come into popular acceptance as psychotomimetic drugs. Pharmacologically, phencyclidine (16a) and ketamine (17) are best classified as parasympatholytics akin to scopolamine and the related JB compounds. Structurally, they are distinct, being extremely lipophilic benzyl amines. Two properties of phencyclidine have contributed to its rapidly increasing popularity: its relatively high potency (5–10 mg), regardless of the route of administration (orally, smoking, injection), and the ease of its synthesis. The social problems associated with its abuse have prompted extensive federal action, both in research (PETERSEN and STILLMAN, 1978) and in legislation. Its original promise as a powerful anesthetic (CHEN et al., 1959) was compromised by bizarre symptoms of delusional and sensorially distorted interpretations upon postoperative recovery (GREIFENSTEIN et al., 1958; JOHNSTONE et al., 1959). It has been just these latter properties that have popularized the drug. The facile synthesis has prompted the exploratory synthesis of numerous analogues, partly to circumvent the law and partly to exploit more readily obtainable starting materials. The thiophene analogue (16b) is easily prepared (KALIR et al., 1969) and has appeared as an illegal drug in street usage. Similarly, the *N*-ethyl analogue (16c, PCE, SMIALEK et al., 1979) and the pyrrolidine analogue (16d, PHP, NAKAMURA et al., 1979) have both been involved in deaths.

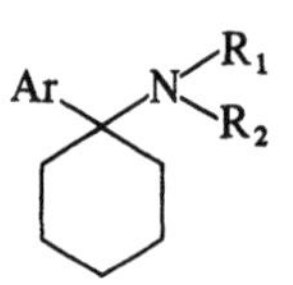

Ar	R_1	R_2	
(16a) Phenyl	$-(CH_2)_5-$		Phencylidine (PCP)
(16b) Thiophene	$-(CH_2)_5-$		Thiophene analogue of phencyclidine (TCP)
(16c) Phenyl	ethyl	H	Cyclohexamine (PCE)
(16d) Phenyl	$-(CH_2)_4-$		Pyrrolidine analogue of phencyclidine (PHP)

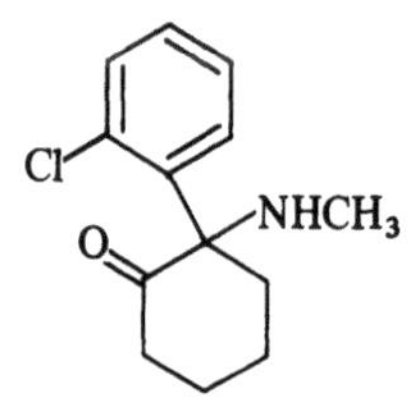

(17) Ketamine

Ketamine (17) is a structural analogue of phencyclidine that has been introduced to bypass some of the limitations of phencyclidine, and it appears clinically effective, although less potent (DOMINO et al., 1965). However, the recovery period was again flawed by bizarre hallucinatory experiences (FINE and FINESTONE, 1973; PEREL and DAVIDSON, 1976). The drug may have a dubious future in clinical practice, but it has appeared broadly in paramedical usage. Its complex synthesis will require that the supply come from diverted legitimate channels; analogues are not likely to appear soon.

III. Ibogaine

Ibogaine (18) is one of the principal alkaloids isolated from the root and bark of the African plant *Tabernanthe iboga*. It has cholinesterase inhibitory properties (VINCENT and SERO, 1942) reminiscent of those mentioned for a similarly complex plant alkaloid harmaline, and its hallucinatory actions, with anxiety and apprehensions (SCHNEIDER and SIGG, 1958), seem to be parallel. A recent report of extensive clinical studies on ibogaine (NARANJO 1973 b) has supported its psychotomimetic potential, at dosages of 300 mg.

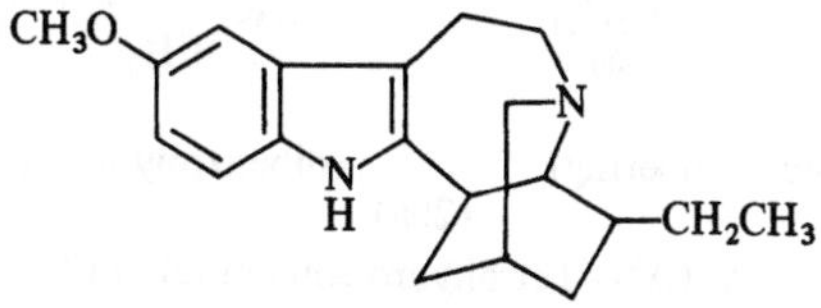

(18) Ibogaine

IV. Kavakava

Another botanical binomial known in psychotropic pharmacology is *Piper methysticum*, the source of the drug kavakava. This plant contains nonnitrogenous components, principally kawain (19 a) and the methylenedioxy analogue methysticin (19 b). Kavakava is used widely throughout the South Pacific as a social intoxicant. These and related isolated lactones have been studied pharmacologically as anticonvulsants (KRETZSCHMAR and MEYER, 1969) and analgetics (BRÜGGEMANN and MEYER, 1963), and there has been extensive synthetic exploration in the preparation and study

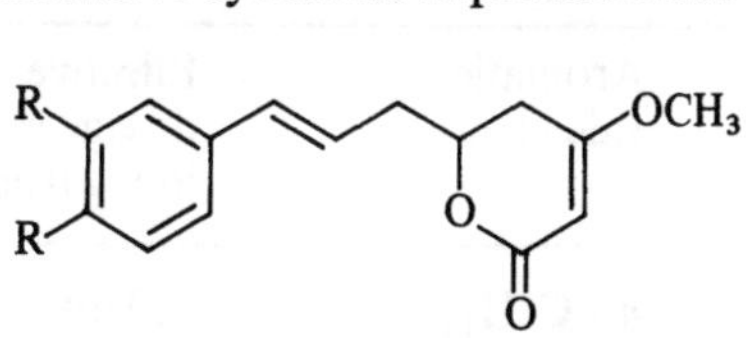

(19a) R = H, H Kawain
(19b) R = –OCH$_2$– Methysticin

of potentially useful analogues. The results have been largely disappointing. It has been observed that the narcotic action of the native plant preparation requires emulsification of the root material (STEINMETZ, 1960), and the natural preparations employ chewing to produce an effective drink. The intrinsic activity of the plant may not be observable in the purified isolated components.

V. Marijuana

The most important and the most extensively studied of the nonnitrogenous psychotomimetics are the terpenic components of the intoxicating plant *Cannabis sativa*. This material has been known since antiquity, and although it may be misleading to classify it as a psychotomimetic drug, it has been widely employed in many forms as an intoxicant, as a therapeutic agent, and as a subtle disinhibitor of sensory stimuli. The active principles are fusion products of a 10-carbon terpene unit and (usually) 5-(*n*)-amylresorcinol. The main active component is Δ^1 (or Δ^9)-tetrahydrocannabinol (THC, 20 a), which is shown in the illustration with its two frequently encountered numbering systems. The first system (terpene-based numbering) reflects the biosynthetic origin, with the numbering of the aliphatic half done in accord with classic ter-

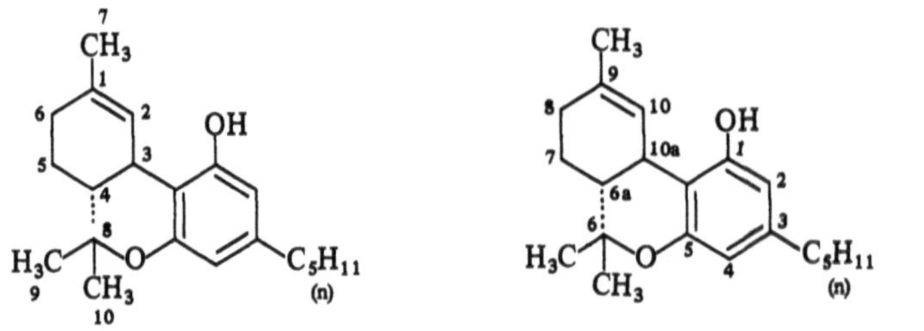

(terpene–based numbering) (dibenzopyran–based numbering)

(20a)

Δ^1 (Δ^9)–Tetrahydrocannabinol (THC)

pene nomenclature. It has the advantage of being applicable (and allowing easy cross-reference) to natural components wherein the pyran ring is opened, but the aromatic moiety must be numbered separately. The second system (dibenzopyran-based numbering) is based upon the intact dibenzopyran nucleus, and although it allows exact assignment in written names (in abstracting), it becomes useless when the pyran ring does not exist. Neither is satisfactory and both are (unfortunately) widely used.

Table 8. Cannabinoids (20a)

Compound	Double-bond position	Aromatic side chain	Effective dosage range in mg (route)	Reference
20a Δ^1-THC	1,2	n—C_5H_{11}	20 (o)	HOLLISTER (1973) HOLLISTER and TINKLENBERG (1973)
			5 (p)	HOLLISTER (1973) ISBELL et al. (1967)
20b Δ^6-THC	6,1	n—C_5H_{11}	20 (o)	HOLLISTER (1973)
20c CBN	Aromatic	n—C_5H_{11}	>400 (o)	HOLLISTER (1973)
			15 (p)	PEREZ-REYES et al. (1973)
20d Δ^3-THC	3,4	n—C_5H_{11}	120 (o)	ADAMS (1942)
			15 (p)	HOLLISTER (1970)
20e Pyrahexyl	3,4	n—C_6H_{13}	60 (o)	ADAMS (1942) WILLIAMS et al. (1946)
20f DMHP	3,4	—$CH(CH_3)CH(CH_3)C_5H_{11}$	5 (o)	ISBELL (1968) SIM (1970)
20g Nabilone	3,4 (carbonyl at C_1)	—$C(CH_3)_2C_6H_{13}$	5 (o)	LEMBERGER and ROWE (1975)
20h 7-OH-Δ^1-THC	1,2 (hydroxy at C_7)	n—C_5H_{11}	3 (p)	PEREZ-REYES et al. (1972)
20i 6(β)OH-Δ^1-THC	1,2 (hydroxy at C_6)	n—C_5H_{11}	4 (p)	WALL et al. (1976)

Although several dozen cannabinoid compounds are now known to be components of the intoxicating resinous extracts of the marijuana plant, only four have been seriously considered as contributors to the overall pharmacologic syndrome of intoxications. Besides Δ^1-THC there is the positional isomer Δ^6-THC (20b), the aromatic counterpart cannabinol (CBN, 20c), and the open-ring counterpart of Δ^1-THC, cannabidiol (CBD). The first three are centrally active, but cannabidiol is not, regardless of the route of administration, either oral (HOLLISTER, 1973; KARNOLL et al., 1975), smoking (ISBELL et al., 1967), or intravenous (PEREZ-REYES et al., 1973).

The published data concerning potency in humans of these natural, as well as synthetic analogues of marijuana, and on human metabilites, are gathered in Table 8. The terpene-based numbering system is employed.

In the earliest synthetic approaches to the THC molecule, the double bond in the terpene ring usually remained at the conjugated position 3,4 (6a, 10a in the dibenzopyran-based system). Three of these synthetic materials (20d, e, f) are orally active in man, the last of these carrying the dimethylheptyl side chain found to be of the greatest animal potency in the seminal studies of ADAMS. A recently proposed pharmaceutical lacks the methyl group at position C1, possessing a carbonyl in its place. This drug, nabilone, is currently in clinical trials as a sedative. Studies on the metabolic fate of THC have shown that hydroxylation is a major pathway. This can occur on the amyl side chain, or in several locations within the terpene moiety. Two of the known human metabolites themselves have intrinsic central action (compounds 20h, i) and have been implicated in the mechanism of action of THC itself.

References

Abood, L.G.: The psychotomimetic glycolate esters. In: Drugs affecting the central nervous system. Burger, A. (ed.), pp. 127–167. New York: Marcel Decker 1968

Abood, L.G., Biel, J.H., Ostfeld, A.M.: The psychotogenic effects of some N-substituted piperidyl benzilates. In: Neuropsychopharmacology. Bradley, P.B., Deniker, P., Radouco-Thomas, C. (eds.), pp. 433–438. Amsterdam: Elsevier 1959a

Abood, L.G., Ostfeld, A.M., Biel, J.H.: Structure-activity relationships of 3-piperidyl benzilates with psychotogenic properties. Arch. Int. Pharmacodyn. Ther. *120*, 185–200 (1959b)

Abramson, H.A.: Lysergic acid diethylamide (LSD-25): XXIX. The response index as a measure of threshold activity of psychotropic drugs in man. J. Psychol. *48*, 65–78 (1959)

Abramson, H.A., Rolo, A.: Comparison of LSD with methysergide and psilocybin on test subjects. In: The use of LSD in psychotherapy and alcoholism. Abramson, H.A. (ed.), pp. 55–73. New York, Bobs-Merrill 1967

Adams, R.: Marihuana. Harvey Lect., Sers. *37*, 168–197 (1942)

Agurell, S., Holmstedt, B., Lindgren, J.-E.: Alkaloid content of *Banisteriopsis rusbyana* (Ndz.) Morton. Am. J. Pharm. *140*, 148–151 (1968)

Aldous, F.A.B., Barrass, B.C., Brewster, K., Buxton, D.A., Green, D.M., Pinder, R.M., Rich, P., Skeels, M., Tutt, K.J.: Structure-activity relationships in psychotomimetic phenylalkylamines. J. Med. Chem. *17*, 1100–1111 (1974)

Alles, G.A.: Some relations between chemical structure and physiological action of mescaline and related compounds. In: Neuropharmacology, Trans. Fourth Conf. Abramson, H.A. (ed.), pp. 181–268. J. Macy Jr. Foundation, 1959

Anderson, G.M. III, Braun, G., Braun, U., Nichols, D.E., Shulgin, A.T.: Absolute configuration and psychotomimetic activity. QuaSAR Research Monograph No. 22. Barnett, G., Trsic, M., Willette, R. (eds.), pp. 8–15. National Institute on Drug Abuse, U.S.G.P.O. 1978

Asatoor, A.M., Dalgleish, C.F.: Amines in blood and urine. Biochem. J. *73*, 26P (only) 1959

Baker, R.W., Chothia, C., Pauling, P., Weber, H.P.: Molecular structures of hallucinogenic stubstances: Lysergic acid diethylamide, psilocybin and 2,4,5-trimethoxyamphetamine. Mol. Pharmacol. *9*, 23–32 (1973)

Barfknecht, C.F., Nichols, D.E., Dunn, W.J.: Correlation of psychotomimetic activity of phenethylamines and amphetamines with 1-octanol-water partition coefficients. J. Med. Chem. *18*, 208–210 (1975)

Benington, F., Morin, R.D., Clark, L.C., Fox, R.P.: Psychopharmacological activity of ring- and side chain-substituted beta-phenethylamines. J. Org. Chem. *23*, 1979–1984 (1958)

Beringer, K.: Der Meskalinrausch, seine Geschichte und Erscheinungsweise, S. 1–315. Berlin: J. Springer 1927

Bigwood, J., Ott, J., Thompson, C., Neely, P.: Entheogenic effects of ergonovine. J. Psychedelic Drugs *11*, 147–149 (1979)

Borison, R.L., Reyes, M., Lemus, F., Havdala, H.S., Diamond, B.I.: Regional localization of 2-phenylethylamine in human brain. Res. Commun. Psych. Psychiat. Behav. *2*, 193–201 (1977)

Braun, U., Braun, G., Jacob, P. III, Nichols, D.E., Shulgin, A.T.: Mescaline analogs: Substitutions at the 4-position. QuaSAR Research Monograph No. 22. Barnett, G., Trsic, M., Willette, R. (eds.), pp. 27–37. National Institute on Drug Abuse, U.S.G.P.O. 1978

Brimblecombe, R.W.: Effects of psychotropic drugs on openfield behaviour in rats. Psychopharmacologia *4*, 139–147 (1963)

Brown, W.T., McGeer, P.L., Moser, I.: Lack of psychotomimetic effect of paramethoxyphenethylamine and 3,4-dimethoxyphenethylamine in man. Can. Psychiat. Assoc. J. *13*, 91–92 (1968)

Brüggemann, F., Meyer, H.J.: Die Analgetische Wirkung der Kawa-Inhaltsstoffe Dihydrokawain und Dihydromethysticin. Arzneim. Forsch. *13*, 407–409 (1963)

Cerletti, A.: Discussion. In: Neuropsychopharmacology. Bradley, P.B., Deniker, P., Radouco-Thomas, C. (eds.), pp. 113–123. Amsterdam: Elsevier 1959

Cerletti, A., Rothlin, E.: Role of 5-hydroxytryptamine in mental diseases and its antagonism to lysergic acid derivatives. Nature *176*, 785–786 (1955)

Chao, J., Der Marderosian, A.H.: Ergoline alkaloidal constituents of Hawaiian Baby Wood Rose, *Argyreia nervosa* (Burm. f.) Bojer. J. Pharm. Sci. *62*, 588–591 (1973)

Chen, G., Ensor, C.R., Russell, D., Bohner, B.: The Pharmacology of 1-(1-Phenylcyclohexyl)-piperidine HCl. J. Pharmacol. Exp. Ther. *127*, 241–250 (1959)

Chilton, W.S.: The course of an intentional poisoning. McIlvania *2*, 17–18 (1975)

Cimbura, G.: PMA deaths in Ontario. Can. Med. Assoc. J. *110*, 1263–1267 (1974)

Cook, L., Fellows, E.J.: Anorexogenic preparation and method of curbing the appitite. U.S. Patent 2,974,148 (1961)

Corne, S.J., Pickering, R.W.: A possible correlation between drug-induced hallucinations in man and a behavoiral response in mice. Psychopharmacology *11*, 65–78 (1967)

Delay, J., Pichot, P., Lemperiere, T., Nicholas-Charles, P.J., Heim, R.: Effects psychophysiologique de la psilocybe. C.R. Acad. Sci. *247*, 1235–1238 (1959)

Der Marderosian, A.H., Youngken, H.W.: The distribution of indole alkaloids among certain species and varities of *Ipomoea*, *Rivea* and *Convolvulus* (Convolvulacae). Lloydia *29*, 35–42 (1966)

Der Marderosian, A.H., Pinkley, H.V., Dobbins, M.F.: Native use and occurence of N,N-dimethyltryptamine in the leaves of *Banisteriopsis rusbyana*. Lloydia *31*, 430 (only) (1968)

Dittrich, A.: Alteration of behavioral changes induced by 3,4,5-trimethoxyphenylethylamine (Mescaline) by pretreatment with 2,4,5-trimethoxyphenylethylamine. A self-experiment. Psychopharmacology *21*, 229–237 (1971)

Domino, E.F., Chodoff, P., Corssen, G.: Pharmacologic effects of CI-581, a new dissociative anesthetic, in man. Clin. Pharmacol. Ther. *6*, 279–291 (1965)

Fabing, H.D., Hawkins, J.R.: Intravenous bufotenine injection in the human being. Science *123*, 886–887 (1956)

Faillace, L.A., Vourlekis, A., Szara, S.: Clinical evaluation of some hallucinogenic tryptamine derivatives. J. Nerv. Ment. Dis. *145*, 306–313 (1967)

Fairchild, M.D.: Some central nervous effects of four phenylsubstituted amphetamine derivatives. Thesis, Ph.D., Calif, U. at Los Angeles 1–147 (1963)

Fine, J., Finestone, S.C.: Sensory disturbances following ketamine anesthesia: Recurrent hallucinations. Anesth. Analg. (Cleve) *52*, 428–430 (1973)

Fischer, E., Spatz, H., Fernández-Labriola, R.S., Rodriguez-Casanova, E.M., Spatz, N.: Quantitative gas-chromatographic determination and infra-red spectrographic identification of urinary phenethylamines. Biol. Psychiatry *7*, 161–165 (1973)

Fischer, R.: Chemistry of the brain. Nature *220*, 411–412 (1968)

Friedhoff, A.J., Van Winkle, E.: Isolation and characterization of a compound from the urine of schizophrenics. Nature *194*, 867–868 (1962)

Genest, K.: A direct densitometric method on thin-layer plates for the determination of lysergic acid amide, isolysergic acid amide and clavine alkaloids in morning glory seeds. J. Chromatog. *19*, 531–539 (1965)

Gogerty, J.H., Dille, J.M.: Pharmacology of d-lysergic acid morpholide (LSM). J. Pharmacol. Exp. Ther. *120*, 340–348 (1957)

Gorodetzky, C.W., Isbell, H.: A comparison of 2,3-dihydrolysergic acid diethylamide with LSD-25. Psychopharmacology *6*, 229–233 (1964)

Greifenstein, F.E., Devault, M., Yoshitake, J., Gajewski, J.E.: A study of 1-arylcyclohexylamine for anaesthesia. Anesth. Analg. (Cleve) *37*, 283–294 (1958)

Grof, S., Soskin, R.A., Richards, W.A., Kurland, A.A.: DPT as an adjunct in psychotherapy of alcoholics. Int. Pharmacopsychiatry *8*, 104–115 (1973)

Heim, R., Wasson, R.G.: Une investigation sur les champignons sacrés des mistèques. Comptes Rend. *254*, 788–791 (1962)

Hofmann, A.: Psychotomimetic drugs. Chemical and pharmacological aspects. Acta Physiol. Pharmacol. Neerl. *8*, 240–258 (1959)

Hofmann, A.: The active principles of the seeds of *Rivea corymbosa* and *Ipomoea violacea*. Bot. Mus. Leafl., Harvard University *20*, 194–212 (1963)

Hofmann, A.: Teonanacatl and Ololiuqui, two ancient magic drugs of Mexico. Bull. Narc. *23*, 3–14 (1971)

Hollister, L.E.: Tetrahydrocannabinol isomers and homologues: Contrasted effects of smoking. Nature *227*, 968–969 (1970)

Hollister, L.E.: Cannabidiol and Cannabinol in man. Experientia *29*, 825–826 (1973)

Hollister, L.E., Tinklenberg, J.R.: Subchronic oral doses of Marijuana extract. Psychopharmacology *29*, 247–252 (1973)

Hollister, L.W., Prusmack, J.M., Paulsen, J.A., Rosenquist, N.: Comparison of three psychotropic drugs (Psilocybin, JB-329 and IT-290). J. Nerv. Ment. Dis. *131*, 428–438 (1960)

Hsu, L.L., Mandell, A.J.: Enzymatic formation of tetrahydro-β-carboline from tryptamine and 5-methyltetrahydrofolic acid in rat brain fractions: Regional and subcellular distribution. J. Neurochem. *24*, 631–636 (1975)

Hylin, J.W., Watson, D.P.: Ergoline alkaloids in tropical wood roses. Science *148*, 499–500 (1965)

Isbell, H.: Discussions on the psychoactive actions of various tryptamine derivatives. In: Ethnopharmacologic search for psychoactive drugs. Efron, D. (ed.), pp. 374–382. U.S.G.P.O. 1967

Isbell, H.: Studies of tetrahydrocannabinol in man. In: Proceedings of the Meeting of the Committee on the Problems of Drug Dependence, National Academy of Sciences, National Research Council, pp. 4832–4847 (1967). *vide* Addendum No. 1 (1968)

Isbell, H., Gorodetsky, C.W., Jasinski, D., Claussen, U., v. Spulak, F., Korte, F.: Effects of (-)Δ^9-trans-tetrahydro-cannabinol in man. Psychopharmacology *11*, 184–188 (1967)

Iversen, L.L.: Biochemical Psychopharmacology of GABA. In: Psychopharmacology: A Generation of Progress. Lipton, M.A., DiMascio, A., Killam, K.F., pp. 25–37. New York: Raven Press 1978

Jacobs, B.L., Trulson, M.E., Stark, A.D., Christoph, G.R.: Comparitive effects of hallucinogenic drugs on the behavior of the cat. Commun. Psychopharmacol. *1*, 243–254 (1977)

Jansen, M.P.J.M.: Beta-2,4,5-trimethoxyphenylethylamine, an isomer of mescaline. Rec. Trav. Chim. *50*, 291–312 (1931)

Johnstone, M., Evans, V., Baigel, S.: Sernyl (CI-395) in clinical anaesthesia. Brit. J. Anaesth. *31*, 433–439 (1959)

Kalir, A., Edery, H., Pelah, Z., Balderman, D., Porath, G.: 1-Phenylcycloalkylamine derivatives. II. Synthesis and pharmacological activity. J. Med. Chem. *12*, 473–477 (1969)
Karnoil, I.G., Shirakawa, I., Takahashi, R.N., Knobel, E., Musty, R.E.: Effects of Δ^9-tetrahydrocannabinol and cannabinol in man. Pharmacology *1975*, 502–512
Keller, K.J., Elliott, G.R., Holman, J.V., Barchas, J.D.: Tryptoline inhibition of serotonin uptake in rat forebrain homogenates. J. Pharm. Exp. Ther. *198*, 619–625 (1976)
Kelley, J.M., Adamson, R.H.: A comparison of common interatomic distances in serotonin and some hallucinogenic drugs. Pharmacology *10*, 28–31 (1973)
Ketchum, J.S., Sidell, F.R., Crowell, E.B., Aghajanian, G.K., Hayes, A.H.: Atropine, Scopolamine, and ditran: Comparative pharmacology and antagonists in man. Psychopharmacology *28*, 121–145 (1973)
Kretzschmar, R., Meyer, H.J.: Vergleichende Untersuchungen über die Antikonvulsive der Pyronverbindungen aus Piper Methysticum Forst. Arch. Int. Pharmacodyn. Ther. *177*, 261–277 (1969)
Kuhn, D.M., White, F.J., Appel, J.B.: Discriminative stimulus properties of hallucinogens: Behavioral assay of drug action. Adv. Behav. Biol. *22*, 137–154 (1977)
Lemberger, L., Rowe, H.: Clinical pharmacology of nabilone, a cannabinol derivative. Clin. Pharmacol. Therap. *18*, 720–726 (1975)
Leuner, H., Baer, G.: Two new short-acting hallucinogens of the psilocybin group. In: Neuropsychopharmacology. Bente, D., Bradley, P.B. (eds.), Vol. 4, pp. 471–474. 1965
Leung, A.Y., Paul, A.G.: Baeocystin, a mono-methyl analog of psilocybin from *Psilocybe baeocystis* Saprophytic culture. J. Pharm. Sci. *56*, 146 (only) (1967)
Leung, A.Y., Paul, A.G.: Bauocystin and norbaeocystin: New analogs of psilocybin from *Psilocybe baeocystis*. J. Pharm. Sci. *57*, 1667–1671 (1968)
MacDougall, T.: *Ipomoea tricolor*, a hallucinogenic plant of the zapotecs. Bol. Cent. Invest. Antropol. Mex. *6*, 6–8 (1960)
McIsaac, W.M.: Formation of 1-methyl-6-methoxy-1,2,3,4-tetrahydro-2-carbolines under physiological conditions. Biochim. Biophys. Acta *52*, 607–609 (1961)
Meller, E., Friedman, E., Schweitzer, J.W., Friedhoff, A.J.: Tetrahydro-β-carbolines: Specific inhibitors of type a monoamine oxidase in rat brain. J. Neurochem. *28*, 995–1000 (1977)
Murphree, H.B., deMarr, E.W.J., Williams, H.L., Bryan, L.L.: Effects of lysergic acid derivatives on man: Antagonism between d-lysergic acid diethylamide and its 2-brom Congener. J. Pharmacol. Exp. Ther. *122*, 55 A–56 A (1958)
Murphree, H.B., Jenner, E.H., Pfeiffer, C.C.: Comparison of the effects of congeners of LSD-25 and tryptophan in normal human volunteers. Pharmacologist *2*, 64 (only) (1960)
Nakamura, G.R., Griesemer, E.C., Joiner, L.E., Noguchi, T.T.: Determination of 1-(1-Phenylcyclohexyl)-pyrrolidine (PHP) in postmortum specimens: a case report. Clin. Toxicol. *14*, 383–388 (1979)
Naranjo, C.: Psychotropic properties of the harmala alkaloids. In: Ethnopharmacologic search for psychoactive drugs. Efron, D. (ed.) pp. 385–391. U.S.G.P.O. 1967
Naranjo, C.: Harmaline and the collective unconscious. In: The healing journey: new approches to consciousness, pp. 124–173. New York: Pantheon Books, Random House 1973 a
Naranjo, C.: Ibogaine: fantasy and reality. In: The healing journey: new approaches of consciousness, pp. 174–228. New York: Pantheon Books, Random House 1973 b
Naranjo, C., Shulgin, A.T., Sargent, T.: Evaluation of 3,4-methylenedioxyamphetamine (MDA) as an adjunct of psychotherapy. Med. Pharmacol. Exp. *17*, 359–364 (1967)
Ostfeld, A.M., Abood, L.G., Marcus, D.A.: Studies with ceruloplasmin and a new hallucinogen. Arch. Neurol. Psychiat. *79*, 317–322 (1958)
Pennes, H.H., Hoch, P.H.: Psychotomimetics, clinical and theoretical considerations: Harmine, Win-2299 and Nalline. Am. J. Psychiatry *113*, 887–892 (1957)
Perel, A., Davidson, J.T.: Recurrent hallucinations following ketamine. Anaesthesia *31*, 1081–1083 (1976)
Peretz, D.I., Smythies, J.R., Gibson, W.C.: A new hallucinogen: 3,4,5-trimethoxyphenyl-beta-aminopropane (with notes on a stroboscopic phenomenon). J. Ment. Sci. *101*, 317–329 (1955)
Perez-Reyes, M., Timmons, M.C., Lipton, M.A., Davis, K.H., Wall, E.M.: Intravenous injection in man of Δ^9-tetrahydrocannabinol and 11-OH-tetrahydrocannabinol. Science *177*, 633–635 (1972)

Perez-Reyes, M., Timmons, M.C., Davis, K.H., Wall, E.M.: A Comparison of the pharmacological activity in man of intravenously administered Δ^9-tetrahydrocannabinol, cannabinol, and cannabidiol. Experientia *29*, 1368–1369 (1973)
Petersen, R.C., Stillman, R.C.: Phencyclidine (PCP) abuse: an appraisal. National Institute on Drug Abuse; Research Monograph No. 21. U.S.G.P.O. 1–313 (1978)
Poisson, J.: Note sur le „Natem" Boisson Toxique Péruvienne et ses Alcaloïdes. Ann. Pharm. Fr. *23*, 241–244 (1965)
Potkin, S.G., Karoum, F., Chuang, L.-W., Cannon-Spoor, H.E., Phillips, I., Whatt, R.J.: Phenylethylamine in paranoid chronic schizophrenia. Science *206*, 470–471 (1979)
Rinkel, M., Atwell, C.R., Dimascio, A., Brown, J.: Experimental psychiatry. V. Psilocybine, a new psychotogenic drug. New Engl. J. Med. *262*, 295–297 (1960)
Rothlin, E.: Lysergic acid diethylamide and related substances. Ann. N. Y. Acad. Sci. *66*, 668–676 (1957)
Schallek, W., Smith, T.H.F.: Electroencephalographic analysis of side effects of spasmolytic drugs. J. Pharmacol. Exp. Ther. *104*, 291–298 (1952)
Schneider, C.W., Chenoweth, M.B.: Effects of hallucinogenic and orther drugs on the nest-building behavior of mice. Nature *225*, 1262–1263 (1970)
Schneider, J.A., Sigg, E.B.: Pharmacologic analysis of tranquilizing and central stimulating effects. In: Psychopharmacology. Pennes, H.H. (ed.) pp. 75–98. New York: Hoeber 1958
Schultes, R.E.: A contribution to our knowledge of *Rivea corymbosa*, the narcotic ololuiqui of the aztecs pp. 15–60. Cambridge, Mass.: Botanical Mus. Leafl. Harvard University 1941
Shulgin, A.T.: Psychotomimetic amphetamines: Methoxy 3,4-dialkoxyamphetamines. Experientia *20*, 366–367 (1964a)
Shulgin, A.T.: 3-Methoxy-4,5-methylenedioxyamphetamine, a new psychotomimetic agent. Nature *201*, 1120–1121 (1964b)
Shulgin, A.T.: Stereospecific requirements for hallucinogenesis. J. Pharm. Pharmacol. *25*, 271–272 (1973)
Shulgin, A.T.: Psychotomimetic agents. In: Psychopharmacological Agents. Gordon, M. (ed.), Volume 4, pp. 59–146. New York: Academic Press 1976
Shulgin, A.T.: Psychotomimetic drugs: Structure-activity relationships. In: Handbook of Psychopharmacology. Iversen, L.L., Iversen, S.D., Snyder, S.H. (eds.), Vol. 11, pp. 243–333. New York: Plenum Press 1978
Shulgin, A.T.: Chemistry of phenethylamines related to mescaline. J. Psychedelic Drugs *11*, 41–52 (1979)
Shulgin, A.T.: Hallucinogens. In: Burger's Medicinal Chemistry: 4th Edition. Wolfe, M.E. (ed.). New York: Wiley 1980 (in press)
Shulgin, A.T., Carter, M.F.: Centrally active phenethylamines. Psychopharmacol. Commun. *1*, 93–98 (1975)
Shulgin, A.T., Dyer, D.C.: Psychotomimetic phenylisopropylamines. V. 4-Alkyl-2,5-dimethoxyphenylisopropylamines. J. Med. Chem. *18*, 1201–1204 (1975)
Shulgin, A.T., Nichols, D.E.: Characteristics of three new psychotomimetics. In: The psychopharmacology of hallucinogens. Willette, R.C., Stillman, R.E. (eds), pp. 74–83. New York: Pergamon Press 1978
Shulgin, A.T., Sargent, T.: Psychotropic phenylisopropylamines derived from apiole and dillapiole. Nature *215*, 1494–1495 (1967)
Shulgin, A.T., Bunnel, S., Sargent, T.: The psychotomimetic properties of 3,4,5-trimethoxyamphetamine. Nature *189*, 1011–1012 (1961)
Shulgin, A.T., Sargent, T., Naranjo, C.: Structure-activity relationships of one ring psychotomimetics. Nature *221*, 537–541 (1969)
Shulgin, A.T., Sargent, T., Naranjo, C.: 4-Bromo-2,5-dimethoxyphenylisopropylamine, a new centrally active amphetamine analog. Pharmacology *5*, 103–107 (1971)
Shulgin, A.T., Sargent, T., Naranjo, C.: Animal pharmacology and human psychopharmacology of 3-methoxy-4,5-methylenedioxyphenylisopropylamine (MMDA). Pharmacology *10*, 12–18 (1973)
Silva, M.T.A., Calil, H.M.: Screening hallucinogenic drugs: Systematic study of three behavioral tests. Psychopharmacologia *42*, 163–171 (1975)
Sim, V.: General discussion concerning psychotomimetic drugs. In: Psychotomimetic drugs. Efron, D. (ed.), pp. 332–338. New York: Raven Press 1970

Slotkin, T.A., Distefano, V., Au, W.Y.W.: Blood levels and urinary excretion of harmine and its metabolites in man and rats. J. Pharmacol. Exp. Ther. *173*, 26–30 (1970)
Slotta, K.H., Müller, J.: Über den Abbau des Mescalins und mescalinähnlicher Stoffe im Organismus. Z. Physiol. Chem. *238*, 14–22 (1963)
Smialek, J.E., Monforte, J.R., Gault, R., Spitz, W.U.: Cyclohexamine ("Rocket Fuel") – phencyclidine's potent analog. J. Anal. Tox. *3*, 209–212 (1979)
Smythies, J.R., Benington, F., Morin, R.: The mechanism of action of hallucinogenic drugs on a possible serotonin receptor in the brain. Int. Rev. Neurobiol. *12*, 207–236 (1970)
Smythies, J.R., Johnson, V.S., Bradley, R.J.: Behavioral models of psychosis. Br. J. Psychiatry *115*, 55–68 (1969)
Snyder, S.H., Merril, C.R.: A relationship between hallucinogenic activity of drugs and their electronic configuration. Proc. Natl. Acad. Sci. USA *54*, 258–266 (1965)
Snyder, S.H., Faillace, L.A., Hollister, L.E.: 2,5-dimethoxy-4-methylamphetamine (STP): A new hallucinogenic drug. Science *158*, 669–670 (1967)
Snyder, S.H., Faillace, L.A., Weingartner, H.: DOM (STP), a new hallucinogenic drug, and DOET: Effects in normal subjects. Am. J. Psychiatry *125*, 357–364 (1968)
Snyder, S.H., Unger, S., Blatchley, R., Barfknecht, C.F.: Stereospecific actions of DOET (2,5-dimethoxy-4-ethylamphetamine) in man. Arch. Gen. Psychiatry *31*, 103–106 (1974)
Soskin, R.A., Grof, S., Richards, W.A.: Low doses of dipropyltryptamine in psychotherapy. Arch. Gen. Psychiatry *28*, 817–821 (1973)
Steinmetz, E.F.: *Piper methysticum* (Kava), pp. 3–46. Dr. E.F. Steinmetz, 347 Keizersgracht, Amsterdam, Netherlands 1960
Stoll, A., Hofmann, A.: Partialsynthese von Alkaloiden von Typus des Ergobasins. Helv. Chim. Acta *26*, 944–965 (1943)
Sung, M.-T., Parker, J.A.: Amphetamines; correlation of activity with stability of molecular complexes. Proc. Natl. Acad. Sci. USA *69*, 1346–1347 (1972)
Szara, S.: Dimethyltryptamine: Its metabolism in man; the relation of its psychotic effect to the serotonin metabolism. Experientia *12*, 441–442 (1956)
Szara, S.: The comparison of the psychotic effect of tryptamine derivatives with the effects of mescaline and LSD-25 in selfexperiments. In: Psychotropic drugs. Garattini, S., Ghetti, V. (eds.), pp. 460–467. Amsterdam: Elsevier 1957
Szara, S., Hearst, E.: The 6-hydroxylation of tryptamine derivatives: A way to produce psychoactive metabolites. Ann. N. Y. Acad. Sci. *96*, 134–141 (1962)
Theobald, W., Büch, O., Kunz, H.A., Krupp, P., Stenger, E.G., Heimann, H.: Pharmakologische und experimentalpsychologische Untersuchungen mit 2 Inhaltsstoffen des Fliegenpilzes *(Amanita Muscaria)*. Arzneim. Forsch. *18*, 311–315 (1968)
Tilson, H.A., Sparber, S.B.: Similarities and differences between mescaline, lysergic acid diethylamide-25 (LSD) and d-amphetamine on various components of fixed interval responding in the rat. J. Pharmacol. Exp. Ther. *184*, 376–384 (1973)
Turek, I.S., Soskin, R.A., Kurland, A.A.: Methylenedioxyamphetamine subjective effects. J. Psychedelic Drugs *6*, 7–14 (1974)
Turner, W.J., Merlis, S.: Effects of some indolealkylamines on man. Arch. Neurol. Psychiatry *81*, 121–129 (1959)
Udenfriend, S., Witkop, B., Redfield, B.C., Weissbach, H.: Studies with reversable inhibitors of monamine oxidase: harmaline and related compounds. Biochem. Pharmacol. *1*, 160–165 (1958)
Usdin, E., Efron, D.H.: (from literature supplied by Sandoz Pharmaceuticals, Hanover, N.J.), *vide*: Psychotropic Drugs and Related Compounds. U.S.G.P.O., 94 only (1972a)
Usdin, E., Efron, D.H.: (from literature supplied by Sandoz Pharmaceuticals, Hanover, N.J.), *vide:* Psychotropic Drugs and Related Compounds. U.S.G.P.O., 101 only (1972b)
Usdin, E., Efron, D.H.: (from literature supplied by Sandoz Pharmaceuticals, Hanover, N.J.), *vide:* Psychotropic Drugs and Related Compounds. U.S.G.P.O., 102 only (1972c)
Vincent, D., Sero, J.: Action inhibitrice de *Tabernanthe iboga* sur la cholinestérase du sérum. C.R. Soc. Biol. *136*, 612–614 (1942)
Vojtěchovský, M., Krus, D.: Psychotropic effects of mescalinelike drugs. Acta Nerv. Sup. *1967*, 381–383
Vojtěchovský, M., Vítec, V., Ryšánek, K., Bultasová, H.: Psychotogenic and hallucinogenic properties of large doses of benactyzine. Experientia *14*, 422–423 (1958)

Wall, M.E., Brine, D.R., Perez-Reyes, M.: Metabolism of cannabinoids in man. In: The pharmacology of marihuana. Braunde, M.C., Szara, S. (eds.), pp. 93–116. New York: Raven Press 1976

Waser, P.G.: The pharmacology of *Amanita muscaria*. In: Ethnopharmacologic search for psychoactive Drugs. Efron, D.H. (ed.), pp. 419–439. U.S.G.P.O. 1967

Williams, E.G., Himmelsbach, C.K., Wikler, A., Ruble, D.C., Lloyd, B.J., Jr.: Studies on marihuana and pyrahexyl compound. Public Health Rep. *61*, 1059–1083 (1946)

Wolbach, A.B., Miner, E.J., Isbell, H.: Comparison of psilocin with psilocybin, mescaline, and LSD-25. Psychopharmacologia *3*, 219–223 (1962)

Wyatt, R.J., Erdelyi, E., Doamaral, J.R., Elliott, G.R., Renson, J., Brachas, J.D.: Tryptoline formation by a preparation from brain with 5-methyltetrahydrofolic acid and tryptamine. Science *187*, 853–855 (1975)

Yensen, I.S., Dileo, F.B., Rhead, J.C., Richards, W.A., Soskin, R.A., Turik, B., Kurland, A.A.: MDA-assisted psychotherapy with neurotic outpatients: a pilot study. J. Nerv. Ment. Dis. *163*, 233–245 (1976)

Zweig, J.S., Castagnoli, N.: Chemical conversion of the psychotomimetic amine 1-(2,5-dimethoxy-4-methylphenyl)-2-aminopropane to 5-hydroxy-2,6-dimethylindole. J. Med. Chem. *17*, 747–749 (1974)

Zweig, J.S., Castagnoli, N.: Metabolic 0-demethylation of the psychotomimetic amine 1-(2,5-dimethoxy-4-methylphenyl)-2-aminopropane. Commun. Psychopharmacol. *1*, 359–371 (1975)

CHAPTER 2

Pharmacology and Toxicology of Psychotomimetics

L. E. HOLLISTER

A. Introduction

During recent years, a number of reviews of psychotomimetic drugs have appeared, covering various aspects of their types, their pharmacologic actions in animals, and their effects in man (FREEDMAN, 1969; COHEN, 1971; BRAWLEY and DUFFIELD, 1972). One multiauthored volume concerned itself primarily with lysergic acid diethylamide (LSD) (SANKAR, 1975), while another concerned itself with psychotomimetics in general (RADOUCO-THOMAS et al., 1974). The subject does not lack interest, although a variety of constraints on human research with these drugs has virtually limited recent literature to accounts of experiences resulting from their illicit use.

B. Definition of a Psychotomimetic Drug

While any definition of the term *psychotomimetic drugs* is bound to be arbitrary, one can limit the field somewhat if the following criteria are used:

1) In proportion to other effects, changes in thought, perception, and mood should predominate.
2) Intellectual or memory impairment should be minimal with doses producing the above mental effects; with large doses these may occur.
3) Stupor, narcosis, or excessive stimulation should not be an integral part of the action.
4) Autonomic nervous system side effects should be neither disabling nor severely disconcerting.
5) Addictive craving should be minimal.

Even with criteria such as these, drugs admissible to the list may vary, depending upon the investigator. Indeed, one can scarcely get any agreement upon the term used to describe this class of drugs, since many objections to the most likely used term, *psychotomimetics*, can be offered. The following terms are often submitted: *hallucinogens*, *phantasticas*, *psychotogens*, *dysleptics*, and *psychedelics*. Nevertheless, psychotomimetic enjoys a broader use and has seniority over most of the alternatives, as well as being about as accurate a designation as any of them.

C. Types of Psychotomimetics

Basing a classification on chemical structures, one can separate seven groups of these drugs: (a) lysergic acid derivatives, of which LSD is the prototype; (b) phenylethylamine derivatives, of which 3,4,5-trihydroxyphenylethylamine (mescaline) is the prototype; (c) indolealkylamines, such as 4-phosphorodimethyltryptamine (psilocybin); (d) other indolic derivatives, such as the harmine alkaloids or ibogaine; (e) piperidyl benzilate esters, such as *N*-ethyl-3-piperidyl cyclopentylphenyl glycolate (JB-329 Ditran); (f) L-phenylcyclohexyl compounds, such as phenylcyclidine (Sernyl); and (g) a miscellaneous group of varying chemical structures. Because the first three groups are virtually identical in their clinical effects, they are often lumped together as the LSD–mescaline–psilocybin group (HOLLISTER, 1968).

D. Epidemiologic Aspects

It is virtually impossible to determine the current frequency of use of psychotomimetics. Epidemiologic studies of drug abuse are fraught with many difficulties. The data obtained are largely anecdotal, that is, what people say, and it is well-known that what people say and what they do may be quite different. To compound the difficulty, even the most honest and cooperative respondent labors under the burden of not really knowing what drug was taken. Mislabeling of street drugs is more common than accurate labeling. Mislabeling of LSD as mescaline may not be of serious consequence for epidemiologic purposes, as the two drugs are quite similar and might well be classified together. On the other hand, mislabeling of THC as phencyclidine (PCP) is of serious consequence as the two categories of drugs are considered to be separate. The only bases that drug users have for correcting for mislabeling are their past experience with similar drugs, the opinions of fellow drug users, or the reputation of their source of drugs. None of these factors are very likely to resolve ambiguity about what they really took. Thus, epidemiologic studies that lack any chemical verification of drugs (and these are virtually impossible to design) will only be crude indices of what drugs are really being used.

Despite these difficulties, the available data in the United States indicate that the rates of psychotomimetic drug use, variable as they may be among separate epidemiologic surveys, have remained relatively constant over the past few years (ABELSON and ATKINSON, 1975). Within this general pattern of use, a substantial change has occurred in regard to the drugs chosen. LSD is less often used (at least so labeled), while PCP use probably has increased in recent years to what is now being called an epidemic. Differences in use by sex are also apparent; more women have tried these drugs than before, their rate of use now approaching that in men. Perhaps this shift is due to the general move toward equality for women. Happily, the rates of frequent use of these drugs, always low in comparison to the number of experimenters with the drug, have not shifted.

E. The LSD–Mescaline–Psilocybin Group

I. Chemistry

Mescaline is a phenylalkylamine, psilocybin is an indolealkylamine, and lysergide has chemical resemblances to both. The structural relationships of members of this group, as well as other related compounds, are shown in Fig. 1.

LSD remains the most potent compound in this series, if not one of the most potent drugs or toxins known. A number of clinical comparisons have been made be-

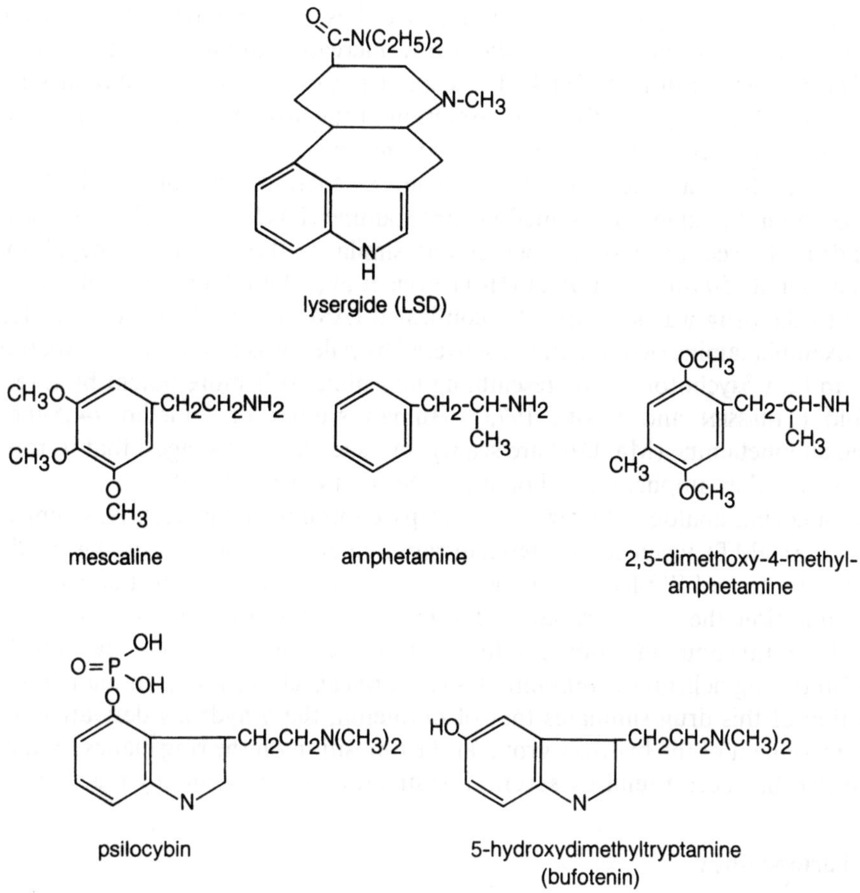

Fig. 1. Structural relationship between lysergide and other psychotomimetics of the phenethylamine and indolealkylamine series

tween LSD and closely related lysergic acid derivatives. One comparison between 2,3-dihydrolysergic acid diethylamide and LSD revealed that the former compound induced LSD-like autonomic and mental changes in man, but was less potent and slower in onset than LSD (GORODETZKY and ISBELL, 1964). Acetylation or methylation of the LSD molecule on the pyrrole nitrogen produces two analogs, L-acetyl lysergic acid diethylamide and L-methyl lysergic acid diethylamide. About 1.5–2.0 times as much of the analogous drugs were required to produce essentially the same clinical reactions with the analogs as with LSD (MALITZ et al., 1960). Replacement of the diethylamine side chain of LSD with a morpholine group results in a compound that has pharmacologic and clinical effects generally similar to those of LSD; potency was probably somewhat less (GOGERTY and DILLE, 1957). In summary, it appears that alterations in the basic structure of LSD may or may not materially change the quality of the clinical effects, but generally tend to reduce potency.

A number of mescaline homologs with psychotomimetic activity have been tested. The amphetamine analog, trimethoxyamphetamine, produces euphoria and a loosening of emotional restraint in doses of 0.8–1.2 mg/kg (PERETZ et al., 1955). Doses in the order of 2.8–3.5 mg/kg evoke tremors, paresthesias, amplified and distorted colors, textures, forms and spatial relationships, increased auditory acuity, and occasional synesthesias (SHULGIN, 1964). The span of action is similar to that of mescaline, lasting about 7 h; the peak of urinary excretion of the drug occurs between 2 and 5 h after a dose, with 20%–35% being excreted unchanged.

Other amphetamine homologs have become popular as street drugs. Most widely used has been 2,5-dimethoxy-4-methylamphetamine (DOM or "STP"). Our studies of the drug showed it to have properties very similar to those of mescaline, although it was about 40–50 times as potent (HOLLISTER et al., 1969). Our report of rapid tolerance to the drug was subsequently confirmed (ANGRIST et al., 1974). 3,4-Methylenedioxamphetamine (MDA), first discovered by Alles, was found by self-experimentation to be a psychotomimetic resembling mescaline. It is more potent by three- to fourfold (THIESSEN and COOK, 1973). Human studies of 3-methoxy-4,5-methylenedioxamphetamine (MMDA) are scanty, but such as exist suggest that it, too, resembles the other amphetamine homologs (SHULGIN et al., 1973).

A psilocybin analog with highly potent psychotomimetic effects, *N,N*-dimethyltryptamine (DMT), when administered intramuscularly in doses of 1 mg/kg, produces a brief but intense LSD-like experience. Because the material is most active by parenteral injection, the onset is rapid, within 15–30 min, but brief, subsiding completely in 1–2 h. Intravenous injection produces an even more precipitous reaction, large doses producing delirium within minutes (ROSENBERG et al., 1964). In many respects the action of this drug simulates that of bufotenin, the 5-hydroxy derivative. Curiously, placement of the hydroxy group at the 6-position on the ring makes for a compound that has been found by several investigators to be essentially inactive.

II. Pharmacology

One of the most distressing aspects of the pharmacology of psychotomimetics has been the difficulty in finding an animal model predictive of psychotomimetic effects of drugs in man. A model that involves two unusual behaviors, limb flick and abortive grooming, in cats has been found to be regularly produced by LSD and other indole hallucinogens (JACOBS, et al., 1976). The limits of this model have not yet been fully tested.

Serotonin has been the neurotransmitter most often studied and implicated in the action of drugs of the LSD group. The exact type of action on serotonin remains controversial. Evidence from a number of studies has been interpreted as indicating that the action of drugs of the LSD group is to stimulate serotonin receptors in the brain, that is, to mimic its action (ANDEN et al., 1971; AGHAJANIAN, 1972). Studies using single neuron preparations produced an opposite conclusion. Drugs of the LSD group specifically antagonized excitation of single neurons by serotonin, even though they may be able to mimic the inhibitory actions of serotonin. Thus, the action of the neurotransmitter may be specific to the location of various types of serotonergic neurons in the brain. This hypothesis is attractive in that one might still explain the reduced turnover of serotonin which has been shown to occur after LSD (BRADLEY and BRIGGS, 1974).

The role of tryptamine as a neurotransmitter is still obscure. Tryptamine mimics LSD in facilitating the flexor reflex of the chronic spinal dog. Both actions are antagonized by cyproheptadine (MARTIN and SLOAN, 1974). Thus, LSD may have a tryptaminergic action, but its relation to clinical manifestations of the drug remains uncertain.

The role of catecholaminergic neurotransmitters in the action of drugs of the LSD group is even more uncertain. Apparently LSD can act as a dopamine agonist in the striatum, but its role as such in other areas of the brain has not been defined (PIERI et al., 1974). A more complex action was suggested by studies showing that LSD can block the interactions between norepinephrine, dopamine, and serotonin with their respective receptors as indicated by the formation of cyclic AMP (VON HUNGEN et al., 1974). Studies of brain norepinephrine metabolism following exposure to various members of the LSD group of hallucinogens revealed differences between them, suggesting that not all of their pharmacologic actions were similar, despite the great similarity of their clinical actions (STOLK et al., 1974).

Autoradiographic studies show that drugs of this class readily penetrate the brain and that the presence of unchanged drug, in this case 2,5-dimethoxy-4-methylamphetamine, correlated with clinical effects. The suggestion was made that termination of the behavioral effects of the drug might be due to a shift in distribution in brain loci rather than to elimination of the drug (IDANPAAN-HEIKKILA et al., 1969).

Humans given doses of 2 µg/kg i.v. had blood specimens taken that were analyzed for LSD using a spectrofluorometric technique. After equilibration had occurred in about 30 min, the plasma level was between 6 and 7 ng/ml. Subsequently, plasma levels gradually fell until only a small amount of LSD was still present after 8 h. The half-life of the drug in humans was calculated to be 175 min (AGHAJANIAN and BING, 1964). Subsequent pharmacokinetic analysis of these data indicated that plasma concentrations of LSD were explained by a two-compartment open model. Performance scores were highly correlated with concentration in the tissue ("outer") compartment, which was calculated at 11.5% of body weight. The new estimation of half-life for loss of LSD from plasma, based on this model, was 103 min (WAGNER et al., 1968).

III. Clinical Effects

Three characteristic types of symptoms – somatic, perceptual, and psychic – have been noted from LSD. In repeated laboratory experiments, subjects report a basic clinical syndrome that might be described as follows:

1) Somatic symptoms: dizziness, weakness, tremors, nausea, drowsiness, paresthesias, and blurred vision.
2) Perceptual symptoms: altered shapes and colors, difficulty in focusing on objects, a sharpened sense of hearing, and, rarely, synesthesias.
3) Psychic symptoms: alterations in mood (happy, sad, or irritable at varying times), tension, distorted time sense, difficulty in expressing thoughts, depersonalization, dreamlike feelings, and visual hallucinations.

Physiologic effects are relatively few. Dilated pupils, hyperreflexia, increased muscle tension, incoordination, and ataxia are common physical signs. Effects on pulse rate, respiration, and blood pressure are so variable that they probably represent varying levels of anxiety of subjects rather than true physiologic effects. Changes in appetite and salivation are inconstant, being increased in some subjects, decreased in others.

The clinical syndrome tends to follow a sequential pattern with somatic symptoms presenting first, perceptual and mood changes next, and finally psychic changes, although there is considerable overlap between these phases. Between 1 and 16 μg/kg, the severity of psychophysiologic effects of LSD in a given subject are proportional to the dose (KLEE et al., 1961). Specific types of reaction, such as paranoid ideation, are more likely a matter of personal predisposition than a function of dose.

Except for the fact that the effective dose of mescaline is one or two of orders of magnitude more than for LSD, there is really little to choose between the two drugs insofar as the clinical effects are concerned. Just as with LSD, there are prominent somatic symptoms, perceptual alterations, and psychic effects. In general, effects of psilocybin strongly resemble those of LSD and mescaline. As with the former drugs, psychotic symptoms were infrequent.

IV. Adverse Effects

The clinical manifestations of adverse psychiatric effects of LSD have been reviewed elsewhere (SARWER-FONER, 1972). In general, not much new has been added over the years. The acute panic reaction is still most common, but of much greater concern has been the prolonged psychosis. The latter is still, fortunately, uncommon. Of 57 patients admitted to a poisoning treatment center in Scotland with reactions due to LSD, only 16 were considered to require psychiatric help. Most were treated with sedation. Men predominated, the mean age being 20 years. Most had previously taken other drugs.

Acute panic reactions to LSD, which are usually of only a few hours duration, may be handled in two ways. One may "talk the patient down," provided staff or friends are available, or one may simply sedate the patient and allow him to sleep off the effects of the drug. In the latter case, recent experience suggests that diazepam or some similar drug is preferable to the antipsychotics (BARNETT, 1971). The latter produce such lasting and noxious side effects that the treatment may ultimately prove to be more disagreeable than the illness.

"Flashbacks" or acute, unpredictable recurrences of phenomena experienced under LSD, have always been a mystery. Because they may occur months later with completely lucid intervals, most of us have subscribed to a psychological theory of causation. They may, of course, be triggered by other drugs that alter consciousness, such as marihuana or, in one unusual case, biperiden given to prevent phenothiazine-induced extrapyramidal reactions (TEC, 1971). Biperiden, being a potent anticholinergic, especially when combined with phenothiazines, may be hallucinogenic in its own right. Although it is difficult to see why it should be effective, haloperidol eliminated flashbacks in four of eight patients treated over a 4-week period and reduced their frequency in the other four patients (MOSKOWITZ, 1971).

Homicides under the influence of LSD continue to be reported. In one tragic case, the homicide occurred soon after the patient had been discharged from psychiatric care following a previous homicidal assault (KLEPTISZ and RACY, 1973). Another patient, with marked homicidal impulses, developed a fairly long-lasting psychosis following use of LSD. While still psychotic, he killed a stranger upon impulse. While recovering from a bullet wound inflicted by a policeman in the fray, his psychosis cleared quickly and he remained free of psychosis for several years (REICH and HEPPS,

1972). During the past several years the author has encountered several instances of persons accused of homicide who claimed that it was perpetrated under the influence of some hallucinogenic drug. Some of these instances strain one's credulity and suggest that this type of plea is often misused.

Self-injury, due to lapses in good judgment, used to be a major danger with the use of these drugs, but is not as big a problem as before. Various speculations have been made about the cause of this change, such as more exact doses, more experienced users, more frequent use in the company of an unintoxicated person, but no specific reason has been found for the diminution of this risk.

Chromosome breaks and gaps are subject to different definitions and to different interpretations when read on slides. Some are to expected as artifacts of the preparation. Consequently, reports on the prevalence of such alterations due to LSD vary greatly. In various studies they have either been the same or more frequent than seen on control preparations, or occur with the same frequency as those from other commonly used drugs. These considerations apply whether or not the tests were done in vitro, or used cells from exposed subjects. At present, the bulk of evidence, as reviewed extensively by two observers, suggests that the burden of proof is still on those who allege that the frequency and severity of chromosomal breaks encountered from LSD exposure is of clinical significance (DISHOTSKY et al., 1971; LONG, 1972). Rather than dismiss the matter out of hand, one should take the stance that harm has not been disproved and try to determine better ways to settle the issue (BERLIN and JACOBSON, 1972).

F. Harmine Alkaloids and Piperidyl Benzilates

Neither of these classes of drugs has much in common except that they are now rarely used as psychotomimetics.

Harmine in doses of 150–200 mg i.v. produced psychotomimetic effects in man. The threshold oral dose was 300 mg. The clinical effects described are distinctly different from those produced by drugs of the LSD group, but no human studies of the drug have been done in over 20 years (PENNES and HOCH, 1957). The drug is supposed to be a potent inhibitor of monoamine oxidase as well as an antagonist of serotonin. It seems unlikely that the first pharmacologic effect could be of major importance in its action (HO et al., 1971).

Early reports of the clinical effects of the piperidyl benzilate esters (JB-318, JB-329) suggested that they were analogous to those of LSD. Further studies have indicated that these central anticholinergics produce a clinical syndrome different from LSD and kindred drugs in a number of respects (DAVIS et al., 1964; OSTFELD et al., 1959). Peripheral anticholinergic effects are more prominent among many of the somatic effects common to the other drugs. Thought processes are much more severely disrupted: disorganization, incoherent speech, confusion, disorientation, and memory loss are striking and comparatively long lasting. They characteristically wax and wane, typical of a true delirium. Tactile, auditory, and visual hallucinations may occur, the latter being less intense than those from comparably disturbing doses of LSD, mescaline, or psilocybin. Mental states produced by the piperidyl benzilates are reminiscent of those from other centrally acting anticholinergics, such as scopolamine or, more recently, benactyzine. These are classical deliria, so there is little wonder that chronic alcoholics react to JB-329 with a delirium tremens syndrome. The analogy of LSD to delirium tremens is less striking.

Usual doses of the piperidyl benzilates range from 5 to 15 mg. Mental disturbance may be quite prolonged at the upper range of dosage, lasting well over 24 h, with mild residual confusion even for days. Unlike the LSD-type drugs, this experience is perceived by most subjects as frightening and distinctly unpleasant. Few subjects claim increased insight; indeed, with larger doses, subjects are unable to remember parts of the experience. Psychological testing of any sort may be completely impossible if the delirium becomes severe enough.

The piperidyl benzilate esters do not interfere with serotonergic mechanisms in the brain. Although they decrease dopamine turnover, this effect is believed to be secondary to their strong antimuscarinic action (ANDEN et al., 1972). The antimuscarinic action is most important in producing the behavioral effects, which strongly resemble those of *Datura stramonium*, a natural plant sometimes used for its psychotomimetic effects. Tetrahydroaminacrin, an anticholinesterase, effectively reverses the behavioral action of the piperdyl benzilate esters. Physostigmine given as intravenous bolus doses of 1 mg every 5–10 min could also be used in cases of severe intoxication (GERSHON and BELL, 1963).

G. Phencyclidine

I. History

The history of PCP is of some interest, as the drug was first thought to be useful for medical practice. It was first studied in 1957 as a potential anesthetic agent ultimately to be marketed under the name "Sernyl" (GREIFENSTEIN et al., 1958). Although it lacked muscle relaxation, it produced a state of analgesia without full loss of consciousness and laryngeal reflexes. By 1959, however, it had become apparent that patients emerging from anesthesia with this drug experienced a mental state that in some ways resembled that of hallucinogenic drugs. As studies of its hallucinogenic effects grew, it became apparent that PCP had such properties, and that these were highly variable depending upon dose and route of administration (LUBY et al., 1959). Further, they were distinctly different from those of LSD. In the opinion of many investigators, the PCP-induced mental state was a better model for schizophrenia than was the mental state produced by LSD. Verification of the hallucinogenic effects of the drug in man led to its withdrawal from the market as an anesthetic in 1965. Its hallucinogenic properties were of less consequence in animals, so that by 1967 it was reintroduced onto the market as an anesthetic for veterinary use under the name "Serylan." This use of the drug has remained to the present, the drug being considered to be quite valuable for anesthesia of primates.

The first street use of the drug occurred in 1967, during the "summer of love," when the drug culture erupted on the streets of San Francisco. The drug's popularity was short-lived, as its unpredictable, unpleasant, and often startling effects gave it a bad reputation. During the next several years PCP was hardly ever used knowingly by drug takers. By 1972 it had become a popular substance for being mislabeled as other drugs, or as an adulterant of other drugs (HART et al., 1972). By 1974, however,

Phencyclidine and Related Compounds

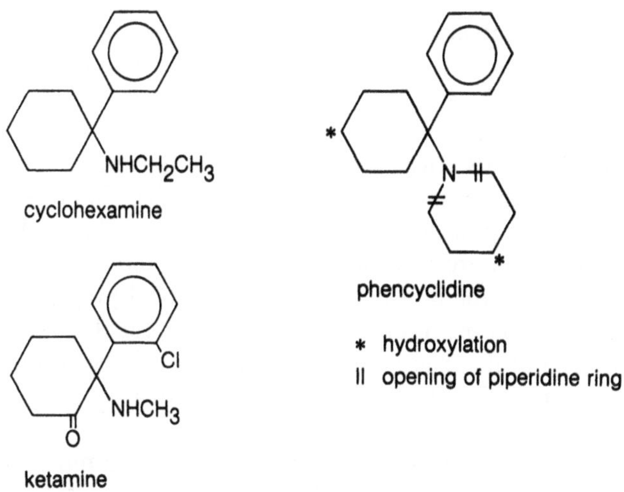

Fig. 2. Structural relationships between phencyclidine and ketamine. Metabolism of phencyclidine includes breaking of piperidine ring as well as possible hydroxylations

the pendulum swung completely back; PCP now became an acceptable drug in its own right, despite its vagaries. From that point on, its use has grown to what is now called epidemic proportions. Because of the frequently dramatic consequence of its use, the actual rate of use may have been overestimated.

The drug is readily synthesized by illicit chemical laboratories and all the evidence suggests that virtually all PCP on the streets comes from such sources. Nonetheless, the panic that its increasing use created has led to the proposal that the drug be rescheduled into a more restricted category of controlled drug. Such rescheduling would make the cost of assuring control of supplies so great that the manufacturer of PCP for veterinary anesthesia seems likely to abandon its sale, much to the concern and consternation of many investigators who rely heavily on it for their work involving primates. The desire to control drugs of abuse often leads to totally inappropriate actions just so long as some action is taken.

II. Chemistry

Phencyclidine is a phenyl cyclohexamine derivative containing a piperidine ring (see Fig. 2). It is closely related to ketamine, a drug currently in clinical use as a dissociative anesthetic. At least one active metabolite of the drug is formed, probably contributing to its long-lived clinical effects.

III. Pharmacology

As is the case with most centrally active drugs, the effects of PCP on various neurotransmitters has been most studied. PCP is believed to act by increasing the availability of dopamine, possibly both by increasing its release as well as by inhibiting its uptake (SMITH et al., 1975). The increased locomotor activity produced by the drug in rodents is characteristic of that induced by other methods of increasing dopaminergic activity. It is enhanced by antimuscarinic drugs and antagonized by cholinergic agents. The effects on acetylcholine are ambiguous. In some situations it seems to be cholinergic and in others, anticholinergic. Many of the latter properties are evident from some of its clinical effects (MAAYANI et al., 1974). The drug blocks uptake of norepinephrine and this action is related to the sympathomimetic effects evident clinically (HITZEMAN et al., 1973). Its effects on serotonin are uncertain.

Neurophysiologic studies indicate that the EEG effects in primates seem to show a possibly characteristic pattern of delta-theta mixed with low voltage fast activity. Sensory evoked potentials are also suppressed, leading to the postulation that the primary site of action is on the nonspecific thalamocortical projection (MIYASAKI and DOMINO, 1968). The impairment of sensation, for pain, touch, and proprioception, is consonant with its clinical use as an anesthetic. It may also be pertinent ot the provocation of a schizophreniclike state, which many investigators have likened to that of sensory deprivation.

The drug is unique among hallucinogens in being self-administered (BALSTER and JOHANSON, 1973). This difference, as well as many clinical and pharmacologic differences from the LSD group of hallucinogens, has led some persons to suggest that PCP be considered as a separate class of drug, similar to the classification of cannabis. However, the definition of hallucinogen is broad enough to include drugs other than the LSD group. So far as the use of the drug on the streets is concerned, it is clearly being used by hallucinogen fanciers. Animals can discriminate the drug apart from morphine, chlorpromazine, tetrahydrocannabinol, ditran, and pentobarbital, again indicating its rather unique set of enteroceptive cues. In man, the effects are said to be similar to those seen in schizophrenic patients, but the closeness of this model psychosis to the real thing has not been studied carefully for many years. It might again be appropriate to do so, for were it to prove to be a viable model, it might be a valuable tool for research into the nature of schizophrenia.

PCP in man is generally considered to be a rather long-acting drug, yet its half-life in plasma is only about 11 h even after large overdoses (MARSHMAN et al., 1976). Due to a high degree of lipid solubility, it moves rapidly into the brain, so that concentrations in brain and in cerebrospinal fluid are more persistent. Thus, the toxicity of the drug may be greatest when the plasma levels are lowest. Some of the drug is secreted from the blood into the stomach, whose acid contents keep the weakly basic drug ionized. As it enters the more alkaline medium of the upper intestine, it again becomes unionized and is reabsorbed. Thus, a certain amount of gastroenteric recycling of the drug occurs. It is likely also that PCP produces active metabolites. Thus, three factors – active metabolites, sequestration in fat, and recycling through the gastrointestinal tract – may account for its long duration of action, which is especially evident in cases of overdose.

IV. Clinical Effects

Distortion of body image, disorientation, detachment from surroundings, and vivid dreaming are some of the most common mental effects of PCP. Those who take it seem to lose the ability to integrate sensory input, especially for touch and proprioception (ROSENBAUM et al., 1959). This effect may, in turn, lead to the analgesia and par-

Table 1. Patterns of clinical effects from increasing oral doses of phencyclidine

Dose	Clinical Effects
5–10 mg	Ataxia, nystagmus, mood changes, hallucinations, vomiting, analgesia, paresthesias Onset, 1–2 h; duration, 4–8 h
10–20 mg	Stupor, eyes open, random movements, resting nystagmus, hyperreflexia, hypertension Onset, $^1/_2$–1 h; duration, 8–24 h
> 50 mg	Deep coma, chills, nystagmus, eyes closed, hypertension, labored breathing, seizures Duration, up to 4 days
>100 mg	Lethal, 3–10 days Respiratory depression, hypertensive crisis, cerebral bleeding, loss of deep tendon reflexes, decreased renal function, decreased liver function

esthesias that are experienced, as well as produce a cataleptic state in some individuals. Such effects are generally produced by doses of the drug of 0.1 mg/kg up to 12 mg single doses, regardless of the route of administration. Some persons develop mania or hostility, but these are generally considered to be side effects, more related to the personality of the subject than to a direct effect of the drug. Although some similarities to the schizophrenic state are obvious, it is not clear that the mental state produced by PCP is an especially good model of that illness.

Physical symptoms include dizziness, dysarthria, ataxia, and nystagmus, lid ptosis, tachycardia, sweating, and increased deep tendon reflexes. Most subjects show some degree of hypertension, associated with increased minute and tidal volumes of respiration, increased formation of urine, and increased muscle tone. The latter may lead to increased serum creatine phosphokinase concentrations. With very large doses, convulsions and respiratory arrest are the terminal events (BURNS et al., 1975). The course of clinical symptoms and signs following various doses of PCP is shown in Table 1.

Most of the experiments with PCP, done in the early 1960s, gave the drug intravenously. On the street, however, the major method of administration is by inhalation (often smoked as a cigarette using parsley as the medium for smoking) or by oral route in a variety of formulations.

V. Overdoses

Overdoses of PCP have been directly fatal, which is somewhat different from the case of other hallucinogens, such as LSD. Hypertensive crises, convulsions, and respiratory arrest are the major causes of death. Indirect fatalities, due to accidents caused by loss of critical judgment, are similar to those known to occur with LSD. For some reason, deaths by drowning are frequent with PCP.

No pharmacologic antidote exists for the effects of the drug. Chlorpromazine aggravates rather than ameliorates the behavioral effects. Diazepam adds to respiratory depression, but may be required for uncontrolled seizures. Experimentally, neither diphenhydramine, droperidol, tetrahydroaminacrine, physostigmine, or scopolamine were useful in reversing the effects of PCP.

Acidification of the urine to pH 5.5, using either ammonium chloride or ascorbic acid, keeps the drug in the ionized form and hastens its excretion (DOMINO and WILSON, 1977). Gastric lavage is useful only when the drug has been taken orally and soon after intake. Continual gastric suction, however, may reduce the gastrointestinal recycling of the drug and is worth doing routinely. General supportive treatment and management of symptoms as they arise is most useful. Reduced sensory stimuli reduce the psychic effects of the drug, so patients should be treated in a quiet room with few extraneous sounds.

H. Conclusions

Psychotomimetic drugs will continue to be used socially in the future as they have been used throughout man's history. Changing fashions may make one or another drug the object of choice for the moment. Many of the currently popular drugs are creations of the laboratory, unknown 30 years ago. It remains to be seen whether still different types of psychotomimetics will be created in the laboratory or, more importantly, become recognized and available to those who would use them socially.

The original hope that these drugs would lead us to a better understanding of naturally occurring mental disorders has not been realized. Neither have they yet proven to be effective therapeutic agents for any mental disorders. Still, the fact that relatively small quantities of these chemicals can so markedly affect mental functions commands our attention. If, by learning how they act, we still remain ignorant of the cause of schizophrenia, we may still learn a lot more about how the brain regulates behavior.

The greatest current challenge is to make experimentation with these drugs more attractive to scientists and less attractive to their social users.

References

Abelson, H.I., Atkinson, R.B.: Public experience with psychoactive substances. Part I: Main findings and Part III: methods and procedures. Report prepared for the National Institute of Drug Abuse, Division of Behavioral and Social Sciences, Rockville, Maryland 1975

Aghajanian, G.K.: LSD and CNS transmission. Annu. Rev. Pharmacol. Toxicol. *12*, 157–168 (1972)

Aghajanian, G.K., Bing, O.H.: Persistence of lysergic acid diethylamide in the plasma of human subjects. Clin. Pharmacol. Ther. *5*, 611–614 (1964)

Anden, N.-E., Corrodi, H., Fuxe, K.: Hallucinogenic drugs of the indolealkylamine type and central monoamine neurons. J. Pharmacol. Exp. Ther. *179*, 236–249 (1971)

Anden, N.-E., Corrodi, H., Fuxe, K.: The effect of psychotomimetic glycolate esters on central monoamine neurons. Eur. J. Pharmacol. *17*, 97–102 (1972)

Angrist, B., Rotrosen, J., Gershon, S.: Assessment of tolerance to the hallucinogenic effects of DOM. Psychopharmacology *36*, 203–207 (1974)

Balster, R.L., Johanson, C.E.: Phencyclidine self-administration in the rhesus monkey. Pharmacol. Biochem. Behav. *1*, 167–172 (1973)

Barnett, B.E.W.: Diazepam treatment for LSD intoxication. Lancet *1971 II*, 270

Berlin, C.M., Jacobson, C.B.: Psychedelic drugs: A threat to reproduction? Fed. Proc. *31*, 1326 (1972)

Bradley, P.B., Briggs, I.: Further studies on the mode of action of psychotomimetic drugs: Antagonism of the excitatory actions of 5-hydroxytryptamine by methylated derivatives of tryptamine. Br. J. Pharmacol. *50*, 345–354 (1974)

Brawley, P., Duffield, J.C.: The pharmacology of hallucinogens. Pharmacol. Rev. *24*, 31–66 (1972)
Burns, R.S., Lerner, S.E., Corrado, R., James, S.H., Schnoll, S.H.: Phencyclidine – states of acute intoxication and fatalities. West. J. Med. *123*, 345–349 (1975)
Cohen, S.: The psychotomimetic agents. Prog. Drug Res. *15*, 68–102 (1971)
Davis, H.K., Fork, H.F., Tupin, J.P., Colvin, A.: Clinical evaluation of JB-329 (Ditran). Dis. Nerv. Syst. *25*, 179–183 (1964)
Dishotsky, N.I., Loughman, W.D., Mogar, R.E., Lipscomb, W.R.: LSD and genetic damage: Is LSD chromosome damaging, carcinogenic, mutagenic, or teratogenic? Science *172*, 431 (1971)
Domino, E.F., Wilson, A.E.: Effects of urine acidification in plasma and urine phencyclidine levels in overdose. Clin. Pharmacol. Ther. *22*, 421–424 (1977)
Freedman, D.X.: The psychopharmacology of hallucinogenic agents. Annu. Rev. Med. *20*, 409–418 (1969)
Gershon, S., Bell, C.: A study of the antagonism of some indole alkaloids to the behavioural effects of "Ditran". Med. Exp. *8*, 15–27 (1963)
Greifenstein, F.E., DeVault, M., Yoshitake, J., Gajewski, J.E.: A study of a 1-aryl cyclo hexyl amine for anesthesia. Anesth. and Analg. (Cleve) *37*, 283–294 (1958)
Gogerty, J.H., Dille, J.M.: Pharmacology of d-lysergic acid morpholide. J. Pharmacol. Exp. Ther. *120*, 340–348 (1957)
Gorodetzky, C.W., Isbell, H.: A comparison of 2,3-dihydrolysergic acid diethylamide with LSD-25. Psychopharmacology *6*, 229–233 (1964)
Hart, J.B., McChesney, J.D., Greis, M., Schulz, G.: Composition of illicit drugs and the use of drug analysis in abuse abatement. J. Psychedelic Drugs *5*, 83–88 (1972)
Hitzeman, R.J., Loh, H.H., Domino, E.F.: Effect of phencyclidine on the accumulation of ^{14}C-catecholamines formed from ^{14}C-tyrosine. Arch. Int. Pharmacodyn. Ther. *202*, 252–258 (1973)
Ho, B.T., Estevez, V., Fritchie, G.E., Iansey, L.W., Idanpaan-Heikkila, J., McIsaac, W.M.: Metabolism of harmaline in rats. Biochem. Pharmacol. *20*, 1313–1319 (1971)
Hollister, L.E.: Chemical psychoses. LSD and related drugs, pp. 190. Springfield: Charles C. Thomas 1968
Hollister, L.E., Magnicol, M.F., Gillespie, H.K.: An hallucinogenic amphetamine analog (DOM) in man. Psychopharmacologia *14*: 62–73 (1969)
Idanpaan-Heikkila, J.E., McIsaac, W.M., Ho, B.T., Fritschie, G.E., Iansey, L.W.: Relation of pharmacological and behavioral effects of a hallucinogenic amphetamine to distribution in cat brain. Science *164*, 1085–1087 (1969)
Jacobs, B.L., Trulson, M.E., Stern, W.C.: An animal behavior model for studying the actions of LSD and related hallucinogens. Science *194*, 741–743 (1976)
Klee, G.D., Bertino, J., Weintraub, W., Gallaway, E.: The influence of varying dosage on the effects of lysergic acid diethylamide (LSD-25) in humans. J. Nerv. Ment. Dis. *132*, 404–409 (1961)
Kleptisz, A., Racy, J.: Homicide and LSD. J. Am. Med. Assoc. *223*, 429 (1973)
Long, S.Y.: Does LSD induce chromosomal damage and malformations? A review of the literature. Teratology *6*, 75 (1972)
Luby, E.D., Cohen, B.D., Roxenbaum, G., Gottlieb, J.S., Kelley, R.: Study of a new schizophrenomimetic drug: Sernyl. Arch. Neurol. Psychiatry. *81*, 363–368 (1959)
Maayani, S., Weinstein, H., Ben-Zvi, N., Cohen, S., Sokolovsky, M.: Psychotomimetics as anticholinergic agents – Biochem. Pharmacol. *23*, 1263–1281 (1974)
Malitz, S., Wilkens, B., Roehrig, W.C., Hock, A.H.: A clinical comparison of three related hallucinogens. Psychiat. Q. *34*, 333–345 (1960)
Marshman, J.A., Ramsay, M.D., Sellers, E.M.: Quantitation of phencyclidine in biological fluids and application to human overdose. Toxicol. Appl. Pharmacol. *35*, 129–136 (1976)
Martin, W.R., Sloan, J.W.: The possible role of tryptamin in brain function and its relationship to the actions of LSD-like hallucinogens. Mt. Sinai J. Med. NY *41*, 276–282 (1974)
Miyasaki, M., Domino, E.F.: Neuronal mechanisms of ketamine-induced anesthesia. Int. J. Neuropharmacol. *7*, 557–573 (1968)
Moskowitz, D.: Use of haloperidol to reduce LSD flashbacks. Milit. Med. *136*, 754 (1971)

Ostfeld, A.M., Visotsky, H., Abood, L., Lebovitz, B.Z.: Studies with a new hallucinogen. Some dosage-response data for JB-318. Arch. Neurol. Psychiatry *81*, 256–263 (1959)
Pennes, H.H., Hoch, P.H.: Psychotomimetics, clinical and theoretical considerations. Harmine, Win-2299, and Nalline. Am. J. Psychiatry *113*, 887–892 (1957)
Peretz, E.I., Smythies, J.R., Gibson, W.C.: A new hallucinogen: 3,4,5-trimethoxyphenyl-b-aminopropane with notes on the stroboscopic phenomenon. J. Ment. Sci. *101*, 317–329 (1955)
Pieri, L., Pieri, M., Haefely, W.: LSD as an agonist of dopamine receptors in the striatum. Nature *252*, 586–588 (1974)
Radouco-Thomas, S., Schwarz, T.H., Michaud, R.: Psychotomimetics and cerebral cations. In: Pharmacology, toxicology and abuse of psychotomimetics (hallucinogens). Radouco-Thomas, S., Villeneuve, A., Radouco-Thomas, C. (eds.), pp. 239–248. Quebec: Les Presses de l'Universite Laval 1974
Reich, P., Hepps, R.B.: Homicide during a psychosis induced by LSD. J.A.M.A. *219*, 869 (1972)
Rosenbaum, G., Cohen, B.D., Luby, E.D., Gottlieb, J.S., Yelen, D.: Comparison of Sernyl with other drugs. Arch. Gen. Psychiatry *1*, 113–118 (1959)
Rosenberg, D.E., Isbell, H., Miner, E.J., Logan, C.R.: The effect of N,N-dimethyltryptamine in human subjects tolerant to lysergic acid diethylamide. Psychopharmacology *5*, 217–227 (1964)
Sankar, D.V. Siva: LSD: A total study pp. 345 Westbury, New York: PJD Publications 1975
Sarwer-Foner, G.J.: Some clinical and social aspects of lysergic acid diethylamide. II. Psychosomatics *13*, 309 (1972)
Shulgin, A.T.: 3-Methoxy-4,5-methylenedioxy amphetamine, a new psychotomimetic agent. Nature *201*, 1120–1121 (1964)
Shulgin, A.T., Sargent, T., Naranjo, C.: Animal pharmacology and human psychopharmacology of 3-methoxy-4,5-methylenedioxyphenylisopropylamine (MMDA). Pharmacology *10*, 12–18 (1973)
Smith, R.C., Meltzer, H., Dekirmenjian, H., Davis, John M.: Effects of phencyclidine on biogenic amines in rat brain. Neurosci. Abstr. *1/468*, 134 (1975)
Stolk, J.M., Barchas, J.D., Goldstein, M., Boggan, W., Freedman, D.X.: A comparison of psychotomimetic drug effects on rat brain norepinephrine metabolism. J. Pharmacol. Exp. Ther. *189*, 42–50 (1974)
Tec, L.: Phenothiazine and biperiden in LSD reactions. J.A.M.A. *215*, 980 (1971)
Thiessen, P.N., Cook, D.A.: The properties of 3,4-methylenedioxy-amphetamine (MDA). I. A review of the literature. Clin. Toxicol. *6*, 45–52 (1973)
von Hungen, K., Roberts, S., Hill, D.F.: LSD as an agonist and antagonist at central dopamine receptors. Nature *252*, 588–589 (1974)
Wagner, J.G., Aghajanian, G.K., Bing, O.H.L.: Correlation of performance test scores with "tissue concentration" of lysergic acid diethylamide in human subjects. Clin. Pharmacol. Ther. *9*, 635–638 (1968)

CHAPTER 3

Psychotomimetics: Behavioral Pharmacology

J. B. APPEL, A. D. POLING, and D. M. KUHN

A. Introduction

This section is concerned with psychotomimetics or hallucinogens such as D-lysergic acid diethylamide (LSD) and its less potent indole and phenylethylamine congeners. In man, low doses of these agents (e.g., 1–5 µg LSD) are said to produce a specific state in which "psychedelic, mystical, or psychotomimetic, perceptions and thought occur in the presence of clear consciousness" (FREEDMAN and HALARIS, 1978). In other animals, psychotomimetics have been reported to produce diverse effects ranging from bizarre alterations in spiders' web building (WITT, 1956) to an elephant's death (WEST and PIERCE, 1962). In more frequently studied species such as rats, LSD increases overall levels of activity (KUHN and APPEL, 1975), prevents the habituation of a startle response (DAVIS and SHEARD, 1974), and causes a characteristic "behavioral syndrome" consisting of tremor, rigidity, Straub trail, hindlimb abduction, lateral head weaving, and reciprocal forepaw treading (TRULSON et al., 1976).

While many of these drug-induced changes in behavior are interesting, they will not be considered further. Instead, this review will focus on those effects of LSD and related compounds that have been analyzed both systematically and objectively within the context of behavioral pharmacology. Thus, we shall be concerned primarily with a few learned behaviors (e.g., bar pressing, key pecking) in pigeons, rats, and monkeys; an attempt will be made, however, to relate drug effects to variables that control the behavior of all organisms (e.g., the relationship between a response and its consequences).

B. The Behavioral Pharmacology of LSD and Related Compounds

I. Operant (Instrumental) Behavior

1. Positive Reinforcement: Schedule-Controlled Behavior

Several years ago the effects of psychotomimetic drugs on behavior maintained by various positive reinforcers (food, water, electrical stimulation of the brain) were reviewed and discussed in detail (APPEL, 1968); the general pattern of results has not changed since that review appeared. In summary, LSD and its congeners, like most psychotropic drugs, have effects that depend upon response rate and the schedule under which behavior is maintained (APPEL, 1968; DEWS and WENGER, 1977; SANGER and BLACKMAN, 1976). For example, sufficiently high doses of LSD (greater than 0.04 mg/kg in the rat) completely disrupt bar pressing maintained under short fixed-ratio (FR) schedules (which generate very high control rates) by inducing periods of pausing or no responding (FREEDMAN et al., 1964). Comparable doses cause less drastic decreases in the relatively high rates maintained under certain variable-interval (VI) or fixed-interval (FI) schedules and increase the low response rates observed under other (FI and Differential Reinforcement of Low Rate, DRL) schedules (APPEL, 1971; ALTMAN and APPEL, 1975; KSIR and NELSON, 1977). The rate-decreasing effects of LSD and related compounds are comparatively greater than the rate-increasing effects of the same doses of the same drugs; high doses of LSD (>0.04 mg/kg) tend to decrease responding regardless of control rates (APPEL, 1971; SANGER and BLACKMAN, 1976). Responding suppressed to a low rate by punishment has been reported to decrease further following high doses of LSD (APPEL, 1971; Barry et al., 1963) and to increase following low doses of both LSD and mescaline (SCHOENFELD, 1976).

Analysis of the effects of psychotomimetic agents on positively reinforced operant behavior has provided useful information about relative potencies (APPEL and FREEDMAN, 1965), time-courses of effect (FREEDMAN et al., 1964; PETERSON, 1966), and dose–response relationships (APPEL et al., 1968; APPEL and FREEDMAN, 1965; FREEDMAN et al., 1964). For instance, measuring the amount of disruption of FR performance has enabled us to determine that, in the rat (APPEL and FREEDMAN, 1965) as in man (ABRAMSON et al., 1960), D-LSD is about 10 times as potent as both psilocybin and D-amphetamine and 100 times as potent as mescaline. It has also enabled us to begin to elucidate the mechanism of action of psychotomimetics in vivo. For example, the finding that the disruptive effects of low doses of LSD are potentiated following pretreatment with reserpine (APPEL and FREEDMAN, 1964) or P-chlorophenylalanine (APPEL et al., 1970a), by raphe lesions (APPEL et al., 1970b), or by intraventricular injections of the specific serotonergic neurotoxin 5,7-dihydroxytryptamine (JOSEPH and APPEL, 1977), along with other pharmacologic evidence (GREENBERG et al., 1975; KUHN et al., 1976, 1977, 1978), suggests that the behavioral effects of LSD are mediated at least in part by serotonergic neural systems. Similar results have also been reported with mescaline (BROWNE, 1978; BROWNE and HO, 1975) and other psychotomimetics (APPEL et al., 1977).

2. Negative Reinforcement: Escape and Avoidance Behavior

Even though LSD has been said to enhance sensitivity to noxious input (FREEDMAN and HALARIS, 1978), the bulk of the literature does not support the hypothesis that this or related compounds has unique effects on behavior maintained by the offset of stimuli (escape behavior); moreover, the effects that have been reported occur only at relatively high doses and depend largely on the specific procedure used (APPEL, 1968). For example, 0.50 mg/kg LSD, a dose much larger than that which reliably disrupts positively reinforced behavior (see above), (1) increases the speed of rats trained to run down an alley to escape from shock (HAMILTON, 1960), (2) has little effect on the speed of turning a wheel to escape from shock (or from a stimulus paired with shock) in an operant chamber (APPEL et al., 1967), and (3) decreases ability to escape from a water-filled T-maze (HAMILTON and WILPIZESKI, 1961). Thus, escape behavior has not been particularly useful in demonstrating selective effects of LSD.

Avoidance behavior (i.e., behavior that is maintained by the response-contingent postponement of a stimulus) is affected unreliably by psychotomimetics (APPEL, 1968). The results seem to depend upon species, dose, and the nature of the avoidance task. In the rat, relatively high doses of LSD (greater than 0.50 mg/kg) decrease responding under various avoidance paradigms (McMILLAN and LEANDER, 1976); lower doses facilitate performance in some situations (JARRARD, 1964), but hinder it in others (McISAAC et al., 1961).

Smythies and his co-workers have reported that the effects of mescaline and its congeners on signaled avoidance responding in a shuttle-box depend upon how long after injection they are measured (SMYTHIES and SYKES, 1964, 1966). Shortly after drug administration, avoidance responding is depressed (relative to controls); that is, reaction times increase and the total number of responses decrease. Over time, these effects are reversed such that avoidance responding is facilitated; that is, mescaline-treated animals avoid shock faster and more often than controls. The authors contend that this biphasic, Bovet-Gatti profile is specific to psychotomimetics and can therefore be useful in drug "screening." However, recent investigations have failed to confirm this reported specificity (CALIL, 1978), and better screening procedures (e.g., procedures involving the discriminative stimulus properties of drugs) are available (APPEL, et al., 1978; BARRY, 1974; CALIL, 1978; KUHN et al., 1976, 1977).

II. Respondent (Pavlovian) Behavior

In the United States and in Western Europe, the effects of psychotomimetic drugs on behavior conditioned by respondent (Pavlovian) techniques, i.e., the contiguous pairing of conditioned (CS) and unconditioned (UCS) stimuli, have not been studied extensively. Recently, however, increasing attention has been paid to this neglected area of behavioral pharmacology.

1. Appetitive Conditioning

In our laboratory, LSD (0.05–0.45 mg/kg) and quipazine (1–8 mg/kg), both of which probably function in vivo as central serotonin agonists (APPEL et al., 1978; APPEL and WHITE, 1978; KUHN et al., 1978; WHITE et al., 1977), have been found to decrease key pecking behavior of pigeons maintained under an automaintenance procedure (in which a CS, brief illumination of a response key, is paired with a UCS, delivery of food). However, this effect was not specific to psychotomimetic (or serotonergic) compounds since various other drugs (e.g., pentobarbital and *d*-amphetamine) also decreased responding (POLING and APPEL, 1978). In a second experiment, both LSD and quipazine were found to have little effect on key pecking maintained under a negative automaintenance procedure, in which food (UCS) was presented following key illumination (CS) only if the lighted key was not pecked; in this situation, both pentobarbital and diazepam increased responding (POLING and APPEL, 1979). Although these initial findings indicate that appetitively conditioned, respondent behavior is not selectively affected by psychotomimetics, the generality of this suggestion remains to be determined.

2. Aversive (Defense) Conditioning

"Aversive" respondent conditioning, i.e., procedures in which a CS (e.g., tone) precedes delivery of a "noxious" UCS (electric shock) regardless of the organism's behavior, have also failed to reveal effects that are specific to psychotomimetics; as is the case with many drugs, high doses apparently interfere with the conditioning of autonomic responses (e. g., "fear") while low doses have few reliable effects (APPEL, 1968).

A study by HILL et al. (1967) was concerned with the effects of LSD and several other drugs on bar-pressing behavior under an ESTES-SKINNER (1941) procedure, in which a tone (CS) paired with unavoidable shock (UCS) was superimposed occasionally on a baseline of positively reinforced responding (VI). It was found that bar pressing, normally suppressed during the presence of the tone, was increased by LSD. It is known, however, that the effects of drugs under aversive conditioning procedures are notoriously sensitive to experimental parameters (APPEL, 1963; MILLENSON and LESLIE, 1974). Thus, the results of Hill and co-workers (1967) do not always obtain. For example, in our laboratory, LSD (0.04–0.36 mg/kg) failed to increase the rate of responding suppressed by either the ESTES-SKINNER procedure or by a stimulus paired with time-out from positive reinforcement (unpublished observations).

III. Perceptual Effects

In 1968, a discussion of the perceptual effects of psychotomimetics concluded:

Low doses of drugs such as LSD ... increase level of physiological arousal or alertness and decrease the ability of an animal to habituate to environmental stimuli which once were, but no longer are, relevant. Behaviorally, increases in amount of generalization to auditory, visual, and other kinds of environmental stimuli and what may be described as enhanced sensory impact occur. Increased arousal and generalization may induce changes in an animal's ability to discriminate events in its environment but whether such changes take the form of increased or diminished accuracy of perception is multi-determinded (e. g., dose, time since the drug is given, and the nature of the task are extremely important) (APPEL, 1968, p. 1219).

Research since the foregoing was written confirms the conclusion that the perceptual effects of psychotomimetics are complex and that few, if any, general conclusions can be drawn from the available data. For example, whether or not LSD increases the generalization of auditory stimuli (pitch) in rats depends (among other things) on the measure of generalization used in a given experiment (APPEL and DYKSTRA, 1977). A dose of 0.16 mg/kg was found to increase the amount of generalization when rate of responding was measured in a free-operant situation similar to that described by GUTTMAN and KALISH (1956), but had no effect on generalization along the same dimension when probability of responding was measured in a discrete-trial, two-choice task (DYKSTRA and APPEL, 1970, 1972).

In an attempt to delineate the extent to which the perceptual effects of various drugs including LSD reflect changes in ability to discriminate stimuli (sensitivity) or changes in some other aspect of the organism's disposition to respond (criterion or bias), the theory of signal detection (GREEN and SWETS, 1966) has recently been used to analyze data obtained in a variety of discrimination situations (APPEL and DYKSTRA, 1977). In contrast to diverse compounds such as morphine, chlorpromazine, and Δ^{-9} tetrahydrocannabinol (THC), LSD has no effect on the ability of either rats or pigeons to discriminate (detect): (1) differences between tones based on frequency (pitch) or duration (DYKSTRA and APPEL, 1974), (2) differences between visual stimuli based on intensity (STRAUB and APPEL, 1975) or duration (ALTMAN et al., 1979), or (3) the presence or absence of either pure tones or mild shock in a background of "white" noise (HERNANDEZ and APPEL, 1979). However, at least some logically complex, conditional visual discriminations may be more susceptible to disruption by LSD than are simple unidimensional tasks (APPEL and DYKSTRA, 1977). In any case, it is clear that LSD does not necessarily alter objectively defined measures of perception in animals, despite the consistency with which humans report that (subjective) perceptual changes occur following ingestion of this compound (SANKAR, 1975).

IV. Tolerance and Related Phenomena

1. Tolerance

Tolerance to the behavioral effects of psychotomimetics develops rapidly in many (e.g., FREEDMAN et al., 1964; BECKER et al., 1967; MAHLER and HUMOLLER, 1959; McGOWAN, 1976), but not all (e.g., FREEDMAN and HALARIS, 1978; HAMILTON, 1960; GILLETT, 1960), situations and is a function of pharmacologic variables such as dose (FREEDMAN et al., 1964) and behavioral variables such as the empirical consequences of altered rates of responding (McGOWAN, 1976).

2. Cross-Tolerance

In general, when tolerance occurs to one psychotomimetic (e.g., LSD) cross-tolerance occurs to other psychotomimetics (e.g., psilocybin) in humans, rats, and birds (ABRAMSON et al., 1960; APPEL and FREEDMAN, 1968; McGOWAN, 1976); however, such relationships have not been examined for all combinations of these pharmacologically related agents and may depend critically upon dose.

While there is evidence that cross-tolerance between LSD and the serotonin precursor 5-HTP occurs, at least in the rat (CARTER and APPEL, 1978), the behavioral effects of LSD and other centrally acting CNS "excitants" such as D-amphetamine, which are mediated by different mechanisms, do not show cross-tolerance (APPEL and FREEDMAN, 1968).

3. Dependence

Psychotomimetics do not induce physical dependence in either humans or other animals, i.e., withdrawal symptoms do not occur when these drugs are witheld following chronic administration (JAFFE, 1965). At least in nonhumans, psychotomimetics do not induce psychological dependence, i.e., there is no evidence that animals will self-administer these compounds (SCHUSTER and JOHANSON, 1974). We discuss psychological dependence in humans elsewhere in this volume (see Chap. 6).

V. Stimulus Properties of Psychotomimetics

In all of the exeriments reviewed thus far, and in most of behavioral pharmacology, the physiologic changes (states) induced by drugs have been analyzed indirectly, in terms of the extent to which they disrupt ongoing activity. Drug states can also be analyzed directly; that is, in terms of the discriminative, reinforcing and other stimulus properties these states might have (THOMPSON and PICKENS, 1971).

1. Discriminative Stimulus Properties

Relatively low doses of LSD, mescaline, and related psychotomimetics have strong discriminative stimulus properties (CAMERON and APPEL, 1973; GREENBERG et al., 1975; HIRSCHHORN and WINTER, 1971; KUHN et al., 1976, 1977; SCHECHTER and ROSECRANS, 1972); i.e., animals readily learn to respond differentially on the basis of whether or not a specific drug state or cue is present. For example, rats trained in a two-choice situation, in which responses on one lever (left) are reinforced intermittently (with water) following i.p. injections of 0.08 mg/kg LSD while responses on the other lever (right) are reinforced following saline, learn within 40 sessions (trials) to respond on the lever appropriate to the substance received (GREENBERG et al., 1975). When doses of the training compound other than the training dose are subsequently administered during sessions in which no reinforcers are delivered, a generalization gradient occurs that is similar to those obtained when other discriminative stimuli (lights, tones, etc.) are used; as the difference between the test and the training stimulus intensity (dose) increases, the proportion of "drug" responses (i.e., those reinforced following drug administration during training) decreases (APPEL et al., 1978).

In general, there is relatively good generalization or cross-transfer between the discriminative effects of LSD, mescaline, psilocybin, and quipazine (APPEL et al., 1978; APPEL and WHITE, 1978). In other words, an animal trained to respond in a particular manner in the presence of one of these agents behaves in a similar manner when one of the other drugs is given. Indeed, transfer studies have been useful in classifying drugs since compounds within a given pharmacologic class appear to have similar discriminative stimulus properties. However, amount of transfer is a function of dose (OVERTON, 1971).

We have argued elsewhere that the drug discrimination procedure, because of its sensitivity and specificity, promises to be very valuable to behavioral pharmacology (KUHN et al., 1976, 1977; APPEL et al., 1978). It has already helped several groups of investigators elucidate the mechanism of action in vivo of diverse compounds including psychotomimetics (APPEL et al., 1978). For example, drugs and other interventions that modify the functional activity of serotonergic neurons, also alter the ability of rats to discriminate low doses of D-LSD (KUHN et al., 1978) and quipazine (APPEL and WHITE, 1978; WHITE et al., 1977). Other transmitter agonists and antagonists do not have this effect. These results, which parallel those of drug-interaction studies utilizing schedule-controlled behavior (see above) and studies involving the stereo-specific binding of D-LSD in vitro (AGHAJANIAN et al., 1975; BENNETT and SNYDER, 1975, 1976; LOVELL and FREEDMAN, 1976), suggest that the behavioral effects of LSD and quipazine are mediated by direct stimulation of (postsynaptic) 5-HT or hallucinogen (LSD) receptors.

2. Reinforcing Properties

Even though most drugs that are self-administered by humans (e.g., opiates, amphetamines, barbiturates) are also self-administered by other animals (THOMPSON and PICKENS, 1975), there is no evidence that psychotomimetics are self-administered (i.e., serve as positive reinforcers) by species other than man. Rather, LSD may have negatively reinforcing properties, since rhesus monkeys respond in order to terminate stimuli associated with the delivery of this compound (HOFFMEISTER, 1975; HOFF-

MEISTER and WUTTKE, 1973). However, it should be noted that whether a given agent is self-administered or avoided depends upon a large number of biochemical, physiologic and behavioral parameters (GOLDBERG, 1976).

3. Unconditioned Stimulus Properties

It has been shown, in a series of experiments, that LSD is one of several psychoactive compounds that can function effectively as a UCS (CAMERON and APPEL, 1972a, 1972b, 1976). That is, when a stimulus such as a light or tone is paried with i. p. injection of LSD and is subsequently presented while a rat is pressing a bar under a VI schedule of food reinforcement, response rate is significantly decreased. This finding has been taken to indicate that LSD may be "aversive," i. e., similar to stimuli such as shock in the ESTES-SKINNER (1941) paradigm. However, this interpretation is open to question in view of recent demonstrations that stimuli paired with the noncontingent presentation of food (a seemingly nonaversive stimulus) may also decrease food-maintained responding (e. g., POLING et al., 1977).

C. Summary and Conclusions

Many of the learned behaviors of nonhumans are affected by relatively low doses of LSD and similar drugs. Within any given paradigm, the effects of these compounds appear to be relatively consistent. However, both behavioral and pharmacologic parameters can influence the magnitude and direction of drug effects. Thus, asking "how do psychotomimetics affect behavior controlled by certain variables (e.g., positively reinforced behavior)?" is much like asking, "how fast do humans run?" The answer to each question depends upon a variety of factors; neither question can be answered meaningfully in the abstract.

Beyond being sensitive to low doses, a behavioral procedure for evaluating drug effects should show selectivity, i. e., not all compounds should produce the same effect. Ideally, drugs that are demonstrated to be similar in other assays (e. g., tests of in vitro activity) should produce similar behavioral effects; drugs with dissimilar effects in other assays should not have the same effects on behavior.

Several behavioral procedures do demonstrate selective effects of LSD, mescaline, psilocybin, and quipazine. For instance, these drugs have uniquely similar discriminative stimulus properties and share similar time-courses of action under certain avoidance schedules. However, selective effects are not so readily demonstrated under some other, commonly used behavioral procedures. For example, responding under a short FR schedule of positive reinforcement may be decreased in dose-dependent fashion by compounds with very different mechanisms of action, such as LSD, D-amphetamine, atropine, and ethanol. A more detailed analysis of drug effects and drug interactions under such a procedure may, nonetheless, disclose selective effects; for instance, the specific manner in which rates are reduced differ following treatment with different combinations of 5-HT, DA, ACh agonists, and nonselective CNS depressants.

Acknowledgement. The preparation of this chapter and some of the research reported herein were supported by USPHS Research Grants MH-24,593, from the National Institute of Mental Health, and 9 RO1 DA-01799, from the National Institute on Drug Abuse.

References

Abrahamson, H.A., Rolo, A., Sklarofsky, B., Stache, J.: Production of cross-tolerance to psychosis-producing doses of lysergic acid diethylamide and psilocybin. J. Psychol. *49*, 151–154 (1960)

Aghajanian, G.K., Haigler, H.J., Bennett, J.L.: Amine receptors in the CNS. III. 5-hydroxytryptamine in the brain. In: Handbook of psychopharmacology. Iversen, L.L., Iversen, S.D., Snyder, S.H. (eds.), pp. 63–69. New York: Plenum 1975

Altman, J.L., Appel, J.B.: LSD and fixed-interval responding in the rat. Pharmacol. Biochem. Behav. *3*, 151–155 (1975)

Altman, J.L., Appel, J.B., Mc Gowan, W.T., III: Drugs and the discrimination of duration. Psychopharmacology *60*, 183–188 (1979)

Appel, J.B.: Drugs, shock intensity, and the CER. Psychopharmacology *4*, 148–153 (1963)

Appel, J.B.: Effects of LSD on time-based schedules of reinforcement. Psychopharmacology **21**, 174–186 (1971)

Appel, J.B.: The effects of "psychotomimetic" drugs on animal behavior. In: Psychopharmacology: A review of progress 1957–1967. Efron, D. (ed.). U.S. Public Health Service Publication *1836*, 1211–1222 (1968)

Appel, J.B., Dykstra, L.A.: Drugs, discrimination and signal detection theory. In: Advances in behavioral pharmacology. Thompson, T., Dews, P.B. (eds.), Vol. I, pp. 139–166. New York: Academic Press 1977

Appel, J.B., Freedman, D.X.: Chemically-induced alterations in the behavioral effects of LSD-25. Biochem. Pharmacol. *13*, 861–869 (1964)

Appel, J.B., Freedman, D.X.: The relative potencies of psychotomimetic drugs. Life Sci. *4*, 2181–2186 (1965)

Appel, J.B., Freedman, D.X., Filby, Y.M.: The effects of three psychoactive drugs on two varieties of escape behavior. Arch. Int. Pharmacodyn. Ther. *167*, 179–193 (1967)

Appel, J.B., Freedman, D.X.: Tolerance and cross-tolerance among psychotomimetic drugs. Psychopharmacology *13*, 267–274 (1968)

Appel, J.B., Joseph, J.A., Utsey, E., Hernandez, L.L., Boggan, W.O.: Sensitivity to psychoactive drugs and the serotonergic neuronal system. Commun. Psychopharmacol. *1*, 541–551 (1977)

Appel, J.B., Lovell, R.A., Freedman, D.X.: Alterations in the behavioral effects of lysergic acid diethylamide by pretreatment with p-chlorophenylalanine and alpha-methyl-p-tyrosine. Psychopharmacology *18*, 387–406 (1970a)

Appel, J.B., Sheard, M.H., Freedman, D.X.: Alterations in the behavioral effects of LSD by midbrain raphe lesions. Commun. Behav. Biol. *5*, 237–241 (1970b)

Appel, J.B., White, F.J.: Behavioral and neuropharmacological aspects of the discriminative stimulus properties of quipazine. Fed. Proc. *37* (1978)

Appel, J.B., White, F.J., Kuhn, D.M.: The use of drugs as discriminative stimuli in behavioral pharmacodynamics. In: Stimulus Properties of Drugs: Ten years of Progress. Colpaert, F.C., Rosecrans, J.A. (eds.), pp. 7–29. Amsterdam–New York: Elsevier/North-Holland 1978

Appel, J.B., Whitehead, W.E., Freedman, D.X.: Motivation and the behavioral effects of LSD. Psychonomic Sci. *12*, 305–306 (1968)

Barry, H., III: Classification of drugs according to their discriminable effects in rats. Fed. Proc. *33*, 1814–1824 (1974)

Barry, H. III, Wagner, S.A., Miller, N.E.: Effects of several drugs on performance in an Approach-Avoidance conflict. Psychol. Rep. *12*, 215–221 (1963)

Becker, D.I., Appel, J.B., Freedman, D.X.: Some effects of LSD on visual discrimination in pigeons. Psychopharmacology *11*, 354–364 (1967)

Bennett, J.P., Snyder, S.H.: Stereospecific binding of d-lysergic acid diethylamide (LSD) to brain membranes: relationship to post-synaptic serotonin receptors. Brain Res. *94*, 523–544 (1975)

Bennett, J.P., Snyder, S.H.: Serotonin and lysergic acid diethylamide binding in rat brain membranes: relationship to post-synaptic serotonin receptors. Mol. Pharmacol. *12*, 373–389 (1976)

Browne, R.G.: The role of serotonin in the discriminative stimulus properties of mescaline. In: Drug discrimination and state dependent learning. Ho, B.T., Richards, D.W., III, Chute, D.L. (eds.). pp. 79–101. New York: Acadmic Press 1978

Browne, R.G., Ho, B.T.: The role of serotonin in the discriminative stimulus properties of mescaline. Pharmacol. Biochem. Behav. *3*, 429–435 (1975)

Calil, H.M.: Screening hallucinogenic drugs. II. Systematic study of two behavioral tests. Psychopharmacology *56*, 87–92 (1978)

Cameron, O.G., Appel, J.B.: Conditioned suppression of bar-pressing behavior by stimuli associated with drugs. J. Exp. Anal. Behav. *17*, 127–137 (1972a)

Cameron, O.G., Appel, J.B.: Generalization of LSD-induced conditioned suppression. Psychonomic Sci. *27*, 302–304 (1972b)

Cameron, O.G., Appel, J.B.: A behavioral and pharmacological analysis of some discriminable properties of d-LSD in rats. Psychopharmacology *33*, 117–134 (1973)

Cameron, O.G., Appel, J.B.: Drug-induced conditioned suppression: specificity due to drug employed as UCS. Pharmacol. Biochem. Behav. *4*, 221–224 (1976)

Carter, R.B., Appel, J.B.: LSD and 5-HTP: Tolerance and cross-tolerance relationships. Eur. J. Pharmacol. *50*, 145–148 (1978)

Davis, M., Sheard, M.H.: Effects of lysergic acid diethylamide (LSD) on habituation and sensitization of the startle response in the rat. Pharmacol. Biochem. Behav. *2*, 675–684 (1974)

Dews, P.B., Wenger, G.R.: Rate-dependency of the behavioral effects of amphetamine. In: Advances in behavioral pharmacology. Thompson, T., Dews, P.B. (eds.), Vol. I, pp. 167–227. New York: Academic Press 1977

Dykstra, L.A., Appel, J.B.: Effects of LSD on auditory generalization. Psychonomic Sci. *21*, 272–274 (1970)

Dykstra, L.A., Appel, J.B.: LSD and stimulus generalization: Rate-dependent effects. Science *177*, 720–722 (1972)

Dykstra, L.A., Appel, J.B.: Effects of LSD on auditory perception: a signal detection analysis. Psychopharmacology *34*, 289–307 (1974)

Estes, W.K., Skinner, B.F.: Some quantitative properties of anxiety. J. Exp. Psychol. *29*, 390–400 (1941)

Freedman, D.X., Appel, J.B., Hartman, F.R., Molliver, M.E.: Tolerance to behavioral effects of LSD-25 in rat. J. Pharmacol. Exp. Ther. *143*, 309–313 (1964)

Freedman, D.X., Halaris, A.E.: Monoamines and the biochemical mode of action of LSD at synapses. In: Psychopharmacology: A generation of progress. Lipton, M.A., DiMascio, A., Killam, K.F. (eds.), pp. 347–359. New York: Raven 1978

Gillett, E.: Effects of chlorpromazine and d-lysergic acid diethylamide on sex behavior of male rats. Proc. Soc. Exp. Biol. Med. *103*, 393 (1960)

Goldberg, S.: The behavioral analysis of drug addiction. In: Behavioral pharmacology. Glick, S.D., Goldfarb, J. (eds.), pp. 283–316. St. Louis: Mosby 1976

Green, D.M., Swets, J.A.: Signal detection theory and psychophysics. New York: Wiley 1966

Greenberg, I., Kuhn, D.M., Appel, J.B.: Behaviorally-induced sensitivity to the discriminable properties of LSD. Psychopharmacology *43*, 229–232 (1975)

Guttman, N., Kalish, H.I.: Discriminability and stimulus generalization. J. Exp. Psychol. *51*, 79–88 (1956)

Hamilton, C.L.: Effects of LSD-25 and amphetamine on a running response in the rat. Arch. Gen. Psychiatry *2*, 104–109 (1960)

Hamilton, C.L., Wilpizeski, C.: Effects of LSD-25 on food intake in the rat. Proc. Soc. Exp. Biol. Med. *108*, 319–321 (1961)

Hernandez, L.L., Appel, J.B.: An analysis of some perceptual effects of morphine, chlorpromazine and LSD. Psychopharmacology *60*, 125–130 (1979)

Hill, H.F., Bell, E.C., Wikler, A.: Reduction of conditioned suppression: actions of morphine compared with those of amphetamine, pentobarbital, nalorphine, cocaine, LSD-25, and chlorpromazine. Arch. Int. Pharmacodyn. Ther. *165*, 212–225 (1967)

Hirschhorn, I.D., Winter, J.C.: Mescaline and lysergic acid diethylamide (LSD) as discriminative stimuli. Psychopharmacology *22*, 64–71 (1971)

Hoffmeister, F.: Negatively reinforcing properties of some psychotropic drugs in drug-naive rhesus monkeys. J. Pharmacol. Exp. Ther. *192*, 468–477 (1975)

Hoffmeister, F., Wuttke, W.: Negative reinforcing properties of morphine antagonists in naive rhesus monkeys. Psychopharmacology *33*, 247–258 (1973)
Jaffe, J.H.: Drug addiction and drug abuse. In: The pharmacological basis of therapeutics. Goodman, L.S., Gilman, A. (eds.), pp. 276–313. New York: Macmillan 1965
Jarrard, L.E.: Effects of d-lysergic acid diethylamide on operant behavior in the rat. Psychopharmacology *5*, 39–46 (1964)
Joseph, J.A., Appel, J.B.: Alterations in the behavioral effects of LSD by motivational and neurohumoral variables. Pharmacol. Biochem. Behav. *5*, 35–37 (1976)
Joseph, J.A., Appel, J.B.: Behavioral sensitivity to LSD: Dependency upon the pattern of central serotonin depletion. Pharmacol. Biochem. Behav. *6*, 499–504 (1977)
Ksir, C., Nelson, S.: LSD and d-amphetamine effects on fixed-interval responding in the rat. Pharmacol. Biochem. Behav. *6*, 269–272 (1977)
Kuhn, D.M., Appel, J.B.: Effect of serotonin agonists and antagonists on motor activity in rats. New York: Society for Neuroscience 1975
Kuhn, D.M., White, F.J., Appel, J.B.: Discriminable stimuli produced by hallucinogens. Psychopharmacol. Commun. *2*, 345–348 (1976)
Kuhn, D.M., White, F.J. Appel, J.B.: Discriminative stimulus properties of hallucinogens: behavioral assay of drug action. In: Discriminative stimulus properties of drugs: Lal, H. (ed.), pp. 137–155. New York: Plenum 1977
Kuhn, D.M., White, F.J., Appel, J.B.: The discriminative stimulus properties of LSD: mechanism of action. Neuropharmacology *17*, 257–263 (1978)
Lovell, R.A., Freedman, D.X.: Stereospecific receptor sites for d-lysergic acid diethylamide in rat brain: effects of neurotransmitters, amine antagonists, and other psychotropic drugs. Mol. Pharmacol. *12*, 620–630 (1976)
Mahler, D.J., Humoller, F.L.: Effect of lysergic acid diethylamide and bufotenine on performance of trained rats. Proc. Soc. Exp. Biol. Med. *102*, 697–701 (1959)
McGowan, W.T., III: Tolerance to LSD and cross-tolerance relationships between LSD and psilocybin. Unpublished thesis. University of South Carolina 1976
McIsaac, W.M., Khairallah, P.A., Page, I.H.: 10-Methoxyharmalan a potent serotonin antagonist which affects conditioned behavior. Science *134*, 674–675 (1961)
McMillan, D.E., Leander, J.D.: Effects of drugs on schedule-controlled behavior. In: Behavioral Pharmacology, Glick, S., Goldfarb, J. (eds.), pp. 85–139. St. Louis: Mosby, 1976
Millenson, J.R., Leslie, J.: The conditioned emotional response as a baseline for the study of anti-anxiety drugs. Neuropharmacology *13*, 1–9 (1974)
Overton, D.A.: Discriminative control of behavior by drug states. In: Stimulus properties of drugs. Thompson T., Pickens R. (eds.), pp. 87–110, New York: Appleton-Century-Crofts 1971
Peterson, N.J.: Some effects of LSD on the control of responding in the cebus monkey by reinforcing and discriminative stimuli. Unpublished thesis. Yale University 1966
Poling, A.D., Appel, J.B.: Drug effects under automaintenance and negative automaintenance procedures. Pharmacol. Biochem. Behav. *9*, 315–318 (1978)
Poling, A.D., Appel, J.B.: Drug effects on the performance of pigeons under a negative automaintenance procedure. Psychopharmacology *60*, 207–210 (1979)
Poling, A., Urbain, C., Thompson, T.: Effects of d-amphetamine and chlordiazepoxide on positive conditioned suppression. Pharmacol. Biochem. Behav. *7*, 233–238 (1977)
Sanger, D.J., Blackman, D.: Rate-dependent effects of drugs: a review of the literature. Pharmacol. Biochem. Behav. *4*, 73–83 (1976)
Sankar, D.V. Siva: LSD – A total study. Westbury, New York: PJD Publications 1975
Schechter, M.D., Rosecrans, J.A.: Lysergic acid diethylamide (LSD) as a discriminative cue: drugs with similar stimulus properties. Psychopharmacology *26*, 313–316 (1972)
Schoenfeld, R.I.: LSD and mescaline induced attenuation of the effect of punishment in the rat. Science *192*, 801–803 (1976)
Schuster, C.R., Johanson, C.E.: The use of animal models for the study of drug abuse. In: Research advances in alcohol and drug problems. Gibbin, R.J., Israel, Y., Popham, R.E., Schmidt, W., Smart, R.G. (eds.), Vol. 1, pp. 1–32. New York: Wiley 1974
Smythies, J.R., Sykes, E.A.: The effect of mescaline upon the conditioned avoidance response in the rat. Psychopharmacology *6*, 163–172 (1964)

Smythies, J.R., Sykes, E.A.: Structure-activity relationship studies on mescaline: the effect of dimethoxyphenylethylamine and N:N-dimethyl mescaline on the conditioned avoidance response in the rat. Psychopharmacology *8*, 324–330 (1966)
Straub, S.A., Appel, J.B.: Signal detection analysis of brightness discrimination following chlorpromazine, LSD and d-amphetamine. Southeastern Psychological Association. Atlanta 1975
Thompson, T., Pickens, R., (eds.): Stimulus properties of drugs. New York: Appleton-Century-Crofts 1971
Thompson, T., Pickens, R.: An experimental analysis of behavioral factors in drug dependence. Fed. Proc. *34*, 1759–1767 (1975)
Trulson, M.E., Ross, C.A., Jacobs, B.L.: Behavioral evidence for the stimulation of CNS serotonin receptors by high doses of LSD. Psychopharmacol. Commun. *2*, 149–164 (1976)
West, L.J., Pierce, C.M.: Lysergic acid diethylamide; its effects on a male asiatic elephant. Science *138*, 1100–1102 (1962)
White, F.J., Kuhn, D.M., Appel, J.B.: Discriminative stimulus properties of quipazine. Neuropharmacology *16*, 827–832 (1977)
Witt, P.N.: Die Wirkung von Substanzen auf den Netzbau der Spinne als biologischer Test. Berlin-Göttingen-Heidelberg: Springer 1956

CHAPTER 4

Biochemical Pharmacology of Psychotomimetics

D.X. FREEDMAN and W.O. BOGGAN

A. Introduction

The long and recently accelerated search for mechanisms of actions of drugs with psychotomimetic effects has utilized a broad array of classic pharmacologic and structure activity approaches (CERLETTI and DOEPFNER, 1958; HOFMANN, 1968), as well as quantitative structure activity relationships linked to molecular and submolecular properties (BARNETT, et al., 1978). Behavioral and psychopharmacologic studies in man (HOLLISTER, 1968; FREEDMAN, 1968) and animal (APPEL, 1968; CAMERON and APPEL, 1973; JACOBS et al., 1977) have appeared. Also utilized have been the techniques of neurophysiology (BRAWLEY AND DUFFIELD, 1972; AGHAJANIAN and WANG, 1978; JACOBS and TRULSON, 1979); and biochemical pharmacology (GIARMAN and FREEDMAN, 1965; BRIMBLECOMBE, 1973; FREEDMAN and HALARIS, 1978) as applied to CNS neurons. Central to this research has been a focus on D-lysergic acid diethylamide (LSD) because of the specificity, high potency, and reliability with which the drug produces a time-limited period of altered mental functioning. Approximately a billionth of a gram of LSD per gram of brain produces a 10-h state in which there is a compelled enhanced attention to subjective experience, a vividness of perception and affectivity (which is labile), and a diminished control over attention to environmental input (to which there is an enhanced but variably sustained reactivity). The experience is a fluid, multipotential one with underlying regularities (FREEDMAN, 1968), beginning with vivid sensory and affective and perceptual changes and continuing to a "postacute" phase that is marked by paranoid cognition and ideas of reference (FREEDMAN, 1968; BRAWLEY and DUFFIELD, 1972). Interestingly, the misinterpretations of reality and heightened subjectivity after LSD are similar to those seen in acute, florid, psychotic states (BOWERS and FREEDMAN, 1966), but not in chronic schizophrenias. It is in contrast to the amnestic and confusional effects of cholinomimetic deliriants; the variable effects of amine precursors or synthesis inhibitors; the very rare and uncertain psychotomimetic effects of *single* doses of stimulants in nonaddicts; the neurologic and performance decrements of the dissociative anesthetics such as phencyclidine; and the toxic confusional or affective states produced variably by a wide range of other drugs and hormones.

This review centers, then, on LSD, the drug which has received the most sustained focus of experimental work. We will refer to the related indolealkylamine psychotomimetics and the phenylethylamine psychotomimetics (epitomized by mescaline), or the methoxylated amphetamines (2,5-dimethoxy-4-methylamphetamine, DOM) primarily as they help to bring into focus mechanisms which clarify our knowledge about LSD or point to experimentally verifiable hypotheses that might elucidate the biochemical mechanisms of action of this class of psychotomimetic effects.

Candid assessment of over 30 years of extensive but rarely sustained and systematic studies of LSD reveals several problems:

1) The nonequivalency and nonselectivity of a vast range of often poorly understood and unreplicated behavioral measures; 2) Studies in a wide range of species (from invertebrates to goats and man) which provide an often uncertain basis upon which inferences about drugs or subclasses of them are frequently based; 3) Failure to note similarities and differences of receptors within the periphery and CNS or to take species differences with regard to this into account; 4) Utilization of agonists and antagonists [especially of serotonin (5-HT)] which are only partially characterized in terms of their pharmacology and physiologic effects, and selected on the basis of various reference systems (e.g., smooth muscles) (DYER and GANT, 1973; GREEN, 1978a; GADDUM, 1957; COSTA, 1956) in order to deduce functional significance or characterize CNS receptor activities of LSD; 5) Imprecision in defining inferred or observed receptor "stimulation", e.g., effects on autoreceptors at the raphe soma versus effects on autoreceptors at nerve endings, or whether postsynaptic effects, are in fact inhibitory or facilitating; 6) The lack of systematic criteria for assessing "low" and "high" doses in human and animal behavioral, electrophysiologic, or biochemical test systems; 7) The failure to utilize both threshold and maximal dosages to determine correlations over time with sequence and duration effects; and 8) Lack of precise statements as to what is sought in experiments.

Remedies to these problems should be apparent. For example a standard array of drugs, of "R" and "S" isomers and equivalent dosages determined on reliable human and animal behavioral, physiologic and receptor assays, might, if applied to brain studies, clarify many of the ambiguities due to sporadic study and interpretation.

If there were a unique biologically measurable response that differentiated psychotomimetics from all other drugs, the tracking of this might provide leads to accountable brain functions and to clinically encountered disorders. But no single molecular, biochemical, receptor, neural, or behavioral event has yet been found to characterize all psychedelic compounds. In fact there are real differences in the biochemical FREEDMAN et al., 1970) and neural response to the structurally different classes of drugs with similar mental effects (e.g., phenylethylamine and indole psychotomimetics). Effects of methoxylated amphetamines in single dosage are unclear (slightly elevated 5-HT and 5-hydroxyindoleacetic acid (5-HIAA), levels that resemble findings with higher doses of mescaline [FREEDMAN et al., 1970]), while depletion of 5-HT after parachlorophenylalanine (PCPA) is reduced by mescaline and DOM (TONGE and LEONARD, 1969; LEONARD and ANDEN et al., 1974). Within a single class, however, LSD, its psychoactive congeners and related indoleamines (such as *N-N*,dimethyltryptamine (DMT), psilocin, and psilocybin), show similarities and can be ranked by potency at the serotonergic dorsal raphe neuron, by their greater sensitivity at the raphe soma than at postsynaptic 5-HT membranes (AGHAJANIAN, this volume), and by their effect on 5-HT metabolism (FREEDMAN et al., 1970). Differences among the indole group are also noted in in vitro receptor binding affinities and in effects on norepinephrine metabolism (STOLK et al., 1974).

Leads sought in the biotransformation of endogenous indoles or tetrohydrocarbolines into psychotomimetically active substances (GIARMAN and FREEDMAN, 1965; BRAWLEY and DUFFIELD, 1972) have not been sustained on further study. Thus while methylated tryptamines (DMT, 5-methoxy-DMT, 5-methoxytryptamine) or phenylethylamines have been identified in human tissue, the monoamines per se have not been shown to be psychotomimetic. Furthermore, even though methylated indoles with psychotomimetic potential (DOMINO, 1975; KOSLOW, 1976) can be generated in mammalian tissue, the data do not link these biotransformations uniquely to schizophrenia (GILLIN et al., 1976) as the methylation hypothesis (BALDESSARINI et al., 1979) predicted. While there has been interest in biotransformation of psychotomimetic drugs as accounting for potency, e.g., HENDLEY and SNYDER (1971), or with respect to diethyltryptamine (SZARA et al., 1962), 6-hydroxylation in man has not been proven accountable (ROSENBERG et al., 1963; SNYDER and RICHELSON, 1968), nor have metabolites of mescaline (*N*-acetylmescaline and 3,4,5-trimethoxyphenylacetic acid) yet been linked with effects in man (CHARALAMPOUS et al., 1966) or animal (SMYTHIES et al., 1967). The mechanisms by which *N*-*N*,dimethylation or O-methylation (DE MONTIGNY and AGHANJANIAN, 1977) of indoles can enhance potency of an indoleamine have not been linked to endogenous metabolic events of clinical significance. All this is not to deny that the duration and onset, as well as potency of some drugs would not be influenced by biotransformations e.g., the in vivo conversion of psilocybin to psilocin (HORITA, 1963).

Structural similarities between phenylethylamines, methoxylated amphetamines, and LSD have been noted by NICHOLS et al. (1978). SHULGIN has noted that the more potent psychotomimetic isomers are those with absolute “R” configuration at the chiral center (ANDERSON et al., 1978), and these and other molecular properties, such as electron-donating capacity or preferred ring formation formed by intramolecular hydrogen binding (by which phenylethylamines might present to receptors as an indole), have been used to predict potencies and receptor characteristics (e.g., KANG and GREEN, 1970). The absolute configuration of optical isomers has indeed proved useful, but predictions utilizing other quantitative parameters have been useful to only a limited extent for some families of compounds. No general theory yet accounts for the unique psychotomimetic property of all psychedelic drugs or receptor characteristics (BRAWLEY and DUFFIELD, 1972).

The search, then, has been for leads, for signs of what components of central nervous system function could be cogently followed to account for psychotomimetic effects, and especially a relatively specific pattern of them. Tryptaminergic (MARTIN and SLOAN, 1977), adrenergic, dopaminergic, histaminergic (GREEN et al., 1978 b), and serotonergic systems have been implicated. Without doubt, serotonergic systems – whatever measures are used – seem most readily to yield evidence of effects of LSD-linked psychotomimetics. But whether one or several of these or other systems is necessary and sufficient for the initiation of effects, or for enhancing or inhibiting the potency and intensity of all or different *components* of effects is unclear.

B. Effects in Man

Obviously required are clear, replicated, reliable, and nonanecdotal observations of the essential components and sequence of psychotomimetic effects in man. Here the extensive studies of, and experience with, effects of LSD in man provide some solid framework for deductions as to mechanisms. However, since the relevant pharmacologic parameters and essential psychopharmacologic effects were not apparent until late in the course of human and animal studies (when human studies were constrained), clearly reliably and replicable cataloguing, quantification, and comparison of effects of the range of relevant drugs in man are still needed if correlational work is to be donse. SHULGIN et al., (1969) have attempted comparative potency estimations across drugs and expressed these as "mescaline units." However, many of the methoxylated amphetamines are known either by anecdotal account or have not been tested for replication by various laboratories. Also needed are unambiguous and clarifying studies concerning antagonists in man; thus, suppression or dampening of LSD effects by dopamine-blocking agents is yet to be distinguished from prevention of effects.

With these ambiguities in view, it is useful to note that the initiation of a *train* of effects ("trip") following LSD must be accounted for. What can be said is that neither the initiation nor the subsequent unfolding effects can be attributed to intermediate metabolites of LSD (NIWAGUCHI et al., 1974). Effects begin within a minute or two following intrathecal injection in man. Brain concentrations of drug peak early in the time course after injection, are always about 1,000-fold less than the plasma (ROSECRANS et al., 1967), and correlate with the onset of behavioral effects of rat (FREEDMAN and BOGGAN, 1974). Within the brain, the drug is preferentially concentrated in optical and limbic areas (and pineal) of the rat (FREEDMAN and COQUET, 1965) and monkey (SNYDER and REIVICH, 1966). A residual drug binding is noted in selective brain areas (DIAB et al., 1971) and the choroid with autoradiographic study. While radioactive LSD in minute amounts can be identified in brain 12 or more hours after injection, systematic correlations with either biochemical or behavioral effects at these extended time intervals are lacking. Clearance from the brain regularly follows the plasma half-life of LSD which marks the termination of acute behavioral effects (about 45 min to a behavioral threshold dose in rat, and between 3 and 4 h in man [AGHAJANIAN and BING, 1964]). Half-life is dose dependent (larger doses slightly extend it) *and* species specific (rapid in mouse and slower in cat and monkey). This *must* be considered when comparing dose and effect across species.

In assessing the relevance of animal data to human mental effects, several criteria should be noted. There is *first* a threshold dose (between 25 and 50 μg) necessary for the psychedelic sequence to be triggered; once triggered, effects thereafter "unfold" (linked to drug clearance). *Secondly*, a concomitant mydriasis is necessary for the triggering of the sequence of psychotomimetic events; this is a dose-dependent response in both magnitude and duration of the effect (see FREEDMAN, 1961 b). *Third*, tolerance to *both* the mental effects *and* mydriasis occurs, appears to be complete after several daily doses, and is lost after 4 days (ISEBELL et al., 1959 a, b; FREEDMAN, 1961 b); in unpublished studies, a degree of acute tolerance was observed (e.g., total duration of the effect is not additive [FREEDMAN, 1968]). *Fourth*, with appropriate dosage regimens, there is a cross tolerance with psilocybin and mescaline (APPEL and FREEDMAN, 1968), as well as with DMT (KOVACIC and DOMINO, 1976), but not with delta-9-tetrahydrocannabinol (Δ^9THC) or amphetamine (BALESTRIERI and FONTANARI, 1959; ISBELL et al., 1964). *Fifth*, several pretreatments with 2-bromo-lysergic acid (BOL) (ISBELL et al., 1959 b) can attenuate the intensity and, probably, the duration of the LSD response. The potency of BOL in high dosage to produce some psychotomimetic effect has been argued (GREEN et al., 1978 a, b), but a clear-cut psychedelic sequence, rather than other subjective effects, is simply not apparent (BERTINO et al., 1959; SCHNECKLOTH et al., 1957). It is not clear whether BOL blocks or attenuates through cross tolerance (CLARK and BLISS, 1957; ISBELL et al., 1959b; BALESTRIERI and FONTANARI, 1959; MURPHREE et al., 1958; ABRAMSON et al., 1958). As has been noted, the issue of blockade and prevention, rather than dampening of LSD effects by neuroleptics and benzodiazepines, simply requires precise clinical investigation (CLARK and BLISS, 1957; ISBELL and LOGAN, 1957). *Sixth*, reserpine pretreatment (ISBELL and LOGAN, 1957), even 48–72 h before LSD (FREEDMAN, 1961b) enhances and prolongs the LSD response in man. On the other hand, chronic, but not acute pretreatment with monoamine oxidase inhibitors has been reported (RESNICK et al., 1964) and noted anecdotally to significantly dampen the LSD effect (whether this is due to a "pan-monoaminergic" subsensitivity has never has been investigated). *Finally*, the "TV show in the head" – the acute phase in man – correlates with the plasma half-life of LSD, about 4 h for a dose of 1 μg/kg (AGHAJANIAN and BING, 1964), while a discernibly altered state (and failure of pupil size to return to normal) continues for a subsequent 4–6 h. These seven characteristics should therefore be accounted for in deducing the array of neurobiological substrates of animal study that may be relevant to the psychedelic drugs.

Keeping in mind the temporal and dosage regimen factors and problems of replicability and reliability of different reported effects, we will review recent developments in the search for accountable mechanisms, summarizing previous data and highlighting more recent work. In overview, the solid and compelling leads have long linked LSD and congeners to central neural and biochemical mechanisms that regulate 5-HT and, to a lesser extent, catecholamines. The effects on norepinephrine (NE) and dopamine (DA) systems and their interactions with adenylate cyclase have been more recently studied (although not at all comprehensively). Perhaps the most extensive recent work has been on the stereospecific, high-affinity binding of ^{3}H-LSD and its interactions with ^{3}H-DA or ^{3}H-5-HT sites and putative dopamine and catecholamine antagonists. Long- and short-term effects on the regulation of the turnover of 5-HT and catechols that may be related to tolerance (possibly to any long-term behavioral aftereffects of LSD) have also been noted. Subcellular investigations with LSD point to the identification in nerve ending mechanisms of endogenous 5-HT carrier systems (FREEDMAN and HALARIS, 1978; HALARIS and FREEDMAN, 1977) or substances (TAMIR et al., 1976; MEHL and GUIARD, 1978; MEHL et al., 1977) regulating the binding and release (HERY et al., 1979) of monoamines. The identification of a nonpsychotomimetic ergoline, lisuride, with potent 5-HT and DA agonist effects poses theoretical problems about the distinctiveness of the LSD effects on biochemical measures (PIERI et al., 1978b). Finally, new information is generated by the hitherto rare availability of coupled behavioral, electrophysiologic and biochemical measures in the same organism (TRULSON and JACOBS, 1979b).

C. 5-HT and LSD

GADDUM (1953) and WOOLLEY and SHAW, (1954) modeled the effects of LSD on its antagonism of peripheral 5-HT systems; agonistic effects at low dosages and antagonistic effects at higher dosages of LSD were later cited (GADDUM, 1957). Since then, three lines of evidence implicate LSD in CNS mechanisms regulating 5-HT. One set comprises effects on 5-HT levels and compartmentalization (FREEDMAN, 1961a; SCHANBERG and GIARMAN, 1962); turnover (ROSECRANS et al., 1967; DIAZ et al., 1968;

ANDEN et al., 1968; ANDEN et al., 1971); synthesis (LIN et al., 1969; SCHUBERT et al., 1970; SHIELDS and ECCLESTON, 1973); inhibition of nerve ending stimulated release (see HERY et al., 1979); and retention of 5-HT taken up by brain slices (ZIEGLER et al., 1973). Secondly, reduction of rat brain 5-HT levels by synthesis inhibition, raphe lesion, or reserpine (APPEL and FREEDMAN, 1964; APPEL et al., 1970a, b) causes a striking reduction (three- or four fold) in the threshold dose of LSD required for behavioral effects. The third is the highly sensitive agonistic effect of LSD on the raphe soma and mixed effects on 5-HT innervated postsynaptic membranes (AGHAJANIAN et al., 1975; DE MONTIGNY and AGHAJANIAN, 1977).

Generally, the biochemical effects of LSD will be found to entail events at the nerve terminal, both unique intrasynaptosomal compartmental effects and effects on the nerve ending membrane. LSD induces inhibition of 5-HT release and retention of 5-HT which is contingent on active, not passive, local membrane processes. LSD also produces an inaccessibility of 5-HT to MAO without directly inhibiting the enzyme (COLLINS et al., 1970). Slowed conversion of tryptophan to 5-HT could be due to LSD as a "false transmitter" at postsynaptic membranes, acting via neural feedback loops, or via local pre- and postsynaptic mechanisms. A presynaptic effect which does not involve a direct effect of LSD on the soluble tryptophan hydroxylase seems probable (HAMON et al., 1976; BOURGOIN et al., 1977), whereas a positive feedback process induced by methiothepin (a neuroleptic *and* 5-HT antagonist that induces synaptic release of 5-HT and increased synthesis) can act via the hydroxylase and be blocked by LSD. The positive feedback mechanism is present in neonatal rats; but the negative feedback on conversion of tryptophan to 5-HT after LSD is not, even though 5-HT effects occur (BOURGOIN et al., 1977). The "signals" regulating these nerve terminal interactions require further dissection and definition. In brief, there are several events which distinctively characterize the effect of LSD and bring a focus on presynaptic, i.e., nerve terminal, events (FREEDMAN, 1961a; FREEDMAN and HALARIS, 1978; HERY et al., 1979). It is therefore useful to focus on different periods in order to clarify the sequence of events after LSD.

I. The First 60 Min

To summarize the effects of LSD as "slowing the turnover of 5-HT" obscures events and mechanisms evident during a close examination of the first 60 min following a behaviorally active dose of LSD. Our laboratory, beginning with rope-climbing behavior and later with positively reinforced operant schedules in the rat (FREEDMAN et al., 1958; APPEL and FREEDMAN, 1965), could meet the criteria for a threshold dose, tolerance to both the sympathomimetic and behavioral effects in the rat with similar time parameters as those observed in man, and the same array of cross-tolerance effects (APPEL and FREEDMAN, 1968). Thus temporal parameters are established for an acute phase of effects in the rat, with which biochemical changes and clearance of drug are correlated with grossly observable and quantifiable behavioral changes (piloerection, EEG alerting, hind limb ataxia, abrupt cessation of bar pressing) (FREEDMAN and GIARMAN, 1963). Following the behaviorally active dose in the rat (and other species [FREEDMAN and GIARMAN, 1962]), a 12%–20% increase in whole brain 5-HT and similar percentage decrease in 5-HIAA are observed (ROSECRANS et al., 1967; DIAZ et al., 1968). The effects are stereospecific; nonpsychoactive congeners did not induce it

(FREEDMAN, 1961 a, b; 1963; FREEDMAN et al., 1970). The peak fall in 5-HIAA occurs first (30 min after 520 μg/kg i.p.) and the peak rise in 5-HT at 45 min, correlating with both the termination of acute behavioral effects and the clearance of the drug to its half-life value. With lower doses, the peak effect on 5-HT occurs earlier, with higher or cumulative doses, later. There is, however, a ceiling (about 100 mμg/gm) on the increase in 5-HT (FREEDMAN, 1961 a, b). This increase in confined largely to the particulate fraction after 100,000 × *g* spin (FREEDMAN, 1961 a, b; SCHANBERG and GIARMAN, 1962). For example, doses of LSD as low as 130 μg/kg at 30 min increase P_2 5-HT by 37%; 45 min after 520 μg/kg the increase is 95%; with osmotic disruption of nerve ending fractions (HALARIS et al., 1972; HALARIS and FREEDMAN, 1977), the increase in 5-HT is almost entirely in the vesicular subfraction (an increase of 50% or more).

This particulate increment is dependent on newly synthesized 5-HT since it does not appear after inhibition of tryptophan hydroxylase or the decarboxylase, or during the period of negative feedback inhibition induced by the reuptake blockade with chlorimipramine (HALARIS et al., 1973; FREEDMAN and HALARIS, 1978). Nevertheless, whole brain 5-HIAA still drops early in the time course. Thus, a dissociation of the 5-HT and 5-HIAA events is evident. The increase of 5-HT and fall of 5-HIAA is apparent after reserpine, even when 5-HIAA levels are markedly elevated. Thus a brief period of inaccessibility of 5-HT to MAO in the absence of inhibition (COLLINS et al., 1970; FREEDMAN et al., 1970) is an early effect of LSD.

Other events during the first 60 min are catecholamine changes (small decreases in NE and tyrosine, and with large doses, a small increase in DA at about 60 min [SMITH et al., 1975]). There is an increase in brain tryptophan (and concomitantly of plasma corticosterone) which peaks at 60 min (FREEDMAN and BOGGAN, 1974). Both the brain tryptophan and plasma steroid effects are abolished with adrenalectomy and to a very great extent after hypophysectomy (HALARIS et al., 1975), procedures that do *not* influence the increase of 5-HT and decrease in 5-HIAA. The slowed in vivo conversion of labeled tryptophan to 5-HT begins as early as 21 min after drug administration (SHIELDS and ECCLESTON, 1973) and probably earlier (FREEDMAN and BOGGAN, 1974), but it is sustained up to 2 or more hours, as are the onset and duration of measures of reduced turnover (ANDEN et al., 1968; ANDEN et al., 1971; DIAZ et al., 1968). Obviously, simply a "slowed-down" turnover does not describe key events.

II. Beyond 60 Min

Analysis of events from 60 to 120 min (FREEDMAN and HALARIS, 1978) shows that the decline of 5-HT toward baseline after 45 min is paralleled by a *further* decline in 5-HIAA. This may possibly reflect an "equilibrium phase" of slowed-down synthesis in which utilization of 5-HT (contingent on nonrelease) is also diminished. The 5-HIAA curve for the feedback period of decreased synthesis induced by chlorimipramine (CMI) is similar to this second phase 5-HT–5-HIAA effect of LSD (HALARIS et al., 1973). Interestingly, the brief and early first 30-min increase in 5-HT produced by CMI does *not* occur in the nerve ending or vesicular fraction (FREEDMAN and HALARIS, unpublished data; HALARIS and FREEDMAN, 1977). If this later, sustained second phase of reduced turnover is produced by negative feedback, it is still unclear if LSD is acting as an agonist (and where), and how and where the early slowed conversion of tryptophan to 5-HT is signaled.

Finally, the effects on 5-HT and 5-HIAA appear to be independent of the direct effect of LSD in inhibiting firing in the raphe soma, since after raphe lesions both 5-HT and 5-HIAA effects were still found in the forebrain (FREEDMAN and HALARIS, 1978). Thus, the early 5-HT and 5-HIAA effects of LSD can be dissociated, but also appear to be nerve terminal events, relatively independent of drug effect on the soma.

The strongest evidence and possible focus on mediating mechanisms for these effects comes from data showing that the release of 5-HT from electrically or K^+-stimulated striatal slices (CHASE et al., 1967; HAMON et al., 1974; BOURGOIN et al., 1977) is inhibited by LSD. The drug also inhibits the uptake of ^{3}H-5-HT into brain slices as well as enhances the retention of intraventricularly applied ^{3}H-5-HT (ZIEGLER et al., 1973). This latter effect can be abolished by depolarization with ouabain. Further, when the efflux of labeled 5-HT and metabolites is measured in ventricular fluid, there is a retention of 5-HT after LSD, but not after CMI. Perhaps the most elegant evidence comes from the use of a push/pull cannula in the head of the caudate nucleus with a release of ^{3}H-5-HT continuously synthesized from labeled tryptophan; this local superfusion technique highlights events at the nerve ending terminal. Thus with local depolarization of 5-HT terminals with KCl or batrachotoxin, a release of ^{3}H-5-HT is seen, and the potassium-evoked release was markedly reduced by LSD (HERY et al., 1979).

Both the effects of LSD in slices or in vivo appear to depend on an active membrane phenomenon; LSD could not prevent release in vivo in the absence of depolarizing stimuli. These effects possibly involve calcium and other ion channels (HERY et al., 1979), and such membrane effects have been adduced with electrophysiologic studies as well (MARRAZZI and HUANG, 1979). It should be noted that the observation by MARCHBANKS (1966; 1967) of substantial inhibition by LSD of 5-HT synaptosomal uptake at 4 °C (a) was nonstereospecific, and (b) could not be replicated when effect were examined at 37 °C (FREEDMAN and HALARIS, 1978).

III. LSD-5-HT Summary

Thus, the four unique effects of LSD on the nerve ending are 1) to inhibit release; 2) to cause an early inaccessibility of intrasynaptosomal 5-HT to MAO; 3) to produce a subsequent retention of newly synthesized 5-HT which is normally stored in reserpine-sensitive vesicles; and 4) to create a later period of sustained, retarded synthesis and turnover and utilization of 5-HT. When vesicular storage is impaired, there is still retention (binding?) in the soluble juxtavesicular compartment leading to the sharp early drop in 5-HIAA. This juxtavesicular retention after LSD can be seen even 15 days after reserpine treatment. It is speculated that this compartment may contain a "carrier" for 5-HT, moving the amine to a vesicle, to terminal membrane, or to mitochondrial MAO. Whether the initial event is at the terminal membrane or at the carrier site, or both, there is somehow a negative feedback which is drug or amine induced and which leads to longer term effects on synthesis. TAMIR et al. (1976) characterized a soluble nerve ending substance capable of binding serotonin, probably an actinlike molecule; however, its drug interaction characteristics are not in accordance with those required from biochemical studies of LSD. On the other side of the coin, MEHL and colleagues (1977, 1978) have reported substances in human cerebrospinal fluid that are capable of displacing LSD from high-affinity binding sites in neuronal membranes. These substances are heat stable, of low molecular weight (500), and anionic at pH 7.4. The continued search for binding and displacing substances or related materials is clearly suggested.

While LSD clearly has electrophysiologic effects on postsynaptic and presynaptic serotonergic neurons, biochemical and membrane effects at the nerve terminal appear to be at least semi-independent of the action potential generated at the raphe. Interference by LSD with normal traffic of 5-HT may lead to less amine available to postsynaptic elements, leaving the drug free to bind to these receptors and to exert its characteristic combined agonistic and antagonistic postsynaptic effects at 5-HT and related acceptor sites. LSD appears very early in its course of action to initiate a sequence of feedback effects that extend beyond the first 60 min that will require focus. Whether the biophysical effects of LSD on nerve terminals, on the raphe soma, and on postsynaptic membranes are identical, is not known.

D. Other Psychotomimetics

An elevation of 5-HT and decrease of 5-HIAA also occurs early in the time course of psilocybin, psilocin, and DMT, but not with behaviorally active doses of mescaline or DOM (FREEDMAN et al., 1970). This is in contrast to the reports of TONGE and LEONARD (1969) that the LSD pattern on 5-HT and 5-HIAA occurred with *all* psychotomimetics (including cholinolytics), an effect we could not replicate even using the same strain of rats (FREEDMAN and HALARIS, 1978). It is not as yet clear whether the unique retention of 5-HT in the vesicular subfraction occurs with all related indoleamine psychotomimetics. We do observe marked and significant increases in the P_2 fraction prior to osmotic disruption with doses of LSD as low as 130 µg/kg at 20 min (37%), an increase of 95% after 520 µg/kg. At 45 min after 50 mg/kg DMT, the increase is 46%; after 25 mg/kg psilocybin, 90%; and after 2 mg/kg BOL, 23%. Yet, after L-LSD and after 50 mg/kg mescaline at 60 min (or CMI), there is no significant effect (FREEDMAN, HALARIS and DEMET, unpublished data).

With respect to mescaline, the data show that low doses, very early in the time course, may slightly elevate 5-HT and decrease 5-HIAA. This is evident also for doses of DOM at 1 mg/kg (FREEDMAN et al., 1970). Interestingly, both inhibit only a subset of dorsal raphe cells and stimulate others. For both drugs, 5-HT and 5-HIAA increases are clearly evident with behaviorally active doses. After the first, but not the second, dose of DOM in the cat, a slight elevation of 5-HT was noted, and the conversion of labeled tryptophan to 5-HT in brain slices of such LSD pretreated cats was *increased* (WALLACH et al., 1972). Yet ANDEN et al. (1974) found slowed turnover after DOM – but not mescaline – while TONGE and LEONARD (1969) found slowed turnover for both. These issues with respect to mescaline and DOM need to be clarified, especially since possible 5-HT links of mescaline are argued by GEYER et al. (1978) and WINTERS (1971).

It is curious that compounds such as amphetamine, which become psychotomimetic in chronic dosage, differ from LSD, which tends to show tolerance with chronic dosage. Although MCLEAN and MCCARTNEY (1961) noted that with increasing and toxic doses of amphetamine, effects on levels of 5-HT and NE resemble those described for LSD (FREEDMAN, 1961 b), TRULSON and JACOBS (1977) have shown a "serotonin hallucinogenic syndrome" and markedly lowered levels of 5-HT and slowed turnover after chronic amphetamine treatment in the cat.

In summary, the paucity of replicated, time-linked studies of amine levels and compartmental events, as well as direct in vivo studies of release or inhibition of release and of 5-HT synthesis and utilization studies is striking as one searches for the data on mescaline and methoxylated amphetamines. Further, study of the release and synthesis and compartmental effects of the indolealkylamine psychotomimetics, and of drugs such as 5-methoxy-*N*,*N*-dimethyltryptamine (utilized in electrophysiologic studies) is largely lacking. Thus, filling these gaps in information would advance our grasp of the field far more than a search of scattered smooth muscle receptors. The precise need is for CNS studies which would allow us to piece together a plausible general 5-HT "story" for the range of psychedelic compounds.

E. LSD and Catecholamines

The lines of evidence implicating noradrenergic and dopaminergic systems in the action of LSD derive from both behavioral and biochemical studies. Behavioral studies show that after lesions the characteristic DA agonist circling behavior is induced by LSD and psychotomimetic congeners (PIERI et al., 1978a; TRULSON et al., 1977b), but not by BOL. Tolerance, however, is not observed with this system. Indeed what is clear is that characteristic DA-mediated stereotypes do not occur with LSD.

After α-methyltyrosine (AMPT) pretreatment, the excitatory effects of LSD in rabbit are diminished and restored with L-Dopa plus a peripheral decarboxylase inhibitor; the LSD-induced pyrexia is not affected (HORITA and HAMILTON, 1969, 1973). In rats, locomotor excitement and hyperthermia are similarly dissociated (BAPNA et al., 1973), but others have not found a striking action of AMPT modifying LSD effects (APPEL et al., 1970b; SUGRUE, 1969). No effects are found in mice (BAPNA et al., 1973; MENON et al., 1977).

Turning to biochemistry most studies replicate the slight decrease in NE originally observed after LSD in rat (FREEDMAN, 1961b; 1963; BARCHAS and FREEDMAN, 1963). In the early phase – the first 60 min – there is thus a fall in NE and brain tyrosine (SMITH et al., 1975; TONGE and LEONARD, 1971) and, at 60 min, an increase in DA levels. Generally, doses of 0.5 mg/kg or higher are required for these DA increases SMITH et al., 1975; PIERI et al., 1978b). An unexplained fall of DA levels in the early time period (30 min) was noted in 12 rats (DIAZ et al., 1968), whereas SMITH et al. (1975), with 1.040 μg/kg, observed a dose-dependent elevation at 30 min. At later time intervals, elevations are not found, e.g., 3.5 h in rats (DAPRADA et al., 1975) or mice (MENON et al., 1977).

If we focus on NE metabolism, data not only on levels, but also on turnover (STOLK et al., 1974) clearly indicate increased release and utilization. BURKI et al. (1978) recently demonstrated both a dose and time-dependent increase in brain stem MOPEG-SO_4, an effect appearing at 60 min (with an $ED_{120\%}$ of 0.5 mg/kg [noted also by PIERI et al., 1978b]) and continuing, after a 10 mg/kg dose (!), to peak at 2 h and to diminish by 8 h. In the vas deferens, the electrically stimulated release of labelled NE and concomitant reduction in smooth muscle response was inhibited by LSD, apparently by interaction with presynaptic α-adrenoreceptors (HUGHES, 1973). Direct in vivo studies of release in brain show similar effects of DOM and amphetamine on in vivo release, and/or blocking of reuptake (VRBANAC et al., 1975), but for LSD we must rely on the turnover studies and measures of substrate and metabolites.

In general, those psychotomimetics that are milder or less potent psychedelic agents than LSD appear to have an even greater and more direct effect than LSD on the synthesis and utilization of NE (STOLK et al., 1974). The pattern of altered NE metabolites after psychotomimetics shows no common mechanism within or across the indole and phenylethylamine groups. Mescaline initially enhances intracellular catabolism of NE, but in subsequent hours there is a significant increase in *O*-methylated metabolites; amphetamine similarly shows increases in *O*-methylated metabolites, as does psilocybin. Both have potent and long-enduring effects (up to 6 h [STOLK et al., 1974]). The sharp fall in NE levels and marked and enduring shift in metabolite pattern after psilocybin raises an unexplored question of an uptake blockade effect in NE terminals. HENDLEY and SNYDER (1971) note a potent normetanephrine reuptake blockade effect for DOM. Unfortunately, comparative data among all related drugs in scarce.

More experimental attention has been focused on DA metabolism. Effects on levels have been noted. With radioactive tyrosine in synthesis studies, the results are not in accord; STOLK et al. (1974) found no significant change in ^{3}H-DA (after 1.300 μg/kg at 1 h), and PERSSON (1970) reported enhanced formation of ^{3}H-DA, but only in the caudate (after 2 mg/kg at 30 min). PERSSON (1978) has focused on studies of Dopa accumulation after decarboxylase inhibition as a measure of synthesis and reports increases in the cerebral cortex, striatum, and brain stem, but not in the olfactory bulb of rats. KEHR and SPECKENBACH (1978) note a forebrain accumulation. The increase in DA synthesis appears to be dose dependent (50 μg/kg–5 mg/kg) and to correlate in time with the effects of LSD on amine concentration (SMITH et al., 1975). This measure of synthesis, however, does not afford a uniform theory of hallucinogenesis, since BOL also increases Dopa accumulation. These effects are characteristic of DA antagonists.

PERSSON and JOHANNSON (1978) attempted to discern if the increased synthesis was contingent on the dorsal or median raphe. Only a combined lesion blocked the LSD effect, but close inspection of the data reveals a trend for the dorsal raphe lesion to reduce the LSD response. 5-HT synthesis inhibitors did not affect it. The dorsal raphe nuclei (B_7), as GEYER et al. (1978) note, contain much more DA than the median, so that drug effects at DA receptors at B_7 might have affected striatal Dopa accumulation. However, the persisting effect of BOL (with its strong DA antagonist effects) after a lesion of B_7 throws some doubt on these interaction hypotheses. The lack of effect of synthesis inhibitors and the lesions do not identify 5-HT systems or the raphe as the "signal" for Dopa accumulation.

Effects of LSD on DA utilization were estimated by the measurement of metabolites or the rate of decline of DA after pretreatment with α-methyltyrosine. With the latter method, *no* effect of LSD was noted (PERSSON, 1978; ANDEN et al., 1972) in whole brain when LSD was given 2–4 h before death, and MENON et al. (1977) saw no effect on turnover at these time intervals in mice. PERSSON found no effect in striatum, and only a 7% effect in the tel-diencephalon was noted at 135 min after LSD – a time when most acute events have subsided (DAPRADA et al., 1975).

Table 1. Biochemical effects of LSD on DA Systems[a]

LSD µg/kg	Synthesis	Decline (αmpt)	HVA	DOPAC	DA Release	
					3 MT	Perfusion
Less than 90 min						
<200	↑[1]		↓[4] 0Δ[5]	↑[7]	↓[8]	
200–500	↑[1]	0Δ[1]		↑[7]		
>500	↑[1,2] 0Δ[3]	0Δ[1]	↑[5]	↑[6,7]	↑[8]	↓[9]
Equal to or greater than 90 min						
<200				↓[6]		
200–500	↓[7]	0Δ[10,1]	↓[9]	↓[6,7]		
>500	0Δ[1]	0Δ[11] ↓[9]		↑[6]		↓[9]

[a] 0Δ = No change
[1] Persson (1978)
[2] Persson (1970)
[3] Stolk et al. (1974)
[4] Pieri et al. (1978)
[5] Keller et al. (1978)
[6] Burki et al. (1978)
[7] Persson (1977)
[8] Kehr (1977)
[9] Da Prada et al. (1975)
[10] Anden et al. (1972)
[11] Menon et al. (1977)

With measures of homovanillic acid (HVA) concentrations in rat brain, a dose- and time-dependence is apparent. Again, if one focuses on the effects within the first 60 min there is but one report (Pieri, et al., 1978b) showing a decrease (20%) in HVA (in whole brain), whereas the same laboratory (Keller et al., 1978) shows slight, but not significant *increases* after 100 µg/kg and marked increases in HVA after 1,000 µg/kg in cortex, limbic, and striatal regions. Yet the only direct release measure (from the perfused head of the caudate) indicates a depressed DA release for 3 h (DaPrada et al., 1975).

DOPAC concentration was reduced in rat brain striatum at doses of LSD below 1 mg/kg and, at higher doses (10 mg/kg), increases were observed at 1 h, returning to normal by 4 h. In contrast, Persson (1977a) finds rat striatal DOPAC values *increased* at *all* doses of LSD – from 50 µg/kg to 4 mg/kg, and this in the first and early phase of LSD effects (at 30 min). A low dose of LSD, 50 µg/kg, given 65 and 35 min before death, decreased 3-methoxytryptamine while a ten-fold increase in dosage increased it. These disparate measures of utilization in general do *not* strongly implicate an agonistic effect of LSD, "turning down" DA synthesis and utilization. A dose effect and time course study of effects with all metabolites would appear, in any event, to be important if further systematic work is to be undertaken (Table 1).

While DA antagonistic effects are implicated in the results with Dopa accumulation (and with the bulk of metabolite findings), examination of LSD effects in perturbed systems, i.e., in animals with either reserpine, cerebral hemisection, or inhibition of impulse flow, shows that LSD acts as an agonist in that it blocks or attenuates the enhanced Dopa accumulation caused by these pretreatments (Persson, 1977a, b). In other words LSD acts to slow synthesis, much as the receptor agonist apomorphine. Kehr and Speckenbach (1978) adduced similar data in the forebrain following axotomy of the ascending monoaminergic tract. The only clear-cut "announcement" of a measure that directly reflects DA agonism in a nonperturbed system are the highly potent effects of LSD on prolactin levels (MELTZER, et al., 1977), which involve pituitary receptors. It is therefore of interest that the structural similarity of LSD to the DA agonist, apomorphine, has been argued (NICHOLS, 1976).

Thus (perhaps with the varying data and clearly with the "perturbed systems"), it is evident that mixed agonist and antagonistic properties of LSD are characteristic and, as PERSSON (1977 a, b) notes, BOL generally is a pure antagonist. To account for these properties CHRISTOPH et al., (1978) postulate a conformational shift in the DA receptor regulated by the availability of agonist or antagonist receptor sites: a prior occupation of antagonist sites would cause LSD to act as an agonist, while prior occupation of agonist sites would cause the drug to look like an antagonist. KEHR and SPECKENBACH (1978) similarly suggest that the amount of occupancy of the receptor by DA determines which state will be manifest. In the nonperturbed system, DA is available at agonist sites, and therefore LSD would likely produce effects characteristic of antagonists. In the perturbed system, with diminished DA at receptors, LSD has ready access to these sites and appears as an agonist. Strikingly, however, the only data available in man show that 48 h after reserpine pretreatment a putative antagonist effect of LSD may have induced the instances of oculogyric crises in three of ten chronically schizophrenic women (FREEDMAN, 1961 b).

LSD appears to have actions both on cell bodies (electrophysiologic data) and nerve ending events (rotational models, effects on synthesis in perturbed systems – during lack of impulse flow – or stimulation of DA-sensitive adenylate cyclase). Perhaps a varied neurochemical picture dependent on both time and dose is inevitable; the reactive and "sensitizing" effects to noxious input noted by AGHAJANIAN for LSD at the locus coeruleus may add further variability. Within short time intervals, primary biochemical actions of LSD would appear, and secondary effects might occur after longer time intervals. Similarly, low doses might produce more selective effects than higher doses. However these data are to be reconciled, it is clear that systematic, fine-grained time and dose studies are needed, and the data with catecholamines are far more complicated to interpret, lacking sufficient direct studies in in vivo and in vitro release, etc., than is the case with 5-HT.

F. Lisuride and LSD

AGHAJANIAN et al. (1975) proposed that psychedelic agents such as LSD produce their psychological effects via inhibition of raphe firing. The fact that lisuride, a *nonhallucinogen* ergoline structurally related to LSD, produces a more powerful suppression of raphe unit spontaneous firing than does LSD calls into question this hypothesis. It also suggests that a comparison of the commonalities and differences in the action of these two compounds may provide a lever for dissecting component mechanisms.

Clinical reports of lisuride indicate a state of enhanced anxiety or fear. Interestingly, similar effects have been noted for piperoxane and yohimbine. LSD can also enhance vigilance and "fear"; however, after LSD these states alternate and coincide with euphoria, a "pleasant-unpleasant" effect accompanied by emotional lability (FREEDMAN, 1968). It may therefore be fruitful to systematically compare these compounds. Furthermore, since an agonist such as clonidine can inhibit the piperoxane effect, it may be a useful tool for dissecting these similar and overlapping mechanisms.

LSD and lisuride (which is more potent and long lasting) induce a haloperidol-antagonizable contralateral turning in chemically lesioned rats (PIERI et al., 1978a) and antagonize reserpine-induced motor depression (HOROWSKI and WACHTEL, 1976) and hypothermia (KEHR, 1977). In the *normal* animal dose-dependent stereotypy (an agonist effect seen with apomorphine) occurs with lisuride but *not* with LSD (HOROWSKI, 1978).

In terms of monoaminergic effects, both lisuride and LSD increase 5-HT and DA in brain, and decrease concentrations of NE and 5-HIAA (PIERI et al., 1978b; KELLER et al., 1978; KEHR, 1977), as well as decrease the formation of 5-HTP KEHR and SPECKENBACH, 1978). Lisuride, but not LSD, antagonizes methiothepin-induced acceleration of 5-HT Turnover as measured by 5-HIAA (PIERI et al., 1978b). Unlike LSD, lisuride does not affect brain levels of tryptophan and tyrosine. Its effects on release and subcellular compartmentation of amines have not been directly examined.

In marked contrast to LSD, lisuride *decreases* Dopa accumulation in both whole brain and in DA-rich regions with doses of 0.1 and 0.3 mg/kg, but not at 1.0 mg/kg. However, in the NE-rich neocortex, 0.3 mg/kg and 1 mg/kg lisuride greatly increase dopa formation. An increase in utilization, as well as in NE synthesis after lisuride is suggested by an accelerated disappearance of NE after AMPT and by the elevations of MOPEG-SO_4 (PIERI, et al., 1978b).

DA disappearance after AMPT (KEHR, 1977) is retarded, unlike LSD (where little if any effect is seen). KELLER et al. (1978) show that 60 min after 100 μg/kg, lisuride, but *not* LSD, markedly reduces HVA concentrations in the cortex, limbic forebrain, and striatum; LSD tends to elevate HVA at the 100 μg/kg dose and markedly so after 1 mg/kg, whereas lisuride markedly *decreases* HVA at both low and high doses. In perturbed systems (after axotomy or reserpine) in which there is a decreased impulse flow leading to increased synthesis, both LSD and lisuride diminsh the increase (as do DA agonists), and the effects of both are antagonized by haloperidol.

LSD stimulation of NE, DA, and 5-HT-sensitive adenylate cyclase (e.g., VON HUNGEN et al., 1974; 1975; SPANO et al., 1975) is known, but no stimulating effects have been reported for lisuride. Both lisuride ($IC_{50} = 1.2 \times 10^{-7}\,M$) and LSD ($IC_{50} = 1 \times 10^{-5}\,M$) inhibit DA-stimulated formation of cyclic AMP in rat striatal homogenates. Also, in limbic slices, the NE-stimulated cyclic AMP formation was inhibited by lisuride ($IC_{50} = 8 \times 10^{-8}\,M$) and LSD ($IC_{50} = 3 \times 10^{-6}\,M$) (KELLER et al., 1978).

In brief, the drugs have both quantitative and qualitative differences and similarities. The longer-lasting, more potent lisuride appears to be a direct and powerful DA agonist and does not appear to act via DA, NE, or 5-HT-sensitive adenylate cyclase on which LSD has both agonist and antagonist properties. One might expect that lisuride would be the more potent psychotomimetic if DA and/or NE systems were of some importance in producing these drug effects.

It is thus curious that LSD, which has long been noted to induce an excitatory and sympathomimetic syndrome, as well as a 5-HT syndrome (JACOBS and TRULSON 1979), is far more complex and less potent in known dopamine-mediated behaviors than lisuride. Perhaps long-term changes in amine regulatory systems, receptors, or the unique interactive combination of physiologic and biochemical events set in motion by LSD account for the differences in these two compounds.

G. Tolerance, Blockade, and Enhancement of LSD Effects

Demonstration of tolerance is critically dependent upon appropriate measures and carefully controlled dosage and time intervals. For example, short-term tolerance occurs with LSD (130 μg/kg) given at hourly intervals (FREEDMAN and AGHAJANIAN, 1959) as well as after daily doses, but dosage of about 520 μg/kg can abscure the effects and restore the initial response. In rat, sympathomimetic effects, EEG alerting and hind limb ataxia showed tolerance; centrally mediated parasympathomimetic effects (salivation and bradycardia, lasting 90 min or more) do not (FREEDMAN et al., 1958). It was frequently noted that tolerance to behavioral effects in rat simply is not evident where noxious reinforcement is entailed, such as escape behavior (APPEL and FREEDMAN, 1968; HAMILTON, 1960).

A decrement in the magnitude and duration not only of physiologic and behavioral, but also biochemical response with several doses of LSD is evident both in measures of 5-HT metabolism in the first 60 min (a diminished magnitude of the 5-HIAA decrement and a shift to the left of the 5-HT peak) and a diminution of both the 60 min tryptophan increase and plasma corticosterone increase (FREEDMAN and BOGGAN, 1974; HALARIS et al., 1975). Similarly, the acute changes in catecholamine concentrations noted by SMITH et al. (1975) show tolerance. Of greater interest are long-term changes in the regulatory processes governing 5-HT and NE metabolism. These have been measured hours after the 60-min acute phase in long-term (14–30 days) low-dosage regimens. Thus 24 h after the last of 14 days of low dosage LSD, NE turnover is increased (PETERS, 1974a). PETERS and TANG (1977) report that 14 days of LSD (100 μg/kg) produce a significant decrease in NE content of the cortex and an increase in tyrosine hydroxylase activity measured 24 h after the last treatment; complex interaction between placebo effects, body weight, and the LSD action with respect to NE is described. DIAZ and HUTTUNEN (1971) show an *increase* in 5-HT turnover 18 h after the last of 28 multiple doses (20 μg/kg). The question is, after one or several episodes of reduced turnover, when do compensatory changes begin and how they are mediated?

It is clear that the effects of LSD in inhibiting the raphe are not modified by any pretreatment or drug interaction (with the exception of the direct iontophoresis of glutamate, which still leaves the effect of 5-HT untouched) BRAMWELL and GOYNE, 1976). Since tolerance and antagonism at the raphe cannot be noted (TRULSON and JACOBS, 1979c), since the behavioral effects in cat long outlast raphe effects (TRULSON and JACOBS, 1979b), and since dosages necessary for behavioral effects (FREEDMAN and HALARIS, 1978) are (as noted below) far greater than maximal concentrations necessary for high affinity binding of LSD, we must conceive of processes beyond the initiation of the LSD effect that are set into motion along with the initial changes. The noted cross tolerances have provoked a search for common receptor sites or mediating processes. Since tolerance is apparently not contingent on drug uptake and clearance (WINTERS, 1971), changes among the component aminergic systems, which have long been thought to modulate *intensity* if not component patterns of LSD effects (FREEDMAN and GIARMAN, 1963), may be sought.

It is difficult to parcel out either the role of specifically involved systems or their link to specific components of the LSD effect. Some dissociation of effects (pretreatment with AMPT in rabbit) involves L-Dopa. Both raphe lesions and raphe stimulation induce enhancement to startle (e.g., DAVIS and SHEARD, 1974), and thus the role of serotonergic systems in enhancing "sensitization" remains to be clarified. At the cellular level, Kandel's group (KLEIN and KANDEL, 1978; BRUNELLI, et al., 1976) show an effect in *Aplysia* in which sensitization and reactivity to input are enhanced; i.e., prolonged enhancement in the behavioral response to one stimulus results from another – typically a noxious or novel one. A prolonged increase in 5-HT release from presynaptic terminals of sensory neurons was implicated in this sensitization, which essentially facilitates transmission between sensory and motor neurons. Facilitating and sensitizing effects of LSD on motor neurons have already been discusses (AGHAJANIAN, this volume); however, it remains to be demonstrated that these are operative in other sensory systems.

LSD "dehabituates" perception; the usual becomes novel. Diminished "barriers" and enhanced arousal, i.e. sensitization, are important components requiring neurobiologic analysis. Serotonin mechanisms affecting arousal have been suggested in mammals (BOWERS, 1975). These questions are fundamental to the flashbacks, aftereffects, and persisting loss of perceptual constancies seen with LSD (FREEDMAN, 1968).

Pretreatment regimens (PCPA, raphe lesion, reserpine) that markedly lower the *thereshold dosage* of LSD (and enhance its effects) may increase *or* decrease actual brain levels of the drug (FREEDMAN and HALARIS, unpublished data; FREEDMAN, et al., 1964); variations in drug plasma levels delivering drugs to critical receptors may possibly be accountable. Pretreatment effects on turnover rates or receptor sensitivity may also be involved. In any event, sensitivity to LSD after 5-HT depletion is apparent as long as 12 days *after* brief treatment with PCPA (APPEL et al., 1970) and with no more than a 15% depletion of the amine after a *single* dose of reserpine (APPEL and FREEDMAN, 1964). As reviewed below, no clear-cut receptor or binding finding unequivocally accounts for these events or tolerance.

Studies of MAO inhibitors and LSD in animals would be needed to elucidate the modulating effect of chronic MAO inhibition noted in man. With respect to antagonism in rat, a dose of 30 μg/kg chlorpromazine (CPZ) can block 130 μg/kg LSD on operant tasks (RAY and MARRAZZI, 1961; APPEL and FREEDMAN, 1964); higher doses of CPZ produce effects of their own. MARRAZZI and HUANG (1979) argue from membrane parameters (spike generation, polarization, transmembrane conduction, and IPSPs) that 5-HT, LSD, and CPZ are qualitatively identical, but quantitatively different; thus the weakest competitive antagonist – CPZ – can substitute for one with a stronger action and thus block LSD, whereas larger doses of CPZ and LSD are cumulative. It would be important to note whether these dosage interactions would in fact prevent the total sequence of LSD effects. To date, only tolerance dosage regimes appear to be so effective and even then, sensitivity to noxious input, or to amphetamine (VAUPEL et al., 1978) may be enhanced in the tolerant animal. The area obviously awaits focused study.

H. Adenylate Cyclase

The use of both receptor binding and adenylate cyclase (AC) as a functionally relevant receptor system has received increasing attention and as such various systems have been sought to model potential events in the brain. MANSOUR and colleagues (1960) demonstrated that $10^{-5} M$ LSD or $10^{-7} M$ 5-HT activated the cyclase in liver fluke and this was followed by a demonstration (BEERNINK et al., 1963) that there was a correlation of muscular contractions of the fluke with hallucinogenic potency. Utilization of this model for studies of receptor interactions and AC systems has continued (NORTHUP and MANSOUR, 1978).

Perhaps the best model system, in terms of relevant concentrations and interactions, has been studied by NATHANSON and GREENGARD (1974) using the thoracic ganglia of the cockroach, in which the cyclase is specifically activated by 5-HT and selectively inhibited by extremely low concentrations of LSD and BOL. Inhibitory constant of LSD was 5 nM similar to the dissociation constant (K_d) of LSD in stereospecific binding studies. The range of inhibitory interactions and potencies is in accord with estimated concentrations of LSD in human brain and with the noted 5-HT-LSD interactions in peripheral smooth muscle (COTTRELL, 1970) or molluscan ganglia (GERSCHENFELD, 1971).

The most direct and current searches are for 5-HT-sensitive enzymes in cell-free preparations in mammalian nervous system and for NE- or DA-activated enzymes affected by very low concentrations of LSD. Micromolar concentrations have, however, generally been required. BOL and LSD, in cell free preparations from rat brain regions, blocked maximal stimulation of AC by NE or DA (VON HUNGEN et al., 1974; 1975). A stereospecific effect of LSD at 10 μM in blocking DA activation was seen in the striatum, and LSD stimulation of the cyclase was observed and blocked not only by BOL, but also by DA blockers. Against a uniform view of psychotomimetic mechanisms, such studies (DAPRADA et al, 1975) show no effect of mescaline, DMT, psilocin, or bufotenin. Nevertheless, LSD is differentiated from its antagonists and nonpsychoactive congeners, and there is antagonism between BOL and LSD. LSD, in contrast to BOL, is an agonist as well as antagonist at the striatal receptors (BOCKAERT et al, 1976). This group, using a punch technique in striatum to correlate the spatial localization of enzymes and transmitters, finds topographic correspondence of DA high affinity uptake, endogenous levels, and the DA-activated cyclase ($10^{-4} M$) in which LSD competitively inhibits (and activates).

There have been recent demonstrations of a postsynaptic 5-HT-sensitive cyclase (ENJALBERT et al, 1978) in the colliculus of neonate rats, stimulated by LSD, in which the 5-HT stimulation is blocked by the drug at higher concentrations (BOURGOIN et al., 1977). AHN and MAKMAN (1979), studying AC of anterior limbic cortex and auditory cortex from monkeys, describe an enzyme stimulated by LSD ($EC_{50} = 0.43$ μM) and mescaline ($EC_{50} = 4.5$ μM). The frontal cortex, caudata, and retina were not stimulated, but LSD could block DA stimulation in all regions. This is the first demonstration that LSD and mescaline may have a common CNS receptor action and the first demonstration of mescaline stimulation. The study suggests the importance of both species differences and regional specificities.

The data with respect to the effects of LSD on other adenylate cyclase systems are minimal. LSD inhibits ($1.6 \times 10^{-7} M$) isoproterenol-activated cyclase in cerebral cortex homogenates, but does not stimulate. Nor inhibit DOLPHIN et al. (1978) the enzyme by itself. BURKI et al. (1978) have indicated that LSD inhibits binding at α-adrenoreceptors ($IC_{50} = 0.2$ μM) with much less effect at β-adrenoreceptors ($IC_{50} = 2.0$ μM). Both LSD and BOL are competitive antagonists at the H_2 receptor linked to AC in the hippocampus and cortes (GREEN et al., 1978a, b).

While adenylate cyclase linked receptors do not describe all the relevant receptor sites for LSD (GREEN et al., 1978a, b) and the action of the range of psychotomimetics in cell free preparations is not as satisfying, there is a growing framework in which AC receptor characteristics, tritiated binding characteristics, and functional effects can be quantitatively compared. The issue still is to relate the effects of LSD at these sites to possible indications of sites and mechanisms related to cross tolerance, blocking, and enhancement of the effects of LSD in man.

1. Stereospecific Binding

The search for 35 years has been for acceptor substances with which both LSD and 5-HT interact. There are studies of LSD binding to an indole-containing moiety of myelin and of proteolipid or protein components derived from nerve endings (CARNEGIE, 1972; FISZER and DEROBERTIS, 1969; MEHL and WEBER, 1974), as well as the soluble 5-HT binding protein which, however, does not show LSD binding (TAMIR et al., 1976). Since stereospecific ^{3}H-LSD high affinity binding was established (BENNETT and AGHAJANIAN, 1974; BENNETT and SNYDER, 1975; LOVELL and FREEDMAN, 1976; BENNETT and SNYDER, 1976), a large number of studies reporting in vitro LSD or ^{3}H-5-HT binding to brain tissues have appeared. LSD binding at DA sites (BURT et al., 1976a, b) (as well as NE) has been established. The fact that ^{3}H-5-HT had a 100-times-greater affinity or ^{3}H-5-HT than for ^{3}H-LSD sites, however, threw doubt on the identity of the two acceptor sites and the lack of correlation of binding, and displacement characteristics with psychotomimetic potency or antagonism of 5-HT, DA, or LSD at ^{3}H-LSD sites was noted (FREEDMAN and HALARIS, 1978).

The in vitro, as well as in vivo, LSD binding assays operate at concentrations too low to be accountable for most of the observed functional effects with the possible exception of effects on the raphe. For example, the raphe are inhibited by 10–20 µg/kg LSD, whereas biochemical and behavioral effects require doses generally from 40–100 µg/kg (ROSECRANS et al., 1967), about the same value can be calculated from a recent in vivo study (KRAUCHI et al., 1978) after 300 µg/kg LSD. Yet, in an in vivo study (KRAUCHI et al., 1978), the displaceable binding sites were saturated after doses as low as 10 µg/kg LSD. The in vivo binding occurs at brain concentrations comparable to those of in vitro binding. Receptors are fully saturated at 17 pmol/gm of tissue, which corresponds to the 15 n*M* in the in vitro assay, assuming homogeneous distribution of LSD. This is the concentration which saturates the LSD displaceable binding sites in the in vitro assay.

Physiologic significance – a correlation between functional and binding potencies – is desirable in validating binding assays (KOSTERLITZ and WATERFIELD, 1975; SEEMAN et al., 1975). Using the data of BENNETT and SNYDER (1975) and mescaline units as a measure of potency in man (BRAWLEY and DUFFIELD, 1972), P. Muller has attempted such correlations for us. However, the correlation of $1/IC_{50}$ is much less than convincing (Table 2). Particularly required are binding data with highly potent LSD congeners such as acetyl lysergic acid diethylamide (CERLETTI and DOEPFNER, 1958). A poor correlation, in part, is due to the high potency of some of the antagonists in the binding assay. A difference is drug kinetics (such as those implicated in discrepancies in correlating analgesic effect and binding potency) could also contribute.

Table 2. Displacement of hallucinogens and derivatives from LSD in vitro binding sites. Comparison with hallucinogenic potency[a]

Drug	BENNETT and SNYDER'S		BRAWLEY and DUFFIELD'S
	^{3}H-LSD-IC_{50} nm	$1/IC_{50}$	Mescaline units Mescaline = 1
Br-LDS	7	1.4×10^{-1}	0
d-LSD	8	1.3×10^{-1}	3,700
d-Lysergic acid monoethylamide	20	5.0×10^{-2}	370
methysergide	100	10^{-2}	0
psilocin	1,000	10^{-3}	31
5-methoxy-dimethyltryptamine	1,000	10^{-3}	31
dimethyltryptamine	2,000	5.0×10^{-4}	4
2,5-dimethoxy-4-methylamphetamine	8,000	1.3×10^{-6}	80
2,5-dimethoxyamphetamine	8,000	1.3×10^{-4}	8
6-trimethoxyamphetamine	30,000	3.5×10^{-5}	10
2-trimethoxyamphetamine	60,000	1.7×10^{-5}	17
4-trimethoxyamphetamine	90,000	1.1×10^{-5}	4

[a] IC_{50} is a concentration of hallucinogen displacing half the displaceable LSD binding. Hallucinogenic potency of various drugs in man is expressed as multiples of mescaline units. Mescaline unit was defined by SHULGIN et al. (1961) and SHULGIN (1963) as a ratio of effective mescaline dose/dose effective dose of the compared drug

An alternative approach in validating radioligand receptor assays is to investigate changes in binding after in vivo treatments which produce known physiologic or functional receptor changes. This strategy has been applied in postmortem investigations of Huntington's chorea (ENNA, et al., 1976; CHIU et al., 1974; MULLER and SEEMAN, 1977, SEEMAN et al. 1978; OWEN et al., 1978, WASTEK et al., 1976). Recently, BENNETT et al. (1979) noted a fall in ^{3}H-LSD binding in the frontal cortex of schizophrenics, but no changes in 5-HT or other neurotransmitter binding; it is uncertain as to whether pretreatment with phenothiazines may not have induced a spectrum of target tissue changes. This has been noted (THESLEFF, 1974), as have changes in more than one receptor system (BANERJEE et al., 1977; MULLER and SEEMAN, 1977). Most observers report no changes in LSD binding following injection of 5,7-dihydroxytryptamine or after raphe lesions. However, 5-HT depletion following daily treatment with reserpine or PCA for 1 or 2 weeks of treatment reportedly produced a rise in LSD binding in certain brain areas (BENNETT and SNYDER, 1976). What is required, however (since these treatments may have changed target tissues), is to account for the fourfold *lowered* threshold dosages of LSD days after a *single* dose of reserpine or PCPA (as previously noted herein). With prolonged treatment, in any event, structural brain changes might make it difficult to standardize results in terms of wet weight of the tissue, or the tissues' protein content. TRULSON and JACOBS (1979a) reported a small reduction in the number of LSD siles in the brain following tolerance dosages. The potential LSD residue in the brains following treatment was not reported, and it is unclear how many separate membrane preparations were needed to establish the Scatchard analysis; a sufficient number of independent determinations on different brain samples is required. Nevertheless, these are interesting possibilities if sufficient specificity and correlations continue to be established.

LOVELL and FREEDMAN (1976) noted that an identity of 5-HT and LSD binding sites, or even an exclusivity of postsynaptic binding sites, could not be supported. Nevertheless, a close relationship in all binding studies between 5-HT and LSD sites is clear (FILLION et al., 1978). It is clear that LSD interacts directly with several neurotransmitters, if not a site of its own. Thus, while dopamine is a weak displacer of ^{3}H-LSD, LSD strongly displaces ^{3}H-DA. Neuroleptics, especially methiothepin, can displace ^{3}H-LSD. The data show that LSD can bind with high affinity and with high steric preference to haloperidol, as well as apomorphine binding sites, to α- and β-adrenergic sites, as well H_2 sites. WHITAKER and SEEMAN (1978), utilizing the principle employed by TITLER et al. (1977), have attempted to produce conditions in which the LSD-5-HT interaction could be studied more selectively. They used phentolamine to prevent binding to α-adrenergic sites, and spiperone and apomorphine to block dopaminergic sites, and they succeeded in reducing the LSD displaceable binding from 1100 fmol/mg protein to 300 fmol/mg protein in the refined assay. The results are clearly dissimilar from the previous LSD binding assays, since *both* LSD and serotonin were more potent (IC_{50} for 5-HT was 35 nM, compared to 200–2000 in previous studies). Furthermore, chlorpromazine and (+) butaclamol retained high potency in this refined system. Recently, WHITAKER and SEEMAN (1979) added phentolamine, 5-HT, and spiperone to the LSD binding assay to study apomorphine-binding sites. This "finetuning" of binding assays for preselected binding properties may make possible different estimates of specificity and potency of the drug with amines.

Regional differences appear to be important as binding studies proceed. LSD, ^{3}H-spiperone, and 5-HT all bind well in both striatum and cortex in both in vivo and in vitro assays (LADURON et al., 1978; BENNETT and SNYDER, 1975; KRAUCHI et al., 1978). The three ligands do not bind to identical receptors. PEROUTKA and SNYDER (1979) now describe two 5-HT receptors (using spiperone) rather than a single one. Thus, a 5-HT_1 receptor is sensitive to tryptamine analogues of 5-HT as well as to LSD, but relatively insensitive to the presence of neuroleptics. In the frontal cortex, the 5-HT_1 receptor is sensitive to LSD and its analogues, as well as to serotonin antagonists (cyproheptidine, mianserine, and cinanserine) and less sensitive to tryptamine analogues of 5-HT. Thus, when spiperone blocks the binding of LSD to 5-HT_2 sites in the cortex, the subsequent binding profile will be closer to that of the 5-HT_1 site. Conversely, blocking 5-HT_1 receptors with serotonin converts the LSD binding closer to 5-HT_2 profile (PEROUTKA and SNYDER, 1979). Whether these refinements will bring into high focus the critical receptor interactions awaits further studies, but quantitative precision appears increasingly possible.

J. Conclusion

It is preposterous but clear that LSD is required to trigger and sustain the sequence of LSD effects (FREEDMAN and HALARIS, 1978). Since the drug concentrations in brain peak early, many of the unfolding effects over time could probably be related to the drug as it is retained and clears from the various affected membranes. Obviously, many elements are involved in the LSD experience, including the drug itself and the pharmacodynamics associated with it, its interaction with various neurotransmitter systems, and the interactions of these systems themselves. Therefore, it seems unlikely that a simple inhibition–disinhibition theory of psychedelic effects can be sustained (Freedman and Halaris, 1978), but if so should be most relevant at the *lowest* brain concentrations (when postsynaptic effects are less apt to seen [Aghajanian et al., 1975]), i.e., at the farthest time point in the LSD experience.

It is not as yet clear what precise biochemical or physiologic changes are necessary to enhance or diminish the LSD effect. However, enhanced sensitivity and reactivity to the environment (Elkes et al., 1954; Bradley and Elkes, 1957) and various different phenomena of sensitization and dehabituation should yield to neurobiologic study. While the psychobiology of the complex of events affecting attentional control and interpretation of reality may prove formidable to pharmacologic analysis, Purpura long ago adduced dimensions requiring further research, i.e., low dose LSD enhancing sensory systems and SIMULTANEOUSLY inhibiting the responsiveness of various cortical systems (Purpura, 1956a, b). The vulnerability of the LSD-treated human and animal to overreact to noxious stimuli and where possible, to disregard reality demands in favor of attending to "private experience," may well be clarified with attention to sensitization, facilitative, and "reactivity" effects at the neural level. With neurophysiologic studies coupled with behavioral and well-established biochemical and pharmacological definitions, and with attention to longer-term compensatory responses of monoaminergic systems, it appears possible to delineate the basis for some of the components of this multifaceted state. The systematic use of an array of drugs and analyses even at the molecular and membrane level, are necessary and possible, and with the use of active and inactive isomers at the appropriate points, we should expect a better grasp of the role of monoaminergic systems, as well as, hopefully, the specificities which underlie the common effects of the array of psychedelic drugs.

Acknowledgment. This work was supported in part by the Louis Block Board Professors Fund and by USPHS grant 5R01 MH13186 to Dr. Daniel X. Freedman and by USPHS grants 5R01 AA01865, 1R01 AA03532 and 1R01 DA0229 to Dr. William O. Boggan. Dr. Pavel Muller is acknowledged for his help in reviewing ligands and calculating data for tabular presentation (USPHS MH-25116). The support of Ms. Marty Lancaster in the final preparation of the manuscript is greatly appreciated.

References

Abramson, H.A., Sklarofsky, B., Baron, M.O., Fremont-Smith, N.: Lysergic acid diethylamide (LSD-25) antagonists. II. Development of tolerance in man to LSD-25 by prior administration of MLD-41 (1-methyl-d-lysergic acid diethylamide). Arch. Neurol. Psychiat. *79*, 201–207 (1958)

Aghajanian, G.K., Bing, O.H.L.: Persistence of lysergic acid diethylamide in the plasma of human subjects. Clin. Pharmacol. Ther. *5*, 611–614 (1964)

Aghajanian, G.K., Haigler, H.J., Bennett, J.L.: Amine receptors in CNS III. 5-hydroxytryptamine in brain. In: Handbook of Psychopharmacology, *6*, ED. Iverson, L.L., Iversen, S.D., Snyder, S.H. (eds.), pp. 63–96 New York: Plenum Press 1975

Aghajanian, G.K., Wang, R.Y.: Physiology and pharmacology of central serotonergic neurons. In: Psychopharmacology: A generation of progress. Lipton, M.A., Dimascio, A., Killam, K.F. (eds.), pp. 171–183, New York: Raven Press 1978

Ahn, H.S., Makman, M.H.: Interaction of LSD and other hallucinogens with dopamine-sensitive adenylate cyclase in primate brain: regional differences. Brain Res. *162*, 77–78 (1979)

Anden, N.E., Corrodi, H., Fuxe, K., Hokfelt, T.: Evidence for a central 5-hydroxy-tryptamine receptor stimulation by lysergic acid diethylamide. Brit. J. Pharmacol. *34*, 1–7 (1968)
Anden, N.E., Corrodi, H., Fuxe, K.: Hallucinogenic drugs of the indolealkyamine type and central monoamine neurons. J. Pharmacol. Exp. Ther. *179*, 236–249 (1971)
Anden, N.E., Corrodi, H., Fuxe, K.: Effect of neuroleptic drugs on central catecholamine turnover assessed using tyrosine and dopamine -β-hydroxylase inhibitors. J. Pharm. Pharmacol. *24*, 177–182 (1972)
Anden, N.E., Corrodi, H., Fuxe, K., Meek, J.L.: Hallucinogenic phenylethylamines: interactions with serotonin turnover and receptors. Eur. J. Pharmacol. *25*, 176–184 (1974)
Anderson, G.M., III, Braun, U., Nichols, D.E., Shulgin, A.: Absolute configuration and psychotomimetic activity. In: Quantitative structure activity relationships of analgesics, narcotic antagonists, and hallucinogens. Barnett,G., Trsic, M., Willette, R.E., (eds.), Washington, D.C.: U.S. Government Printing Office, NIDA Research Monograph 22 (1978) (Stock No. 017-024-00786-2; (pp. 8–15)
Appel, J.B., Freedman, D.X.: Chemically-induced alterations in the behavioral effects of LSD-25. Biochem. Pharmacol. *13*, 861–869 (1964)
Appel, J.B., Freedman, D.X.: The relative potencies of psychomimetic drugs. Life Sci. *4*, 2181–2186 (1965)
Appel, J.B.: The effects of "psychotomimetic" drugs on animal behavior. In: Psychopharmacology: A Review of Progress, 1957–1967. Efron D.H. (ed.) Washington, D.C.: U.S. Government Printing Office 1968
Appel, J.B., Freedman, D.X.: Tolerance and cross-tolerance among psychotomimetic drugs. Psychopharmacology *13*, 267–274 (1968)
Appel, J.B., Sheard, M.H., Freedman, D.X.: Alterations in the behavioral effects of LSD by mid-brain raphe lesions. Commun. Behav. Biol. (Part A) *5*, 237–241 (1970a)
Appel, J.B., Lovell, R.A., Freedman, D.X.: Alterations in the behavioral effects of LSD by pretreatment with p-chloro-phenylalanine and alpha-methyl-p-tyrosine. Pschopharmacology *18*, 387–406 (1970b)
Apter, J.T.: Anaeptic action of lysergic acid diethylamide [LSD-25] against pentobarbital. Arch. Gen. Psychiatry *79*, 711–715 (1958)
Axelrod, J., Brady, R.O., Witkop, B., Evarts, E.V.: The distribution and metabolism of lysergic acid diethylamide. Ann. N.Y. Acad. Sci. *66*, 435–444 (1957)
Balestrieri, A., Fontanari, D.: Acquired and crossed tolerance to mescaline, LSD-25, and BOL-148. Arch. Gen. Psychiatry *1*, 279 (1959)
Baldessarini, R.J., Stramentinoli, G., Lipinski, J.F.: Methylation hypothesis. Arch. Gen. Psychiatry *36*, 303–307 (1979)
Banerjee, S.P., Sharma, V.K., Kung, L.S.: B-adrenergic receptors in innervated and denervated skeletal muscle. Biochim. Biophysica Acta *470*, 123–127 (1977)
Bapna, J.S., Dandiya, P.C., Kulkarni, S.L.: Dissociation of excitatory and hyperpyrexic effects of LSD in rats treated with α-methyl-tyrosine. Jpn. J. Pharmacol. *23*, 735–737 (1973)
Barchas, J.D., Freedman, D.X.: Brain amines: response to physiological stress. Biochem. Pharmacol. *12*, 1225 (1963)
Barnett, G., Trsic, M., Willette, R.E., EDS. QuaSAR: Quantitative Structure Activity Relationships of Analgesics, Narcotic Antagonists, and Hallucinogens. Washington, D.C., U.S. Government Printing Office, NIDA Research Monograph 22 1978 (Stock No. 017-024-00786-2)
Beernink, K.D., Nelson, S.D., Mansour, T.E.: Effect of lysergic acid derivatives on the liver fluke, Fasciola hepatica. Int. J. Neuropharmacol. *2*, 105–112 (1963)
Bennett, J.L., Aghajanian, G.K.: LSD binding to brain homogenates: possible relationship to serotonin receptors. Life Sci. *15*, 1935–1944 (1974)
Bennett, J.P., Snyder, S.H.: Stereospecific binding of d-lysergic acid diethylamide (LSD) to brain membranes: relationship to serotonin receptors. Brain Res. *94*, 523–544 (1975)
Bennett, J.P., Jr., Snyder, S.H.: Serotonin and lysergic acid diethylamide binding in rat brain membranes: relationship to postsynaptic serotonin receptors. Molec. Pharmacol. *12*, 373–389 (1976)
Bennett, J.P., Jr., Salvatore, J.B., Bylund, C.B., Gillin, J.C., Wyatt, R.F., Snyder, S.H.: Neurotransmitter receptors in frontal cortex of schizophrenies. Arch. Gen. Psychiatry *36*, 927–924 (1979)

Berridge, M.J., Prince, W.T.: The nature of the binding between LSD and a 5-HT receptor: a possible explanation for hallucinogenic activity. Brit. J. Pharmacol. *51*, 269–278 (1974)
Bertino, J.R., Klee, G.D., Weintraub, M.D.: Cholinesterase, d-lysergic acid diethylamide, and 2-bromolysergic acid diethylamide. J Clin. Exp. Psychopathol. *20*, 218–227 (1959)
Bock, E., Braestrup, C.: Regional distribution of the synaptic membrane proteins: synaptin, D1, D2 and D3. J. Neurochem. *30*, 1603–1607 (1978)
Bockaert, J., Premont, J., Glowinski, J., Thierry, A.M., Tassin, J.P.: Topographical distribution of dopaminergic innervation and of dopaminergic receptors in the rat striatum. II. Distribution and characteristics of dopamine adenylate cyclase. Interaction of LSD with dopaminergic receptors. Brain Res. *107*, 303–315 (1976)
Boggan, W.O., Freedman, D.X., Appel, J.B.: p-chlorophenylalanine-induced alterations in the behavioral effects of 5-hydroxytryptophan. Psychopharmacology *33*, 293–298 (1973)
Bourgoin, S., Faivre-Bauman, A., Benda, P., Glowinski, J., Hamon, M.: Plasma tryptophan and 5-HT metabolism in the CNS of the newborn rat. J. Neurochem. *23*, 319–327 (1974)
Bourgoin, S., Artaud, F., Enjalbert, A., Hery, F., Glowinski, J., Hamon, M.: Acute changes in central serotonin metabolism induced by the blockade or stimulation of serotonergic receptors during ontogenesis in the rat. J. Pharmacol. Exp. Ther. *202*, 519–531 (1977)
Bowers, M.B., Freedman, D.X.: "Psychedelic" experiences in acute psychoses. Arch. Gen. Psychiatry *15*, 240–248 (1966)
Bowers, M.B., Jr.: Serotonin (5-HT) systems in psychotic states. Psychopharmac. Commun. *1*, 655–662 (1975)
Bradley, P.B., Elkes, J.: The effects of some drugs on the electrical activity of the brain. Brain *80*, 77–117 (1957)
Bramwell, G.J., Goyne, T.: Responses of midbrain neurones to microion tophoretically applied 5-hydroxytryptamine: comparison with the response to intravenously administered lysergic acid diethylamide. Neuropharmacology *15*, 457–461 (1976)
Brawley, P., Duffield, J.C.: The pharmacology of hallucinogens. Pharmacol. Rev. *24*, 31–66 (1972)
Brimblecombe, R.W.: Psychotomimetic drugs: biochemistry and pharmacology. In: Advances in drug research. Simmonds, A.B., (ed.), pp. 165–206, Vol. VII, London: Academic Press 1973
Brimblecombe, R.W, Pinder, R.M.: Hallucinogenic agents. Bristol: Wright-Scientechnica 1975
Brown, W.A., Krieger, D.T., van Woert, M.H., Ambani, L.M.: Dissociation of growth hormone and cortisol release following apomorphine. J. Clin. Endocrin. *38*, 1127–1129 (1974)
Brunelli, M., Castellucci, V., Kandel, E.R.: Synaptic facilitation and behavioral sensitization in aplysia: possible role of serotonin and cyclic AMP. Science *194*, 1178–1180 (1976)
Burki, H.R., Asper, H., Ruch, W., Zuger, P.B.: Bromocriptine, dihydroergotoxine, methysergide, LSD, CF 25-397, and 29-712: effects on the metabolism of the biogenic amines in the brain of the rat. Psychopharmacology *57*, 227–337 (1978)
Burt, D.R., Creese, I., Snyder, S.H.: Antischizophrenic drugs: chronic treatment elevates dopamine receptor binding in brain. Science *196*, 326–328 (1976a)
Burt, D.R., Creese, I., Snyder, S.H.: Binding interactions of lysergic acid diethylamide and related agents with dopamine receptors in the brain. Molec. Pharmacol. *12*, 631–638 (1976b)
Burt, D.R., Creese, I. Snyder, S.H.: Properties of (^{3}H) haloperidol and (^{3}H) dopamine binding associated with dopamine receptors in calf brain membranes. Molec. Pharmacol. *12*, 800–812 (1976c)
Cameron, O.G., Appel, J.B.: A behavioral and pharmacological analysis of some discriminable properties of LSD in rats. Psychopharmacology *33*, 117–134 (1973)
Carnegie, P.R.: Interaction of 5-hydroxytryptamine with the encephalitogenic protein of myelin. In: The Neurosciences: Third Study Program. Schmitt, F.O., Worden, F.G. (eds.), pp. 925–928, Cambridge: MIT Press 1972
Cerletti, A., Doepfner, W.: Comparative study on the serotonin antagonism of amide derivatives of lysergic acid and of ergot alkaloids. J. Pharmacol. Exp. Ther. *188*, 124–136 (1958)
Charalampous, K.D., Walker, K.E., Kinross-Wright, J.: Metabolic fate of mescaline in man. Psychopharmacology *9*, 48–63 (1966)
Chase, T.N., Breese, G.R., Kopin, I.J.: Serotonin release from brain slices by electrical stimulation: regional differences and effect of LSD. Science *157*, 1461–1463 (1967)

Chiu, T.H., Lapa, A.J., Barnard, E.A., Albuquerque, E.X.: Binding of d-Tubocurarine and a-Bungarotoxin in normal and denervated mouse muscles. Exp. Neurol. *43*, 399–413 (1974)
Christian, S.T., Harrison, R., Pagel, J.: Evidence for dimethyltryptamine (DMT) as a naturally-occurring transmitter in mammalian brain. Ala. J. Med. Sci. *13*, 162–165 (1976)
Christian, S.T., Harrison, R., Quayle, E., Pagel, J., Monti, J.: The in vitro identification of dimethyltryptamine (DMT) in mammalian brain and its characterization as a possible endogenous neuroregulatory agent. Biochem. Med. *18*, 164–183 (1977)
Christoph, G.R., Kuhn, D.M., Jacobs, B.L.: Dopamine Agonist pretreatment alters LSD's electrophysiological action from dopamine agonist to antagonist. Life Sci. *23*, 2099–2110 (1978)
Clark, L.D., Bliss, E.L.: Psychopharmacological studies of lysergic acid diethylamide (LSD-25) intoxication. Effects of premedication with BOL-148 (2-bromo-d-lysergic acid deithylamide), mescaline, atropine, amobarbital, and chlorpromazine. Arch. Neurol. Psychiat. *78*, 653–655 (1957)
Collins, B.J., Lovell, R.A., Boggan, W.O., Freedman, D.X.: Effects of hallucinogens on rat brain monoamine oxidase activity. Pharmacologist *12*, 256 (1970)
Consroe, P., Jones, B., Martin, P.: Lysergic acid diethylamide antagonism by chlorpromazine, haloperidol, diazepam, and pentobarbital in the rabbit. Toxicol. Appl. Pharmacol. *42*, 45–54 (1977)
Costa, E.: Effects of hallucinogenic and tranquilizing drugs on serotonin evoked uterine contractions. Proc. Soc. Exp. Biol. *91*, 39–41 (1956)
Cottrell, G.A.: Direct postsynaptic responses to stimulation of serotonin-containing neurones. Nature *225*, 1060–1062 (1970)
DaPrada, M., Saner, A., Burkard, W.P., Bartholini, G., Pletscher, A.: Lysergic acid diethylamide: Evidence for stimulation of cerebral dopamine receptors. Brain Res. *94*, 67–73 (1975)
Davis, M., Sheard, M.H.: Habituation and sensitization of the rat startle response: effects of raphe lesions. Physiol. Behavior *12*, 425–431 (1974)
de Montigny, C., Aghajanian, G.K.: Preferential action of 5-methoxytryptamine and 5-methoxydimethyltryptamine on presynaptic serotonin receptors: a comparative iontophoretic study with LSD and serotonin. Neuropharmacology *16*, 811–818 (1977)
Diab, I.M., Roth, L.J., Freedman, D.X.: [3_H] lysergic acid diethylamide: cellular audoradiographic localization in rat brain. Science *173*, 1022–1024 (1971)
Diag, J.L., Huttunen, M.O.: Persistent increase in brain serotonin turnover after chronic administration of LSD in the rat. Science *174*, 62–64 (1971)
Diaz, P.M., Ngai, S.H., Costa, E.: Factors modulating brain serotonin turnover. In: Advances in Pharmacology vol. 6B, pp. 75–92, New York, Academic Press 1968
DiPaolta, T., Hall, L.H., Kier, L.B.: Structure-activity studies on hallucinogenic amphetamines using model interaction calculations. J. Theor. Biol. *71*, 295–309 (1978)
Dolphin, A., Enjalbert, A., Tassin, J., Lucas, M., Bockaert, J.: Direct interaction of LSD with central "beta"-adrenergic receptors. Life Sci. *22*, 345–352 (1978)
Domino, E.F.: The indole hallucinogen model: Is it worth pursuing? In: Predictability in psychopharmacology. Preclinical and clinical correlations. Sudilovsky, A., Gershon, S., Beer, B. (eds.), pp. 247–268, New York: Raven Press 1975
Dyer, D.C., Gant, D.W.: Vasoconstriction produced by hallucinogens on isolated human and sheep umbilical vasculature. J. Pharmacol. Exp. Ther. *184*, 366–375 (1973)
Elkes, J., Elkes, C., Bradley, P.B.: The effect of some drugs on the electrical activity of the brain and on behavior. J. Ment. Sci. *100*, 125–141 (1954)
Enjalbert, A., Bourgoin, S., Hamon, M., Adrien, J., Bockaert, J.: Postsynaptic serotonin-sensitive adenylate cyclase in the central nervous system: I. Development and distribution of serotonin and dopamine-sensitive adenylate cyclases in rat and guinea pig brain. Molec. Pharmacol. *14*, 2–10 (1978)
Enna, S.J., Bird, E.D., Bennett, J.P., Bylund, D.B., Yamamura, H.I., Iversen, L.I., Snyder, S.H.: Huntington's chorea: changes in neurotransmitter receptors in the brain. New Engl. J. Med. *294*, 1305–1309 (1976)
Fillion, G., Fillion, M.-P., Spirakis, C., Bahers, J.-M., Jacob, J.: 5-Hydroxytryptamine binding to synaptic membranes from rat brain. Life Sci. *18*, 65–74 (1976)

Fillion, G.M.B., Rousselle, J.D., Fillion, M.P., Beaudoin, D.M., Goiny, M.R., Deniau, J.M., Jacob, J.J.: High affinity binding of [^{3}H]5-hydroxytryptamine to brain synaptosomal membranes: comparison with [^{3}H] lysergic acid diethylaminde binding. Molec. Pharmacol. *14*, 50–59 (1978)
Fiszer, S., De Robertis, E.: Subcellular distribution and chemical nature of the receptor for 5-hydroxytryptamine in the central nervous system. J. Neurochem. *16*, 1201–1209 (1969)
Freedman, D.X., Aghajanian, G.K., Ornitz, E.M., Rosner, B.S.: Patterns of tolerance to lysergic acid diethylamide and mescaline in rats. Science *127*, 1173–1174 (1958)
Freedman, D.X., Aghajanian, G.L.: Time parameters in acute tolerance, cross tolerance, and antagonism to psychotogens. Fed. Proc. *18*, 390 (1959)
Freedman, D.X.: Effects of LSD on brain serotonin. J. Pharmacol. Exp. Ther. *134*, 160–166 (1961a)
Freedman, D.X.: Studies of LSD-25 and serotonin in the brain. Proc. 3rd World Congress of Psychiat. *1*, 653 (1961b)
Freedman, D.X., Giarman, N.J.: LSD-25 and the status and level of brain serotonin. Ann. N.Y. Acad. Sci. *96*, 98–106 (1962)
Freedman, D.X.: Psychotomimetic drugs and brain biogenic amines. Am. J. Psychiatr. *119*, 843–850 (1963)
Freedman, D.X., Giarman, N.J.: Brain amines, electrical activity, and behavior. In: EEG and Behavior, (ed.) Glaser, G.H., pp. 198–243. New York: Basic Books 1963
Freedman, D.X., Effect of reserpine on plasma binding and brain uptake of LSD-25. Fed. Proc. *23*, 147 (1964)
Freedman, D.X., Coquet, C.A.: Regional and subcellular distribution of LSD and effects on 5-HT levels. Pharmacologist *7*, 183 (1965)
Freedman, D.X.: On the use and abuse of LSD. Arch. Gen. Psychiatr. *18*, 330–347 (1968)
Freedman, D.X., Gottlieb, R., Lovell, R.A.: Psychotomimetic drugs and brain 5-hydroxytryptamine metabolism. Biochem. Pharmacol. *19*, 1181–1188 (1970)
Freedman, D.X., Halaris, A.E.: The role of serotonin in the action of psychotomimetic drugs. (Abstract). Presented at 3rd Ann. Meeting Society for Neurosci. (1973)
Freedman, D.X., Boggan, W.O.: In: Serotonin – New Vistas: Histochemical and Pharmacology (Advances in Biochemical Psychopharmacology), Costa, E., Gessa, G.L., Sandler, M. (eds.), Vol. 10, pp. 151–157, New York: Raven Press 1974
Freedman, D.X., Halaris, A.E.: Monoamines and the biochemical mode of action of LSD at synapses. In: Psychopharmacology: A generation of progress, Lipton, M.S., Dimascio, A., Killam, K.F. (eds.), pp. 347–359, New York: Raven Press 1978
Freedman, D.X.: The mode of action of hallucinogenic drugs. In: Handbook of Biological Psychiatry. van Praag, Rafaelsen, Lader, Sacher (eds.), Vol. 2., New York: Marcel Dekker Inc. (in Press)
Fuxe, K., Fredholm, B.B., Ogren, S.O., Agnati, L.F., Hokfelt, T., Gustafsson, J.A.: Ergot drugs and central monoaminergic mechanisms: a histochemical, biochemical and behavioral analysis. Fed. Proc. *37*, 2128–2191 (1978a)
Fuxe, K., Orgen, S.O., Aganti, L.F., Jonsson, G., Gustaffson, J.A.: 5,7-dihydroxytryptamine as a tool to study the functional role of central 5-hydroxytryptamine neurons. Ann. N.Y. Acad. Sci. *305*, 346–369 (1978b)
Gaddum, J.H.: Antagonism between lysergic acid diethylamide and 5-hydroxytryptamine. J. Physiol. *121*, 15 (1953)
Gaddum, J.H.: Serotonin-LSD interactions. Ann. N.Y. Acad. Sci. *66*, 643–648 (1957)
Gerschenfeld, H.M.: Serotonin: Two different inhibitory actions on snail neurons. Science *171*, 1252–1254 (1971)
Geyer, M.A., Dawsey, W.J., Mandell, A.J.: Fading: a new cytofluorimetric measure quantifying serotonin in the presence of catecholamines at the cellular level in brain. J. Pharmacol. Exp. Ther. *207*, 650–667 (1978)
Giarman, N.J., Freedman, D.X.: Biochemical aspects of the actions of psychotomimetic drugs. Pharmacol. Rev. *17*, 1–25 (1965)
Gillin, J.C., Kaplan, J., Stillman, R., Wyatt, R.J.: The psychedelic model of schizophrenia: the case of N,N-dimethyltryptamine. Am. J. Psychiat. *133*, 203–208 (1976)
Goodwin, J.S., Katz, R.I., Kopin, I.J.: Effect of bromide on evoked release of monoamines from brain slices and intact atria. Nature *221*, 556–557 (1969)

Green, J.P., Johnson, C.L., Weinstein, H., Kang, S., Chou, D.: Molecular determinants for interaction with the LSD receptor: biological studies and quantum chemical analysis. In: The psychopharmacology of hallucinogens. Willette, R.E., Stillman, R.C. (eds.), pp. 28–60, New York: Pergamon Press (1978a)
Green, J.P., Weinstein, H., Maayant, S.: Defining the histamine H_2-receptor in brain: the interaction with LSD. In: Quantitative structure activity relationships of analgesics, narcotic antagonists, and hallucinogens. Barnett, G., Trsic, M., Willette, R.E. (eds.), pp. 38–59, Washington, D.C.: U.S. Government Printing Office, NIDA Research Monograph 22 1978b (Stock No. 017-024-00786-2)
Greenberg, D.A., U'Prichard, D.C., Snyder, S.H.: Alpha-noradrenergic receptor binding in mammalian brain: differential labeling of agonist and antagonist states. Life Sci. *19*, 69–76 (1976)
Greiner, T., Burch, N.R., Edelbert, R.: Psychopathology and psychophysiology of minimal LSD-25 dosage. Arch. Neurol. Psychiat. *79*, 208–210 (1958)
Guilbaud, G., Besson, J.M., Oliveras, J.L., Liebeskind, J.C.: Suppression by LSD of the inhibitory effect exerted by dorsal raphe stimulation on certain spinal cord interneurons in the cat. Brain Res. *61*, 417–422 (1973)
Halaris, A.E., Lovell, R.A., Freedman, D.X.: Subcellular studies on the effect of LSD in rat brain serotonin. Soc. Neurosci, 2nd Annu. Meet. p. 114 (Abstr.) (1972)
Halaris, A.E., Lovell, R.A., Freedman, D.X.: Effect of chlorimipramine on the metabolism of 5-hydroxytryptamine in the rat brain. Biochem. Pharmacol. *22*, 2200–2202 (1973)
Halaris, A.E., Freedman, D.X., Fang, V.S.: Plasma corticoids and brain tryptophan after acute and tolerance dosage of LSD. Life Sci. *17*, 1467–1472 (1975)
Halaris, A.E., Freedman, D.X.: Vesicular and juxtavesicular serotonin: effects of lysergic acid diethylamide and reserpine. J. Pharmacol. Exp. Ther. *203*, 575–586 (1977)
Hamilton, C.L.: Effects of LSD-25 and amphetamine on a running response in the rat. Arch. Gen. Psychiatry *2*, 104–109 (1960)
Hamon, M., Bourgoin, S., Jagger, J., Glowinski, J.: Effects of LSD on synthesis and release of 5-HT in rat brain slices. Brain Res. *69*, 265–280 (1974)
Hamon, M., Bourgoin, S., Enjalbert, A., Bockaert, J., Hery, F., Ternaux, J.P., Glowinski, J.: The effect of quipazine on 5-HT metabolism in the rat brain. Arch. Pharmacol. *294*, 99–108 (1976)
Hashimoto, H., Hayashi, M. Nakahara, Y., Niwaguchi, T., Ishii, H.: Hyperthermic effects of d-lysergic acid diethylamide (LSD) and its derivatives in rabbits and rats. Arch. Int. Pharmacodyn. *228*, 314–321 (1977)
Hendley, E., Snyder, S.H.: Correlation between psychotropic potency of psychotomimetic methoxyamphetamines and their inhibition of ^{3}H-normetanephrine uptake in rat cerebral cortex. Nature *229*, 264–266 (1971)
Hery, F., Simonnet, G., Bourgoin, S., Soubrie, P., Artaud, F., Hamon, M., Glowinski, J.: Effect of nerve activity on the in vivo release of [^{3}H] serotonin continuously formed from L-[^{3}H]tryptophan in the caudate nucleus of the cat. Brain Res. *169*, 317–334 (1979)
Hofmann, A.: Psychotomimetic agents. In: Drugs affecting the central nervous system, Medical research series. Burger, A. (ed.), Vol.II, Chapter 5, pp. 169–236, New York: Marcel Dekker 1968
Hollister, L.E.: Some human pharmacological studies of three psychotropic drugs: thiothixine, molidone and w-1867. J. Clin. Pharmacol. *8*, 95–101 (1968)
Hollister, L.E., Macnicol, M.F., Gillespie, H.K.: An hallucinogenic amphetamine analog (DOM) in man. Psychopharmacology *14*, 62–73 (1969)
Horita, A.: Some biochemical studies on psilocybin and psilocin. J. Neuropsychiat. *4*, 270–273 (1963)
Horita, A., Hamilton, A.E.: Lysergic acid diethylamide: dissociation of its behavioral and hyperthermic actions of DL-α-methyl-p-tyrosine. Science *164*, 78–79 (1969)
Horita, A., Hamilton, A.E.: The effects of DL-α-methyltyrosine and L-dopa on the hyperthermic and behavioral actions of LSD in rabbits. Neuropharmacology *12*, 471–476 (1973)
Horowski, R., Wachtel, H.: Direct dopaminergic actions of lisuride hydrogen maleate, an ergot derivative in mice. Eur. J. Pharmacol. *36*, 373–383 (1976)

Horowski, R.: Differences in the dopaminergic effects of the ergot derivatives bromocriptine, lisuride and LSD as compared with apomorphine. Eur. J. Pharmacol. *51*, 157–166 (1978)

Hughes, J.: Inhibition of noradrenaline release by lysergic acid diethylamide. Brit. J. Pharmacol. *49*, 706–708 (1973)

Isbell, H., Logan, C.R.: Studies on the diethylamide of lysergic acid (LSD-25). II. Effects of chlorpromazine, azacyclonol, and reserpine on the intensity of the LSD-reaction. Arch. Neurol. Psychiat. *77*, 350–358 (1957)

Isbell, H., Logan, C.R., Miner, E.J.: Relationships of psychotomimetic to anti-serotonin potencies of congeners of lysergic acid diethylamide (LSD-25). Psychopharmacology *1*, 20–28 (1959a)

Isbell, H., Miner, E.J., Logan, C.R.: Cross tolerance between d-2-Bromlysergic acid diethylamide (BOL-148) and d-diethylamide of lysergic acid (LSD-25). Psychopharmacology *1*, 109–116 (1959b)

Isbell, H., Wolbach, A.B., Wikler, A., Miner, E.J.: Cross tolerance between LSD and psilocybin. Psychopharmacology *2*, 147–159 (1964)

Jacobs, B.L., Trulson, M.E., Stern, W.C.: Behavioral effects of LSD in the cat: Proposal of an animal behavioral model for studying the actions of hallucinogenic drugs. Brain Res. *132*, 301–314 (1977)

Jacobs, B.L., Trulson, M.E.: Mechanisms of action of LSD. Am. Sc. *67*, 396–404 (1979)

Jonsson, G., Pollare, T., Hallman, H., Sachs, C.H.: Developmental plasticity of central serotonin neurons after 5,7-dihydroxytryptamine treatment. Ann. N.Y. Acad. Sci. *305*, 328–345 (1978)

Kang, S., Green, J.P.: Steric and electronic relationships among some hallucionogenic compounds. Proc. Natl. Acad. Sci. USA *67*, 62–67 (1970)

Katz, R.I., Kopin, I.J.: Effect of LSD and related compounds on release of norepinephrine-^{3}H and serotonin-^{3}H evoked from brain slices by electrical stimulation. Pharmacol. Res. Commun. *1*, 54–62 (1969)

Kehr, W.: Effect of lisuride and other ergot derivatives on monoaminergic mechanisms in rat brain. Eur. J. Pharmacol. *41*, 261–273 (1977)

Kehr, W., Speckenbach, W.: Effect of lisuride and LSD on monoamine synthesis after axotomy or reserpine treatment in rat brain. Naunyn-Schmiedeberg Arch. Pharmacol. *301*, 163–169 (1978)

Keller, H.H., Burkhard, W.P., Lieri, L., Bonetti, E.P., DaPrada, M. Lisuride and LSD-induced changes of monoamine turnover in the rat brain. Adv. Biochem. Psychopharmacol. *19*, 393–396 (1978)

Kier, L.B., Glennon, R.A.: Progress with several models for the study of the SAR of hallucinogenic agents. In: Quantitative structure activity relationships of analgesics, narcotic antagonists, and hallucinogens. Barnett, G., Trsic, M., Willette R.E. (eds.), pp. 149–185, Washington, D.C.: U.S. Government Printing Office, NIDA Research Monograph 22 1978 (Stock No. 017-024-00786-2)

Klein, M., Kandel, E.R.: Presynaptic modulation of voltage-dependent Ca^{2+} current: mechanism for behavioral sensitization of aplysia californica. Proc. Natl. Acad. Sci. U.S.A. *75*, 3512–3516 (1978)

Koslow, S.H.: The biochemical and biobehavioral profile of 5-methoxytryptamine. In: Trace amines and the brain. Usdin, E., Sandler, M. (eds.), pp. 103–130, New York: Marcel Dekker 1976

Kosterlitz, H.W., Waterfield, A.A.: In vitro models in the study of structure-activity relationships of narcotic analgesics. Ann. Rev. Pharmacol. *15*, 29–47 (1975)

Kovacic, B., Domino, E.F.: Tolerance and limited cross-tolerance to the effects of N, N-dimethyltryptamine (DMT) and lysergic acid diethylamide-25 (LSD) on food-rewarded bar pressing in the rat. J. Pharmacol. Exp. Ther. *197*, 495–502 (1976)

Kräuchi, K., Feer, H., Lichtsteiner, M., Wirz-Justice, A.: Specific in vivo binding of LSD in rat brain. Experientia *34*, 761–762 (1978)

Laduron, P.M., Janssen, P.F.M., Leysen, J.E.: Spiperone: ligand of choice for neuroleptic receptors. Biochem. Pharmacol. *27*, 317–321 (1978)

Lin, R.C., Ngai, S.H., Costa, E.: Lysergic acid diethylamide: Role in conversion of plasma tryptophan to brain serotonin (5-hydroxy-tryptamine). Science *166*, 237–239 (1969)

Lovell, R.A., Freedman, D.X.: Stereospecific receptor sites for d-lysergic acid diethylamide in rat brain: effects of neurotransmitters, amine antagonists and other psychotropic drugs. Molec. Pharmacol. *12*, 620–630 (1976)

Mandell, A.J., Geyer, M.A.: Hallucinations: chemical and physiological. In: Biological foundations of psychiatry. Grenell, R.G., Gabay, S. (eds.), pp. 729–753, New York: Raven Press 1976

Mansour, T.E., Sutherland, E.W., Rall, T.W., Bueding, E.: The effect of serotonin (5-hydroxytryptamine) on the formation of adenosine 3', 5'-Phosphate by tissue particles from the liver fluke, Fasciola hepatica. J. Biol. Chem. *235*, 466–470 (1960)

Marchbanks, R.M.: Serotonin binding to nerve ending particles and other preparations from rat brain. J. Neurochem. *13*, 1481–1493 (1966)

Marchbanks, R.M.: Inhibitory effects of lysergic acid derivatives and reserpine on 5-HT binding to nerve ending particles. Biochem. Pharmacol. *16*, 1971–1979 (1967)

Marrazzi, A.S., Huang, C.C.: Qualitative identity of cerebral neuronal membrane actions of 5-HT, LSD, and CPZ. Biol. Psychiatry *14*, 637–644 (1979)

Martin, W.R., Sloan, J.W.: Pharmacology and classification of LSD-like hallucinogens. In: Drug addiction. Martin, W.R. (ed.), pp. 305–368, Berlin-Heidelberg-New York: Springer Verlag 1977

Martin, W.R.: The nature of opioid and LSD receptors: structural activity relationship implications. In: Quantitative structure activity relationships of analgesics, narcotic antagonists, and hallucinogens. Barnett, G., Trsic, M., Willette, R.E., (eds.), pp. 60–69, Washington, D.C.: U.S. Government Printing Office, NIDA Research Monograph 22 1978 (Stock No. 017-024-00786-2)

McLean, J.R., McCartney, M.: Effect of d-amphetamine on rat brain noradrenaline and serotonin. Proc. Soc. Exp. Biol. Med. *107*, 77–79 (1961)

Mehl, E., Weber, L.: Affinity chromatography for subfractionation of 5-hydroxytryptamine, LSD-binding proteins from cerebral and nerve ending membranes. Adv. Biochem. Psychopharmacol. *11*, 105–108 (1974)

Mehl, E., Ruther, E., Redemann, J.: Endogenous ligands of a putative LSD-serotonin receptor in the cerebrospinal fluid: Higher level of LSD-displacing factors (LDF) in unmedicated psychotic patients. Psychopharmacology *54*, 9–16 (1977)

Mehl, E., Guiard, L.: Physiological ligands of putative LSD-serotonin receptors: Heterogeneity of LSD-displacing factors in human body fluids and nervous tissue. Hoppe-Seyler's Z. Physiol. Chem. *359*, 539–542 (1978)

Meltzer, H.Y., Fessler, R.G., Simonovic, M., Doherty, J., Fang, V.S.: Lysergic acid diethylamide: evidence for stimulation of pituitary dopamine receptors. Psychopharmacology *54*, 39–44 (1977)

Menon, M.K., Clark, W.G., Masuoka, D.T.: Possible involvement of the central dopaminergic system in the antireserpine effect of LSD. Psychopharmacology *52*, 291–297 (1977)

Muller, P., Seeman, P.: Brain neurotransmitter receptors after long-term haloperidol: dopamine, acetylcholine, serotonin, α-noradrenergic and naloxone receptors. Life Sci. *21*, 1751–1758 (1977)

Murphree, H.B., DeMaar, E.W.J., Williams, H.L., Bryan, L.L.: Effects of lysergic acid derivatives on man: antogonism between d-lysergic acid diethylamide and its 2-brom congener. J. Pharmacol. Exp. Ther. *122*, 55A (1958)

Nathanson, J.A., Greengard, P.: Serotonin-sensitive adenylate cyclase in neural tissue and its similarity to the serotonin receptor: a possible site of action of lysergic acid diethylamide. Proc. Natl. Acad. Sci. U.S.A. *71*, 797–801 (1974)

Nichols, D.E.: Structural correlation between apmorphine and LSD: involvement of dopamine as well as serotonin in the actions of hallucinogens. J. Theor. Biol. *59*, 167–177 (1976)

Nichols, D.E., Pfister, W.R., Yim, G.K.W.: LSD and phenethylamine hallucinogens: new structural analogy and implications for receptor geometry. Life Sci. *22*, 2165–2170 (1978)

Niwaguchi, T., Inoue, T., Sakai, T.: Studies on the *in vitro* metabolism of compounds related to lysergic acid diethylamide (LSD). Biochem. Pharmacol. *23*, 3063–3066 (1974)

Northup, J.K., Mansour, T.E.: Adenylate cyclase from *Fasciola Hepatica:* 2. Role of guanine nucleotides in coupling adenylate cyclase and serotonin receptors. Molec. Pharmacol. *14*, 820–833 (1978)

Owen, F., Crow, T.J., Poulter, M., Cross, A.J., Longden, A., Riley, G.J.: Increased dopamine-receptor sensitivity in schizophrenia. Lancet *1978 II*, 223–225

Palmer, G.C., Burks, T.F.: Central and peripheral adrenergic blocking actions of LSD and BOL. Eur. J. Pharmacol. *16*, 113–116 (1971)

Paul, S.M., Halaris, A.E., Freedman, D.X., Hsu, L.L.: Rat brain aryl acylamidase: stereospecific inhibition by LSD and serotonin related compounds. J. Neurochem. *27*, 625–627 (1976)

Peroutka, S.J., Snyder, S.H.: Multiple serotonin receptors: differential binding of [^{3}H]5-hydroxytryptamine, [^{3}H]lysergic acid diethylamide and [^{3}H]spiroperidol. Molec. Pharmacol. *16*, 687–699 (1979)

Persson, S.-A.: Effects of lysergic acid diethylamide (LSD) and 2-bromolysergic acid diethylamide (BOL) on central catecholaminergic pathways – A biochemical study. UMEA University Medical Dissertations No 32, University of Umeą, Sweden (1977a)

Persson, S.-A.: The effect of LSD and 2-bromo LSD on the striatal dopa accumulation after decarboxylase inhibition in rats. Eur. J. Pharmacol. *43*, 73–83 (1977b)

Persson, S.A., Johansson, H.: The effect of lysergic acid diethylamide (LSD) and 2-bromolysergic acid diethylamide (BOL) on the striatal dopa accumulation: influence of central 5-hydroxytryptaminergic pathways. Brain Res. *142*, 505–513 (1978)

Persson, S.-A.: Effects of LSD and BOL on the catecholamine synthesis and turnover in various brain regions. Psychopharmacology *59*, 113–116 (1978)

Persson, T.: Drug induced changes in ^{3}H-catecholamine accumulation after ^{3}H-tyrosine. Acta Pharmacol. Toxicol. *28*, 378–390 (1970)

Peters, D.A.V.: Comparison of the chronic and acute effects of d-lysergic acid diethylamide (LSD) treatment on rat brain serotonin and norepinephrin. Biochem. Pharmacol. *23*, 231–237 (1974a)

Peters, D.A.V.: Chronic lysergic acid diethylamide administration and serotonin turnover in various regions of rat brain. J. Neurochem. *23*, 625–627 (1974b)

Peters, D.A.V., Tang, S.: Persistent effects of repeated injections of D-lysergic acid diethylamide on rat brain 5-hydroxytryptamine and 5-hydroxyindoleacetic acid levels. Biochem. Pharmacol. *26*, 1085–1086 (1977)

Pieri, L., Pieri, M., Hafeley, W.: LSD as an agonist of dopamine receptors in the striatum. Nature *252*, 586–588 (1974)

Pieri, M., Schaffner, R., Pieri, L., DaPrada, M., Hafeley, W.: Turning in MFG-lesioned rats and antagonism of neuroleptic-induced catalepsy after lisuride and LSD. Life Sci. *22*, 1615–1622 (1978a)

Pieri, L., Keller, H.H., Burkard, W., DaPrada, M.: Effects of lisuride and LSD on cerebral monoamine systems and hallucinosis. Nature *272*, 278–280 (1978b)

Prozialeck,W.C., Vogel, W.H.: MAO inhibition and the effects of centrally administered LSD, serotonin, and 5-methoxy-tryptamine on the conditioned avoidance response in rats. Psychopharmacology *60*, 309–310 (1979)

Purpura, D.: Electrophysiological analysis of psychotogenic drug action. I. Effect of LSD on specific systems in the cat. Arch. Neurol. Psychiat. *75*, 122–131 (1956a)

Purpura, D.: Electrophysiological analysis of psychotogenic drug action. II. General nature of lysergic acid diethylamide (LSD) action on central synapses. Arch. Neurol. Psychiat. *75*, 132–143 (1956b)

Ray, O.S., Marrazzi, A.S.: A quantifiable behavioral correlate of psychotogen and tranquilizer actions. Science *133*, 1705–1706 (1961)

Resnick, O., Krus,D.M., Ruskin, M.: LSD-25 action in normal subjects treated with a monoamine oxidase inhibitor. Life Sci. *3*, 1207–1214 (1964)

Rosecrans, J.A., Lovell, R.A., Freedman, D.X.: Effects of lysergic acid diethylamide on the metabolism of brain 5-hydroxytryptamine. Biochem. Pharmacol. *16*, 2011–2021 (1967)

Rosenberg, D.E., Isbell, H., Miner, E.J.: Comparison of a placebo, N-dimethyltryptamine, and 6-hydroxy-N-dimethyltryptamine in man. Psychopharmacology *4*, 39–42 (1963)

Rosenberg, D.E., Isbell, H., Miner, E.J., Logan, C.R.: The effect of N,N-dimethyltryptamine in human subjects tolerant to lysergic acid diethylamide. Psychopharmacology *5*, 217–227 (1964)
Sai-Halász, A.: The effect of MAO inhibition of the experimental psychosis induced by dimethyltryptamine. Psychopharmacology *4*, 385–388 (1963)
Schanberg, S.M., Giarman, N.J.: Drug-induced alterations in the subcellular distribution of 5-hydroxytryptamine in rat's brain. Biochem. Pharmacol. *11*, 187–194 (1962)
Schneckloth, R., Page, I.H., DelGreco, F., Corcoran, A.C.: Effects of serotonin antagonists in normal subjects and patients with carcinoid tumors. Circulation *16*, 523–532 (1957)
Schubert, J., Nyback, H., Sedvall, G.: Accumulation and disappearance of ^{3}H-5-hydroxytryptamine formed from ^{3}H-tryptophan in mouse brain; effect of LSD-25. Eur. J. Pharmacol. *10*, 215–224 (1970)
Seeman, P., Chau-Wang, M. Tedesio, J., and Wang, K.: Brain receptors for antipsychotic drugs and dysamine: Direct binding assays. Proc. Natl. Acad. Sci. U.S.A. *72*, 4376–4380 (1975)
Seeman, P., Tedesco, J.L., Lee, T.; Chau-Wong, M., Muller, P., Bowles, J., Whitaker, P.M., McManus, C., Tittler, M., Weinreich, P., Friend, W.C., Brown, G.M.: Dopamine receptors in the central nervous system. Fed. Proc. *37*, 130–136 (1978)
Shields, P.J., Eccleston, D.: Evidence for the synthesis and storage of 5-hydroxytryptamine in two separate pools in the brain. J. Neurochem. *20*, 881–888 (1973)
Shulgin, A.T.: Psychotomimetic drugs: structure-activity relationships. In: Handbook of psychopharmacology. Iversen, L.L., Iversen, S.D., Snyder, S.H. (eds.), pp. 243–333, Vol. II, New York: Plenum 1978
Shulgin, A.T., Sargent, T., Naranjo, C.: Structure-activity relationships of one-ring psychotomimetics. Nature *221*, 537–541 (1969)
Shulgin, A.T., Sargent, T., Naranjo, C.: 4-Bromo-2,5-diemethoxyphenyl-isopropylamine, a new centrally active amphetamine analog. Pharmacology *5*, 103–107 (1971)
Smith, R.C., Boggan, W.O., Freedman, D.X.: Effects of single and multiple dose LSD on endogenous levels of brain tyrosine and catecholamines. Psychopharmacology *42*, 271–276 (1975)
Smythe, G.A.: The role of serotonin and dopamine in hypothalamic-pituitary function. Clin. Endocr. *7*, 325–341 (1977)
Smythies, J.R., Johnson, V.S., Bradley, R.J.: Alteration by pretreatment with iproniazid and an inactive mescaline analogue for a behaviour change induced by mescaline. Nature *216*, 196–197 (1967)
Snyder, S.H., Merril, C.R.: A relationship between the hallucinogenic activity of drugs and their electronic configuration. Proc. Natl. Acad. Sci. U.S.A. *54*, 258–266 (1965)
Snyder, S.H., Reivich, M.: Regional localization of lysergic acid diethylamide in monkey brain. Nature *209*, 1093–1095 (1966)
Snyder, S.H., Richelson, E.: Psychedelic drugs: steric factors that predict psychotropic activity. Proc. Natl. Acad. Sci. U.S.A. *60*, 206–213 (1968)
Snyder, S.H., Weingartner, H., Faillace, L.A.: DOET (2,5-Dimethoxy-4-Ethylamphetamine), a new psychotropic drug: effects of varying doses in man. Arch. Gen. Psychiatry *24*, 50–55 (1971)
Snyder, S.H.: Neurochemical actions of psychotropic drugs. Psychopharmacol. Bull. *11*, 62 (1975a)
Snyder, S.H.: The opiate receptor. Neurosci. Res. Progr. Bull. *13*, Suppl., 1–27 (1975b)
Soskin, R.A., Grof, S., Richards, W.A.: Low doses of dipropyltryptamine in psychotherapy. Arch. Gen. Psychiatry *28*, 817–821 (1973)
Spano, P.F., Kumakura, K., Tonon, G.C., Govoni, S., Trabucchi, M.: LSD and dopamine-sensitive adenylate-cyclase in various rat brain areas. Brain Res. *93*, 164–167 (1975)
Stolk, J.M., Barchas, J.D., Goldstein, M., Boggan, W.O., Freedman, D.X.: A comparison of psychotomimetic drug effects of rat brain norepinephrine metabolism. J. Pharmacol. Exp. Ther. *189*, 42–50 (1974)
Sugrue, M.F.: A study of the role of noradrenaline in behavioral changes produced in the rat by psychotomimetic drugs. Br. J. Pharmacol. *35*, 243–252 (1969)
Szara, S.: Dimethyltryptamine: its metabolism in man; the relation of its psychotic effects to the serotonin metabolism. Experientia *12*, 441–442 (1956)

Szara, S., Hearst, E., Putney, F.: Metabolism and behavioral action of psychotropic tryptamine homologues. Int. J. Neuropharmacol. *1*, 111–117 (1962)
Tamir, H., Klein, A., Rapport, M.M.: Serotonin binding protein: enhancement of binding by Fe^{2+} and inhibition of binding by drugs. J. Neurochem. *26*, 871–878 (1976)
Thesleff, F.: Physiological effects of denervation of muscle. New York Acad. Sci. *228*, 89–104 (1974)
Tilson, H.A., Sparber, S.B.: Studies on the concurrent behavioral and neurochemical effects of psychoactive drugs using the push-pull cannula. J. Pharmacol. Exp. Ther. *181*, 387–398 (1972)
Tittler, M., Weinreich, P., Seeman, P.: New detection of brain dopamine receptors with [^{3}H]dihydroergocryptine (neuroleptics/ergots/ neurotransmitters/norepinephrine/schizophrenia). Proc. Natl. Acad. Sci. U.S.A. *74*, 3750–3753 (1977)
Tonge, S.R., Leonard, B.E.: The effects of some hallucinogenic drugs upon the metabolism of 5-hydroxytryptamine in the brain. Life Sci. *8*, 805–814 (1969)
Tonge, S.R., Leonard, B.E.: Hallucinogens and non-hallucinogens: a comparison of the effects on 5-hydroxytryptamine and noradrenaline. Life Sci. *10*, 161–168 (1971)
Trulson, M.E., Eubanks, E.E., Jacobs, B.L.: Behavioral evidence for supersensitivity following destruction of central serotonergic nerve terminals by 5,7-dihydroxytryptamine. J. Pharmac. Exp. Ther. *198*, 23–32 (1976)
Trulson, M.E., Jacobs, B.L.: Usefulness of an animal behavioral model in studying the duration of action of LSD and the onset and duration of tolerance to LSD in the cat. Brain Res. *132*, 315–326 (1977)
Trulson, M.E., Ross, C.A., Jacobs, B.L.: Lack of tolerance of the depression of raphe unit activity by lysergic acid diethylamide. Neuropharmacology *16*, 771–774 (1977a)
Trulson, M.E., Stark, A., Jacobs, L.: Comparative effects of hallucinogenic drugs on rotational behavior in rats with unilateral 6-hydroxydopamine lesions. Eur. J. Pharmaol. *44*, 113–119 (1977b)
Trulson, M.E., Jacobs, B.L.: Alterations of serotonin and LSD receptor binding following repeated administration of LSD. Life Sci. *24*, 2053–2062 (1979a)
Trulson, M.E., Jacobs, B.L.: Dissociations between the effects of LSD on behavior and raphe unit activity in freely moving cats. Science *205*, 515–518 (1979b)
Uzonov, P. Weiss, B.: Psychopharmacological agents in the cyclic AMP system of rat brain. In: Advances in Cyclic Nucleotide Research, Vol. I. Greengard, P., Paoletti, R., Robeson, G.A. (eds.), pp. 435–453. New York: Raven Press 1972
Van Loon, G.R., Scapagnini, V. Moberg, G.P., Ganong, W.F.: Evidence for central adrenergic neural inhibition of ACTH secretion in the rat. Endocrinology *89*, 1464–1469 (1971)
Vaupel, D.B., Nozaki, M., Martin, W.R., Bright, L.D.: Single dose and cross tolerance studies of B-phenethylamine, d-amphetamine and LSD in the chronic spinal dog. Eur. J. Pharmacol. *48*, 431–437 (1978)
von Hungen, K., Roberts, S., Hill, D.F.: LSD as an agonist and antagonist at central dopamine receptors. Nature *252*, 588–589 (1974)
von Hungen, K., Roberts, S., Hill, D.F.: Interactions between lysergic acid diethlylamide and dopamine-sensitive adenylate cyclase systems in rat brain. Brain Res. *94*, 57–66 (1975)
Vrbanac, J.J., Tilson, H.A., Moore, K.E., Rech, R.H.: Comparison of 2,5-Dimethoxy-4-Methylamphetamine (DOM) and d-amphetamine for in vivo efflux of catecholamines from rat brain. Pharmacol. Biochem. Behav. *3*, 57–64 (1975)
Wallach, M.B., Friedman, E., Gershon, S.: 2,5-Dimethoxy-4-methylamphetamine (DOM), a neuropharmacological examination. J. Pharmacol. Exp. Ther. *182*, 145–154 (1972)
Wastek, G.J., Stern, L.Z., Johnson, P.C., Yamamura, H.I.: Huntington's disease: regional alteration in muscarinic cholinergic receptor binding in human brain. Life Sci. *19*, 1033–1040 (1976)
Weinstein, H., Green, J.P., Osman, R., Edwards, W.E.: Recognition and activation mechanisms on the LSD/serotonin receptor: the molecular basis of structure activity relationships. In: Quantitative structure activity relationships of analgesics, narcotic antagonists, and hallucinogens. Barnett, G., Trsic, M., Willette, R.E. (eds.), pp. 333–35 Washington, D.C.: U.S. Government Printing Office, NIDA Research Monograph 22 1978 (Stock No. 017-024-00786-2

Whitaker, A.E., Lovell, R.A., Freedman, D.X.: Effect of chlorimipramine on the metabolism of 5-hydroxytryptamine in the rat brain. Biochem. Pharmacol. *22*, 2200–2202 (1973)
Whitaker, P.M., Seeman, P.: Selective labelling of serotonin receptors by ^{3}H-LSD in calf caudate. Proc. Natl. Acad. Sci. U.S.A. *75*, 5783–5787 (1978)
Whitaker, P.M., Seeman, P.: Selective labelling of apomorphine receptors by ^{3}H-LSD. Eur. J. Pharmacol. *56*, 269–271 (1979)
Winters, J.C.: Tolerance to a behavioral effect of lysergic acid diethylamide and cross-tolerance to mescaline in the rat: absence of a metabolic component. J. Pharmacol. Exp. Ther. *178*, 625–630 (1971)
Woolley, D.W., Shaw, E.: A biochemical and pharmacological suggestion about certain mental disorders. Proc. Natl. Acad. Sci. U.S.A. *40*, 228–231 (1954)
Wyatt, R.J., Cannon, E.H., Stoff, D.M., Gillin, J.C.: Interactions of hallucinogens at the clinical level. Ann. N.Y. Acad. Sci. *281*, 456–486 (1976)
Ziegler, M.G., Lovell, R.A., Freedman, D.X.: Effects of lysergic acid diethylamide on the uptake and retention of brain 5-hydroxytryptamine in vivo and in vitro. Biochem. Pharmacol. *22*, 2183–2193 (1973)

CHAPTER 5

Neurophysiologic Properties of Psychotomimetics

G. K. AGHAJANIAN

A. Introduction

In recent years, physiologic studies on psychotomimetic drugs (e.g., psychedelics, stimulants, and deliriants) have focused increasingly upon actions at the single neuron level. This trend has been fostered by the mapping of a number of neuronal systems in the central nervous system according to neurotransmitter content. Of prime importance to investigations on psychedelic and stimulant drugs has been the mapping of monoaminergic neurons in the brain by the formaldehyde-condensation histochemical method of FALCK and HILLARP (DAHLSTRÖM and FUXE, 1965). By means of this and related methods it has been possible to identify the location of the cell bodies, axons, and terminal fields of the major monoaminergic pathways (i.e., noradrenergic, dopaminergic, and serotonergic). Similarly, the mapping of central cholinergic pathways has been crucial to investigating the actions of the antimuscarinic drugs, which produce a state of delirium.

This emerging histochemical knowledge has had an inevitable impact on physiologic approaches to the investigation of psychotomimetic drugs. Many psychotomimetic drugs are closely related in chemical structure to known neurotransmitters in the brain (e.g., the monoamines or acetylcholine). This review will place emphasis on single-cell recording studies dealing with the actions of psychotomimetic drugs on chemically related, histochemically identified neuronal systems. Wherever possible an effort will be made to establish correlations between the single-cell studies and relevant biochemical and behavioral data. The more general physiologic actions of psychotomimetic drugs have been reviewed by BRAWLEY and DUFFIELD (1972).

As defined above, the scope of this review is limited by the fact that several psychotomimetic drugs (e.g., the tetrahydrocannabinols and phencyclidine) have no obvious chemical relationship to any known neurotransmitters. On the other hand, major sections will be devoted to the indoleamine and phenethylamine group of psychedelic drugs and the stimulant drugs; these drugs are chemically related to the monoamines and have been studied extensively within histochemically identified monoaminergic systems. The delirium-inducing anticholinergic (antimuscarinic) drugs also will be considered since their actions have been studied within identified central cholinergic pathways by single-cell recording techniques.

B. Psychotomimetic Drugs and Related Neurotransmitters

I. Psychedelics

The psychedelic class includes D-lysergic acid diethylamide (LSD), the O- and *N*-methylated indoleamines, mescaline, the methoxyamphetamines, and several marijuana derivatives (e.g., Δ^9-tetrahydrocannabinol). These drugs, which are sometimes referred to as "hallucinogens," produce an altered state of perception, cognition, and affect without inducing the profound confusion and disorientation which are typical of a "toxic" or "organic" psychosis. It has been proposed that the psychedelic state represents an appropriate model for incipient phases of certain acute psychosis but not for chronic stages of schizophrenia (BOWERS and FREEDMAN, 1966).

On a single-cell level, LSD and the simple indoleamine hallucinogens will be discussed together as they appear to have many actions in common. Mescaline and the methoxyamphetamines will be considered separately as they differ from the indoleamine group in many of their cellular actions despite their similar overall effects on behavior. A similar analysis of the sites of action of the tetrahydrocannabinols is not possible since these compounds have not been linked as yet to any specific neurotransmitter systems.

1. LSD and the Simple Indoleamines

a) Background

Partly because of its structural similarity to the endogenous indoleamine serotonin (5-hydroxytryptamine; 5-HT), it has been thought that LSD might act upon 5-HT receptors in the CNS (GADDUM, 1953; WOOLLEY and SHAW, 1954; FREEDMAN, 1961). More recently, it has been found by single-cell recording and microiontophoretic techniques that there are at least three types of central 5-HT receptors in the mammalian brain: inhibitory postsynaptic, facilitatory postsynaptic, and autoreceptors (AGHAJANIAN et al., 1975; AGHAJANIAN and WANG, 1978; MCCALL and AGHAJANIAN, 1979). The actions of hallucinogenic drugs at each type of 5-HT receptor will be reviewed.

b) Actions at Autoreceptors and Inhibitory Postsynaptic Receptors

The first direct evidence for an effect of LSD on the physiologic activity of a histochemically identified neuronal system came with the demonstration that small intravenous doses of LSD inhibit the firing of 5-HT neurons in the raphe nuclei of rats (AGHAJANIAN et al., 1968; AGHAJANIAN et al., 1970). Initially, it was suggested that LSD might inhibit 5-HT neurons through a negative feedback circuit by acting as an agonist on postsynaptic neurons (AGHAJANIAN et al., 1968; ANDÉN et al., 1968). However, subsequent studies have shown that LSD has a powerful direct inhibitory action upon 5-HT neurons in the raphe when applied by microiontophoresis (AGHAJANIAN et al., 1972; BRAMWELL and GONYE, 1976). Moreover, the inhibition of 5-HT neurons by LSD is more pronounced than its inhibitory effect upon neurons receiving an identified serotonergic input in several visual and limbic areas (HAIGLER and AGHAJANIAN, 1974a; DEMONTIGNY and AGHAJANIAN, 1977). In contrast, 5-HT itself shows no such preferential activity. The 2-bromo derivative of LSD, which has minimal hallucinogenic effects, also fails to show such preferential action (AGHAJANIAN, 1976). By inhibiting 5-HT neurons directly, LSD could release postsynaptic neurons from a tonic inhibitory 5-HT influence; such a release or disinhibition might account for the sensory, cognitive, and other disturbances caused by LSD. The finding of increased activity of some neurons in the lateral geniculate nucleus, amygdala, and other areas after low doses of LSD is consistent with this idea (MOURIZ-GARCIA et al., 1969; GUILBAUD et al., 1973; HORN and MCKAY, 1973; HAIGLER and AGHAJANIAN, 1974a).

Three simple indoleamine hallucinogenic drugs, psilocin (4-hydroxy-*N*,*N*-dimethyltryptamine), DMT (*N*,*N*-dimethyltryptamine), and 5-methoxy-*N*,*N*-dimethyltryptamine also have a preferential inhibitory action upon 5-HT neurons as compared to postsynaptic neurons in the lateral geniculate (ventral nucleus) and amygdala (AGHAJANIAN and HAIGLER, 1975; DEMONTIGNY and AGHAJANIAN, 1977). On the other hand, there is only a slight difference between the pre- und postsynaptic actions of bufotenine (5-hydroxy-*N*,*N*-dimethyltryptamine). In general, these results parallel the known hallucinogenic (or psychotogenic) actions of these compounds. Except for LSD and some of its congeners, psilocin is the most potent of the indoleamine hallucinogens that have been tested in human subjects (WOLBACH et al., 1962). The effects of another powerful indoleamine hallucinogen, psilocybin (4-phosphoryl-*N*,*N*-dimethyltryptamine) are most probably mediated through its rapid metabolic conversion to psilocin (HORITA, 1963). The physiologic effects of DMT are similar to those of LSD and psilocin except for its lesser potency (SZARA, 1956; ROSENBERG et al., 1964). On the other hand, even high doses of bufotenine have little hallucinogenic action (FABING and HAWKINS, 1956; TURNER and MERLIS, 1959). Perhaps part of the reason for bufotenine's low hallucinogenic activity is the fact that is penetrates the brain poorly (SANDERS and BUSH, 1967). It is also possible that bufotenine has low activity as an hallucinogen because it differentiates less well between pre- and postsynaptic serotonergic sites than do psilicin, DMT, and 5-methoxy-*N*,*N*-dimethyltryptamine.

In general, these results are compatible with the hypothesis that LSD and the simple indoleamine hallucinogens could produce their hallucinogenic effects by acting preferentially upon 5-HT autoreceptors on or near the soma 5-HT neurons in the raphe nuclei. Two possible physiologic functions can be suggested for 5-HT autoreceptors. The autoreceptors could mediate the effects of 5-HT axon collaterals (or dendrodendritic junctions) within or between the various raphe nuclei. Recently, direct physiologic evidence for recurrent or collateral inhibition has been provided by studies in which the major ascending 5-HT pathway was activated antidromically during the recording of 5-HT cells which originate in the raphe (WANG and AGHAJANIAN, 1977, 1978). Another possible function of 5-HT autoreceptors is suggested by the finding that LSD blocks 5-HT release from isolated brain slices (CHASE et al., 1967; FARNEBO and HAMBERGER, 1971; HAMON et al., 1974). Thus, the autoreceptors that are sensitive to LSD may be involved in a local negative feedback regulation of 5-HT release from serotonergic terminals.

Figure 1 summarizes the differential actions of indoleamine hallucinogens at autoreceptors and postsynaptic inhibitory 5-HT receptors.

c) Actions at Facilitatory Postsynaptic 5-HT Receptors

Motoneurons of the brain and spinal cord receive a dense 5-HT input (DAHLSTRÖM and FUXE, 1965). Recently, it has been found that excitation of facial and other motoneurons by various means (e.g., stimulation of motor cortex, iontophoresis of glutamate) is markedly facilitated by 5-HT (MCCALL and AGHAJANIAN, 1979). By itself 5-HT has no excitatory action on the normally quiescent motoneurons. The facilitatory action of 5-HT is characterized by a long latency of onset and persistence for extended periods beyond the cessation of iontophoresis. The interpretation of this data for fa-

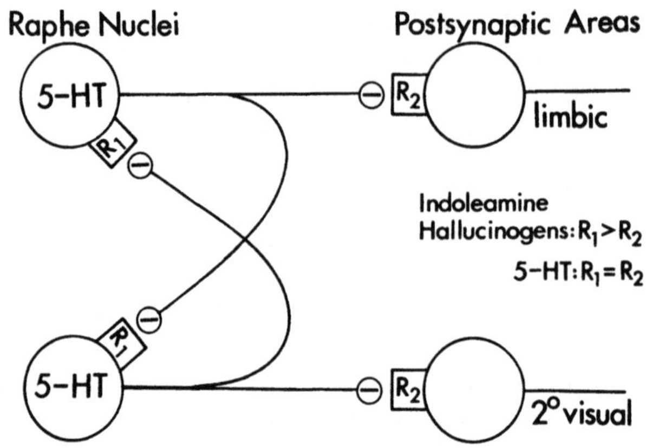

Fig. 1. A hypothetical circuit diagram of the differential localization of 5-HT autoreceptors R_1 and inhibitory (−) postsynaptic 5-HT receptors R_2. 5-HT autoreceptorts are shown in relation to inhibitory 5-HT axon collaterals within the raphe nuclei; postsynaptic 5-HT receptors are shown in relation to postsynaptic neurons in limbic and 2° visual areas

cial motoneurons is simplified by the fact that there are no interneurons within the facial nerve nucleus itself. Thus, 5-HT presumably facilitates through an action on synaptic inputs or on the motoneuron itself. The classic 5-HT antagonists (e.g., methysergide and cyproheptadine), which are not consistently or selectively effective at inhibitory 5-HT receptors (CURTIS and DAVIS, 1962; BLOOM et al., 1972; HAIGLER and AGHAJANIAN, 1974b; SEGAL, 1976), selectively and powerfully block the facilitatory effects of 5-HT on facial motoneuron excitation. Norepinephrine (NE) also facilitates motoneuron excitation, but via a different receptor as its effect is blocked by α-adrenoceptor antagonists but not by 5-HT antagonists (MCCALL and AGHAJANIAN, 1979). Previous studies have reported "excitatory" actions of 5-HT on unidentified spontaneously active brain stem neurons (e.g., BOAKES et al., 1970). In the latter area, as in the facial nerve nucleus, responses to 5-HT tended to be delayed and prolonged. Based on the facial nerve studies, these apparent excitations induced by 5-HT could be interpreted alternatively as representing a facilitation of tonic excitatory inputs. The excitatory effects of 5-HT on brain stem neurons have been reported to be blocked by LSD (BOAKES et al., 1970). However, since the existence of a 5-HT input to the latter neurons has not been established, the physiologic relevance of these findings must await further study. In contrast, the facilitation of facial neuron excitation by 5-HT as well as by NE is greatly enhanced by low intravenous doses of LSD (e.g., 10 μg/kg) (MCCALL and AGHAJANIAN, 1980). The iontophoresis of LSD at low currents, which by themselves have no effect, also enhances 5-HT facilitation; at higher currents LSD temporarily antagonizes the response. Thus, in small amounts LSD appears to sensitize these receptors to the facilitatory effects of 5-HT. Interestingly, mescaline also sensitizes and/or acts as an agonist at motoneuron 5-HT receptors despite the fact that it acts differently from LSD at certain other 5-HT receptors (see below). These sensitizing or facilitating effects on motoneuron excitability could account for the enhancement of certain spinal reflexes by LSD (ANDÉN et al., 1968) and mescaline (MAJ et al., 1977). The interaction of hallucinogenic drugs with the facilitation of motoneuron excitability by 5-HT is depicted in Fig. 2.

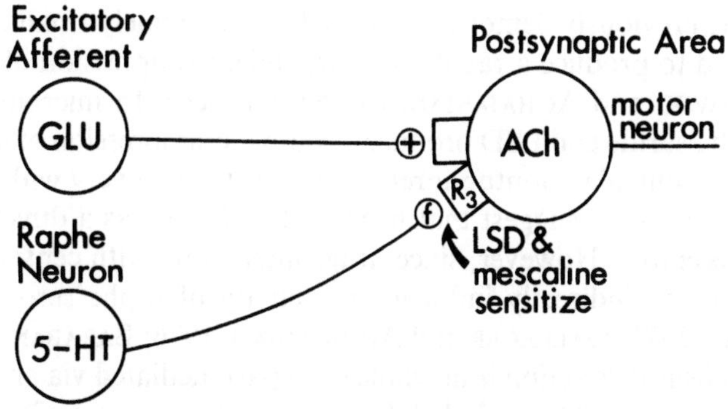

Fig. 2. A diagrammatic representation of the interaction between a hypothetical excitatory (+) glutaminergic *GLU* input to a cholinergic motor neuron *ACh* and a facilitatory 5-HT input *f* acting at a receptor R_3 on the motor neuron. The facilitatory R_3 receptor could also be located presynaptically (i.e., on the excitatory nerve terminal). LSD and mescaline are shown to sensitize the facilitatory 5-HT receptor R_3

d) Indoleamine Hallucinogens, 5-HT Neurons, and Behavior

Recently, Trulson and Jacobs (1978, to be published, a) have examined the behavioral effects of hallucinogenic drugs in awake, freely moving cats, while simultaneously recording the activity of 5-HT neurons. Both LSD and 5-methoxy-*N*,*N*-dimethyltryptamine decreased the activity of 5-HT neurons in a dose-dependent manner in association with increases in behaviors that are characteristically produced by hallucinogenic drugs in cats (e.g., the limb flick response). In the case of 5-methoxy-*N*,*N*-dimethyltryptamine, the onset, offset, and peak of the behavioral effects were temporally correlated with changes in neural activity. The results with LSD were in general similar to those seen with 5-methoxy-*N*,*N*-dimethyltryptamine. However, in the case of LSD the behavioral effects outlasted the depression in 5-HT neuronal activity. Furthermore, when LSD was readministered the next day, it produced little or no behavioral effect, but the depression in 5-HT cell activity was as large as that on the first day. Thus, it appears that while LSD may be having its primary effect by depressing the firing of 5-HT neurons, it might also produce changes in postsynaptic neurons that can both outlast the primary effect and modify responses to subsequent injections. Such changes could involve alterations in the sensitivity of postsynaptic 5-HT receptors to LSD, 5-HT, or both (Trulson et al., 1977; Trulson and Jacobs, to be published, b).

e) Comparison of LSD with Lisuride, a Nonhallucinogenic ergoline

Lisuride is an ergoline derivative which is structurally similar to LSD. However, unlike LSD, lisuride does not produce hallucinations in man and, in fact, has recently been evaluated for use in the prophylaxis of migraine headache (Herrmann et al., 1977) and in the treatment of hyperprolactinemic states (Liuzzi et al., 1978; Horowski et al., 1978). In common with some but not all chemically related ergot alkaloids (Burki et al., 1978; Fuxe et al., 1978), lisuride reduces 5-HT and dopamine (DA) turnover and, at higher doses, increases NE turnover (Kehr, 1977; Pieri et al., 1978). These and other biochemical observations have led to the conclusion that lisuride is a potent 5-HT and DA receptor agonist and a somewhat weaker NE receptor antagonist.

Recently, as previously demonstrated for LSD, extremely small doses of lisuride have been found to produce a rapid, dose-dependent suppression of 5-HT neuronal activity (Rogawski and Aghajanian, to be published). In microiontophoretic experiments, both lisuride and LSD produce a complete suppression of most raphe units studied, but, for equivalent iontophoretic currents, the recovery with lisuride is more prolonged. These results suggest that lisuride, like LSD, has a direct agonist action at 5-HT autoreceptors. However, since drugs interacting with central adrenoceptors have been found to indirectly influence to activity of raphe serotonergic neurons (Svensson et al., 1975; Gallager and Aghajanian, 1976; Baraban et al., 1978), the possibility that lisuride's action is in whole or in part mediated via an action at adrenergic receptor sites cannot be excluded. In any case, the response of raphe neurons appears to be highly selective since units in the locus ceruleus are not depressed by the drug.

In contrast to its depressant effects in the raphe, lisuride, in somewhat higher doses, causes an activation of noradrenergic neurons in the locus ceruleus. This activation is consistent with the increased turnover of NE reported after corresponding higher doses in biochemical studies. Pharmacologic agents with α-adrenoceptor blocking properties, such as piperoxan, which activate the locus ceruleus (Cedarbaum and Aghajanian, 1976) have been reported to produce anxiety or fear in human subjects (Goldenberg et al., 1947; Soffer, 1954). It is therefore of interest to note that one of the most prominent side effects of lisuride is its anxiety-producing or "dysphoric" action (Itil et al., 1975). LSD also causes an activation of locus ceruleus neurons and has been reported to decrease NE levels and accelerate NE turnover (Freedman, 1963; Diaz et al., 1968; Leonard and Tonge, 1969; Stolk et al., 1974), but both the physiologic and biochemical effects are less pronounced than with lisuride (Pieri et al., 1978).

Lisuride's action on dopaminergic neurons is not as clear-cut as its effects on the other two monoaminergic systems. The majority of cells tested are depressed by low doses of the drug, but in many cases this response is only partial and a small proportion of the cells were excited (Rogawski and Aghajanian, to be published). Similar effects of LSD on dopamine cells have been reported (Christoph et al., 1977).

In summary, lisuride resembles LSD in its effects on 5-HT and other monoaminergic neurons, except for a more prominent effect of lisuride on noradrenergic neurons.

f) Conclusions

Considerable evidence has now accumulated that LSD and the simple indoleamine hallucinogens can inhibit directly the firing of 5-HT neurons through a preferential action on 5-HT autoreceptors. In general, the first-dose effect of these drugs on hallucinogen-specific behaviors in cats correlates well with their ability to suppress 5-HT cell activity, although the behavioral effects of LSD seem to outlast changes in firing rate. In any case, by directly suppressing 5-HT cell activity these drugs could produce a psychedelic–hallucinatory state by disinhibiting postsynaptic neurons in various postsynaptic areas where 5-HT is inhibitory (e.g., in limbic and 2° visual nuclei of the brain; Haigler and Aghajanian, 1974a). One problem with this hypothesis is the fact that ergoline drug lisuride, which is even more powerful than LSD in inhibiting 5-HT neurons, is not hallucinogenic. However, lisuride might share some properties with indirectly acting agents that suppress 5-HT cell firing (e.g., α-adrenergic antagonists) and therefore would not express hallucinogenic activity. In any case, it will be of theoretical interest to further investigate pharmacologic differences between lisuride and LSD which could reveal drug actions critical for psychotomimetic activity.

Finally, the discovery of receptors at which LSD and mescaline can sensitize the facilitatory action of 5-HT opens a new approach to the study of these drugs on single cells. Thus far, these sensitizing effects of psychedelic drugs have been observed directly only on motoneurons. If similar effects can be found in sensory pathways, then sensitization, in distinction to disinhibition, might account for the altered perceptual reactivity induced by this drug.

2. Mescaline and Methoxyamphetamines

a) Background

As the effects of LSD and mescaline (3,4,5-trimethoxyphenylethylamine) on autonomic function and behavior are similar (WOLBACH et al., 1962), it generally has been assumed that these two drugs share a common site of action. In various species, cross tolerance occurs between LSD and mescaline (BALESTRIERI and FONTANARI, 1959; APPEL and FREEDMAN, 1968). A metabolic mechanism does not seem to account for such cross tolerance since prior treatment with mescaline does not reduce brain levels of LSD (WINTERS, 1971). Several investigators (SNYDER and RICHELSON, 1968; KANG and GREEN, 1970; NICHOLS et al., 1977) have proposed that mescaline may assume a conformation resembling a portion of the LSD molecule. Taken together, these data suggest that LSD and mescaline may act on the same receptor site in the CNS. Single-cell studies to test this hypothesis have dealt mainly with actions in the serotonergic and noradrenergic systems.

b) Mescaline, Methoxyamphetamines, and 5-HT Neurons

Systemic administration of mescaline (2–4 mg/kg, i.v.) has been found to inhibit a subpopulation of 5-HT neurons located within the ventral portion of the dorsal raphe nucleus and adjacent areas of the median raphe nucleus (AGHAJANIAN et al., 1970). A similar subpopulation of raphe neurons are inhibited by 2,5-dimethoxy-4-methylamphetamine (DOM). When LSD is administered systemically in doses comparable to those that produce behavioral effects, the firing of serotonergic neurons in the raphe nuclei of the brain stem is reversibly inhibited (see above). When LSD is administered microiontophoretically a similar inhibition is obtained (AGHAJANIAN et al., 1972). These data, coupled with the fact that after the systemic administration of mescaline a subpopulation of raphe neurons is inhibited (AGHAJANIAN et al., 1970), indicate that there may exist a subpopulation of raphe neurons that would be inhibited by the microiontophoretic application of mescaline. However, this expectation is not borne out by studies in which the effects of microiontophoretically and systemically applied mescaline are compared (HAIGLER and AGHAJANIAN, 1973). Although some raphe neurons are partially depressed by the microiontophoretic application of mescaline, this effect may represent a local anesthetic action and is not correlated with the inhibition produced by mescaline given intravenously. On the other hand, some raphe cells are unaffected by the microiontophoretic application of mescaline but are completely inhibited by the systemic administration of mescaline. The failure to obtain a response to mescaline, even under extreme conditions, from cells that are very sensitive to systemic mescaline does not support the view that the action of systemic mescaline on these raphe neurons is a direct one. In contrast, certain cortical neurons are highly responsive to the direct application of mescaline with no reported local anesthetic effect (BRADSHAW et al., 1971). In the raphe there is no correlation between response to mescaline and NE administered microiontophoretically (HAIGLER and AGHAJANIAN, 1973) as has been reported for cortical cells (BRADSHAW et al., 1971). Moreover, in the raphe there is no relationship between responses to i.v. mescaline and responses to NE given iontophoretically.

A possible explanation for the lack of correlation between the effect of mescaline given systemically or microiontophoretically would be that an active metabolite is formed in the periphery when the drug is given by the systemic route. Therefore, when mescaline is applied very close to the cell it would be relatively ineffective since there would be no opportunity for it to be metabolized. Two metabolites of mescaline that have been studied in man (i.e., *N*-acetylmescaline and 3,4,5-trimethoxyphenylacetic acid) do not produce physiologic and psychological effects (CHARLAMPOUS et al., 1966). The primary metabolite of mescaline in rats is 3,4,5-trimethoxyphenylacetic acid (MUSACCHIO and GOLDSTEIN, 1967). The possibility that mescaline must be converted to this metabolite in rats before it is effective on raphe cells has not been ruled out. However, the blockade of mescaline metabolism by iproniazid does not prevent certain of its behavioral effects (SMYTHIES et al., 1967). Moreover, in the single-cell experiments, the onset of the inhibition of firing in the raphe cells is within 30–40 s after the i.v. injection of mescaline, suggesting that if an active metabolite is formed this must occur extremely rapidly to be responsible for the inhibition.

In conclusion, it would appear that the effects of systemically administered mescaline upon 5-HT cells are via an indirect mechanism since the only direct mescaline effect obtainable was of a local anesthetic type. Furthermore, it appears that responses to mescaline by either route are unrelated to response to NE. As both LSD and mescaline can inhibit cells in the raphe nuclei when given systemically, but only LSD readily produces an inhibition in these cells when applied microiontophoretically, it would appear that they differ in their mode of action upon raphe cells. On a biochemical level, LSD and mescaline also differ as LSD but not mescaline depresses the metabolism of brain serotonin (FREEDMAN et al., 1970). The possibility remains that LSD and mescaline share a common site of action in some other area of the CNS.

c) Mescaline, Methoxyamphetamines, and Noradrenergic Transmission

In the periphery, mescaline can have both agonistic and antagonistic actions on adrenergic receptors (CLEMENTE and LYNCH, 1968). When applied to unidentified brain stem neurons, mescaline at high iontophoretic currents blocks responses to catecholamines (GONZALEZ-VEGAS, 1971). In the cerebral cortex, mescaline (again at high iontophoretic currents) exerts both excitatory and depressant actions (BRADSHAW et al., 1971; BEVAN et al., 1974). Regardless of the direction of change, the effects of mescaline have a higher correlation with the effects produced by NE than with those produced by 5-HT. However, mescaline is a much weaker "agonist" than either of the endogenous amines and its effects are not antagonized in a specific way by adrenergic or serotonergic antagonists.

Of course, it is possible that mescaline and methoxyamphetamine have their effects on monoamine transmission through an indirect action, such as on uptake (DENGLER et al., 1961) or release of endogenous transmitter (TILSON and SPARBER, 1972), rather than through a direct action on receptors. Mescaline, as well as LSD and the simple indoleamine hallucinogens, induces a decrease in levels of NE in brain (BARCHAS and FREEDMAN, 1963; DIAZ et al., 1968; LEONARD and TONGE, 1969). However, NE metabolite patterns are not altered in a consistent fashion, indicating that the various psychotomimetic drugs may not share a common effect on brain NE neurons (STOLK et al., 1974).

Recently, the effects of mescaline on the firing pattern of single NE neurons of the locus ceruleus have been studied in rats (AGHAJANIAN, 1980). In low systemic doses (1–4 mg/kg) mescaline has a dual action on these neurons. It induces a suppression of baseline firing rate while reactivity to peripheral stimuli remains the same or increases. NE neurons of the locus ceruleus respond to a noxious stimulus applied anywhere on the body by an initial activation followed by a period of suppressed activity (CEDARBAUM and AGHAJANIAN, 1978 a). The activation appears to be via direct spinal afferents, although some relay neurons may be involved (CEDARBAUM and AGHAJANIAN, 1978 a and b). There is evidence that the postactivation suppression in firing is mediated by NE released from a direct axon-collateral negative feedback system (AGHAJANIAN et al., 1977; CEDARBAUM and AGHAJANIAN, 1978 a). Mescaline prolongs the period of postactivation inhibition and thus behaves like desipramine, an inhibitor of NE uptake (AGHAJANIAN et al., 1978). As in the case of desipramine, the extended postactivation suppression induced by mescaline can be reversed by the presynaptic ($\alpha 2$) adrenoceptor antagonist piperoxan (AGHAJANIAN, in preparation). However, mescaline differs from desipramine, amphetamine, and the $\alpha 2$-agonist clonidine as the latter drugs depress reactivity to peripheral stimuli (AGHAJANIAN, 1980). Mescaline also differs from the $\alpha 2$-antagonist piperoxane; the latter diminishes postactivation collateral inhibition, but does not increase the initial reactivity to peripheral stimuli. Thus, mescaline possesses a unique action upon NE neurons which cannot be classified according to simple agonism or antagonism. Microiontophoretic results are consistent with this view: mescaline does not directly depress the firing of NE neurons (except at high iontophoretic currents), nor does it antagonize the depressant effects of NE.

d) Conclusions

Mescaline and the methoxyamphetamines do not fit into any simple category as agonists or antagonists with respect to either 5-HT or NE neurons. Indeed, the enhancement of NE-neuronal reactivity in relation to a reduction in baseline activity which is produced by mescaline represents an effect unlike that seen with known adrenergic agonists or antagonists that act at that site. Recent single-cell recording studies show that low doses of LSD (5 µg/kg, i.v.) also enhance reactivity of NE neurons to peripheral stimuli (AGHAJANIAN, in preparation). These findings are reminiscent of the earlier studies that show an activating effect of low doses of LSD on evoked potentials in specific sensory systems (PURPURA, 1956). Moreover, the activation of EEG by LSD is enhanced by increased external stimuli (BRADLEY and KEY, 1958). Similarly, clinical reports show that the subjective effects of LSD are accentuated with increased environmental stimulation (ELKES et al., 1954; COHEN and EDWARDS, 1964). Furthermore, the ECoG-activating effect of the psychedelic drugs differs from the stimulants, such as amphetamine, that activate the ECoG independently of the level of ambient stimulation (BRADLEY and ELKES, 1957). More recently, it has been shown that LSD (DAVIS and SHEARD, 1974; MILIARESSIS and ST-LAURENT, 1974) and mescaline (GEYER et al., 1978) enhance startle responses to acoustic and tactile stimuli, respectively. Thus, the mechanisms by which LSD or mescaline enhance NE-cell reactivity to peripheral stimuli may offer a clue to an understanding of mechanisms these psychedelic drugs may have in common.

II. Stimulants

In large doses, the amphetamine and other stimulants can induce a psychosis that bears a close clinical resemblance to spontaneous paranoid psychoses or paranoid schizophrenia (CONNELL, 1958; BEAMISH and KILOH, 1960; BELL, 1965; ELLINWOOD, 1967). Because of their obvious similarity in chemical structure to the catecholamines, the amphetamines have long been presumed to act via these neurotransmitters (SNYDER, 1972). Single-cell recording and microiontophoretic studies support the concept that amphetamine acts indirectly through the release or blockade of reuptake of endogenous catecholamines (e.g., BOAKES et al., 1972; BUNNEY et al., 1973; GROVES et al., 1976).

Several studies have indicated that paranoid symptoms can be elicited in human subjects with similar doses of L- and D-amphetamine (ANGRIST et al., 1971; JANOWSKY and DAVIS, 1976). These results suggest that brain systems in which the two isomers have nearly equal actions may be involved in mediating the psychotomimetic effects of these drugs. Thus, a major strategy in approaching their biochemical, behavioral, and physiologic actions on catecholaminergic neurons has been to compare relative potencies of the amphetamine isomers in various test systems (SNYDER et al., 1974).

1. Comparison of Amphetamine Isomers on the Activity of NE and DA Neurons

Most (SVENSSON, 1971; COSTA et al., 1972; FERRIS et al., 1972; SCHEEL-KRÜGER, 1972; HARRIS and BALDESSARINI, 1973; JORI et al., 1973; THORNBURG and MOORE, 1973; HOLMES and RUTLEDGE, 1976; PETERSON and SPARBER, 1976) but not all (ROFFMANN et al., 1978) recent biochemical and behavioral studies have indicated that D- and L-amphetamine are approximately equipotent in the NE system, but that D-isomer is much more potent than the L-isomer in the DA system. Similar differences have been found in single-cell recording studies (BUNNEY et al., 1975). DA neurons of the substantia nigra (zona compacta) are 5–20 times more sensitive to the depressant effect of D- and L-amphetamine given intravenously. On the other hand, the potency of L-amphetamine in depressing the firing of NE neurons is equal to that of D-amphetamine. From these results it would appear that low doses of L-amphetamine have a preferential action on the firing of NE as opposed to DA neurons. There is evidence from single-cell studies that the depression of DA cell firing by D-amphetamine is mediated indirectly by a postsynaptic neuronal feedback circuit (BUNNEY and AGHAJANIAN, 1976). An alternative view is that D-amphetamine depresses the firing of DA neurons by releasing DA locally from dendrites (GROVES et al., 1975). In this case, the local "self-inhibitory" effect of DA could be mediated by DA autoreceptors (AGHAJANIAN and BUNNEY, 1977). In either case, the much greater effect of D-amphetamine on DA cells firing correlates with the greater potency of this isomer in affecting the firing of postsynaptic striatal neurons innervated by the DA neurons of the zona compacta (REBEC and GROVES, 1975). Comparisons between D- and L-amphetamine have been made on NE-innervated postsynaptic neurons in the cerebellum (WISE and HOFFER, 1977); the two isomers have an equal ability to inhibit Purkinje cell discharge in this region. If D- and L-amphetamine prove to have equal actions at other postsynaptic NE sites as well, then the NE rather than DA system would seem more likely to be responsible for the amphetamine-induced paranoid psychosis. However, new data on differential actions of D- and L-amphetamine within subgroups of DA neurons necessitates a modification of this conclusion (see below).

2. Differential Actions of Amphetamine Isomers on Striatal and Nonstriatal DA Systems

It hat been proposed by a number of investigators that while the nigrostriatal DA system is involved in extrapyramidal motor functions, the nonstriatal mesocortical and mesolimbic DA projection systems, which arise in the ventral tegmental area, may be involved in schizophrenia (COSTA and GESSA, 1977). In a recent single cell recording study, the potencies of L- and D-amphetamine in decreasing the firing of DA neurons in both the substantia nigra (A9) and the ventral tegmentum area (A10) were compared (BROWDER et al., to be published). In agreement with previous results (BUNNEY et al., 1975), the firing rate of A9 neurons is much more sensitive to D- and than L-amphetamine. In addition, the dose-response of A10 cells to D-amphetamine is comparable to that of A9 cells.

Surprising, however, A10 cells are at least as sensitive to the depressant action of L- as D-amphetamine. These data show that the various DA nuclei are not pharmacologically homogenous. Moreover, as the two amphetamine isomers have similar potencies on A10 neurons, the mesolimbic and mesocortical DA systems represent a possible site through which the stimulant drug could produce a paranoid psychosis.

III. Deliriants

A delirious state (or toxic psychosis) is characterized by confusion, disorientation, memory deficits, and hallucinations. When produced by nonspecific toxic agents the delirium is often accompanied by generalized metabolic dysfunctions. The antimuscarinic drugs (e.g., atropine and scopolamine), which block cholinergic transmission at muscarinic receptor sites, are of particular pharmacologic interest as model psychotomimetic agents since they can reliably induce a delirious state in normal subjects without also inducing concomitant metabolic disturbances (e.g., KETCHUM et al., 1973). As the antimuscarinic drugs have a structural relationship to the neurotransmitter acetylcholine (ACh) (ABOOD and BIEL, 1962), it may be hypothesized that the antimuscarinic drugs act upon cholinergic receptors in the brain, as they do in the periphery. A further clue about central mechanisms of action comes from the fact that anticholinesterase agents such as physostigmine, which block the hydrolysis of ACh, are able to reverse the delirium produced by antimuscarinic drugs (KLEINWACHTER,

1864; FORRER and MILLER, 1958; CROWELL and KETCHUM, 1967; GOLDNER, 1967; DUVOISIN and KATZ, 1968; HEISER and GILLIN, 1971; KETCHUM et al., 1973). These clinical findings clearly link the psychotomimetic effects of the antimuscarinic drugs to cholinergic mechanisms.

With the discovery of presumptive cholinergic pathways in the brain by means of acetylcholinesterase (AChE) straining (SHUTE and LEWIS, 1963) combined with more specific biochemical assays (LEWIS et al., 1967) it has become possible to apply single-cell recording techniques to the investigation of the actions of antimuscarinic drugs on central cholinergic neurotransmission.

1. Antimuscarinic Drugs and Central Cholinergic Pathways

Perhaps the best-characterized cholinergic pathway in brain lies within the septohippocampal projection. Some of the evidence is as follows: (1) ACh is located in the hippocampus and ACh levels are greatly reduced following lesions of the medial septum that interrupt the septohippocampal tract (KUHAR et al., 1973); (2) stimulation of the medial septal nucleus results in the release of ACh from the dorsal hippocampus (ROMMELSPRACHER and KUHAR, 1974; SMITH, 1974; DUDAR, 1975); (3) choline acetyltransferase, the enzyme necessary for the synthesis of ACh, is localized to the neuropil adjacent to the pyramidal cell layer of the hippocampus (FONNUM, 1970); (4) the activity of this enzyme in the hippocampus is decreased by medial septal lesions (LEWIS et al., 1967; KUHAR et al., 1973); (5) AChE, the enzyme responsible for the degradation of ACh, is localized to the neuropil adjacent to the pyramidal cells (SHUTE and LEWIS, 1966; STORM-MATHISEN and BLACKSTAD, 1964); and (6) septal lesions result in a marked decrease in AChE activity in the hippocampal cell layer (LEWIS et al., 1967; STORM-MATISEN, 1972; MELLGREN and SREBRO, 1973). It should be noted, however, that there is not as yet a universally accepted histochemical method for cholinergic neurons (e.g., by using choline acetyltransferase as a marker).

The hippocampus has been linked with the functions of memory (SCOVILLE, 1957; VICTOR et al., 1961), learning (MEISSNER, 1966), and spatial orientation (OLTON and ISSACSON, 1968; O'KEEFE and DOSTROVSKY, 1971; MAHUT and ZOLA, 1973). As these are major functions disrupted by the antimuscarinic drugs, the hippocampus represents a relevant system for exploring the mechanism of action of their drugs. Hippocampal pyramidal cells are exceedingly sensitive to the excitatory action of ACh and muscarinic agonists, but not to nicotinic agonists applied by microiontophoresis (HERZ and NACIMENTO, 1965; BISCOE and STRAUGHAN, 1966; BIRD and AGHAJANIAN, 1975 and 1976; SEGAL, 1978). Muscarinic antagonists (i.e., atropine, scopolamine, and quinuclidinyl benzylate) totally and selectively block ACh excitation of hippocampal cells. Some but not all nicotinic antagonists are also effective, suggesting cholinergic receptors of the hippocampus are of the mixed type (BIRD and AGHAJANIAN, 1976; SEGAL, 1978). Similar findings have been reported for the cerebral cortex (KRNJEVIĆ and PHILLIS, 1963), which also receives a cholinergic projection from the septal area. Excitatory responses to ACh are also blocked by antimuscarinic drugs in the lateral geniculate nucleus (PHILLIS et al., 1967). The latter observation may be of interest in relation to the visual hallucinatory phenomenon induced by these drugs. Taken together, these studies establish that antimuscarinic drugs have powerful anticholinergic actions in identified or presumed central cholinergic pathways.

2. Action of Physostigmine in Cholinergic Pathways

Since physostigmine, a AChE inhibitor, can reverse the delirium produced by antimuscarinic drugs, its effect on transmission in known central cholinergic systems may be relevant to its clinical action. In normal animals, physostigmine greatly enhances the excitatory effect of ACh on neurons in several brain regions such as the lateral geniculate nucleus (PHILLIS et al., 1967) and the hippocampus (BIRD and AGHAJANIAN, 1975). When the septohippocampal pathway is lesioned, causing a depletion of AChE, a marked increase occurs in sensitivity to ACh but not carbachol (which is resistant to hydrolysis by AChE). In the lesioned animals, with the loss of presynaptic AChE, physostigmine no longer enhances ACh excitation (BIRD and AGHAJANIAN, 1975). These results show that denervation supersensitivity to ACh in the septohippocampal pathway is due primarily to decreased inactivation of ACh by presynaptic AChE. An implication of this finding is that AChE inhibitors can substantially increase the amounts of ACh at physiologically active sites. The therapeutic effect of physostigmine and other AChE inhibitors in reversing the delirium induced by antimuscarinic drugs may thus be explained by the fact that the action of ACh in the hippocampus and possibly other areas of the brain is so critically modulated by AChE.

3. Deliriants as a Model for Human Memory Disorders

Based on the fact that antimuscarinic drugs impair memory processes and anticholinergic drugs improve certain aspects of memory function, it has been suggested that diminished cholinergic transmission may underlie certain human memory disorders (DAVIS and YAMAMURA, 1978, for review). In support of this hypothesis, an age-related decrease in the central cholinergic enzymes choline acetyltransferase and AChE has been observed (MCGEER and MCGEER, 1976). These decrements are more severe in patients with Alzheimer's type senile dementia (PERRY et al., 1977). Thus, the possibility arises that drugs or precursors that enhance central cholinergic transmission might be useful in patients with senile or presenile dementias.

C. General Conclusions

As can be seen from the foregoing review, drugs within each of the major subgroups of psychotomimetics have dramatic effects on single-cell activity in chemically identified neuronal systems. Furthermore, each major subgroup appears to be separable according to transmitter-specific actions as follows:

I. Stimulants

Based on a large body of biochemical, behavioral, and physiologic evidence, the effects of stimulants (e.g., D- and L-amphetamine) within catecholaminergic systems can be attributed to a single overall action: the enhancement of the synaptic availability of NE or DA through a release and/or block of the reuptake of these catecholamines. However, a major question remains as to which of the several neuronal systems in which the stimulants have actions are most responsible for the psychotomimetic effects of these drugs. The noradrenergic system and the mesolimbic and mesocortical

DA systems have been implicated in the psychotomimetic effects of D- and L-amphetamine by virtue of the fact that they affect neuronal activity in these systems to a similar degree and have approximately equal effects in eliciting a paranoid psychosis. On the other hand, D-amphetamine, which has much greater activity than the L-isomer in the nigrostriatal DA system, can be linked to disturbances in extrapyramidal motor functions. However, several caveats should be mentioned. Knowledge about relative psychotomimetic potencies of D- and L-amphetamine is based on clinical studies involving relatively few subjects; ultimately further confirmation will be required. Furthermore, even if the nigrostriatal DA system could be ruled out in psychotogenesis, the remaining catecholamine pathways (both NE and DA) project so extensively within the brain that a multitude of other sites remain to be considered. Thus, much work needs to be done to define more precisely which brain systems are most closely involved in the psychotomimetic effects of the stimulant drugs.

II. Deliriants

As in the case of the stimulants, the central effects of the delirium-inducing antimuscarinic drugs can be attributed to a single action: the blockade of cholinergic transmission at muscarinic receptors. Moreover, certain of the major cholinergic pathways in the brain project to regions whose presumed functions are similar to functions that are disturbed in states of delirium. For example, the hippocampus, which receives the cholinergic septohippocampal projection, has been implicated in aspects of memory and orientation. However, the precise manner in which the cholinergic inputs modulate hippocampal function is not known. Moreover, the complete delineation of cholinergic systems in the brain has been hampered by the lack of a workable, specific histochemical method for mapping. A more complete picture of central cholinergic pathways will be needed to assess all possible sites at which the antimuscarinic drugs could be acting to induce the multiple disturbances seen in delirium.

III. Psychedelic Drugs

In contrast to the stimulants and deliriants, the effects of psychedelic drugs cannot as yet be attributed to a single action. In fact, at least two different types of mechanisms have been hypothesized by which the psychedelic drugs could act. The first can be termed the "5-HT disinhibitory" hypothesis, which applies best to LSD and the simple indoleamine hallucinogens. According to this hypothesis these hallucinogens, by directly inhibiting 5-HT neurons, would release postsynaptic neurons (e.g., in limbic or 2° visual areas) from tonic 5-HT influences, allowing hallucinatory and other psychedelic phenomena to emerge. However, there are seeming difficulties with the disinhibitory hypothesis as a unitary explanation. First, lisuride also appears to inhibit 5-HT neurons by acting at autoreceptors, yet it is not an hallucinogenic drug. Secondly, despite the fact that mescaline and the methoxyamphetamines have psychedelic effects that are very similar to those of LSD, they do not act upon 5-HT autoreceptors. On the other hand, both LSD and mescaline are similar in enhancing the responsivitity of noradrenergic neurons to peripheral stimuli. Furthermore, in some recent single-cell studies it has been observed that mescaline and LSD do share certain facilitatory actions. For example, they both directly sensitize facilitatory 5-HT receptors found on motoneurons. Thus, the psychedelic drugs can have a facilitatory as well as inhibitory and disinhibitory actions on a single-cell level. It remains for future research to ascertain the degree to which each of these mechanisms contributes to the final common behavioral effects of the two major classes of psychedelic drugs.

Acknowledgments. Supported in part by USPHS Grants MH-17871, MH-14459 and the State of Connecticut. I thank Ms. Leslie Fields, Ms. Annette Lorette, and Ms. Nancy Margiotta for their invaluable assistance in preparing this chapter.

References

Abood, L.G., Biel, J.H.: Anticholinergic psychotomimetic agents. Int. Rev. Neurobiol. *4*, 217–273 (1962)

Aghajanian, G.K.: LSD and 2-Bromo-LSD: Comparison of effects on serotonergic neurones and on neurones in two serotonergic projection areas, the ventral lateral geniculate and amygdala. Neuropharmacology *15*, 521–528 (1976)

Aghajanian, G.K.: Mescaline and LSD facilitate the activation of locus coeruleus neurons by peripheral stimuli. Brain Res.

Aghajanian, G.K., Bunney, B.S.: Dopamine "autoreceptors": pharmacological characterization by microiontophoretic single cell recording studies. Naunyn Schmiedbergs Arch. Pharmacol. *297*, 1–7 (1977)

Aghajanian, G.K., Cedarbaum, J.M., Wang, R.Y.: Evidence for norepinephrine-mediated collateral inhibition of locus coeruleus neurons. Brain Res. *136*, 570–577 (1977)

Aghajanian, G.K., Foote, W.E., Sheard, M.H.: Lysergic acid diethylamide: sensitive neuronal units in the midbrain raphe. Science *161*, 706–708 (1968)

Aghajanian, G.K., Foote, W.E., Sheard, M.H.: Action of psychotogenic drugs on single midbrain raphe neurons. J. Pharmacol. Exp. Ther. *171*, 178–187 (1970)

Aghajanian, G.K., Haigler, H.J.: Hallucinogenic indoleamines: preferential action upon presynaptic serotonin receptors. Psychopharmacol. Commun. *1*, 619–629 (1975)

Aghajanian, G.K., Haigler, H.J., Bennett, J.L.: Amine receptors in brain-111-5-hydroxytryptamine. In: Handbook of psychopharmacology. Iversen, L.L., Snyder, S.H. (eds.), pp. 63–96. New York: Plenum 1975

Aghajanian, G.K., Haigler, H.J., Bloom, F.E.: Lysergic acid diethylamide and serotonin: direct actions on serotonin-containing neurons. Life Sci. *11*, 615–622 (1972)

Aghajanian, G.K., Wang, R.Y.: Physiology and pharmacology of central serotonergic neurons. In: Psychopharmacology: generation of progress. Lipton, M.A., Dimascio, A., Killam, K.F. (eds.), pp. 171–182. New York: Raven 1978

Andén, N.E., Corrodi, H., Fuxe, K., Hökfelt, T.: Evidence for a central 5-hydroxytryptamine receptor stimulation by lysergic acid diethylamide. Br. J. Pharmacol. *34*, 1–7 (1968)

Angrist, B., Shopsin, B., Gershon, S.: The comparative psychotomimetic effects of stereoisomers of amphetamine. Nature *234*, 152–154 (1971)

Appel, J.B., Freedman, D.X.: Tolerance and cross-tolerance among psychotomimetic drugs. Psychopharmacology *13*, 267–274 (1968)

Balestrieri, A., Fontanari, D.: Acquired and crossed tolerance to mescaline, LSD-25 and BOL-148. Arch. Gen. Psychiatry *1*, 279 (1959)

Baraban, J.M., Wang, R.Y., Aghajanian, G.K.: Reserpine suppression of dorsal raphe neuronal firing: mediation by adrenergic system. Eur. J. Pharmacol. 52, 27–36 (1978)

Barchas, J.D., Freedman, D.X.: Brain amines: response to physiological stress. Biochem. Pharmacol. *12*, 1225–1235 (1963)

Beamish, P., Kiloh, L.G.: Psychoses due to amphetamine consumption. J. Ment. Sci. *106*, 337–343 (1960)

Bell, D.S.: A comparison of amphetamine psychosis and schizophrenia. Br. J. Psychiatry *111*, 701–707 (1965)

Bevan, P., Bradshaw, C.M., Roberts, M.H.T., Szabadi, E.: The effect of microelectrophoretically applied mescaline on cortical neurones. Neuropharmacology *13*, 1033–1045 (1974)

Bird, S.J., Aghajanian, G.K.: Denervation supersensitivity in the cholinergic septohippocampal pathway: a microiontophoretic study. Brain Res. *100*, 355–370 (1975)

Bird, S.J., Aghajanian, G.K.: The cholinergic pharmacology of hippocampal pyramidal cells: a microiontophoretic study. Neuropharmacology *15*, 273–282 (1976)

Biscoe, T.J., Straughan, D.W.: Microelectrophoretic studies of neurons in the cat hippocampus. J. Physiol. (Lond.) *183*, 341–359 (1966)

Bloom, F.E., Hoffer, B.J., Siggins, G.R., Barker, J.L., Nicoll, R.A.: Effects of serotonin on central neurons: microiontophoretic administration. Fed. Proc. *31*, 97–106 (1972)

Boakes, R.J., Bradley, P.B., Briggs, I., Dray, A.: Antagonism of 5-hydroxytryptamine by LSD 25 in the central nervous system: a possible neuronal basis for the actions of LSD 25. Br. J. Pharmacol. *40*, 202–218 (1970)

Boakes, R.J., Bradley, P.B., Candy, J.M.: A neuronal basis for the alerting action of (+)-amphetamine). Br. J. Pharmacol. *45*, 391–403 (1972)

Bowers, M.B., Freedman, D.X.: "Psychedelic" experience in acute psychoses. Arch. Gen. Psychiatry *15*, 240–248 (1966)

Bradley, P.B., Elkes, J.: The effects of some drugs on the electrical activity of the brain. Brain *80*, 77–117 (1957)

Bradley, P.B., Key, B.J.: The effect of drugs on arousal responses produced by electrical stimulation of the reticular formation of the brain. Electroencephalogr. Clin. Neurophysiol. *10*, 97–110 (1958)

Bradshaw, C.M., Roberts, M.H.T., Szabdi, E.: Effect of mescaline on single cortical neurones. Br. J. Pharmacol. *43*, 871–873 (1971)

Bramwell, G.J., Gonye, T.: Response of midbrain neurones to microiontophoretically applied 5-hydroxytryptamine: comparison with the response to intravenously administered lysergic acid diethylamide. Neuropharmacology *15*, 457–461 (1976)

Brawley, P., Duffield, J.C.: The pharmacology of hallucinogens. Pharmacol. Rev. *24*, 31–66 (1972)

Browder, S., German, D.C., Kiser, R.S., Shore, P.A.: Differential actions of amphetamine isomers on A 9 and A 10 dopamine neurons: correlation with psychotogenic effects. In: Catecholamines: basic and clinical frontiers. Usdin, E. (ed.). New York: Pergamon, to be published

Bunney, B.S., Aghajanian, G.K.: d-Amphetamine-induced inhibition of central dopaminergic neurons: mediation by a striato-nigral feedback pathway. Science *192*, 391–393 (1976)

Bunney, B.S., Aghajanian, G.K., Roth, R.H.: Comparison of effects of L-dopa, amphetamine and apomorphine on firing rate of rat dopaminergic neurones. Nature *245*, 123–125 (1973)

Bunney, B.S., Walters, J.R., Kuhar, M.J., Roth, R.H., Aghajanian, G.K.: D and L amphetamine stereoisomers: comparative potencies in affecting the firing of central dopaminergic and noradrenergic neurons. Psychopharmacol. Commun. *1*, 177–190 (1975)

Burki, H.R., Asper, H., Ruch, W., Zuger, P.B.: Bromocriptine, dihydroergotoxine, methysergide, d-LSD, CF 25–397, and 29–712: effects on the metabolism of the biogenic amines in the brain of the rat. Psychopharmacology *57*, 227–337 (1978)

Cedarbaum, J.M., Aghajanian, G.K.: Noradrenergic neurons of the locus coeruleus: inhibition by epinephrine and activation by the α-antagonist piperoxane. Brain Res. *112*, 413–419 (1976)

Cedarbaum, J.M., Aghajanian, G.K.: Activation of locus coeruleus neurons by peripheral stimuli: modulation by a collateral inhibitory mechanism. Life Sci. *23*, 1383–1392 (1978a)

Cedarbaum, J.M., Aghajanian, G.K.: Afferent projections to the rat locus coeruleus as determined by a retrograde tracing technique. J. Comp. Neurol. *178*, 1–15 (1978b)

Charlampous, K.D., Walker, K.E., Kinross-Wright, J.: Metabolic fate of mescaline in man. Psychopharmacology *9*, 48–63 (1966)

Chase, T.N., Breese, G.R., Kopin, I.J.: Serotonin release from brain slices by electrical stimulation: regional differences and effect of LSD. Science *157*, 1461–1463 (1967)

Christoph, G.R., Kuhn, D.M., Jacobs, B.L.: Electrophysiological evidence for a dopaminergic action of LSD: depression of unit activity in the substantia nigra of the rat. Life Sci. *21*, 1585–1596 (1977)

Clemente, E., Lynch, V.P.: In vitro action of mescaline: possible mode of action. J. Pharm. Sci. *57*, 72–78 (1968)

Cohen, S., Edwards, A.E.: The interaction of LSD and sensory deprivation: physiological considerations. Recent Adv. Biol. Psychiatry *6*, 139–144 (1964)
Connell, P.H.: Amphetamine Psychosis. London: Chapman and Hall 1958
Costa, E., Gessa, G.L. (eds.): Nonstriatal dopaminergic neurons. In: Advances in biochemical psychopharmacology. E. Costa, P. Greengard (eds.), Vol. 16, pp. 108. New York: Raven 1977
Costa, E., Groppetti, A., Naimzada, M.K.: Effects of amphetamine on the turnover rate of brain catecholamines and motor activity. Br. J. Pharmacol. *44*, 742–751 (1972)
Crowell, E.G.Jr., Ketchum, J.S.: The treatment of scopolamine-induced delirium with physostigmine. Clin. Pharmacol. Ther. *8*, 409–414 (1967)
Curtis, D.R., Davis, R.: Pharmacological studies upon neurones of the lateral geniculate nucleus of the cat. Br. J. Pharmacol. *18*, 217–246 (1962)
Dahlström, A., Fuxe, K.: Evidence for the existence of monoamine-containing neurons in the central nervous system. I. Demonstration of monoamines in the cell bodies of brain stem neurons. Acta Physiol. Scand. [Suppl. 232] *62*, 1–155 (1965)
Davis, K.L., Yamamura, H.I.: Cholinergic underactivity in human memory disorders. Life Sci. *23*, 1729–1734 (1978)
Davis, M., Sheard, M.H.: Effects of lysergic acid diethylamide (LSD) on habituation and sensitization of the startle response in the rat. Pharmacol. Biochem. Behav. *2*, 675–683 (1974)
deMontigny, C., Aghajanian, G.K.: Preferential action of 5-methoxytryptamine and 5-methoxydimethyltryptamine on presynaptic serotonin receptors: a comparative iontophoretic study with LSD and serotonin. Neuropharmacology *16*, 811–818 (1977)
Dengler, H.J., Spiegel, H.E., Titus, E.O.: Effects of drugs on uptake of isotopic norepinephrine by cat tissues. Nature *191*, 816–817 (1961)
Diaz, P.M., Ngai, S.H., Costa, E.: Factors modulating brain serotonin turnover. In: Advances in pharmacology. Garattini, S., Shore, P.A. (eds.), Vol. 6, pp. 15–92. New York: Academic Press 1968
Dudar, J.D.: The effect of septal nuclei stimulation on the release of acetylcholine from the rabbit hippocampus. Brain Res. *83*, 123–133 (1975)
Duvoisin, R.C., Katz, R.: Reversal of central anticholinergic syndrome. J. Am. Med. Assoc. *206*, 1963 (1968)
Elkes, J., Elkes, C., Bradley, P.B.: The effect of some drugs on the electrical activity of the brain and on behaviour. J. Ment. Sci. *100*, 125–141 (1954)
Ellinwood, E.H., Jr.: Amphetamine psychosis I: Description of the individuals and process. J. Nerv. Ment. Dis. *144*, 273–283 (1967)
Fabing, H.D., Hawkins, R.J.: Intravenous bufotenine injection in human being. Science *123*, 886–887 (1956)
Farnebo, L.O., Hamberger, B.: Drug-induced changes in the release of ^{3}H-monoamines from field stimulated rat brain slices. Acta Physiol. Scand. *371*, 35–44 (1971)
Ferris, R.M., Tang, F.L.M., Maxwell, R.A.: A comparison of the capactities of isomers of amphetamine, deoxypipradrol and methylphenidate to inhibit the uptake of tritiated catecholamines into rat cerebral cortex slices, synaptosomal preparations of rat cerebral cortex, hypothalamus and striatum and into adrenergic nerves of rabbit aorta. J. Pharmacol. Exp. Ther. *181*, 407–416 (1972)
Fonnum, F.: Topographical and subcellular localization of choline acetyltransferase in rat hippocampal region. J. Neurochem. *17*, 1029–1037 (1970)
Forrer, G.R., Miller, J.J.: Atropine coma: a somatic therapy in psychiatry. Am. J. Psychiatry *115*, 455–458 (1958)
Freedman, D.X.: Effects of LSD-25 on brain serotonin. J. Pharmacol. Exp. Ther. *134*, 160–166 (1961)
Freedman, D.X.: Psychotomimetic drugs and brain biogenic amines. Am. J. Psychiatry *119*, 843–850 (1963)
Freedman, D.X., Gottlieb, R., Lovell, R.A.: Psychotomimetic drugs and brain 5-hydroxytryptamine metabolism. Biochem. Pharmacol. *19*, 1181–1188 (1970)
Fuxe, K., Fredholm, B.B., Ogren, S.O., Agnati, L.F., Hökfelt, T., Gustafsson, J.A.: Ergot drugs and central monoaminergic mechanisms: a histochemical, biochemical and behavioral analysis. Fed. Proc. *37*, 2181–2191 (1978)
Gaddum, J.H.: Antagonism between lysergic acid diethylamide and 5-hydroxy-tryptamine. J. Physiol. (Lond.) *121*, 15 (1953)

Gallager, D.W., Aghajanian, G.K.: Effect of antipsychotic drugs on the firing of dorsal raphe cells. I. Role of adrenergic system. Eur. J. Pharmacol. *39*, 341–355 (1976)
Geyer, M.A., Petersen, L.R., Rose, G.J., Horwitt, D.D., Light, R.K., Adams, L.M., Zook, J.A., Hawkins, R.L., Mandell, A.J.: The effects of lysergic acid diethylamide and mescaline-derived hallucinogens on sensory-integrative function: tactile startle. J. Pharmacol. Exp. Ther. *207*, 837–847 (1978)
Goldenberg, M., Snyder, S.H., Aranow, H., Jr.: A new test for hypertension due to circulating epinephrine. J. Am. Med. Assoc. *135*, 971–976 (1947)
Goldner, R.D.: Scopolamine sleep treatment in private practice. Int. J. Neuropsychiatry *3*, 234–247 (1967)
Gonzalez-Vegas, J.A.: Antagonism of catecholamine inhibition of brain stem neurones by mescaline. Brain Res. *35*, 264–267 (1971)
Groves, P.M., Young, S.J., Wilson, C.J.: Self-inhibition by dopamine neurones: disruption by (±)-α-methyl-p-tyrosine pretreatment or anterior diencephalic lesions. Neuropharmacology *15*, 755–762 (1976)
Groves, P.M., Wilson, C.J., Young, S.J., Rebec, G.V.: Self-inhibition by dopaminergic neurons. Science *190*, 522–529 (1975)
Guilbaud, G., Besson, J.M., Oliveras, J.L., Liebeskind, J.C.: Suppression by LSD of the inhibitory effect exerted by dorsal raphe stimulation on certain spinal cord interneurons in the cat. Brain Res. *61*, 417–422 (1973)
Haigler, H.J., Aghajanian, G.K.: Mescaline and LSD: direct and indirect effects on serotonin-containing neurons in brain. Eur. J. Pharmacol. *21*, 53–60 (1973)
Haigler, H.J., Aghajanian, G.K.: Lysergic acid diethylamide and serotonin: a comparison of effects on serotonergic neurons and neurons receiving a serotonergic input. J. Pharmacol. Exp. Ther. *188*, 688–699 (1974a)
Haigler, H.J., Aghajanian, G.K.: Peripheral serotonin antagonists: failure to antagonize serotonin in brain areas receiving a promiment serotonergic input. J. Neural. Trans. *35*, 257–273 (1974b)
Hamon, M., Bourgoin, S., Jagger, J., Glowinski, J.: Effects of LSD on synthesis and release of 5-HT in rat brain slices. Brain Res. *69*, 265–280 (1974)
Harris, J.E., Baldessarini, R.J.: Uptake of [^{3}H]-catecholamines by homogenates of rat corpus striatum and cerebral cortex: effects of amphetamine analogues. Neurophormacology *12*, 669–679 (1973)
Heiser, J.F., Gillin, J.C.: The reversal of anticholinergic drug-induced delirium and coma with physostigmine. Am. J. Psychiatry *127*, 1050 (1971)
Herrmann, W.M., Horowski, R., Dannehl, U., Kramer, U., Lurati, K.: Clinical effectiveness of lisuride hydrogen maleate: a double-blind trial versus methysergide. Headache *17*, 54–60 (1977)
Herz, A., Nacimiento, A.C.: Über die Wirkung von Pharmaka auf Neurone des Hippocampus nach mikroelektrophoretischer Verabfolgung. Naunyn Schmiedbergs Arch. Pharmacol. *251*, 295–314 (1965)
Holmes, J.C., Rutledge, C.O.: Effects of the d- and l-isomers of amphetamine on uptake, release and catabolism of norepinephrine, dopamine and 5-hydroxytryptamine in several regions of rat brain. Biochem. Pharmacol. *25*, 447–451 (1976)
Horita, A.: Some biochemical studies on pilocybin and psilocin. J. Neuropsychiatry *4*, 270–273 (1963)
Horn, G., McKay, J.M.: Effects of lysergic acid diethylamide on the spontaneous activity and visual receptive fields of cells in the lateral geniculate nucleus of the cat. Exp. Brain Res. *17*, 271–284 (1973)
Horowski, R., Wendt, H., Graf, K.J.: Prolactin-lowering effect of low doses of lisuride in man. Acta Endocrinol. (Kbh.) *87*, 234–240 (1978)
Itil, T.M., Herrmann, W.M., Akpinar, S.: Prediction of psychotropic properties of lisuride hydrogen maleate by quantitative pharmaco-electroencephalogram. Int. J. Clin. Pharmacol. Biopharm. *12*, 221–233 (1975)
Janowsky, D.S., Davis, J.M.: Methylphenidate, dextroamphetamine and levamfetamine. Effects on schizophrenic symptoms. Arch. Gen. Psychiatry *33*, 304–308 (1976)

Jori, A., Dolfini, E., Tognoni, G., Garattini, S.: Differential effects of amphetamine, fenfluramine and norfenfluramine stereoisomers on the increase of striatum homovanillic acid in rats. J. Pharm. Pharmacol. *25*, 315–318 (1973)
Kang, S., Green, J.P.: Steric and electronic relationships among some hallucinogenic compounds. Proc. Natl. Acad. Sci. U.S.A. *67*, 62–67 (1970)
Kehr, W.: Effect of lisuride and other ergot derivatives on monoaminergic mechanisms in rat brain. Eur. J. Pharmacol. *41*, 261–273 (1977)
Ketchum, J.S., Sidell, F.R., Crowell, E.B.Jr., Aghajanian, G.K., Hayes, A.H.Jr.: Atropine, scopolamine, and ditran: comparative pharmacology and antagonists in man. Psychopharmacology *28*, 121–145 (1973)
Kleinwachter, I.: Observations concerning the effectiveness of extract of calabar against atropine poisoning. Berl. Klin. Wochenschr. *1*, 369–377 (1864)
Krnjević, K., Phillis, J.W.: Pharmacological properties of acetylcholine sensitive cells in the cerebral cortex. J. Physiol. (Lond.) *166*, 328–350 (1963)
Kuhar, M.J., Sethy, V.H., Roth, R.H., Aghajanian, G.K.: Choline: selective accumulation by central cholinergic neurons. J. Neurochem. *20*, 581–593 (1973)
Leonard, B.E., Tonge, S.R.: The effects of some hallucinogenic drugs upon the metabolism of noradrenaline. Life Sci. *8*, 815–825 (1969)
Lewis, P.R., Shute, C.C.D., Silver, A.: Confirmation from choline acetylase analyses of a massive cholinergic innervation to the rat hippocampus. J. Physiol. (Lond.) *191*, 215–224 (1967)
Liuzzi, A., Chiodini, P.G., Oppizzi, G., Botalla, L., Verde, G., Destefano, L., Colussi, G., Graff, K.J., Horowski, R.: Lisuride hydrogen maleate: evidence for a long lasting dopaminergic activity in humans. J. Clin. Endocrinol. Metab. *46*, 196–202 (1978)
Mahut, H., Zola, S.M.: A nonmodality specific impairment in spatial learning after fornix lesions in monkeys. Neuropsychologia *11*, 225–269 (1973)
Maj, J., Palider, W., Rawlów, A.: The influence of mescaline on the flexor reflex of the limb of the spinal rat. J. Pharm. Pharmacol. *29*, 177–178 (1977)
McCall, R.B., Aghajanian, G.K.: Serotonergic facilitation of facial motoneuron excitation. Brain Res. *169*, 11–27 (1979)
McCall, R.B., Aghajanian, G.K.: Hallucinogens sensitize serotonin and norepinephrine receptors in the facial motor nucleus. Life Sci.
McGeer, P.L., McGeer, E.G.: Enzymes associated with the metabolism of catecholamines, acetylcholine and GABA in human controls and patients with Parkinson's disease and Huntington's chorea. J. Neurochem. *26*, 65–76 (1976)
Meissner, W.W.: Hippocampal functions in learning. J. Psychiatr. Res. *4*, 235–304 (1966)
Mellgren, S.I., Srebro, B.: Changes in acetylcholinesterase and distribution of degenerating fibers in the hippocampal region after septal lesions in the rat. Brain Res. *52*, 19–36 (1973)
Miliaressis, T.E., St-Laurent, J.: Effets of de l'amide de l'acid lysergique-25 sur la réaction de sursant chez le rat. Can. J. Physiol. Pharmacol. *52*, 126–129 (1974)
Mouriz-Garcia, A., Schmidt, R., Arlazoroff, A.: Effects of LSD on the spontaneous and evoked activity of retinal and geniculate ganglion cells. Psychopharmacology *15*, 382–391 (1969)
Musacchio, J.M., Goldstein, M.: The metabolism of mescaline-^{14}C in rats. Biochem. Pharmacol. *16*, 963–970 (1967)
Nichols, D.E., Pfister, W.R., Yim, G.K.W., Cosgrove, R.J.: A new view of the structural relationship between LSD and mescaline. Brain Res. Bull. *2*, 169–171 (1977)
O'Keefe, J., Dostrovsky, J.: The hippocampus as a spatial map, preliminary evidence from unit activity in the freely moving rat. Brain Res. *34*, 171–175 (1971)
Olton, D.S., Issacson, R.L.: Hippocampal lesions and active avoidance. Physiol. Behav. *3*, 719–724 (1968)
Perry, E.K., Perry, R.H., Blessed, G., Tomlinson, B.E.: Necropsy evidence of central cholinergic deficits in senile dementia (letter). Lancet *1977 I*, 189
Peterson, D.W., Sparber, S.B.: Differential actions of D- and L-amphetamine on the metabolism of ^{3}H-norepinephrine in rat brain. Pharmacol. Biochem. Behav. *4*, 545–549 (1976)
Pieri, L., Keller, H.H., Burkhard, W., Daprada, M.: Effects of lisuride and LSD on cerebral monoamine systems and hallucinosis. Nature *272*, 278–280 (1978)
Phillis, J.W., Tebècis, A.K., York, D.H.: A study of cholinoceptive cells in the lateral geniculate nucleus. J. Physiol. (Lond.) *192*, 695–713 (1967)

Purpura, D.: Electrophysiological analysis of psychotogenic drug action. I. Effect of LSD on specific systems in the cat. Arch. Neurol. Psychiatr. *75*, 122–131 (1956)
Rebec, G.V., Groves, P.M.: Differential effects of the optical isomers of amphetamine on neuronal activity in the reticular formation and caudate nucleus of the rat. Brain Res. *83*, 301–318 (1975)
Roffmann, M., Cassens, G., Schildkraut, J.J.: Effects of the D- and L-isomers of amphetamine on the levels of 3-methoxy-4-hydroxyphenylglycol sulfate in whole ratbrain and rat brain regions. Biochem. Pharmacol. *27*, 1774–1777 (1978)
Rogawski, M.A., Aghajanian, G.K.: Response of central monoaminergic neurons to lisuride: comparison with LSD. Life Sci., to be published
Rommelspacher, H., Kuhar, M.J.: Effects of electrical stimulation of acetylcholine levels in central cholinergic nerve terminals. Brain Res. *81*, 243–251 (1974)
Rosenberg, D.E., Isbell, H., Miner, E.J., Logan, C.R.: The effect of N,N-dimethyltryptamine in human subjects tolerant to lysergic acid diethylamide. Psychopharmacology *5*, 217–227 (1964)
Sanders, E., Bush, M.T.: Distribution, metabolism and excretion of bufotenine in the rat with preliminary studies on its o-methyl derivative. J. Pharmacol. Exp. Ther. *148*, 340–352 (1967)
Scheel-Krüger, J.: Behavioral and biochemical comparisons of amphetamine derivatives, benztropine and tricyclic antidepressant drugs. Eur. J. Pharmacol. *18*, 63–73 (1972)
Scoville, W.B., Milner, B.: Loss of recent memory after bilateral hippocampal lesions. J. Neurol. Neurosurg. Psychiatry *20*, 11–21 (1957)
Segal, M.: 5-HT antagonists in rat hippocampus. Brain Res. *103*, 161–166 (1976)
Segal, M.: The acetylcholine receptor in the rat hippocampus; nicotinic, muscarinic or both? Neuropharmacology *17*, 619–623 (1978)
Shute, C.C.D., Lewis, P.R.: Cholinesterase-containing systems of the brain of the rat. Nature *199*, 1160–1164 (1963)
Shute, C.C.D., Lewis, P.R.: Electron microscopy of cholinergic terminals and acetylcholinesterase-containing neurones in the hippocampal formation of the rat. Z. Zellforsch. *69*, 334–343 (1966)
Smith, C.M.: Acetylcholine release from the cholinergic septohippocampal pathway. Life Sci. *14*, 2159–2166 (1974)
Smythies, J.R., Johnston, V.S., Bradley, R.J.: Alteration by pre-treatment with iproniazid and an inactive mescaline analogue of a behaviour change induced by mescaline. Nature *216*, 196–197 (1967)
Snyder, S.H.: Catecholamines in the brain as mediators of amphetamine psychosis. Arch. Gen. Psychiatry *27*, 169–179 (1972)
Snyder, S.H., Banerjee, S.P., Yamamura, H.I., Greenberg, D.: Drugs, neurotransmitters and schizophrenia. Science *184*, 1243–1253 (1974)
Snyder, S.H., Richelson, E.: Psychedelic drugs: steric factors that predict psychotropic activity. Proc. Natl. Acad. Sci. U.S.A. *60*, 206–213 (1968)
Soffer, A.: Symposium on efficacy of new drugs; regitine and benodaine in diagnosis of pheochromocytoma. Med. Clin. North Am. *38*, 375–384 (1954)
Stolk, J.M., Barchas, J.D., Goldstein, M., Boggan, W.O., Freedman, D.X.: A comparison of psychotomimetic drug effects on rat brain norepinephrine metabolism. J. Pharmacol. Exp. Ther. *189*, 42–50 (1974)
Storm-Mathisen, J., Blackstad, T.W.: Cholinesterase in the hippocampal region. Acta. Anat. (Basel) *56*, 216–253 (1964)
Storm-Mathisen, J.: Glutamate decarboxylase in the rat hippocampal region after lesions of the afferent fibre systems. Evidence that the enzyme is localized in intrinsic neurones. Brain Res. *40*, 215–235 (1972)
Svensson, T.H.: Functional and biochemical effects of D- and L-amphetamine on central catecholamine neurons. Naunyn Schmiedbergs Arch. Pharmacol. *271*, 170–180 (1971)
Svensson, T.H., Bunney, B.S., Aghajanian, G.K.: Inhibition of both noradrenergic and serotonergic neurons in brain by the α-adrenergic agonist clonidine. Brain Res. *92*, 291–306 (1975)

Szara, S.: Dimethyltryptamine: its metabolism in man; the relation of its psychotic effect to the serotonin metabolism. Experientia *12*, 441–442 (1956)
Thornburg, J.E., Moore, K.E.: The relative importance of dopaminergic and noradrenergic neuronal systems for the stimulation of locomotor activity induced by amphetamine and other drugs. Neuropharmacology *12*, 853–866 (1973)
Tilson, H.A., Sparber, S.B.: Studies on the concurrent behavioral and neurochemical effects of psychoactive drugs using the push-pull cannula. J. Pharmacol. Exp. Ther. *181*, 387–398 (1972)
Trulson, M.E., Jacobs, B.L.: Effects of LSD on behavior and raphe unit activity in freely moving cats. Fed. Proc. *37*, 346 (1978)
Trulson, M.E., Jacobs, B.L.: Effects of 5-methoxy-N,N-dimethyltryptamine on behavior and raphe unit activity in freely-moving cats. Eur. J. Pharmacol., to be published, a
Trulson, M.E., Jacobs, B.L.: Alterations of serotonin and LSD receptor binding following repeated administration of LSD. Life Sci., to be published, b
Trulson, M.E., Ross, C.A., Jacobs, B.L.: Lack of tolerance of the depression of raphe unit activity by lysergic acid diethylamide. Neuropharmacology *16*, 771–774 (1977)
Turner, W.J., Merlis, S.: Effect of some indolealkylamines on man. Arch. Neurol. Psychiatry *81*, 121–129 (1959)
Victor, M., Angevine, J.B., Mancall, E.L., Fisher, C.M.: Memory loss with lesions of hippocampal formation. Report of a case with some remarks on the anatomical basis of memory. Arch. Neurol. *5*, 244–263 (1961)
Wang, R.Y., Aghajanian, G.K.: Antidromically identified serotonergic neurons in the rat midbrain: evidence for collateral inhibition. Brain Res. *132*, 186–193 (1977)
Wang, R.Y., Aghajanian, G.K.: Collateral inhibition of serotonergic neurones in the rat dorsal raphe nucleus: pharmacological evidence. Neuropharmacology *17*, 819–825 (1978)
Winters, J.C.: Tolerance to a behavioral effect of lysergic acid diethylamide and cross-tolerance to mescaline in the rat: absence of a metabolic component. J. Pharmacol. Exp. Ther. *178*, 625–630 (1971)
Wise, R.A., Hoffer, B.J.: Equal suppression of cerebellar Purkinje cells activity by amphetamine stereo-isomers. Physiol. Behav. *18*, 1005–1009 (1977)
Wolbach, A.B., Jr., Miner, E.J., Isbell, H.: Comparison of psilocin with psilocybin, mescaline and LSD-25. Psychopharmacology *3*, 219–223 (1962)
Woolley, D.W., Shaw, E.: A biochemical and pharmacological suggestion about certain mental disorders. Proc. Natl. Acad. Sci. U.S.A. *40*, 228–231 (1954)

CHAPTER 6

Dependence-Producing Liability of LSD and Similar Psychotomimetics

A. D. POLING [1] and J. B. APPEL

A. Introduction: Definition of Drug Dependence

The WORLD HEALTH ORGANIZATION (1975) has defined dependence as "a state, psychic and sometimes also physical, resulting in the interaction between a living organism and a drug, characterized by behavioural and other responses which will always include a compulsion to take the drug on a continuous or periodic basis in order to experience its psychic effects and sometimes to avoid the discomfort of its absence." In behavioral terms, this definition seems to imply that any agent that consistently acts as a positive reinforcer, i.e., maintains behavior leading to its delivery, induces dependence. If a compound acts as a positive reinforcer and the physiologic syndrome of "withdrawal" occurs when the compound is withheld after chronic administration, the dependence is termed "physical"; a compound that acts as a positive reinforcer and does not produce withdrawal effects causes "psychological" dependence (SCHUSTER and JOHANSON, 1974).

An organism that is psychologically dependent upon a drug is not necessarily debilitated: some drugs – such as caffeine in our morning coffee and afternoon tea – are self-administrated over long periods without obviously deleterious consequences. Nevertheless, dependence on many drugs is demonstrably harmful either to the dependent individual, to society, or to both, and the understanding and control of dependence ("drug abuse") is of worldwide concern. Therefore, the purpose of this section is to briefly consider the dependence-producing liability of the psychotomimetic LSD; much of what follows also holds true for psychotomimetics that are pharmacologically related to LSD (e.g. mescaline, psilocybin) although not necessarily for other psychoactive agents.

B. Discovery of and Effects of LSD

The story of the discovery of LSD (D-lysergic acid diethylamide) in 1939 is well-known. This indole alkaloid (Fig. 1) was initially synthesized by Albert Hofmann from the brown protrusions (ergot) formed on rye and certain other grains by the fungus *Claviceps purpurea*. The discovery was not "accidental" as is sometimes alleged, but occurred as part of a systematic investigation of the analeptic and other properties of partially synthetic amides of lysergic acid (HOFMANN, 1975). However, Hofmann's ingestion of the compound on the afternoon of 6 April 1943 was in fact unplanned.

1 Presently at the Department of Psychology, Western Michigan University, Kalamazoo, MI 49008.

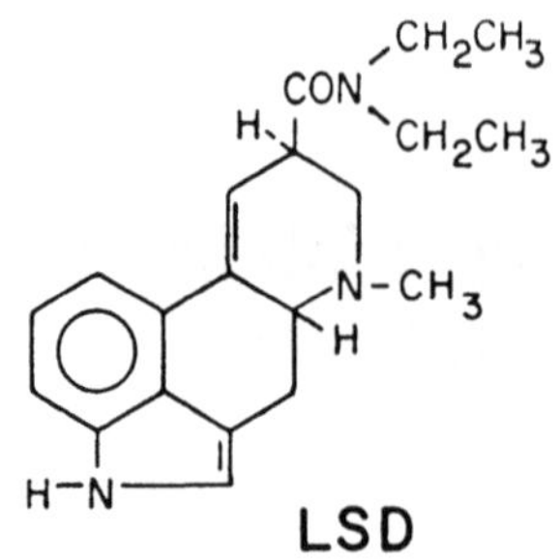

Fig. 1. Lysergic acid diethylamide (D-LSD)

The subjective effects experienced on that occasion led him to take intentionally 0.25 mg LSD, about five times the normal effective dose (in humans); his description of the resultant drug state reads in part as follows (HOFMANN, 1975, p. 114):

"As far as I remember, the following were the most outstanding symptoms: vertigo; visual disturbances; the faces of those around me appeared as grotesque, colored masks; marked motoric unrest, alternating with paralysis; an intermittent heavy feeling in the head, limbs and the entire body, as if they were filled with lead; dry constricted sensation in the throat; feeling of choking; clear recognition of my condition, in which state I sometimes observed, in the manner of an independent observer, that I shouted half insanely... Occasionally I felt as if I were out of my body.

...Six hours after ingestion of the LSD my condition had already improved considerably. Only the visual disturbances were still pronounced... At about one o'clock (nine hours after taking the drug) I fell asleep and awoke next morning feeling perfectly well."

Following this first planned exposure to LSD, subsequent experiments on humans in the Sandoz laboratories confirmed the hallucinatory potency of LSD. A series of nonhuman studies designed to explore the other effects and mechanisms of action of the drug was also begun. Such research has continued to the present day and considerable information concerning the physiologic, pharmacologic, and behavioral effects of LSD has been garnered (e.g., APPEL et al., to be published; CASHMAN, 1966; HOFFER and OSMOND, 1967; SANKAR, 1975). While it is beyond the scope of the present paper to even begin to review these effects – one such attempt covers 960 pages (SANKAR, 1975) – it is worth noting that LSD is a relatively nontoxic drug (i.e., the lethal dose/effective dose ratio is quite low) that probably exerts both central and peripheral effects by altering the functioning of serotonin-containing neurons in a manner not yet fully understood. The compound does not produce obvious tissue damage when given either chronically or acutely, although LSD-induced chromosomal alterations have been reported by some but no means all investigators (see SANKAR, 1975, p. 471ff.).

In humans and nonhumans alike, tolerance develops rapidly with repeated exposure to LSD, but LSD does not cause physical dependence (JAFFEE, 1965; MCISAAC et al., 1970). The drug induces some degree of psychological dependence at least in humans (see below); certain groups of individuals have self-administrated LSD since it was first synthesized in spite (or because) of the fact that governments regularly have attempted to control this behavior via legislation. For example, it was estimated in 1970 that 7,500,000 Americans had tried LSD on at least one occasion (NATIONAL RESEARCH COUNCIL ON MARIJUANA AND DRUG ABUSE, 1970); in the United States LSD is a Schedule 1 drug, the unlicensed possession or sale of which is accompanied by severe penalties.

C. Problems in Assessing Dependence-Producing Liability

It is not easy to quantify the dependence-producing liability (abuse potential) of LSD or, indeed, of other drugs. Part of the difficulty concerns the lack of a satisfactory operational definition of "drug dependence". As noted previously, dependence involves a "compulsion to take a drug on a continuous basis," but what frequency and time course of intake define a compulsion? Thus, investigators often present data gathered from human drug users as number of administrations during some arbitrary period (e.g., 10% of the subjects took LSD more than 10 but less than 20 times during the past year), or as less-than-nominal self-evaluations (e.g., 50% of the subjects took LSD "very frequently" during the past year), and leave the issue of dependence to the reader. In this manner some consensually validated criterion of dependence (e.g., at least one incident of self-administration per week over 1 year) can be selected and applied to the reported data and a relative index of dependence-producing liability can be obtained from actuarial statistics (by calculating the number of individuals who have taken the drug on at least one occasion and dividing this by the number of individuals who are dependent upon the drug). The higher the resultant ratio, the greater the dependence-producing liability of the substance in question.

While this approach to measuring relative dependence-producing liability is fine in theory, it is difficult to use successfully in practice, first of all because such use rests upon the dubious assumption that a single index can categorize meaningfully compounds that differ widely in potency, behavioral effects, and characteristic patterns of self-administration. Further, acquiring reliable data from (or about) human drug users poses a major problem. In most countries the possession of LSD and other abused substances is illegal, and subjects may be unwilling to report illegal experiences; on the other hand, individuals who perceive themselves as members of drug-using subcultures may exaggerate the extent of their involvement with certain compounds that are, at least momentarily, "in." Moreover, the true identity of illicit drugs may not be known by their users (or sellers); "street" LSD can be any of a number of substances. Finally, there is a problem in choosing an appropriate sample of subjects. As will be discussed subsequently, drug dependence reflects social as well as pharmacologic factors. Therefore, it is misleading to speak of the potential of a drug for producing psychological dependence without specifying the group of individuals under consideration; statements about the dependence-producing liability of LSD and other drugs derived from data involving both one-time and repeated users are, at best, of limited value.

For all of these and, no doubt, many other reasons, researchers have attempted to devise animal models for assessing dependence-producing liability (e.g., SCHUSTER and THOMPSON, 1969). These models have been used to evaluate a given drug's ability to produce both physical or psychological dependence, although primary emphasis has been directed toward the former. Tests for physical-dependence liability involve exposing rodents or other animals to a chronic drug regimen, terminating the regimen, then determining whether physiologic or behavioral signs of withdrawal appear. In such tests there is no evidence that LSD produces physical dependence.

Nonhuman procedures for evaluating dependence-producing liability usually involve as a first step a demonstration that the compound acts as a positive reinforcer under at least one set of conditions. If so the drug, by definition, produces psychological dependence, although further manipulations may be needed to evaluate the drug's efficacy in so doing. In general, those classes of drugs that are abused by humans serve as positive reinforcers for rats and monkeys; a partial listing of such compounds includes ethanol, Δ^9THC, nicotine, phencyclidine, cocaine, barbiturates, opiates, and amphetamines (POLING and APPEL, 1979; THOMPSON and PICKENS, 1970). Notably lacking from the list is LSD, which to the best of our knowledge has never been demonstrated to serve as positive reinforcer for nunhumans and in actuality has been shown to function as a negative reinforcer (HOFFMEISTER, 1975; HOFFMEISTER and WUTTKE, 1973). This suggests that the pharmacologic properties of the compound are aversive to animals other than man, although it is possible that the drug might be established as a positive reinforcer for nunhuman species under certain, presently unknown, circumstances. In any case, animal models do not predict any dependence-producing liability of LSD. The finding that nonhumans do not self-administer the drug suggests that uniquely human, social factors may be of primary importance in determining its consumption by humans.

D. Social Factors and the Dependence-Producing Liability of LSD

By social factors, we mean the contingencies that a group arranges for its members; i. e., the consequences that are made to follow actions such as drug-taking. The social environment determines in part the history of an individual, as well as the events that occur immediately before, during, and after a drug experience; it has been convincingly demonstrated within and outside the laboratory that both past experience and current circumstances exert powerful control over drug-taking behavior (e. g., HARRIS et al., 1970; WEEKS, 1975; THOMPSON and PICKENS, 1970; POLING and APPEL, 1979). For example, a drug may be self-administered in order to avoid an aversive consequence, e. g., electric shock in the laboratory and social ostracism in society, or to gain access to a reward, e. g., food or social interaction. Although drug taking in this sense is an operant response maintained by nondrug stimuli, repeated pairings of a drug state with positive consequences may serve to establish the drug as a positive (conditioned) reinforcer such that drug-taking behavior is maintained by the drug alone. Further, in practice it matters little and is seldom possible to tell whether drug intake is controlled by the direct pharmacologic effects produced by a substance, by social variables, or, as is usually the case, by some combination of pharmacologic and social factors.

In any event, LSD self-administration traditionally has been associated with a social movement. In the eastern part of the United States, such a movement was initiated (or reawakened from relative quiescence) by Timothy Leary and associates during the late 1950s (LEARY, 1968). The incidence of LSD use spread among hippies during the following decade, and seemed to reach a peak on the West Coast in the late 1960s. Although reliable figures are difficult to obtain (see above), the relative frequency of LSD use in America reportedly has decreased since that time (SANKAR, 1975, p. 277ff.), perhaps due to the fragmentation or reorientation of the social groups that once supported its use and the increased popularity of other substances, such as marijuana and, more recently, phencyclidine (PCP).

E. Summary and Conclusions

Even during the height of LSD's popularity, it is generally accepted that, with some notable exceptions, few individuals ingested LSD on a regular basis (WILLIS, 1970); the predominant pattern of LSD intake seemingly involves a relatively small number of exposures (often, one) over a brief span of time, followed by complete or nearly complete abstinence. This suggests that the dependence-producing liability of LSD is lower than that of other commonly abused substances (e.g., ethanol, opiates, barbiturates, amphetamines) which, unlike LSD, regularly maintain a great deal of drug-seeking and drug-taking behavior even in animals. This conclusion is strengthened by the absence of programs and procedures specifically designed to treat LSD dependence; interest has centered on dealing with the effects of acute, not chronic, exposure to LSD.

However, it must be emphasized that some persons, particularly those involved with groups that condone and support illicit drug use, have taken LSD on a regular basis for several years (e.g., LEARY, 1968; WILLIS, 1974), and it is not possible to quantify the dependence-producing liability of LSD among such persons. Further, even if the dependence-producing liability of the substance is low, as it seems to be, this is in no sense tantamount to saying that LSD is a safe compound. LSD is extremely potent and its effects are striking and potentially dangerous. For example, WILLIS (1974) notes that adverse reactions to the drug are common and may involve an acute psychotic reaction characterized by thought disturbance, delusion, and perceptual disturbances; a chronic condition characterized by high anxiety and depression; or chronic and severe feelings of unreality and depersonalization. Each of these conditions can be decidedly unpleasant, and may also be associated with the emission of behaviors that are dangerous to the affected individual and to those around him. Thus, LSD may be "behaviorally toxic." This is true not only when the compound produces adverse effects, but also when the usual hallucinogenic effects occur: an individual who is hallucinating may be rendered incapable of safely perfoming a variety of acts, such as driving a car, yet may attempt to do so – with potentially tragic results.

Nonetheless, it has been argued that exposure to LSD under certain conditions, which may or may not prevent the occurence of harmful overt acts, can be beneficial: the drug, for instance, has been claimed to be useful for inducing "religious" experiences, and as an adjunct to psychotherapy (SANKAR, 1975, p. 651ff). Despite the mass of data collected, debate continues among laymen and professionals alike over the legitimacy of such claims; we expect that such debates will not soon end.

Acknowledgment. Preparation of this chapter was supported by USPHS Research Grants MH-24, 593, from the National Institute of Mental Health, and 9 ROI DA-01799 from the National Institute on Drug Abuse.

References

Appel, J.B., Poling, A.D., Kuhn, D.M.: Psychotomimetics: Behavioral pharmacology. In: Handbook of experimental pharmacology. Hoffmeister, F. (ed.), Vol. II, Berlin-Heidelberg-New-York: Springer, to be published

Cashman, J.: The LSD story. Greenwich: Fawcett 1966

Harris, R.T., McIsaac, W.M., Schuster, C.R.: Drug-dependence. Austin: Capital 1970

Hoffmeister, F.: Negatively reinforcing properties of some psychotropic drugs in drug-naive rhesus monkeys. J. Pharmacol. Exp. Ther. *192*, 468–477 (1975)
Hoffmeister, F., Wuttke, W.: Negatively reinforcing properties of morphine antagonists in naive rhesus monkeys. Psychopharmacology *33*, 247–258 (1973)
Hoffer, A., Osmond, H.: The hallucinogens. New York: Academic Press 1967
Hofmann, A.: Chemistry of LSD. In: LSD – A total study. Sankar, D.V. (ed.), pp. 107–140. Westbury, New York: PJD 1975
Jaffee, J.H.: Drug addiction and drug abuse. In: The pharmacological basis of therapeutics. Goodman, L.S., Gilman, A. (eds.), pp. 276–313. New York: Macmillan 1965
Leary, T.: High priest. New York: World Publishing 1968
McIsaac, W.M., Harris, R.T., Ho, B.T.: The indole hallucinogens. In: Drug dependence. Harris, R.T., McIsaac, W.M., Schuster, C.R. (eds.), pp. 41–54. Austin, Capital 1970
National Research Council on Marijuana and Drug Abuse Report (U.S.A.). Washington: Government Printing Office 1970
Poling, A., Appel, J.B.: Procedures for reducing drug intake: Non-human studies. In: Advances in behavioral pharmacology. Thompson, T., Dews, P.B. (eds.), Vol. II, pp. 209–227. New York: Academic Press 1979
Sankar, D.V.: LSD – A total study. Westbury, New York: PJD Publications 1975
Schuster, C.E., Johanson, C.E.: The use of animal models for the study of drug abuse. In: Research advances in alcohol and drug problems. Gibbin, R.J., Israel, Y., Popham, R.E., Schmidt, W., Smart, R.G. (eds.), Vol. II, pp. 1–31. New York: Wiley 1974
Schuster, C.E., Thompson, T.: Self-administration of and behavioral dependence on drugs. Annu. Rev. Pharmacol. Toxicol. *9*, 483–501 (1969)
Thompson, T., Pickins, R.: Behavioral variables influencing drug self-administration. In: Drug dependence. Harris, R.T., McIsaac, W.M., Schuster,C.E. (eds.), pp. 143–157. Austin: Capital 1970
Weeks, J.R.: Environmental influences affecting the boluntary intake of drugs: An overview. Fed. Proc. *34*, 1755–1758 (1975)
Willis, R.H.: Drug dependence. London: Faber & Faber 1970
World Health Organization Technical Report Series, Number 577. Evaluation of dependence liability and dependence potential of drugs. New York: World Health Organization 1975

Cannabis

CHAPTER 7

Chemistry of Cannabis

R. MECHOULAM

A. Introduction

The aim of this chapter is to present a short summary of cannabinoid [1] chemistry with emphasis on those aspects which have pharmacological relevance. A comprehensive chemical review is beyond the scope of this handbook. Since 1964, when the active principle of cannabis, Δ^1-tetrahydrocannabinol (Δ^1-THC), was identified (GAONI and MECHOULAM, 1964a), nearly 5,000 scientific articles on cannabis, Δ^1-THC and other cannabinoids have appeared; approximately 1,000 of these articles are chemically oriented. For this reason alone the present review will have to be selective.

The only natural source of cannabinoids is the dioecious plant *Cannabis sativa*. Both male and female plants produce cannabinoids, in approximately equal concentrations. Botanists recognize numerous "chemotypes" of *C. sativa*, which differ mainly in the ratio of the cannabinoids present in them. Usually chemotypes growing in Mexico, Lebanon, India, Indochina and Africa contain considerable amounts of Δ^1-THC, which in the pure resin (hashish, chagas) may vary between 3% and 10%. The total dried tops (in the Americas called "marihuana") contains ca. 0.5%–1% Δ^1-THC. The chemotypes grown in colder climates generally have low amounts of Δ^1-THC. The differences seem to depend on genetic, climatic and ecological factors. Some chemotypes lack certain constituents. For example, South African *C. sativa*, the source of dagga, does not contain cannabidiol (CBD), which is the major neutral cannabinoid in Lebanese hashish (for a recent review on the pharmacognosy of cannabis, see FAIRBAIRN, 1976).

Two numbering systems for the cannabinoids are in use today. In one of them the formal chemical rules for numbering of pyran type of compounds are used. This system is used by *Chemical Abstracts*. The second nomenclature has a biogenetic basis; the cannabinoids are regarded as substituted monoterpenoids. The latter system is used in the present review.

The vast literature on cannabis and cannabinoids has been the object of several books, reviews and annotated bibliographies. The chemistry, pharmacology, metabolism and clinical effects have been reviewed in two books (MECHOULAM, 1973; NAHAS, 1972). In the first of these considerable emphasis is placed on the chemical aspects, including structure–activity relationships; it has since been updated (chemistry: MECHOULAM et al., 1967; pharmacology: PATON, 1975). The chemistry of cannabis has also been reviewed by RAZDAN, 1973. The analytical problems in this field are discuss-

---

1 The term "cannabinoids" was introduced (MECHOULAM and GAONI, 1967a) to embrace the group of C_{21} compounds characteristically present in *Cannabis sativa*, their carboxylic acids, analogues, homologues and transformation products

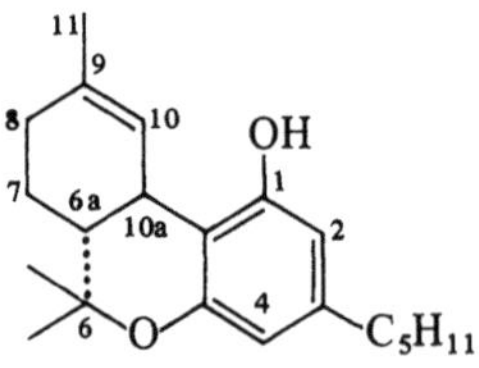

≡

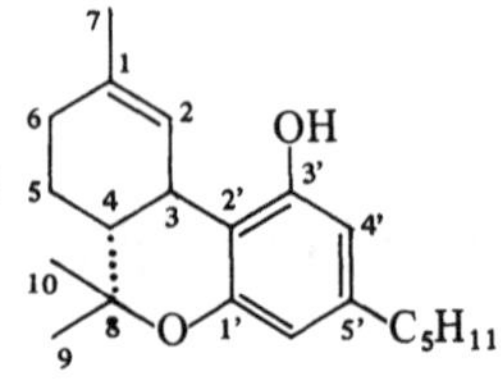

Δ^9–THC Δ^1–THC

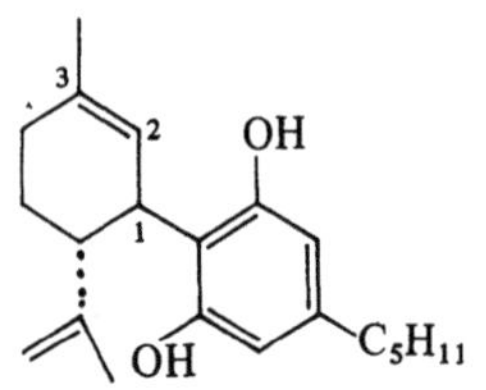

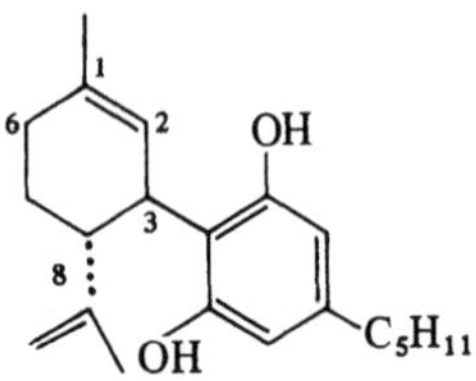

Formal numbering

Monoterpenoid numbering (used in this review)

ed in a book published by the U.S. National Institute for Drug Abuse (WILLETTE, 1976). A chapter in the book of LEMBERGER and RUBIN, 1976 and several in those of BRAUDE and SZARA, 1976 and NAHAS, 1976 are devoted to cannabinoid metabolism. The medicinal chemistry aspects of cannabinoids, both natural and synthetic, have been reviewed (COHEN and STILLMAN, 1976; ARCHER, 1974; MECHOULAM and CARLINI, 1978; BHARGAVA, 1978). An annotated bibliography covering the years 1964 to 1974 has been published (WALLER et al., 1976). Work on this valuable bibliographic tool is continuing and further volumes are expected.

B. Naturally Occurring Cannabinoids

I. Isolation and Structure

The early attempts to isolate the natural cannabinoids was by fractional distillation or crystallization. Both methods failed as cannabinoids generally boil within the same temperature range (ca. 155 °C 0.05 mm) and are mostly oily materials which are difficult to crystallize. The advent of chromatography bypassed cannabinoid chemistry by nearly 30 years and it was only in the 1960s that serious attempts to separate the constituents of marihuana and hashish were recorded. Up till 1964 only two (or possibly three) components had been isolated in pure form. The structure of only one compound, cannabinol (CBN) had been established. The pure constituents isolated did not include compounds with psychotropic activity. An impure mixture apparently containing a high percentage of what was later recognized to be Δ^1-THC was isolated in 1942 (WOLLNER et al., 1942). Work reported by several groups since 1964 has led to the isolation of numerous new cannabinoids which today number 56. The structure of these was determined mainly by the use of physical methods such as mass spectrometry and nuclear magnetic resonance. Figure 1 presents the structures of the predominant natural cannabinoids with references to the original reports of their isolation or structure elucidation.

Most natural cannabinoids belong to several basic structural types: THC (including CBN), cannabigerol, CBD, cannabichromene, cannabicyclol and cannabielsoin.

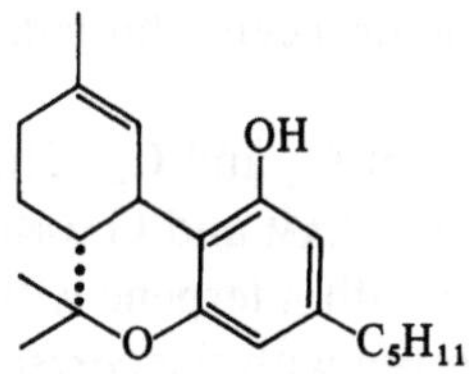

Δ^1–Tetrahydrocannabinol
(Δ^1–THC, also named Δ^9–THC)
(GAONI and MECHOULAM, 1964a)

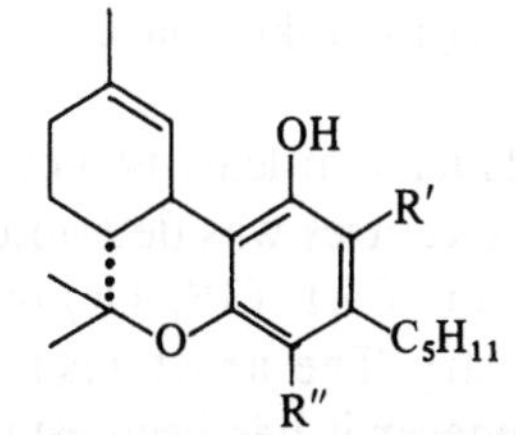

Δ^1–THC acid A
R′ = COOH, R″ = H
(KORTE et al., 1965)
Δ^1–THC acid B
R′ = H, R″ = COOH
(MECHOULAM et al., 1969)

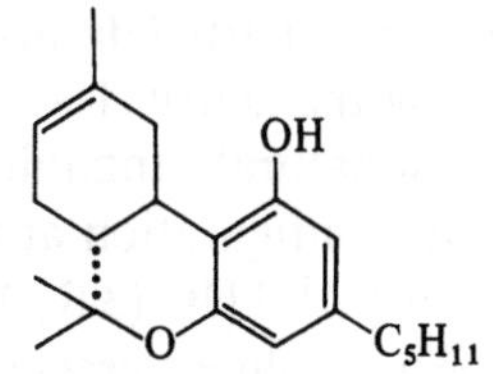

Δ^6–THC
(also named Δ^8–THC)
(HIVELY et al., 1966)

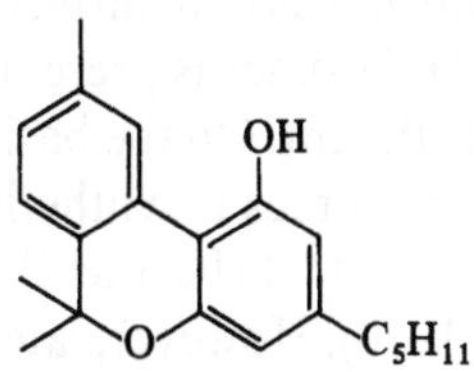

Cannabinol (CBN)
(ADAMS et al., 1940)

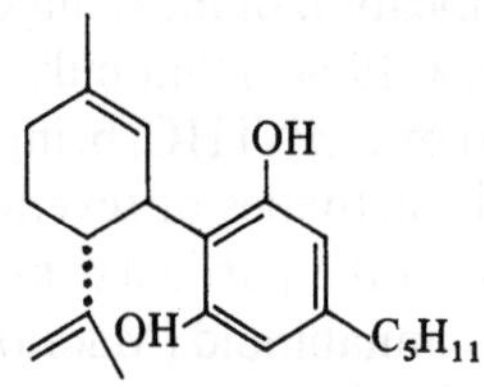

Cannabidiol (CBD)
(MECHOULAM and SHVO, 1963)

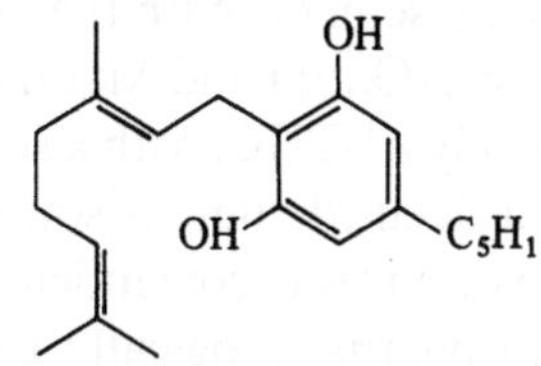

Cannabigerol
(GAONI and MECHOULAM, 1964b)

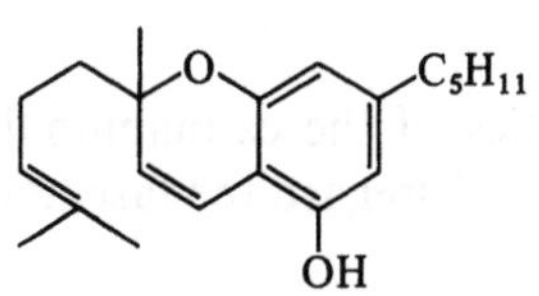

Cannabichromene
(CLAUSSEN et al., 1966;
GAONI and MECHOULAM, 1966)

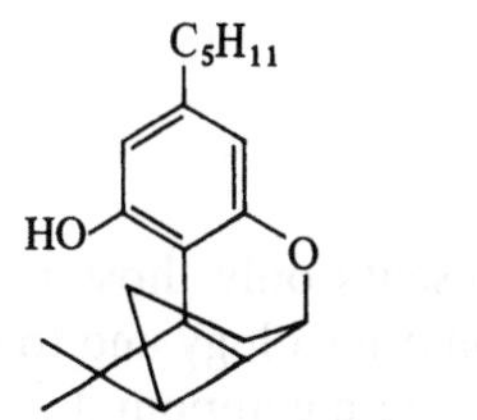

Cannabicyclol
(CROMBIE et al., 1968)

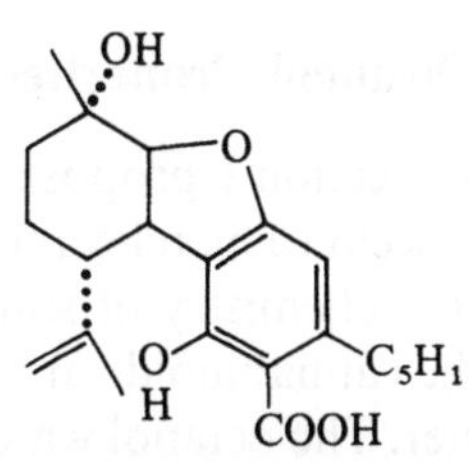

Cannabielsoic acid A
(SHANI and MECHOULAM, 1974)

Fig. 1. Representative natural cannabinoids

Additional, usually very minor constituents belonging to related structural types have been shown to be present. They include cannabicitran (BERCHT et al., 1974), cannabitriol (CHAN et al., 1976), cannabichromanons (GROTTE and SPITELLER, 1978) and a dimeric cannabinoid (SPULAK et al., 1968). The variations on the basic types are standard: a carboxyl group on the phenolic ring (e.g. Δ^1-THC acid A, Δ^1-THC acid B); a methyl, propyl or butyl side chain replacing the pentyl one or dehydrogenation of the terpene moiety to an aromatic ring (e.g. CBN).

The cannabinoids in the growing plant are present mostly, or exclusively, as the pharmacologically inactive acids (i.e. Δ^1-THC acids A and B rather than Δ^1-THC). However, during the preparation of the illegal materials – hashish, chagas or even marihuana – partial decarboxylation takes place leading to the neutral cannabinoids, including the active Δ^1-THC.

Most natural cannabinoids have at least two chiral centres – at C_3 and C_4. The absolute configuration at these centres was determined by MECHOULAM and GAONI, 1967b for Δ^1-THC (3R, 4R) and CBD (3S, 4R) by correlation with a terpene with a known absolute stereochemistry. The structures in Fig. 1 are given with the correct absolute stereochemistry, whenever it has been established.

In addition to cannabinoids, numerous terpenes, phenolic compounds, alkaloids, flavonoids and other natural products have been isolated from *C. sativa* (MECHOULAM, 1973; TURNER et al., 1976; EL-FERALY et al., 1977; SEGELMAN et al., 1978). These non-cannabinoids do not seem to contribute to the typical cannabis-type activity. However, this point needs further substantiation.

Early work on cannabis claimed that the activity was due to a mixture of (unidentified) isomers. With the identification of most major constituents it was conclusively shown (GAONI and MECHOULAM, 1964a) that only one major THC isomer is present, namely Δ^1-THC, with a second one, Δ^6-THC, being a minor constituent. On the basis of a detailed comparison of the activities of several cannabinoids versus a synthetic mixture it was concluded that, in the particular monkey test used, Δ^1-THC was the only pharmacologically active cannabinoid (MECHOULAM et al., 1970). However, later reports have brought evidence that in rodent tests Δ^1-THC cannot always account for all the activity (KARNIOL and CARLINI, 1972). Whatever should be the chemical basis for these observations (synergism or additional active constituents) and its possible relevance to cannabis activity in humans, further research is urgently needed to clarify this important point.

II. Chemical Properties

In this section I propose to discuss only those characteristics of the cannabinoids which seem to be relevant to pharmacology and to reluctantly disregard the fascinating pure chemistry of some of these compounds.

The cannabinoids are lipid soluble compounds which are practically non-soluble in water. The octanol water partition coefficient of Δ^1-THC was reported to be of the order of 6,000 (GILL and JONES, 1972). For administration to animals, therefore, it is always necessary to use a non-aqueous solvent or to add a dispersing agent. The most commonly used vehicles have been olive oil (given intraperitoneally), polyethylene glycol or Tween 80-saline given by any route. Dimethyl formamide, dimethylsulphoxide, gum arabic, serum albumin and polyvinylpyrrolidone have also been employed. The suspensions prepared by dissolving the cannabinoid in a dispersing agent and diluted with water are not stable and should be used shortly after preparation. However, solutions of cannabinoids in ethanol kept at 0 °C in the dark are stable for months or years.

Neither CBD, which has two phenolic groups, nor Δ^1-THC, which has one such group, are soluble in dilute base. The pKa' value of Δ^1-THC has been shown to be 10.6 (GARRETT and HUNT, 1974). This paper also gives detailed information on solubility, partitioning and stability of Δ^1-THC.

Δ^1-THC is very susceptible to oxidation. On exposure to air it slowly converts into CBN. This is due to the lability of the C_3 hydrogen, which is both allylic and benzylic.

Δ^6-THC is considerably more stable and needs very strong oxidation conditions for dehydrogenation to CBN. As Δ^6-THC is active in essentially all animal models used for Δ^1-THC testing it is convenient to employ the Δ^6 isomer for preliminary work.

CBD is easily oxidized, in the presence of base, to coloured quinonic compounds (MECHOULAM et al., 1968). In the crystal form or in ethanolic solution it is, however, quite stable. The same applies for cannabigerol. Little is known about the susceptibility to oxidation of the other cannabinoids. However, in view of the presence of phenolic groups some oxidation on the aromatic rings is to be expected. Allylic oxidation is also possible. Some of the cannabinoids (especially those present in illegal preparations) may in fact be artefacts formed on oxidation. Thus cannabichromene (which has no optical activity, a feature associated with enzymatic synthesis) may be formed by oxidation of cannabigerol followed by cyclization.

Most cannabinoids are stable to heat in the absence of air. Thus the neutral cannabinoids can be distilled at up to 200 °C (at a reduced pressure) or analysed by gas chromatography at 250 °C. However, the cannabinoid acids undergo decarboxylation at ca. 120 °–150 °C. Therefore on smoking (but not on oral consumption), the amount of available neutral cannabinoids including THC is potentially higher than in the crude material. One has, however, to take into account that on smoking, only ca. 20%–25% of the neutral cannabinoids (including those formed on decarboxylation) enter the body; the rest is burned or lost. SPRONG and SALEMINK, 1978 have investigated the reactions taking place on pyrolysis (a smoking model). Most of these involve cleavage of the molecule followed by further modifications leading to non-active molecules. In several cases modifications of the cannabinoid molecule take place. The cleavage and transformation products seem to be inactive, but at present limited pharmacological work on these products has been reported. The quantitative aspects of these transformations are not clear; the impression is that while Δ^1-THC is relatively stable, giving some CBN on smoking, CBD is cleaved or cyclized (possibly partly to Δ^1-THC) or oxidized (to cannabielsoin-type products) with relative ease.

In the presence of acids many cannabinoids undergo transformations (MECHOULAM, 1973). Δ^1-THC with strong acids is easily isomerized into Δ^6-THC. CBD is converted by boron trifluoride into Δ^1-THC, accompanied by Δ^8-iso-THC; with p-toluene sulphonic acid it gives Δ^6-THC in essentially quantitative yield (Fig. 2). Cannabigerol and cannabichromene undergo complicated cyclizations. However, Δ^6-THC and cannabicyclol are relatively stable. In the presence of water or alcohols and mineral acids, additions to the double bonds may occur (MECHOULAM 1973; GARRETT and TSAU, 1974). Are the cannabinoids stable in the acid milieu of the stomach? There is indirect evidence, based on the activity of orally administered Δ^1-THC, that to a large extent no major changes occur. However, one can expect some isomerization to Δ^6-THC, or possibly additions to the double bond. The oral activity of CBD (in antiepileptic studies) and lack of psychotropic effects indicate that it is not transformed to Δ^1 or Δ^6-THC in the stomach. However, direct experimental evidence is needed.

The cannabinoids are photolabile compounds. CBD can cyclize to Δ^1-THC or isocannabinoids (SHANI and MECHOULAM, 1971). This reaction may have biogenetic significance. It has recently been reported that when a growing cannabis plant is exposed the sunlight it contains more Δ^1-THC and less cannabichromene than a non-irradiated plant (VALLE et al., 1978; this observation contradicts previous results, FAIRBAIRN and LIEBMAN, 1974). CBD can also undergo reduction of the Δ^8 double bond

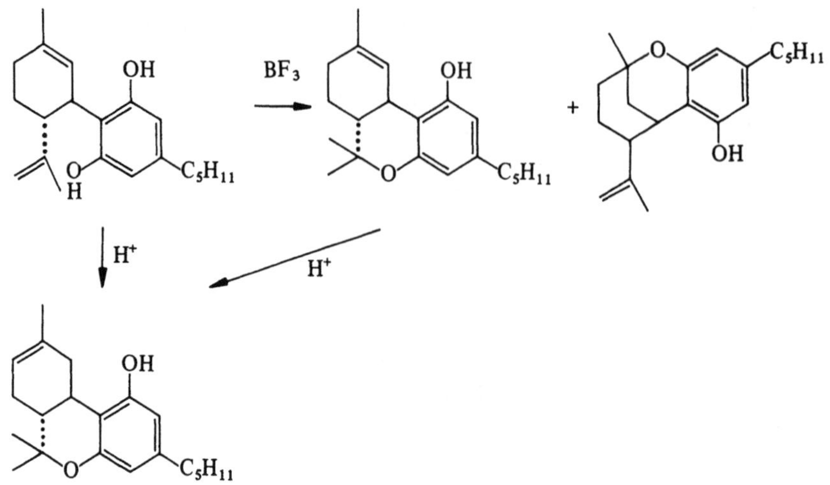

Fig. 2. Some transformations of cannabinoids in acids

or addition of solvent to the aromatic ring. In the presence of oxygen, reactions leading to cannabielsoic-type compounds are observed (SHANI and MECHOULAM, 1974). No detailed work on Δ^1-THC has been reported, but one can expect addition reactions as well as dimerizations through the aromatic ring.

The psychoactive cannabinoids may be classified as partial anaesthetics producing the same perturbation of the membrane structure as that caused by sub-anaesthetic doses of general anaesthetics (LAWRENCE and GILL, 1975). This was determined by estimation of the degree of disorder of the hydrocarbon chain in phospholipid liposomes. Introduction of various cannabinoids altered the order parameters within the hydrophobic core of the liposome, and the change in this factor correlated qualitatively with psychotropic potency.

Cannabinoids bind to serum proteins (WAHLQVIST et al., 1970). Albumin appears to bind Δ^1-THC much less avidly than α-lipoprotein, which in turn shows a slightly reduced avidity compared to β-lipoprotein (MCCALLUM and EASTWOOD, 1978). Δ^1-THC binds to glass or membranes (GARRETT and HUNT, 1974) and the possibility that there is competition by these surfaces for Δ^1-THC during in vitro experiments cannot be ignored.

III. Syntheses

It is beyond the scope of this review to describe all the synthetic routes used to prepare the various natural cannabinoids. These have been reviewed in considerable detail (MECHOULAM, 1973; MECHOULAM et al., 1976). It should be pointed out that facile syntheses for most cannabinoids are available. Δ^1-THC can be prepared in high yield and with high stereospecificty by several methods. The ones generally employed are presented in Fig. 3. They are based on condensation of a suitable monoterpene with olivetol (5-penthylresorcinol) to yield Δ^6-THC which can easily be converted into Δ^1-THC. RAZDAN et al., 1974 have found that the Petrzilka synthesis can be improved to yield directly Δ^1-THC if magnesium sulphate is added to the reaction mixture.

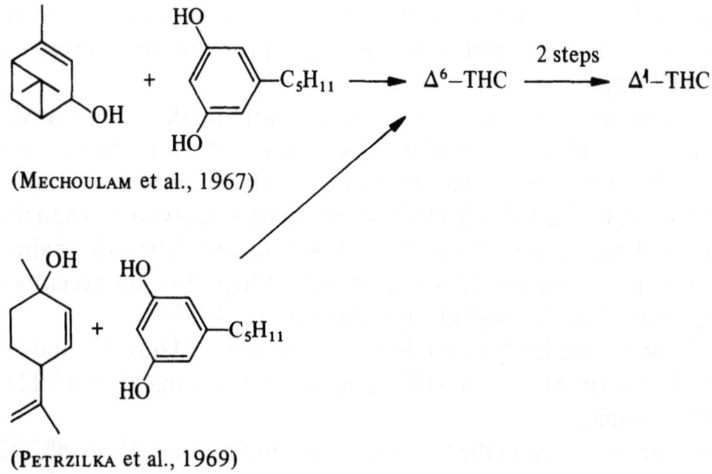

Fig. 3. Some syntheses of Δ^1-THC

(+)-Δ^1-THC can be obtained from the synthesis based on verbenol (MECHOULAM et al., 1972) as the latter compound is obtainable in both (+) and (−) forms. The (+) (unnatural) cannabinoids are of importance as control compounds in pharmacological and biochemical work in order to ascertain that effects observed with natural (−) cannabinoids are specific and are not due to the general liposolubility of this group of compounds.

The above syntheses have been employed for the preparation of labelled material. BURSTEIN, 1973 has presented a list of methods used for this purpose. More recent developments are a detailed report on the syntheses of numerous labelled cannabinoids (PITT et al., 1975), the syntheses of labelled cannabinoid acids (SHOYAMA et al., 1978) and the publication of the method of HOELLINGER et al., 1977 leading to Δ^1-THC with a specific activity of 50 Ci/mmol.

C. Structure-Activity Relationships (SARs)

These relationships, mainly as regards the typical cannabis activity, have been surveyed previously (MECHOULAM, 1973; MECHOULAM et al., 1976). These data, together with newly published results, can be summarized as follows:

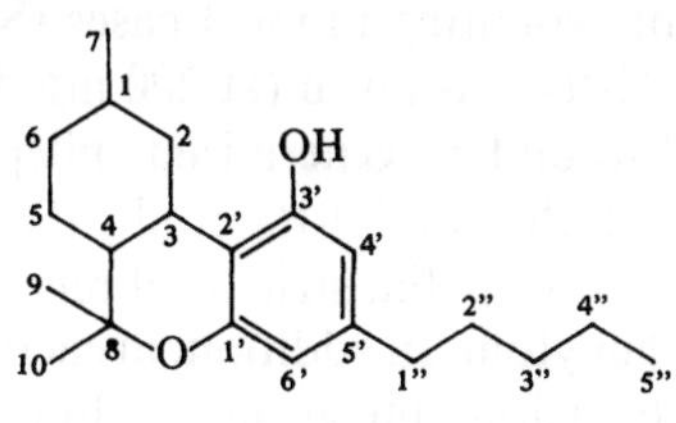

1) A tricyclic (preferably benzopyran)-type structure with a hydroxyl group at the 3′ aromatic position and an alkyl group on the 5′ aromatic position seems to be a requirement. Opening of the pyran ring leads to loss of activity.

2) The phenolic group has to be free. Blocking of this group as an ether causes complete inactivation while esterfication does not, probably because esters can be hydrolysed in the body.

3) Electronegative groups (such as carboxyl, carbomethoxyl or acetyl) on the aromatic ring eliminate activity. Alkyl groups on the C-4′ aromatic position cause no change in activity, while such a substitution on C-6′ eliminates activity.

4) The minimal C-5′ alkyl side chain seems to be a pentyl one (though little work has been reported on the propyl and butyl homologues). The side chains leading to highest activity apparently are 1,1 or 1,2-dimethyl heptyl or the recently discovered 1-methyl-4-(*p*-flurophenyl)-butyl groups (PARS et al., 1977).

5) Not all the theoretically possible THCs are active. Thus Δ^1- and Δ^6-THC are active in the 3 R, 4 R series only; Δ^5-THC and Δ^7-THC are inactive; Δ^3-THC is active; Δ^1-3,4-*cis*-THC is inactive.

6) Monohydroxylation on the C-7 methyl group, in either Δ^1- or Δ^6-THC, the C-6 position on Δ^1-THC, or on the C-2″, C-3″, C-4″ or C-5″ position of the side chain leads to active compounds; C-1″-hydroxy-Δ^6-THC is, however, inactive. Hydroxylation of the C-9 methyl group in Δ^1-THC also gives an active compound.

7) In the hexahydrocannabinol series the methyl group (or hydroxymethyl group) on C-1 has to be equatorial, i.e. essentially in the same plane as the phenolic hydroxyl. The axial methyl isomer is much less active.

8) The terpenoid and pyran rings may be modified considerably. These modifications do not seem to follow a regular pattern, and even tentative rules cannot yet be put forward.

Detailed SAR studies of synthetic N-containing cannabinoids as regards various pharmaceutically important parameters have been published (PARS et al., 1977; RAZDAN et al., 1976b).

Several cannabinoids have shown considerable clinical promise (for recent reviews see MECHOULAM and CARLINI, 1978; BHARGAVA, 1978). Δ^1-THC in humans exhibits anti-asthma, analgetic, antiglaucoma, antihypertensive and anti-emetic properties. The analgetic, antiglaucoma and antihypertensive effects cannot be exploited due to the CNS side-effects. However, they can serve as synthetic leads. The anti-asthma effect is observed at doses considerably lower than those at which CNS effects are present (HARTLEY et al., 1978). Further clinical work is certainly warranted. The most promising results are in the use of Δ^1-THC as an anti-emetic drug during cancer chemotherapy or irradiation therapy. Repeated vomiting is a serious side-effect of such therapy and it is not always improved by existing anti-emetic drugs during cancer chemotherapy or irradiation therapy. Oral administration of Δ^1-THC, ca. 2 h before the anticancer treatment prevents vomiting in most cases (SALLAN et al., 1975).

In a double-blind study CBD was given (at 200 mg daily doses for 3 months) to epileptics with uncontrolled secondary generalized epilepsy with temporal foci. Very significant improvement was noticed (CUNHA et al., 1980). Further research is indicated. It is of interest that a close spatial structural relationship exists between CBD and the anti-epileptic drug phenytoin. In addition, in each of these compounds the distance between their two electron donating groups is almost the same. It seems possible that the two compounds act on the same, or a similar, receptor (TAMIR et al., 1980).

The synthetic cannabinoid, nabilone, developed by the American firm Ely Lilly, is being clinically tested mainly as an anti-emetic in cancer chemotherapy and as an anti-anxiety agent (HERMAN et al., 1977; NAKANO et al., 1978). Nabilone is apparently not as good a tranquillizer as diazepam; however, it seems to be a good anti-emetic agent.

Clinical trials with the nitrogen-containing cannabinoid shown below have demonstrated its effectiveness as an analgetic (ca. ten times more active than codeine); however, the side-effects observed make it a poor candidate for further work in man (STAQUET et al., 1978).

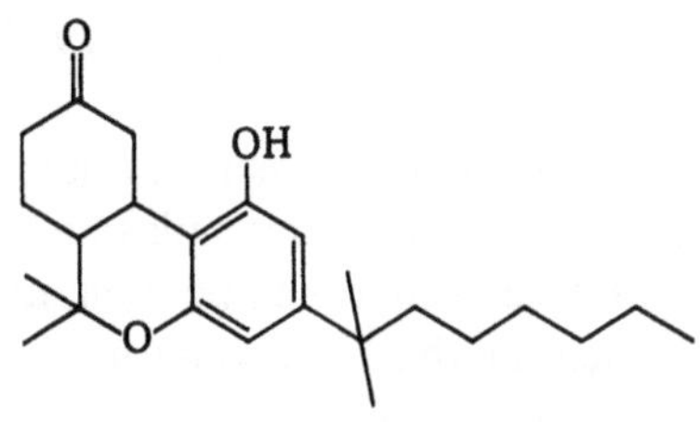

Nabilone

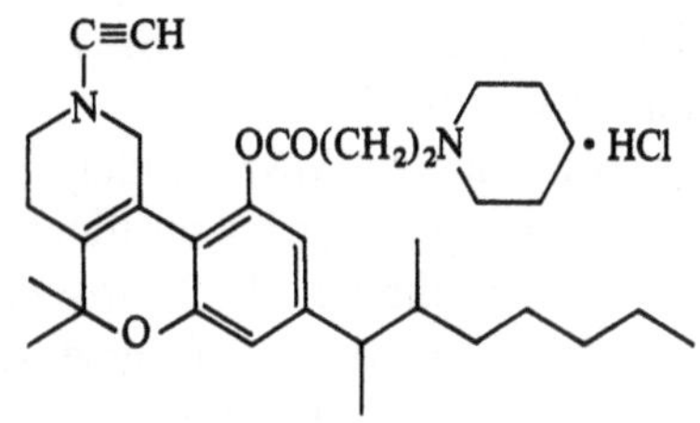

D. Cannabinoid Analysis

The identification of crude cannabis is routine in forensic laboratories. It is usually done by a combination of colour tests (Duquenois, Beam etc.) and chromatographic ones [thin layer chromatography (TLC), gas chromatography (GC) etc.]. These have been reviewed in detail elsewhere (MECHOULAM, 1973; MECHOULAM et al., 1976; CROMBIE, 1976). A problem which has not yet found a fully satisfactory solution is the analysis of cannabinoids in body fluids, in particular urine. The main reasons for this difficulty are the low amounts usually consumed by man and the extensive rapid metabolism (VINSON, 1979).

The most widely used method for detecting cannabinoids on TLC is by spraying with a feshly prepared solution of di-*o*-anisidine tetrazolium chloride (fast blue salt B), which offers both excellent sensitivity of detection (to approximately 50 ng) and different colour reactions for different components.

By the fluorescent method of FORREST et al., 1971, in which the cannabinoids are converted to 1-dimethyl-aminoaphthalene sulphonates, cannabinoids may be detected on TLC down to levels of 0.5 ng. VINSON et al., 1977 have developed on alternative facile fluorescent method.

Gas chromatography is the method of choice for rapid qualitative and quantitative identifications. A large variety of stationary phases have been found to provide excellent separations of the cannabinoids on packed columns, and the use of capillary columns has been found to improve separations considerably (NOVOTNY and LEE, 1973; GROTTE and SPITELLER, 1978). Flame ionization detection, normally used with GLC, gives a maximum sensitivity of approximately 50 ng. The formation of trimethylsilyl derivatives increases the maximum sensitivity of detection to about 10 ng.

The use of electron capture detection for suitably derivatized cannabinoids has improved detection sensitivity. SCHOU et al., 1971 report that the use of chloroacetyl derivatives gives maximum sensitivity of approximately 0.04 ng and have applied this method ot urinalysis. GARRETT and HUNT, 1973 demonstrate a maximum sensitivity of detection of approximately 5 pg for Δ^1-THC pentafluorobenzoate, whereas 1 pg Δ^1-THC heptafluorobutyrate can be detected when a capillary column and low volume coaxial electron capture detector are used (FENIMORE et al., 1973).

To overcome the necessity of purification, McCALLUM et al., 1978 have developed a method involving GLC with flame ionization detection of cannabinoid phosphate esters. This method has a sensitivity of 0.5 ng/ml of whole blood. The detection is so specific that preliminary clean-up procedures are unnecessary.

High pressure liquid chromatographic (HPLC) methods for the separation of cannabinoids have been developed (SMITH and VAUGHAN, 1976; KNAUS et al., 1976; GARRETT and HUNT, 1977).

Mass spectrometry (MS) is widely employed in cannabis analysis. AGURELL et al., 1973 report that a preliminary purification of the extract from human plasma by chromatography on Sephadex LH-20 provides adequate clean-up for subsequent quantification of the Δ^1-THC by mass fragmentometry. Their method has been found suitable for measuring Δ^1-THC down to levels of 0.3 ng/ml when fragmentograms of the 299 and 314 mass fragments (at 50 eV) are used. Improvements of this method have been reported by ROSENFELD, 1977. A facile GLC–MS method has been described by ROSENTHAL et al., 1978.

A number of laboratories have developed immunoassay methods. TEALE et al., 1975, GROSS and SOARES, 1978 and others (see WILLETTE, 1976) have reported practical procedures. Recently a combined HPLC–radio-immunoassay was described (WILLIAMS et al., 1978) which is capable of quantifying 0.1 ng of a cannabinoid in 1 ml plasma. CAIS et al., 1975 have developed a free radical immunoassay (comparable to the one available for morphine).

E. Cannabinoid Metabolites*

Early in 1970 several groups almost simultaneously identified the major primary route of cannabinoid metabolism – hydroxylation at the allylic C_7 position (BURSTEIN et al., 1970; BEN-ZVI et al., 1970; NILSSON et al., 1970; WALL et al., 1970; FOLTZ et al., 1970). Intensive ongoing work by several groups, mainly in Sweden, United States, Israel and the United Kingdom, has shown that Δ^1-THC, Δ^6-THC, CBD and CBN are hydroxylated (or oxygenated) by many animal species, including man, at most allylic positions as well as on the side chain. The relevant positions are indicated by arrows in Fig. 4.

A further minor primary route (which apparently takes place only very early after administration of the drug) is dehydrogenation of Δ^1-THC and Δ^6-THC to CBN (McCALLUM et al., 1977). It is usually accompanied by further hydroxylation. Metabolic reduction of the Δ^1 double bond has been recorded (HARVEY et al., 1977a). Epoxidation of this double bond has also been observed.

The monohydroxylated products can undergo further hydroxylations as well as oxidations to the corresponding 7-oic acids. The side chain can also be cleaved and oxidized giving mono- or polycarboxylic acids. Recent publications identifying numerous new metabolites (generally along the above-described pathway) are those by

* Due to the large number of publications on metabolism and metabolites in this area, most of the pre-1976 work is not given in any detail or referenced. The reader should consult the reviews cited in the introduction for full coverage

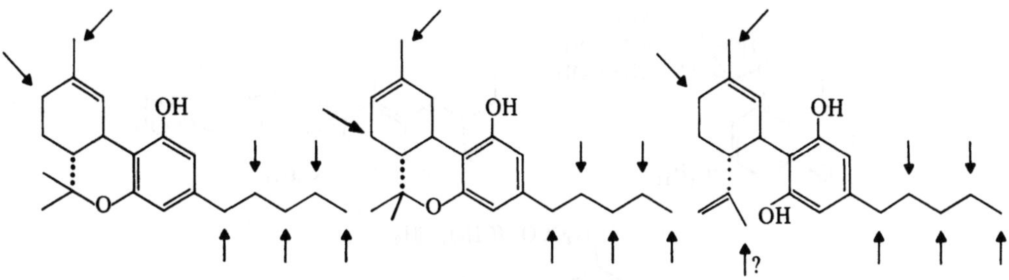

Fig. 4. Positions of phase I oxidations in cannabinoid metabolism

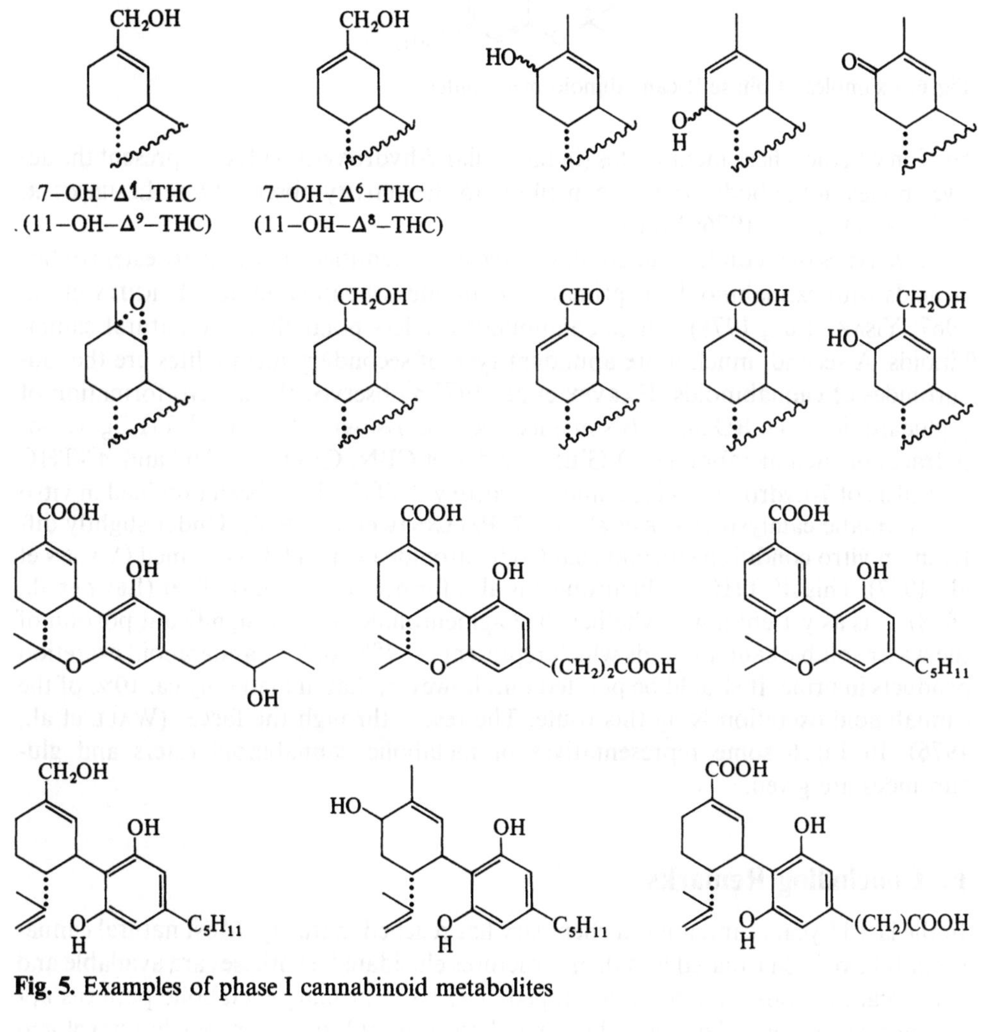

Fig. 5. Examples of phase I cannabinoid metabolites

HARVEY et al., 1977b; MARTIN et al., 1976, and MARTIN et al., 1977. Some cannabinoid metabolites, excluding conjugates, are given in Fig. 5. It should be pointed out that considerable metabolic species specificity exists, although the general pathways apparently are similar.

As already mentioned in Sect. C, most monohydroxylated (or mono-oxygenated) THC metabolites are pharmacologically active. It is still a question of heated dis-

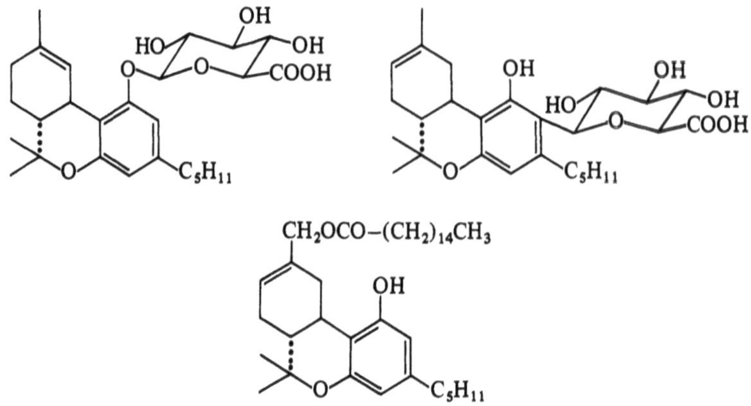

Fig. 6. Examples of phase II cannabinoid metabolites

cussion whether these metabolites (in particular 7-hydroxy-Δ^1-THC) represent the active species in the body or even contribute to the activity observed (see LEMBERGER, 1976; WALL et al., 1976; MARTIN et al., 1978).

Two types of secondary metabolites have been identified. The first are esters of fatty acids with cannabinoids or primary metabolites of cannabinoids (LEIGHTY et al., 1967; YISAK et al., 1978). These compounds are less polar than the natural cannabinoids. A second, much more abundant type of secondary metabolites are the glucuronides of cannabinoids. HARVEY et al., 1977b observed the in vivo formation of 0-glucuronides of CBD and CBN in mice liver. Suprisingly, Δ^6- and Δ^1-THC gave only traces of such metabolites. O-Glucuronides of CBN, CBD, Δ^1-THC and Δ^6-THC as well as of 7-hydroxy-Δ^1-THC and 5′-hydroxy Δ^1-THC have been obtained in vitro by enzymatic catalysis (LYLE et al., 1977; PALLANTE et al., 1978). Under slightly different in vitro conditions the unusual C-glucuronide of Δ^6-THC is formed (YAGEN et al., 1977). This Δ^6-THC C-glucuronide is also formed in vivo in rat liver (LEVY et al., 1978). It is as yet unknown whether the C-glucuronides form a significant portion of the water soluble cannabinoids which represent ca. 75% of the cannabinoid excretion products in urine. It should be pointed out, however, that in man only ca. 10% of the cannabinoid excretion is by this route. The rest is through the faeces (WALL et al., 1976). In Fig. 6 some representatives of metabolic cannabinoid esters and glucuronides are given.

F. Concluding Remarks

In the last 15 years cannabinoid chemistry has reached maturity. Most natural cannabinoids have been isolated and their structures elucidated, syntheses are available and analytical methods have been developed. The basic primary metabolic patterns apparently are known. The secondary metabolism is still, however, partly unexplored territory.

I believe that now the trend is towards development of new drugs based on the cannabinoid nucleus. It has been shown that separation between the various activities is possible. We may look forward to new analgetic, anti-emetic, antiglaucoma, anti-asthma and anti-epileptic compounds which cause little or no THC-type effects.

References

Adams, R., Baker, B.R., Wearn, R.B.: Synthesis of cannabinol, 1-hydroxy-3 n-amyl-6,6,9-trimethyl-6-dibenzopyran. J. Am. Chem. Soc. *62*, 2204–2207 (1940)

Agurell, S., Gustafsson, B., Holmstedt, B., Leander, K., Lindgren, J.-E., Nilsson, I., Sandberg, F., Asberg, M.: Quantitation of Δ^1-THC in plasma from cannabis smokers. J. Pharm. Pharmacol. *25*, 554–558 (1973)

Archer, R.A.: The cannabinoids: Therapeutic potential. Ann. Rep. Med. Chem. *9*, 253–259 (1974)

Ben-Zvi, Z., Mechoulam, R., Burstein, S.: Identification through synthesis of an active Δ^6-THC metabolite. J. Am. Chem. Soc. *92*, 3468 (1970)

Bercht, C.A.L., Lousberg, R.J.J.C., Küppers, F.J.E.M., Salemink, C.A.: Cannabicitran: A new naturally occurring tetracyclic diether from Lebanese Cannabis sativa. Phytochemistry *13*, 619–621 (1974)

Bhargava, N.H.: Potential therapeutic applications of naturally occurring and synthetic cannabinoids. Gen. Pharmacol. *9*, 195–213 (1978)

Braude, M.C., Szara, S. (eds.): The pharmacology of marihuana. New York: Raven 1976

Burstein, S.H.: Labeling and metabolism of the THC's. In: Marijuana. Chemistry, pharmacology, metabolism and clinical effects. Mechoulam, R. (ed.), pp. 167–190. New York, London: Academic Press 1973

Burstein, S.H., Menezes, F., Williamson, E., Mechoulam, R.: Metabolism of Δ^6-THC, an active marihuana constituent. Nature *225*, 87–88 (1970)

Cais, M., Dani, S., Josephy, Y., Modiano, A., Gershon, H., Mechoulam, R.: Studies of cannabinoid metabolites – a free radical immunoassay. FEBS Lett. *55*, 257–260 (1975)

Chan, W.R., Magnus, K.E., Watson, H.A.: The structure of cannabitriol. Experientia *32*, 283 (1976)

Claussen, U., Spulak, F. v., Korte, F.: Cannabichromene, ein neuer Haschisch Inhaltstoff. Tetrahedron *22*, 1477–1479 (1966)

Cohen, S., Stillman, R.C. (eds.): The therapeutic potential of marihuana. New York: Plenum 1976

Crombie, L., Ponsford, R., Shani, A., Yagnitinsky, B., Mechoulam, R.: Photochemical production of cannabicyclol from cannabichromene. Tetrahedron Letters *55*, 5771–5772 (1968)

Crombie, W.M.L.: The analysis of cannabis. In: Cannabis and health. Graham, J.D.P. (ed.) pp. 21–41. London: Academic Press 1976

Cunha, I.M., Carlini, E.A., Pereira, A.E., Ramos, O.L., Gagliardi, R., Sanvito, W.L., Lander, N., Mechoulam, R.: Chronic administration of cannabidiol to healthy volunteers and epileptic patients. Pharmacology *21*, 175–185 (1980)

El-Feraly, F.S., Elsohly, M.A., Boeren, E.G., Turner, C.E., Ottersen, T., Aasen, A.: Crystal and molecular structure of cannabispiran and its correlation to dehydrocannabispiran. Tetrahedron *33*, 2373–2387 (1977)

Fairbairn, J.W.: The pharmacognosy of Cannabis. In: Cannabis and Health. Graham, J.D.P. (ed.), pp. 3–19. London: Academic 1976

Fairbairn, J.W., Liebman, J.A.: The cannabinoid content of Cannabis sativa L. grown in England. J. Pharm. Pharmacol. *26*, 413–419 (1974)

Fenimore, D.C., Freeman, R.R., Loy, P.R.: Determination of Δ^9-THC in blood by electron capture gas chromatography. Anal. Chem. *45*, 2331–2335 (1973)

Foltz, R., Fentiman, A.F., Leighty, E.G., Walter, J.L., Drewes, H.R., Schwartz, W.E., Page, T.F.Jr., Truitt, E.F.Jr.: Metabolite of Δ^8-THC: Identification and synthesis. Science *168*, 844–855 (1970)

Forrest, I.S., Green, D.E., Rose, S.D., Skinner, G.C., Torres, D.M.: Fluorescentlabeled cannabinoids. Res. Commun. Chem. Pathol. Pharmacol. *2*, 787–792 (1971)

Gaoni, R., Mechoulam, R.: Isolation, structure and partial synthesis of an active constituent of hashish. J. Am. Chem. Soc. *86*, 1646–1647 (1964a)

Gaoni, Y., Mechoulam, R.: The structure and synthesis of cannabigerol. Proc. Chem. Soc. *82*, (1964b)

Gaoni, Y., Mechoulam, R.: Cannabichromene, a new active principle in hashish. Chem. Commun. *20* (1966)

Garrett, E.R., Hunt, C.A.: Picogram analysis of THC and application to biological fluids. J. Pharm. Sci. *62*, 1211–1214 (1973)
Garrett, E.R., Hunt, C.A.: Physiochemical properties, solubility and protein binding of Δ^9-THC. J. Pharm. Sci. *63*, 1056–1064 (1974)
Garrett, E.R., Hunt, C.A.: Separation and analysis of Δ^9-THC in biological fluids using HPLC and GLC. J. Pharm. Sci. *66*, 20–26 (1977)
Garrett, E.R., Tsau, J.J.: Stability of THC's. J. Pharm. Sci. *63*, 1563–1574 (1974)
Gill, E.W., Jones, G.: Brain levels of Δ^1-THC and its metabolites in mice. Biochem. Pharmacol. *21*, 2237–2248 (1972)
Gross, S.J., Soares, J.R.: Validated direct blood Δ^9-THC radioimmune quantitation. J. Anal. Toxicol. *2*, 98–100 (1978)
Grotte, H., Spiteller, G.: Neue Cannabinoide. J. Chromatogr. *154*, 13–23 (1978)
Hartley, J.P.R., Nogrady, S.G., Seaton, A., Graham, J.D.P.: Bronchodilator effect of Δ^1-THC. Br. J. Clin. Pharmacol. *5*, 523–525 (1978)
Harvey, D.J., Martin, B.R., Paton, W.D.M.: Identification of metabolites of Δ^1 and Δ^6-THC containing a reduced double bond. J. Pharm. Pharmacol. *29*, 495–497 (1977a)
Harvey, D.J., Martin, B.R., Paton, W.D.M.: Identification of di and tri-substituted hydroxy and ketone metabolites of Δ^1-THC in mouse liver. J. Pharm. Pharmacol. *29*, 482–486 (1977b)
Herman, T.S., Jones, S.E., Dean, J., Leigh, S., Dorr, R., Moon, T.E., Salmon, S.E.: Nabilone, a potent antiemetic cannabinol with minimal euphoria. Biomedicine *27*, 331–334 (1977)
Hivley, R.L., Mosher, W.A., Hoffmann, F.W.: Isolation of Δ^6-THC from marijuana. J. Am. Chem. Soc. *88*, 1832–1833 (1966)
Hoellinger, H., Nam, N.H., Decauchereux, J.F., Pichat, L.: Synthese de Δ^8 et Δ^9-THC deuteries et tritiés. J. Label. Compounds Radiopharm. *13*, 401–415 (1977)
Karniol, I.G., Carlini, E.A.: The content of Δ^9-THC does not explain all biological activity of some Brazilian marihuana samples. J. Pharm. Pharmacol. *24*, 833–835 (1972)
Knaus, E.E., Coutts, R.T., Kozakoff, C.W.: The separation, identification and quantitation of cannabinoids and their derivatives using HPLC. J. Chromatogr. Sci. *14*, 525–530 (1976)
Korte, F., Haag, M., Claussen, U.: Tetrahydrocannabinol carboxylic acid, a component of hashish. Angew. Chem. [Engl.]. *4*, 872 (1965)
Lawrence, D.K., Gill, E.W.: The effects of Δ^1-THC and other cannabinoids on spin labeled liposomes and their relationship to mechanisms of general anesthesia. Mol. Pharmacol. *11*, 595–602 (1975)
Leighty, E.G., Fentiman, A.F.Jr., Foltz, R.L.: Long-retained metabolites of Δ^9 and Δ^8-THC identified as novel fatty acid conjugates. Res. Commun. Chem. Pathol. Pharmacol. *14*, 13–28 (1976)
Lemberger, L.: The pharmacokinetic of Δ^9-THC and its metabolites. In: Marihuana. Chemistry, biochemistry and cellular effects. Nahas, G.G. (ed.), pp. 169–178. Berlin, Heidelberg, New York: Springer 1976
Lemberger, L., Rubin, A.: Physiologic disposition of drugs of abuse. New York: Spectrum 1976
Levy, S., Yagen, B., Mechoulam, R.: Identification of a C-glucuronide of Δ^6-THC in a mouse liver. Science *200*, 1391–1392 (1978)
Lyle, M.A., Pallante, S., Head, K., Fenselau, C.: Synthesis and characterization of glucuronides of cannabinol, cannabidiol, Δ^9-THC and Δ^8-THC. Biomed. Mass. Spectrom *4*, 190–196 (1977)
Martin, B., Agurell, S., Nordqvist, M., Lindgren, J.-E.: Dioxygenated metabolites of cannabidiol formed by rat liver. J. Pharm. Pharmacol. *28*, 603–608 (1976)
Martin, B.R., Harvey, D.J., Paton, W.D.M.: Biotransformation of cannabidiol in mice. Identification of new acid metabolites. Drug. Metab. Dispos. *5*, 259–267 (1977)
Martin, B.R., Carney, J.M., Balster, R.L., Harris, L.S.: Behavioral activity, distribution and metabolism of ^3H-Δ^9-THC in monkey brain following an intraventricular injection. Fed. Proc. *37*, 164 (1978)
McCallum, N.K., Eastwood, M.E.: In vivo binding of Δ^1-THC and CBN to rat serum proteins. J. Pharm. Pharmacol. *30*, 384–386 (1978)
McCallum, N.K., Gugelmann, A., Brenninkmeijer, C.A.M., Mechoulam, R.: Isotope effect studies in the dehydrogenation of Δ^1-THC in the rat. Experientia *33*, 1012–1014 (1977)

McCallum, N.K., Cairns, E.R., Ferry, D.G., Wong, R.J.: A simple GLC method for routine Δ^1-THC analyses of blood and brain. J. Anal. Toxicol. *2*, 89–92 (1978)
Mechoulam, R. (ed.): Marijuana. Chemistry, pharmacology, metabolism and clinical effects. New York, London: Academic 1973
Mechoulam, R., Carlini, E.A.: Toward drugs derived from Cannabis. Naturwissenschaften *65*, 174–179 (1978)
Mechoulam, R., Gaoni, Y.: Recent advances in the chemistry of hashish. In: Fortschritte Chemisch Organischer Naturstoffe. Zechmeister, L. (ed.), Vol. 25, pp. 175–213. Wien: Springer 1967a
Mechoulam, R., Gaoni, Y.: The absolute configuration of Δ^1-THC. Tetrahedron Letters *12*, 1109–1111 (1967b)
Mechoulam, R., Shvo, Y.: The structure of cannabidiol. Tetrahedron *19*, 2073–2078 (1963)
Mechoulam, R., Ben-Zvi, Z., Gaoni, Y.: On the nature of the Beam test. Tetrahedron *24*, 5615–5624 (1968)
Mechoulam, R., Ben-Zvi, Z., Yagnitinsky, B., Shani, A.: A new THC acid, Tetrahedron Letters *28*, 2339–2341 (1969)
Mechoulam, R., Braun, P., Gaoni, Y.: A stereospecific synthesis of Δ^1-THC and $\Delta^{1(6)}$-THC. J. Am. Chem. Soc. *89*, 4552–4554 (1967)
Mechoulam, R., Braun, P., Gaoni, Y.: Syntheses of Δ^1-THC and related cannabinoids. J. Am. Chem. Soc. *94*, 6159–6165 (1972)
Mechoulam, R., McCallum, N.K., Burstein, S.: Recent advances in the chemistry and biochemistry of Cannabis. Chem. Rev. *76*, 75–112 (1976)
Mechoulam, R., Shani, A., Edery, H., Grunfeld, Y.: Chemical basis of hashish activity. Science *169*, 611–612 (1970)
Nahas, G.G.: Marihuana – deceptive weed. New York: Raven 1972
Nahas, G.G. (ed.): Marihuana. Chemistry, biochemistry and cellular effects. Berlin, Heidelberg, New York: Springer 1976
Nakano, S., Gillespie, H.K., Hollister, L.E.: A model for evaluation of antianxiety drugs with the use of experimentally induced stress: comparison of nabilone with diazepam. Clin. Pharmacol. Ther. *23*, 54–62 (1978)
Nilsson, I.M., Agurell, S., Nilsson, J.L.G., Ohlsson, A., Sandberg, F., Wahlqvist, M.: Δ^1-THC: Structure of a major metabolite. Science *168*, 1228–1229 (1970)
Novotny, M., Lee, M.L.: Detection of marijuana smoke in the atmosphere of a room. Experientia *29*, 1038–1039 (1973)
Pallante, S., Lyle, M.A., Fenselau, C.: Synthesis and characterization of glucuronides of 5′-OH-Δ^9-THC and 11-OH-Δ^9-THC. Drug Met. Dispos. *6*, 389–395 (1978)
Pars, H.G., Razdan, R.K., Howes, J.F.: Potential therapeutic agents derived from the cannabinoid nucleus. Adv. Drug Res. *11*, 97–189 (1977)
Paton, W.D.M.: Pharmacology of marijuana. Annu. Rev. Pharmacol. *15*, 191–220 (1975)
Petrzilka, T., Haefliger, W., Sikemeier, C.: Synthese von Haschisch – Inhaltsstoffen. Helv. Chim. Acta *52*, 1102–1134 (1969)
Pitt, C.G., Hobbs, D.T., Schran, H., Twine, C.E.Jr., Williams, D.L.: The synthesis of deuterium, carbon-14 and carrier-free tritium labeled cannabinoids. J. Label. Compounds Radiopharm. *11*, 551–575 (1975)
Razdan, R.K.: Recent advances in the chemistry of cannabinoids. Prog. Org. Chem. *8*, 78–101 (1973)
Razdan, R.K., Dalzell, H.C., Handrick, G.R.: A simple one-step synthesis of Δ^1-THC from p-mentha-2,8-diene-1-ol and olivetol. J. Am. Chem. Soc. *96*, 5860–5865 (1974)
Razdan, R.K., Howes, J.F., Uliss, D.B., Dalzell, H.C., Handrick, G.R., Dewey, W.L.: 8β-Hydroxymethyl-Δ^1-THC, a novel physiologically active analog of Δ^1-THC. Experientia *32*, 416–417 (1976a)
Razdan, R.K., Terris, B.Z., Pars, H.G., Plotnikoff, N.P., Dodge, P.W., Dren, A.T., Kyncl, J., Somani, P.: Drugs derived from cannabinoids. 2. Basic esters of N- and carbocyclic analogs. J. Med. Chem. *19*, 454–461 (1976b)
Rosenfeld, J.: The simultaneous determination of Δ^9-THC and 11-hydroxy-Δ^9-THC in plasma. Anal. Lett. *10*, 917–930 (1977)

Rosenthal, D., Harvey, T.M., Bursey, J.T., Brine, D.R., Wall, M.E.: Comparison of GC-MS methods for the determination of Δ^9-THC in plasma. Biomed. Mass. Spectrom *5*, 312–316 (1978)
Sallan, S.E., Zinberg, N.E., Frei, E.: Antiemetic effect of Δ^9-THC in patients receiving cancer chemotherapy. N. Engl. J. Med. *293*, 795–797 (1975)
Schou, J., Steentoft, A., Worm, K., Andersen, J.M., Nielsen, E.: Highly sensitive method for gas chromatography of THC and CBN. Acta Pharmacol. Toxicol. (Kbh). *30*, 480–482 (1971)
Segelman, A.B., Segelman, F.P., Star, A.E., Wagner, H., Seligman, O.: Structure of two C-diglycosyl-flavones from Cannabis sativa. Phytochemistry *17*, 824–826 (1978)
Shani, A., Mechoulam, R.: Photochemical reactions of CBD. Tetrahedron *27*, 601–606 (1971)
Shani, A., Mechoulam, R.: Cannabielsoic acids. Isolation and synthesis by a novel oxidative cyclization. Tetrahedron *30*, 2437–2446 (1974)
Shoyama, Y., Hirano, H., Nishioka, I.: Synthesis of cannabigerorcinic-carboxyl-^{14}C acid, cannabigerovarinic-carboxyl-^{14}C-acid and cannabichromevarinic-carboxyl-^{14}C-acid. J. Label. Comp. Radiopharm. *14*, 835–842 (1978)
Smith, R.M., Vaughan, C.G.: High pressure liquid chromatography of Cannabis. J. Chromatogr. *129*, 347–354 (1976)
Spronck, H.J., Salemink, C.A.: Isolation and synthesis of olivetol derivatives formed in the pyrolysis of CBD. Rec. Trav. Chim. Bays-Bas. *97*, 187–190 (1978)
Spulak, F.v., Claussen, U., Fehlhaber, H.W., Korte, F.: Cannabidiolcarbonsaure-tetra hydrocannabitriol-ester, ein neuer Haschisch-Inhaltsstoff. Tetrahedron *24*, 5379–5383 (1968)
Staquet, M., Gantt, C., Machin, D.: Effect of a nitrogen analog of THC on cancer pain. Clin. Pharmacol. Ther. *23*, 397–401 (1978)
Tamir, I., Mechoulam, R., Meyer, A.Y.: Cannabidiol and phenytoin, a structural comparison. J. Med. Chem. *23*, 220–223 (1980)
Teale, J.D., Forman, E.J., King, L.J., Piall, E.M., Marks, V.J.: The development of a radio immunoassay for cannabinoids in blood and urine. J. Pharm. Pharmacol. *27*, 465–472 (1975)
Turner, C.E., Hsu, M.H., Knopp, J.E., Schiff, P.L., Slatkin, D.J.: Isolation of cannabisativine, an alkaloid from Cannabis sativa L. J. Pharm. Sci. *65*, 1084–1085 (1976)
Valle, J.R., Viera, J.E.V., Aucelio, J.G., Valio, I.F.M.: Influence of photoperiodism on cannabinoid content of Cannabis sativa L. Bull. Narcotics *30/1*, 67–68 (1978)
Vinson, J.A. (ed.): Cannabinoid analysis in physiological fluids. Washington, D.C.: American Chemical Society 1979
Vinson, J.A., Patel, D.D., Patel, A.H.: Detection of THC in blood and serum using a fluorescent derivative and TLC. Anal. Chem. *49*, 163–165 (1977)
Wahlqvist, M., Nilsson, I.M., Sandberg, F., Agurell, S., Granstrand, B.: Binding of Δ^1-THC to human plasma proteins. Biochem. Pharmacol. *19*, 2579–2589 (1970)
Wall, M.E., Brine, D.R., Brine, G.A., Pitt, G.G., Freudenthal, R.I., Christensen, A.D.: Isolation, structure and biological activity of several metabolites of Δ^9-THC. J. Am. Chem. Soc. *92*, 3466–3468 (1970)
Wall, M.E., Brine, D.R., Perez-Reyes, M.: Metabolism of cannabinoids in man. In: The pharmacology of marihuana. Braude, M.C., Szara, S. (eds.), pp. 93–113. New York: Raven 1976
Waller, C.W., Johnson, J.J., Buelke, J., Turner, C.E.: Marihuana: An annotated bibliography. New York: MacMillan 1976
Williams, P.L., Moffat, A.C., King, L.J.: Combined HPLC and radio immunoassay for the quantitation of Δ^9-THC and some of its metabolites in human plasma. J. Chromatogr. *155*, 273–283 (1978)
Willette, R.E. (ed.): Cannabinoid assays in humans. Rockville: National Institute on Drug Abuse 1976
Wollner, H.J., Matchett, J.R., Levine, J., Loewe, S.: Isolation of a physiologically active tetrahydrocannabinol from Cannabis sativa resin. J. Am. Chem. Soc. *64*, 26–29 (1942)
Yagen, B., Levy, S., Mechoulam, Ben-Zvi, Z.: Synthesis and enzymatic formation of a C-glucuronide of Δ^6-THC. J. Am. Chem. Soc. *99*, 6444–6446 (1977)
Yisak, W., Agurell, S., Lindgren, J.-E., Widman, M.: In vivo metabolites of CBN identified as fatty acid conjugates. J. Pharm. Pharmacol. *30*, 462–463 (1978)

CHAPTER 8

Pharmacology and Toxicology of Cannabis

H. COPER

A. Introduction

The chemistry, pharmacology, and toxicology of cannabis were described in details in the Handbook of Experimental Pharmacology, Vol. 54/2 (1977). The purpose of this article is not to repeat that information, but to supplement it and present other points of view, as well as to summarize new aspects, e.g., the interaction of cannabis with other drugs. In addition, attempts to provide explanations for certain phenomena that cannot be definitely interpreted owing to contradictory findings (mostly resulting from the diverse methodologies used) are perhaps not only of heuristic value.

The history, epidemiology, and chemistry of cannabinoids were also treated in the aformentioned handbook and consequently will not be discussed here. Rather, this article will focus on the pharmacokinetic and pharmacodynamic effects of cannabis and cannabinoids, aspects of tolerance, and the interaction of these substances with other drugs.

B. Pharmacokinetic Effects

I. Absorption

It may be considered as proven that cannabinoids are absorbed rapidly and easily and that the onset of the effect of equivalent doses is greater in inhaling than after oral application. Inadequate attention was drawn to the finding that the vehicle in which Δ-9-tetrahydrocannabinol (THC) is administered has a significant influence on the kinetics and also on the effectivity of the drug.

AGURELL et al. (1969), for example, injected ^{3}H-labeled THC into rats in a 10% sesame oil-saline emulsion (1:9) and found an elimination of less than 50% of the radioactivity within 1 week. On the contrary, KLAUSNER and DINGELL (1971) described for the same species a nearly complete elimination of ^{14}C-labeled THC within a period of 6 days. In these investigations, a mixture of propylene glycol and rat serum served as vehicle (30:70).

In rats, the same dose of THC administered in polyethylene glycol evokes a decrease in body temperature of more than 3 °C, whereas after administration of THC dissolved in rape oil no hypothermia occurred. Similar observations were made in respect of cataleptic effects. THC in Cremophor may cause a prolongation of hexobarbital-induced sleep for some hours, an effect which is less pronounced after administration of THC in rape oil, but, nevertheless, persists for 2 days (COPER et al., 1971; FERNANDES and COPER, 1971).

Using the disruption of food-reinforced operant behavior of rats as the test-system for cannabinoid activity, a polyvinylpyrrolidone dispersion had the most rapid onset of action while the polysorbate-65-sorbitan monolaurate combination had the longest duration of action. An olive oil solution had little effect (BORGEN and DAVIS, 1973).

When injected intraperitoneally, THC was most effective in delaying convulsions when given in a propylene glycol/Tween 80 (PPG) mixture, fairly effective in polyvinylpyrrolidone (PVP), and almost ineffective in bovine serum albumin (BSA) or saline / Tween 80 (TW) (SOFIA, et al., 1974).

Higher ^{14}C plasma concentrations were seen 1 h after intravenous injection of THC with PPG than with TW and BSA. BSA produced lower values than did PPG and TW. However, the ^{14}C lung concentration was four times higher with BSA than with PPG and TW. There were no significant differences in ^{14}C brain concentrations 4 h after intravenous administration of THC with TW, BSA, or PPG. However, TW with THC produces significantly higher ^{14}C brain values 1 h after intravenous injection. Concentration of ^{14}C in all tissues was significantly lower after intraperitoneal or oral administration of THC in corn oil than after TW (MANTILLA-PLATA and HARBISON, 1975).

From these findings it may be deduced that there exists a complex equilibrium between the water-insoluble cannabinoids, certain vehicles, plasma proteins, especially α- and β-lipoproteins, as well as tissue constituents (MCCALLUM and EASTWOOD, 1978). Therefore, the affinity of the drugs for these various retaining or uptake sites and their amount play an important role in the intensity and duration of the different effects of the cannabinoids. This factor explains many discrepancies in the literature concerning the effectiveness of THC.

II. Distribution

In principle, the distribution of cannabinoids and their active metabolites takes place like that of every other drug, namely in accordance with physical and chemical properties, especially the lipid solubility, the blood circulation, and the space and medium of diffusion. The situation concerning cannabinoids is particularly complicated, because THC, for example, is obviously transformed relatively quickly into active and inactive metabolites not only hepatically but also extrahepatically. The velocity whith which the metabolism in the various tissues takes place and the simultaneous concentration of the respective substances over a time course cannot yet be taken for granted. It must also be realized that measurement of radioactivity in different tissues or subcellular particles does not reflect the content of the active compounds and gives only limited information about dose-response relationship. Most of the studies of tissue distribution correspond roughly to this deficient pattern. In acute experiments with injection of ^{3}H-as well as ^{14}C-labeled drugs, activity is high in lung, liver, and kidney; moderate in heart, spleen, and some endocrine glands; and relatively low in the brain, particularly in the gray area. The time course of rise and fall of radioactivity in the various organs and tissues closely resembled that of thiopental and other strongly lipophilic substances. Relatively high levels persisted in fat at 48 h, but levels in brain were quite low (WILLINSKY et al., 1974). There is no doubt that THC and the active metabolite are concentrated to a high degree in the synaptosomal fraction of the cells, but it is a nonspecific binding and is carried out mainly by simple diffusion and not by an active process (COLBURN et al., 1974; DEWEY et al., 1976; ROTH and WILLIAMS, 1979).

HARRIS et al. (1978) presented some evidence utilizing hepatoma cells that a high degree of binding is associated with the crude nuclear fraction. In the brain, it was shown that binding depends on protein concentration and that a portion of this binding is temperature dependent. The authors concluded from their experiment that specific binding of the cannabinoids may occur in certain cells or cell fractions and that this binding may have stereospecificity. But they stress that they do not know whether such binding has any relevance to the pharmacologic effect of this class of drugs.

It has largely been accepted that the site of action of THC and other cannabinoids is the lipid phase of the cell membrane. All psychoactive compounds are very lipophilic, oxygenated hydrocarbons and are devoid of any ionic or strongly bipolar substituent groups. At low concentrations the molecular pertubation is related to an increase in the molecular disorder of the liposome. At high concentrations, the effects level off to a more or less constant value. This phenomenon is explained by limited solubility of THC in phospholipid bilayers (LAWRENCE and GILL, 1975; GILL, 1976).

III. Elimination

Many investigations have confirmed that cannabinoids are metabolized rapidly, mainly by hydroxylation into mono- and dihydroxylated compounds. Unmodified THC or 11-OH-THC were not detected in urine and feces. Thus, elimination takes place exclusively by metabolism. The particular steps of transformation are described by MECHOULAM (see Chap. 7). A special aspect in this connection is the interaction of cannabinoids with other drugs in the microsomal drug-metabolizing enzyme system. Δ-9-THC, Δ-8-THC, cannabidiol (CBD), and cannabinol (CBN) produce type I spectral changes in rat liver chromosomes, indicating the formation of the enzyme-substrate complex with cytochrome P_{450}.

Treatment of rats with SKF-525-A prior to administration of tritium-labeled (-)-Δ-9-THC resulted in a decrease of nearly 50% of 11-OH-THC and Δ-9-THC in both the brain and liver as compared with the animals without SKF-525-A pretreatment. The microsomal oxidation inhibitor also caused a reduction of the dihydroxylated metabolite, 8, 11-$(OH)_2$-Δ-9-THC, to 14% of control values. The large reduction of the acid metabolite in the brain (65% of controls) and the liver (16% of controls) by SKF-525-A indicates that the oxidative pathway producing the acid is a microsomal process (ESTEVEZ et al., 1974).

Pentobarbital, phenobarbital, and amphetamine also produce in vitro an apparently noncompetitive inhibition of THC metabolism. The inhibition engendered by meprobamate was at least partly competitive. Morphine and mescaline had no evident effect. With the exception of SKF-525-A none of the drugs tested in vivo influenced the biliary ^{14}C excretion or metabolite pattern or the final tissue levels. (SIEMENS et al., 1975).

Finally, CBD is a strong inhibitor of microsomal drug metabolism and is therefore capable of suppressing THC metabolic degradation (JONES and PERTWEE, 1972; FERNANDES et al., 1973; BORYS and KARLER, 1979). Thus, using a cannabis extract, the elimination and, partly, the effect of THC and obviously of other pharmacologically active cannabinoids such as tetrahydrocannabivarol depends on the amount of CBD. Using pure substances it depends on the affinity with which the competing compounds are bound to the microsomal oxygenase system.

Excluding the influence of different perfusion conditions, there is no doubt that THC is also metabolized extrahepatically, for example, by isolated perfused lungs of rabbit and dog. At least five metabolites were shown to be present in lung tissue and perfusate (WIDMAN et al., 1975; LAW, 1978). THC is also obviously metabolized in brain. COLBURN et al. (1974) reported that most of the radioactivity in brain supernatant fraction (^{3}H THC metabolites) was not extractable in heptane 2.5 h after intracisternal injection of 20 µg ^{3}H-Δ-9-THC in rats. BEN-ZVI et al. (1976) found as well that Δ-9-THC could be 7-hydroxylated in the intact monkey brain following an intraventricular injection of radiolabeled Δ-9-THC. On the other hand, MARTIN et al. (1977) found no evidence for metabolism of Δ-9-THC by perfusion of the isolated rat brain with ^{14}C-Δ-9-THC.

MAGOUR et al. (1976) have shown that after the intraperitoneal injection of 10 mg/kg ^{3}HΔ-9-THC, the relatively specific activity of Δ-9-THC and 11-OH-THC is diminished in each subcellular fraction of the rat brain. Meanwhile, the concentration of highly polar metabolites which cannot be totally transported from liver increases in all subfractions, especially in the cytosol, so that net radioactivity in the whole brain within 12 h is decreased only to a minor extent.

C. Pharmacodynamic Effects

I. In Information-Bearing Macromolecules

Indications that cannabinoids, especially Δ-9-THC, inhibit DNA, RNA, and protein synthesis, have led to the study of their cytostatic, anti-immune, and chromosome-damaging effects in vitro and in vivo (STRENCHEVER et al., 1972; BLEVINS and REGAN, 1976; CARCHMAN et al., 1976; HARRIS et al., 1976; MON et al., 1978). These investigations have been carried out with quite different schedules and in various systems. Thus, no clear statements can be made about the conditions under which cannabinoids interfere with the metabolism of macromolecules.

Damaged or broken chromosomes are not typical in cannabis users, and they also occur after various other external chemical stimuli. Moreover, findings on the mutagenicity of THC were not reproducible (HERHA and OBE, 1974; COHEN, 1976; VAN WENT, 1978). Genetic damage by use of cannabis cannot be excluded with certainty. However, this risk is probably not more significant than that occuring with other unphysiological environmental stimuli. A review of the literature (FLEISCHMAN et al., 1975) which describes the results of 25 experiments conducted in rats, mice, hamsters, rabbits and chimpanzees indicates, with just a few exceptions, a general lack of teratogenesis following subcutaneous, intraperitoneal or oral administration of marihuana extract of pure THC. These results are confirmed recently by SOFIA et al. (1979) in New Zealand rabbits.

There is no doubt that immune suppressive effects are demonstrable in vitro depending on the structure of the compounds, but to evoke these effects in vivo considerable doses are needed (GAUL and MELLORS, 1975; LEFKOWITZ and KLAGER, 1978; SMITH et al., 1978). In such high doses, Δ-9-THC also suppresses the induction of arylhydrocarbon hydroxylase and aminopyrine demethylase by phenobarbital or 3-methylcholanthrene. RNA synthesis is the probable site of action. (FRIEDMAN, 1976), since Δ-9-THC interfered with phenobarbital stimulation of nuclear RNA synthesis, but had no effect on protein synthesis. Similarly, retardation of Lewis lung adenocarcinoma growth and of Friend leukemia virus-induced splengomegaly occurs only with very high doses (MUNSON et al., 1975).

II. In Functional Macromolecules

The mechanism of interaction between two different substances on the microsomal oxygenase system clearly indicates that the net effect does not take a single pathway to an inhibition of THC by the other drug. The cannabinoids, especially CBD, are able to suppress in vitro and partly in vivo the metabolism of typical type I compounds. The hydroxylation of testosterone is inhibited competitively also by Δ-9-THC and Δ-8-THC. The effect is dose dependent over the dose range tested (25–100 μ*M*) (CHAN and TSE, 1978). Testosterone synthesis is also markedly reduced by cannabinoids (DALTERIO et al., 1977; BURSTEIN et al. 1978 and 1979a).

Aminopyrine demethylation is competitively diminished by Δ-9-THC, Δ-8-THC, CBN, and CBD, by the latter in concentrations below 10 μ*M*. The inhibitor constants were found to be 58, 68, 80, and 5 μ*M*, respectively. In a similar way, morphine demethylation was also inhibited. Δ-8-THC, however, did not suppress this reaction, and inhibition of CBD was mixed at all concentrations. These inhibitory potencies of cannabis constituents on drug metabolism in vitro parallel the results obtained in vivo by interaction studies with hexobarbitone (FERNANDES et al., 1973). PATON and PERTWEE (1972) reported that CBD is a stronger inhibitor of phenazone metabolism in mouse liver supernatant than THC.

Thus, it must be concluded that CBD, which is by far more potent in inhibiting drug metabolism than other cannabinoids, contributes significantly to the effects of crude cannabis preparations, at least in rodents.

Induction of some enzymes by THC has also been noted. WITSCHI and SAINT-FRANCOIS (1972) first described a dose-dependent enhancement of benzpyrene hydroxylase activity in lung and liver 24 h after treatment of male rats with high doses of crude cannabis resins. After exposure to smoke produced by burning cigarettes made from cannabis sativa the activity of pulmonary aryl-hydrocarbon hydroxylase is enhanced. But it needs to be considered that the activity of the enzyme is also increased 6–24 h after inhalation of cigarettes from which the cannabinoids have been extracted (MARCOTTE and WITSCHI, 1972). Enhanced biotransformation of theophylline in marihuana and tobacco smokers is described by JUSKO et al. (1978). HO et al. (1973) have shown that chronic administration of THC to rats increases the metabolism of the compound in the liver but not in the lungs. On the other hand, KUPFER et al. (1973) found no effect of the vitro microsomal demethylation of aminopyrine and p-chloro-*N*-methyl-aniline or the oxidative metabolism of Δ-9-THC. Recently, WRENN and FRIEDMAN (1978) have described a dose-related stimulation of tyrosine aminotransferase 12 h after Δ-9-THC.

In contrast to prior results (CHARI-BITRON and BINO, 1971; JAIN et al., 1974), Δ-9-THC produces a dose-dependent (2.5–40 μ*M*) inhibition of $Na^{+}K^{+}$ and Mg^{2+} Ca^{2+} (adenosine triphosphatase, ATPase) in all subcellular particles without Mg^{2+} ATPase in the crude mitochondrial fractions (BLOOM et al., 1978a; HERSHKOWITZ et al., 1977).

Another membrane-bound enzyme inhibited by Δ-9-THC, the acyl coenzyme A from brain synaptosomes, was detected by GREENBERG and co-workers in 1978.

Monoamine oxydase (MAO) activity is slightly suppressed by THC, CBD, and hashish extract, in enzyme preparations from which the phospholipids were extracted, the sensitivity to Δ-9-THC essentially disappeared. Sensitivity could be regained upon addition of phosphatidylcholine (SCHURR et al., 1978; STILLMAN et al., 1978). In apparent contrast to these findings are the results of BANERJEE et al. (1975a) who reported that the intraperitoneal administration of 10 mg/kg and 50 mg/kg Δ-9-THC increased the activity of MAO in blood platelets in whole brain, and in hypothalamus and heart mitochondria. They discussed an increased accessibility and/or permeability of the mitochondrial membrane lipid component.

Low doses of THC (0.1–1.0 mg/kg) caused 50%–160% elevations of cAMP levels in mouse brain, whereas higher THC concentrations depressed cAMP levels (DOLBY and KLEINSMITH, 1974). A similar biphasic effect has been reported in cultured human lung cells (KELLY and BUTCHER, 1979).

Pharmacologic evidence that THC causes an increase of the biosynthesis of prostaglandins was given by KAYMAKCALAN et al. (1975), who found that THC has diuretic and vasodilatory effects on isolated perfused rabbit kidney, which are inhibited by acetylsalicylic acid but not by atropine, phenylbutazone, or mepyramine. On the other hand, JACKSON et al. (1976) found a dose-related antagonism between THC and prostaglandin E_1 in the abdominal constriction response.

BURSTEIN and HUNTER (1978) confirmed enhancement of prostaglandin production in intact cells by THC, whereas in earlier investigations the authors found an inhibition of prostaglandin synthesis in all microsome preparations (BURSTEIN et al., 1973).

In addition to reports on cannabis-induced inhibition of spermatogenesis and steroidogenesis as well as suppression of growth hormone (GH), luteinizing hormone (LH), and follicle-stimulating hormone (FSH) secretion in animals (DIXIT et al., 1974; COLLU et al., 1975; DALTERIO et al., 1977; BURSTEIN et al., 1979a, b); SMITH et al., 1979), KOLODNY et al. (1974, 1976) described low plasma testosterone levels in heavy marihuana smokers. But testing of this observation by MENDELSON et al. (1978) yielded no confirmation. KUBENA et al. (1971), as well as KOKKA and GARCIA (1974), demonstrated that in rats THC in doses of 2–16 mg/kg or 5–20 mg/kg, respectively, increased plasma corticosterone concentrations. CBD was inactive. Recently, JACOBS et al. (1979) have shown that the combination of stress and 5 mg/kg THC results in higher corticosterone values than either stress or THC alone. CBD acts opposite to THC.

All these effects are not related to psychoactive properties of the drugs. It must be kept in mind that independent of apparently specific or nonspecific effects of cannabinoids, all their actions on structural of functional macromolecules, including intervention in the immune system, are attributed to an interaction with the phospholipids of the different cell membranes (LAWRENCE and GILL, 1975; BACH et al., 1976; KALOFOUTIS et al., 1978).

III. In Functional Systems

1. Neurotransmission

The effects of cannabinoids upon biogenic amines are not yet established firmly. The numerous data about the involvement of cannabinoids in transmitter level and turnover rate are to some extent documented by HARRIS et al. (1977). Most of the described changes were slight and occurred only with extremely high doses. Fundamental new judgments are not available. Inhibition of amine uptake, decrease in acetylcholine release, and depression of presynaptic cholinergic transmission seem to be reproducible effects of THC (CAVERO et al., 1972; GRAHAM et al., 1974; BENSEMANA and GASCON, 1974; BANERJEE et al. 1975b; MCCONNELL et al., 1978; ROTH, 1978). REVUELTA et al. (1979) gave some evidence that THC causes reduction of turnover rates of acetylcholine in the cholinergic septalhippocampal pathway by increasing the release of γ-aminobutyric acid (GABA) from septal GABAergic interneurons. In addition to these direct, obvious effects on membranes, THC acts indirectly on amine-mediated functions such as lipolysis (MALOR et al., 1978; WING and PATON, 1978).

The effect of THC in suppressing signs of the quasi-morphine withdrawal syndrome (COLLIER et al., 1974) is presumably not connected to the opiate receptor, dopaminergic mechanisms or sedation (ZALUZNY et al., 1979).

2. Cardiovascular and Respiratory Systems

The most distinct, dose-related effect of hashish extract, Δ-8-THC, or Δ-9-THC upon the cardiovascular system is tachycardia (JOHNSON and DOMINO, 1971; WEISS et al., 1972; CLARK et al., 1974; PRAKASH et al., 1975; COHEN, 1976; KANAKIS et al., 1976). The increased heart rate is accompanied by a shortened preejection period and a prolonged left ventricular ejection time with no change in afterload. The peak heart rate increase after THC is attenuated by atropine and propranolol and nearly abolished by atropine-propranolol pretreatment. Changes in forearm blood flow and vascular resistance are also reduced. Under the chosen conditions, propranolol has no substantial influence on psychomotor performance (MARTZ et al., 1972; SULKOWSKI et al., 1977; BENOWITZ et al., 1979). The data suggest that THC induces sympathetic stimulation and parasympathetic inhibition of cardiovascular control pathways. But using a cross-circulation preparation in dogs, CAVERO et al. (1973) found some evidence that THC also induces cardiovascular alterations by central mechanisms.

The same is valid for the antagonism between THC and phentolamine after intraventricular perfusion of cats (LOKHANDWALA et al., 1977). Moreover, Δ-9-THC (0.2–1 mg/kg) blocks the cardiac conditioned response (tachycardia as well as bradycardia) in monkeys in a dose-related manner. The effects were similar to those of diazepam (MCLENDON et al., 1976), and it has to be taken into consideration that the animals show some sedation.

In man, hypertension with bradycardia occurred when the blood pressure control was challenged by a change in posture or blood volume (PEREZ-REYES et al., 1973). A significant decrease in the systolic pressure and heart rate by THC was also observed in hypertensive rats and dogs (CAVERO et al., 1973; VARMA and GOLDBAUM, 1975).

In urethane-anesthetized rats, Δ-8-THC and Δ-THC produce a dose-related transient increase in blood pressure followed by prolonges hypotensive response and bradycardia (ADAMS et al., 1976). In a single- and double-blind trial, CLARK et al. (1974) recorded forearm venous and arterial pressure, forearm blood flow, and heart rate while the subject was supine. Again, tachycardia was the most consistent cardiovascular response to marihuana inhalation (600 mg). But they also found increased venous pressure and increased peripheral resistance as well as decreased reflex sympathetic response. In contrast to the effect of single doses, prolonged ingestion of THC slows heart rate, reduces supine and standing blood pressure, and impairs circulatory response to exercise (BENOWITZ and JONES, 1975). Under these conditions, atropine elevates systolic and diastolic blood pressure as well as heart rate (BENOWITZ and JONES, 1977). Thus, the effects of cannabis compounds upon the cardiovascular system are not uniform, but always suggest some disturbance in homeostatic mechanism. Moreover, they vary with species, particular compound (cannabinol and cannabidiol are ineffective) and vehicle used, dose, frequency, and duration of application, the route of administration, and finally, the condition of measuring (whether the subject was anesthetized, supine or upright, etc.).

Concerning respiration, it has been confirmed more than once that smoked or orally applied Δ-9-THC reduces airway resistance, without alteration of functional residual air or carbon dioxide sensitivity (VACHON et al., 1973; TASHKIN et al., 1973). These findings are similar to those obtained with isoproterenol. However, THC does not operate as a β-adrenergic agonist (SHAPIRO and TASHKIN, 1976). Intravenous injection of 0.5 mg/kg Δ-9-THC in anesthetized dogs resulted in an increase of lung resistance, which appeared to be vagally mediated and was not accompanied by a decrease in lung compliance or blood gas changes (BRIGHT et al., 1975). In a recent placebo study, it was again ascertained that smoking marihuana significantly increases ventilation and hypercapnic ventilatory response. Blood pH, pCO_2, and ventilatory response to hypoxia were unchanged. Propranolol completely abolished the increase in hypercapnic ventilatory response, but did not affect the other changes (ZWILLICH et al., 1978). Also, COHEN (1976) found that, unlike isoproterenol, the THC-induced increase in specific airway conductance is not blocked by propranolol. In contrast to atropine, the effect of THC on bronchial diameter is also not influenced by metacholine. Therefore, THC apparently works independently of β-adrenergic or muscarinic mechanisms (DAVIES et al., 1975; SHAPIRO and TASHKIN, 1976). In asthmatic patients, Δ-9-THC produces bronchiodilatation (HARTLEY et al., 1978). The rate of onset, magnitude, and duration of the effect were dose related.

3. Food Consumption and Temperature Regulation

THC exerts a dose-dependent depressant effect on water and food intake (FERNANDES et al., 1974; JOHANSSON et al., 1975). Since the reduction in food consumption exactly parallels the reduction in motility (running wheel, activity, and crossings), it is assumed that the changed pattern of feeding following Δ-9-THC may be a direct consequence of the rats' alterated state of arousal. This hypothesis is consistent with the action of tranquilizers and barbiturates (DREWNOWSKI and GRINKER 1978).

Similar to morphine, THC at low doses produces hyperthermia, and, at higher doses, hypothermia. Depending on the ambient temperature, the decrease in body temperature is dose related (HAAVIK and HARDMAN, 1973a, b; FERNANDES et al., 1974; JOHANSSON et al., 1974; HATTENDORF et al., 1977; HAAVIK and HARDMAN, 1979; TAYLOR and FENNESSY, 1977; BLOOM and DEWEY, 1978; BLOOM et al., 1978b). In all effects on autonomically regulated functions such as food intake or body temperature, cannabidiol and cannabinol are ineffective. But in combination with CBD, the actions of THC are prolonged.

4. Analgetic and Anticonvulsant Effects

Marihuana produces analgesic activity in animals (SOFIA et al., 1975; BLOOM and DEWEY, 1978) and man (MILSTEIN et al., 1974). THC, 11-OH-THC, and cannabinol work dose dependently; CBD is inactive (WILSON and MAY, 1975; WELBURN et al., 1976). In the hot plate test, however, there exists a synergism between CBD and THC (TAKAHASHI and KARNIOL, 1975).

In the mouse, the abdominal constriction response induced by formic acid, phenylquinone, 5-HT, prostaglandin E_1, and bradykinin is antagonized by THC (ED_{50} between 1.0 and 2.6 mg/kg) (JACKSON et al., 1976; SANDERS et al., 1979). Certainly, it remains to be considered whether THC also produces an attenuation of the escape response. PARKER and DUBAS (1973) have discussed the extent to which altered qualities of perception are related to the analgesic effects of THC.

Using the method of limited ascending and descending thresholds for painful and nonpainful stimulation, HILL et al. (1974) have some evidence that smoked marihuana (14 mg THC) has no analgesic properties. NOYES et al. (1975) demonstrated a mild analgesic effect of THC in patients with cancer. But in a dose of 20 mg, the drug induces severe side-effects that prohibit its wide therapeutic use.

Since those first observations of LOEWE and GOODMAN (1947), dose-related anticonvulsant effects of Δ-9-THC and CBD have been well documented in laboratory animals (FRIED and MACINTYRE, 1973; CORCORAN et al., 1973; CONSROE et al., 1976c; CONSROE and WOLKIN, 1977). Interestingly, in New Zealand white rabbits Δ-9-THC and cannabinol in low doses (0.5 mg/kg) produce seizures which are antagonized by CBD and anticonvulsants such as carbamazepine, diazepam, and phenytoin (CONSROE et al., 1977).

5. Motor System, Psychomotor Performance Tasks, and EEG

Hashish, like most of the psychoactive drugs, has depressant as well as excitatory effects. Depending on the dosage, both actions can be present in parallel (HOLLISTER and GILLESPIE, 1973; HILL et al., 1974). In man, after 5–7 mg Δ-9-THC, the sedative component predominates, at higher doses (15 mg and more), stimulating symptoms prevail. In animals, cannabis and THC mainly tend to suppress spontaneous and exploratory locomotion. Higher doses were necessary for rodents than for other species. A summary of findings on the effect of THC on the motor system of behavioral effects in animals is given by MILLER and DREW (1974).

In rats, THC induces dose-related catalepsy. The effect is triggered by intracisternal but not by intrapallidal injections. CBD is not effective, but extends the cataleptic response of THC. Amphetamine attenuates Δ-9-THC catalepsy, whereas intrapallidal administration of amphetamine potentiates the effect (FERNANDES et al., 1974; GOUGH and OLLEY, 1978).

In general, cannabis inhibits aggressive response. Shock- and isolation-induced aggressive activities, as well as predatory aggression, are inhibited by doses that do not impair motor function (MICZEK, 1978). The mouse- and frog-killing activity of rats is blocked (ABEL, 1975; MICZEK, 1976a), but under starvation and sleep deprivation, non-mouse killers developed muricidal behavior (FUJIWARA and UEKI, 1978).

THC disrupts performances on Rotarod and an established conditioned avoidance response (CAR) in rats and monkeys as well as the acquisition and extinction of reinforcement schedule behavior in a dose-related fashion. Maze learning is also impaired under the influence of THC (KILBEY et al., 1973; MCDONOUGH et al., 1972; PRYOR et al., 1976).

In man, too, THC produces decrements in general performance (reaction speed, cognition, and psychomotor coordination), including the ability to perceive emotions in others (BELGRAVE et al., 1979; CLOPTON et al., 1979). Handling performance in automobile driving and psychomotor tracking is decreased by cannabis in the relatively high dose of 5.9 mg/kg THC (HANSTEEN et al., 1976). Memory is influenced in the sense that marihuana obviously affects storage processes but not perception, registration, and retrieval (ABEL, 1971; DARLEY et al., 1973; DORNBUSH et al., 1971).

WIKLER and LLOYD (1945) were one of the first who described a decrease in EEG α-activity and an increase in the fast frequencies. Later, EEG frequency changes were carefully quantified by power density spectral analysis. The results were inconsistent. FINK (1976) studied EEG profiles in occasional cannabis users in New York and long-term, high-dose hashish users in Athens. The EEG effects of enhanced α-activity, decreased β-activity, and decreased mean frequency were dose dependent, both in intensity and in duration. The behavioral measures, particularly selfratings of euphoria ("high" or "mastura") and heart rate, were also dose dependent and interrelated with the EEG measures. Similar results are described by KOUKKOU and LEHMANN (1978) in an acute trial with volunteers who were abstinent during the 3 months prior to the study. In the report of COHEN (1976), marihuana smoking is associated with downward alpha shift and a narrowing of band width.

D. Aspects of Tolerance

Since the fundamental considerations of KALANT et al. (1971), it is well known that tolerance can be quantified only by measuring the parallel shift of dose-response curves for acute and chronic drug treatment. The usual procedure for measuring tolerance ensuing from a fixed dose leads to a high probability of error. If a test is carried out constantly in a maximum effective dose range, tolerance to the action examined is hardly perceptible. The same can happen if the dose is below the tolerance-inducing level. Moreover, with a single dose, the parallelism of the shift to the right cannot be evaluated.

This statement is valid not only for functional tolerance where development of tolerance to some effects is different in time and intensity at various doses, but also for dispositional tolerance, where in principle all effects of the drug are diminished after chronic administration. In that case, some effects can yet be realized in spite of a forced metabolism, if only a sufficient amount of the drug remains for those reactions. On the other hand, effects which require comparatively higher concentrations can decrease under the threshold of effectiveness.

Because these basic facts are often ignored, it is not yet determined whether tolerance to cannabis is caused metabolically or functionally, or if both phenomena are of relevance.

In their review of 1978, LEMBERGER and RUBIN argue that in animals tolerance is not due to alterations in the disposition of the drug with chronic administration since apparently no major differences were seen in absorption, distribution, metabolism, or excretion of cannabinoids. In humans, however, differences were observed between naive subjects and chronic marihuana smokers in plasma half-lives of Δ-9-THC as well as in its metabolism. But the authors question whether dispositional alterations could be solely responsible for tolerance in man. In their opinion, it is more likely that tolerance is related to an adaptation by the cells of the CNS.

The synopsis in the review of HARRIS et al. (1977) may indicate dispositional tolerance, because all of the more than ten different effect listed are reduced. Distinctly differentiated tolerance to depressive effects and not to excitatory ones, as seen in chronic opioid use, apparently has not yet been established.

The favored assumption that tolerance to cannabis is not mediated by forced metabolism is not totally convincing. As indicated in the discussion of pharmacokinetic effects, especially for cannabinoids it is not valid to use measurements of radioactivity to assess the proportion and intensity of drug metabolism. The occurrence of enhanced transformation in animals was shown by HO et al. (1973) and confirmed by MAGOUR et al. (1977). The discrepancy between the results concerning distribution of THC in animals after subchronic treatment may be caused also by the vehicle used. MARTIN et al. (1976) found after intravenous injection of Emulphor EL-620:ethanol: saline (5:5:490) that the distribution of Δ-9-THC in the organism was not significantly different in tolerant and nontolerant animals. (A marked reduction, however, was found in the gray area of the brain in tolerant rats.) PRYOR et al. (1976) even demonstrated an accumulation of radioactivity following subacute treatment with Δ-9-THC dissolved in sesame oil and given orally. In their investigations, subacute pretreatment with 10 mg/kg Δ-9-THC for 6 days caused significant tolerance to all five measures (CAR, photocell activity, heart rate, body temperature, and time on Rotarod).

Moreover, daily 12 mg/kg intraperitoneal injections of THC produced tolerance during a 9-day drug series on a number of behavioral measures in rats performing on a discriminated-Sidman avoidance schedule and reversed completely during a similar period under vehicle-only injections (WEBSTER et al., 1973).

Important evidence for the mechanism of functional tolerance is provided by the mouse-killing behavior. THC or cannabis extracts consistently suppress predatory, attack, and killing behavior in rats and cats after acute administration. But daily administration of high doses induces mouse-killing behavior (MICZEK et al., 1976a and b, 1979). Thus, after depressive effects have diminished, the excitatory ones, e. g., killing behavior, prevail. However, it must be pointed out that this kind of aggression is connected with special conditions. In aggressive behavior induced by tactile and visual isolation, TEN HAM and DEJONG (1974) found no attenuation although tolerance to hypothermia was seen.

Another indicator for functional tolerance may be temporally different attenuation of hypothermia, intestinal motility, and spontaneous locomotor activity after chronic THC administration (ANDERSON et al., 1975). Lack of tolerance to a negative chronotropic effect of THC in rats has been described by KAYMAKCALAN et al. (1974).

Further arguments for the existence of functional tolerance are the results of investigations on cross-tolerance between THC and ethanol. In agreement with the findings of SPRAGUE and CRAIGMILL (1976), SIEMENS and DOYLE (1979), using Rotarod performance, demonstrated cross-tolerance which was not a function of changes in drug degradation.

Some of the inconsistency in the preceding report about tolerance to cannabis in humans is based on a simple but important fact, often overlooked or forgotten. In

1963, SEEVERS and DENEAU pointed out that the development of tolerance requires "continual neuronal exposure" to the drug without interruption. Failure to recognize this requirement has led to "erroneous conclusions from poorly designed experiments." Therefore, it is not quite correct to compare the results of experiments in which volunteers have smoked varying amounts of hashish cigarettes under standardized conditions with defined substances, doses, and kind and frequency of application to data obtained from occasional or chronic hashish users.

In agreement with most other authors, JONES et al. (1976) found that tolerance developed to many physiologic effects of cannabis in humans. The changes followed a time course similar to that of subjective intoxication judgements and are listed below (see also LIAKOS et al., 1976; GIBBINS et al., 1976; NOWLAN and COHEN, 1977).

Mood changes	EEG slowing
Tachycardia	EEG evoked potential alterations
Orthostatic hypotension	Sleep EEG changes
Skin temperature decrease	Sleep time and quality
Body temperature increase	Eye tracking
Salivary flow decrease	Psychomotor tast performance
Intraocular pressure decrease	Ward behavior alterations

Obviously, the effect depends on the dose and frequency of consumption. BABOR et al. (1975) found that heavy users indicated a progressive decline in ratings of intoxication and duration of pulse rate effect; moderate users showed no changes in either of these reactions. COHEN (1976) found disappearance of tachycardia after chain smoking of marihuana cigarettes; PEREZ-REYES et al. (1974; 1976) documented that marihuana does not produce tolerance to accelerated heart rate. RENAULT et al. (1974) demonstrated in man that tolerance does not develop to the two most reliable indexes of marihuana intoxication, the heart rate increase and subjective feelings of highness, unless rather heavy doses of Δ-9-THC are self administered repeatedly.

MENDELSON et al. (1976) tried to study behavioral and social reactions to marihuana when smoked under conditions that approached typical social usage. He found in casual and heavy users a significantly declined activity level; this decline is reflected in the subject's tendency to prefer more passive activities. But the relationship between marihuana and physical activities seems not to be causative, because subjects smoked at those times when they would ordinarily be inactive. Behavioral tolerance in heavy smokers suggests that some of the effects are pharmacologic rather than learned.

There is no doubt that in the establishment of tolerance to the psychomotor effects of Δ-9-THC, the influence of learning is a special problem. It was again KALANT et al. (1971) who showed that in animal behavior, e.g., lever pressing in some difficult task, the disturbance in function produced by a drug may not be present unless the animal attempts to perform the task. Therefore, it is not surprising to find that tolerance to a drug develops more rapidly if the animal performs or attempts to perform the function while under the influence of the drug. Using numerous examples, WIKLER (1976) has discussed this aspect thoroughly. He concluded that tolerance at all levels of complexity in the brain involves "learning" in the sense of the acquisition of compensatory adaptations to the consequences of the presence of a drug-produced disturbance in function. Depending on the function tested, species and dose of cannabis used, tolerance, behaviorally augmented (to induce disturbed function) or not, develops at different rates or not at all, e.g., to impairment of the logical sequence of thoughts, to which tolerance has yet been demonstrated.

LARSEN and PRYOR (1977) showed attenuation of the impairing effect of Δ-9-THC on the avoidance task when the drug was given independent of the opportunity to perform the conditioned avoidance response (pole climb). These results differ from those of MANNING (1976), who found that independent exposure was insufficient to induce tolerance to the impairing effect of Δ-9-THC. But he used another operant schedule that required a low rate of spaced responding (30–s reduction of food reinforcement).

JÄRBE (1978) treated rats with Δ-9-THC for 14 days and found tolerance to THC-induced hypothermia and depression of CAR in shuttle box. The noncontingent exposure also produced tolerance to spontaneous (unlearned) behavior as measured in an open field test. He concluded from this data that there is no essential role of learned tolerance under the influence of THC.

E. Interactions with Other Drugs

Interactions of cannabis and other drugs have to be differentiated in metabolic and functional interactions.

Concerning functional interactions of cannabis and other drugs, general problems in this field must be remembered. THC interferes with several centrally regulated motoric, sensory, and vegetative functions. The linear part of the log-dose response curve of the various effects does not proceed in a simple additive and parallel manner. Thus, variation of the dose does not only change the intensity of the single partial actions to a different degree, but also can modify the whole profile of action. Therefore, depending on dose, the steepness of the dose-response curve, and the duration of treatment, THC in combination with other drugs, which dispose also of large spectrum of action, may lead to different results, especially if the effects of the two substances occur in different systems and receptors (LEVY 1976; MITCHELL, 1976; COPER, 1979).

In earlier investigations, KUBENA and BARRY (1970) reported that a dose of 4 mg/kg THC antagonized the stimulating effect of 2 mg/kg methamphetamine, whereas a dose of 16 mg/kg THC failed to diminish the stimulant effect of 0.5 mg/kg methamphetamine. On the other hand, PIRCH et al. (1973) found a dose-related antagonism of the stimulation caused by amphetamine. In aggregated mice, THC augmented the locomotor activity produced by 0.5 mg/kg methamphetamine. The effect was dose related and lasted for 2 h (EVANS et al. 1976a).

With the aid of reciprocal dose-response curves, PRYOR et al. (1978) studied the interaction of THC with D-amphetamine, cocaine, and nicotine in rats on conditioned avoidance response (CAR), photocell activity, heart rat, temperature, and Rotarod performance. Neither the two stimulants nor nicotine influenced CAR performance, but the increased intertrial response with amphetamine and cocaine was partially antagonized by THC. The cannabinoid completely blocked the stimulated photocell activity of amphetamine, whereas there was mutual antagonism between Δ-9-THC and cocaine. Nicotine markedly potentiated the THC-mediated depression. Amphetamine and cocaine tended to offset the impairment of Rotarod performance caused by Δ-9-THC, whereas this performance was augmented by nicotine. THC-induced bradycardia and hypothermia were increased by the stimulants and by nicotine.

Also CONSROE et al. (1976a) gave evidence for the concept that depending upon the parameters being investigated, the interaction of THC with catecholaminergic drugs (amphetamine, cocaine, and apomorphine) may result in an antagonism or potentiation of the effect. In another study CONSROE et al. 1975; (1976b) described in rabbits an antagonism between caffeine and THC in cortical and hippocampal EEG, whereas nicotine reversed the EEG alterations. But this combination caused behavioral collapses preceded by behavioral disturbances.

Under a double-blind, randomized, complete block design, subjects were given either placebo or 10 mg/70 kg dextroamphetamine sulfate orally, followed 1.5 h later with a marihuana cigarette prepared to deliver 25 μg/kg THC. The evaluation of subsequent psychomotor performance showed an impairment which was related to smoking marihuana. No difference could be distinguished between marihuana alone and marihuana-dextroamphetamine sulfate combination. Subjective evaluations as measured by the modified Cornell Medical Index demonstrated only additive effects for the combination (EVANS et al., 1976b).

PRYOR et al. (1976) showed that an ineffective dose of phenobarbital in combination with THC increases impairment of CAR performance and vice versa. The dose-related results suggest that a critical level of either THC or phenobarbital is sufficient to trigger the impairment of CAR performance. The results for ethanol show a somewhat different pattern. The interaction appears to be more critically dependent on the dose of ethanol than on that of Δ-9-THC. A third pattern is illustrated by the results for phenycyclidin caused a graded dose-related increase of impairment. With the lower doses of phenycyclidin, the potentiation was more than additive, whereas with the highest dose it was less. All these studies strengthen the notion that the interactions between THC and other drugs are the result of a complex interplay involving various receptor sites and neurohumoral systems.

Without interference with the metabolism of ethanol in rats, THC but not CBD enhanced the depressant action of ethanol, although ethanol reduced THC-affected brain and Blood levels (SIEMENS and KHANNA, 1977).

CHESHER et al. (1976, 1977) investigated the effects in man of THC alone and in combination with ethanol on perceptual and cognitive motor functions. Both THC (0.14 mg/kg) and ethanol (0.54 mg/kg) have little effect when administered alone. The combination of the drugs, however, induced a significant decrement in performance and was considered to be at least additive. The peak blood ethanol concentration was higher when the subjects received both drugs. If the dose of THC was increased to 0.21 mg/kg, THC alone produced markedly decrements.

When this dose was combined with 0.14 mg/kg ethanol, an additive effect appeared in the first part of the investigation, but later there was a suggestion of antagonism. Subjects who received the drugs in combination performed better than those who received only the high dose of THC.

THC significantly prolonged the anesthesia induced by cetamin, pentobarbitone, thiopentone, and propanidid in a dose-dependent manner. Cannabinol and cannabidiol prolonged pentobarbitone-induced anesthesia (FRIZZA et al., 1977). This interaction is obviously metabolically and not centrally mediated, as confirmed by former investigations by CHESHER et al. (1974) and FERNANDES et al. (1974) who demonstrated that CBD prolonged hexobarbital-induced sleep by inhibition of the metabolic degradation of the anesthetic.

As described in Sect. III, cannabinoids, especially CBD, suppress the metabolism of phenazone, aminopyrine, and other drugs (PATON and PERTWEE, 1972; FERNANDES et al., 1973).

In rodents, CBD also inhibits the degradation of THC. But in man, this mechanism obviously is without relevance, because a combination of THC (20 mg) with CBD (40 mg) produces no detectable changes in quality, intensity, or duration of the effect of THC alone (HOLLISTER and GILLESPIE, 1975).

F. Conclusion

During the past 10 years much has been learned about the pharmacology and toxicology of cannabis and from that about the therapeutic potency of its pure constituents (TASHKIN et al. 1978). But balancing benefit against risk, the therapeutical value of cannabinoids remains small. Bronchodilation, reversal of bronchospasm and a decrease in airway resistance after THC for example, are advantageous. These effects were the basis for the study of marihuana in asthma therapy. However, the smoke has a directly irritating effect on the lungs, and chronic inhalation is associated with impairment of pulmonary functions, including slight respiratory depression and respiratory disorders such as laryngitis, pharyngitis, bronchitis, and their consequences BELLVILLE et al., 1975; VACHON, 1976; FLEISCHMAN et al., 1979).

Due to disturbances in the homeostatic mechanism of the cardiovascular system THC has no therapeutic value in subjects with heart or circulatory insufficiency. In patients with coronary artery disease, marihuana-smoking decreased myocardial oxygen delivery and the exercise time until the onset of anginal pain and increased myocardial oxygen demand. In addition, it significantly enhanced the cognitive impairment of subjects, as measured by the content of speech, and blocked the usual, nondrug psychocardiovascular correlations. Therefore, for anginal patients marihuana is more a medical hazard than a help (GOTTSCHALK et al., 1977).

The efficacy of cannabinoids as an anticonvulsant drug has been investigated mainly in animals. Information about its antiepileptic properties in man is insufficient (COHEN and STILLMAN, 1976).

Reduction of intraocular pressure after oral or inhaled THC is undisputed (GREEN, 1975). In the meantime it could be shown in rabbits that after topically applied THC intraocular pressure diminished. No tolerance has been noted (GREEN et al., 1977). Thus, in the future cannabinoids may offer an alternative medication for glaucoma.

All other efforts to take cannabinoids for the treatment of various disorders or disease symptoms (anxiety, depression, nausea, pain, and cancer, or even infectious diseases) were not successful until recently now (COHEN, 1978).

Sensational news about the therapeutic possibilities of the "devil's weed", cannabis, is obviously not to be expected. Nevertheless, many important unsettled questions, especially about the basic mechanisms of action, have to be solved and make it necessary to continue research on cannabinoids.

References

Abel, E.L.: Marihuana and memory: Acquisition or retrieval? Science *173*, 1038–1040 (1971)
Abel, E.L.: Cannabis and aggression in animals. Behav. Biol. *14*, 1–20 (1975)
Adams, M.D., Earnhardt, J.T., Dewey, W.L., Harris, L.S.: Vasoconstrictor actions of Δ^8- and Δ^9-tetrahydrocannabinol in the rat. J. Pharmacol. Exp. Ther. *196*, 649–656 (1976)
Agurell, S., Nilsson, U.M., Ohlsson, A., Sandberg, F.: Elimination of tritium-labelled cannabinols in the rat with special reference to the development of tests for the identification of cannabis users. Biochem. Pharmacol. *18*, 1195–1201 (1969)
Anderson, P.F., Jackson, D.M. Chesher, G.B., Maler, R.: Tolerance to the effects of Δ^9-tetrahydrocannabinol in mice on intestinal motility, temperature and locomotor activity. Psychopharmacology *43*, 31–36 (1975)
Babor, T.F., Mendelson, J.H., Greenberg, I., Kuehnle, J.C.: Marijuana consumption and tolerance to physiological and subjective effects. Arch. Gen. Psychiat. *32*, 1548–1552 (1975)
Bach, D., Raz, A., Goldman, R.: The interaction of hashish compounds with planar lipid bilayer membranes (BLM). Biochem. Pharmacol. *25*, 1241–1244 (1976)
Banerjee, A., Poddar, M.K., Saha, S., Gosh: J.J.: Effect of Δ^9-tetrahydrocannabinol on monoamine oxidase activity of rat tissues in vivo. Biochem. Pharmacol. *24*, 1435–1436 (1975a)
Banerjee, S.P., Snyder, S.H., Mechoulam, R.: Cannabinoids: Influence on neurotransmitter uptake in rat brain synaptosomes. J. Pharmacol. Exp. Ther. *194*, 74–81 (1975b)
Belgrave, B.E., Bird, K.D., Chesher, G.B., Jackson, D.M., Lubbe, K.E., Stramer, G.A., Theo, R.K.: The effect of (–) trans-Δ^9-tetrahydrocannabinol, alone and in combination with ethanol, on human performance. Psychopharmacology *62*, 53–60 (1979)
Bellville, J.W., Swanson, G.D., Aqleh, K.A.: Respiratory effects of delta-9-tetrahydrocannabinol. Clin. Pharmacol. Ther. *17*, 541–548 (1975)
Benowitz, N.L., Jones, R.T.: Cardiovascular effects of prolonged Δ^9-tetrahydrocannabinol ingestion in man. Clin. Pharmacol. Ther. *18*, 287–297 (1975)
Benowitz, N.L., Jones, R.T.: Prolonged delta-9-tetrahydrocannabinol ingestion. Effects of sympathomimetic amines and autonomic blockades. Clin. Pharmacol. Ther. *21*, 336–342 (1977)
Benowitz, N.L., Rosenberg, J., Rogers, W., Bachman, J., Jones, R.T.: Cardiovascular effects of intravenous delta-9-tetrahydrocannabinol: Autonomic nervous mechanisms. Clin. Pharmacol. Ther. *25*, 440–446 (1979)
Bensemana, D., Gascon, A.L.: Effect of Δ-9-THC on the distribution uptake and release of catecholamine in rats. Rev. Can. Biol. *33*, 269–278 (1974)
Benz-Zvi, Z., Bergen, J.R., Burstein, S., Sehgal, P.K., Varanelli, C.: In: The Pharmacology of Marihuana. Braude, M.C., Szara, S. (eds.), p. 63. New York: Raven Press 1976
Blevins, R.D., Regan, J.D.: Δ-9-tetrahydrocannabinol: Effect on macromolecular synthesis in human and other mammalian cells. Arch. Toxicol. *35*, 127–135 (1976)
Bloom, A.S., Dewey, W.L.: A comparison of some pharmacological actions of morphine and Δ-9-tetrahydrocannabinol in the mouse. Psychopharmacology *57*, 243–248 (1978)
Bloom, A.S., Haavik, C.O., Strehlow, D.: Effects of Δ-9-tetrahydrocannabinol on ATPases in mouse brain subcellular fractions. Sciences *23*, 1399–1404 (1978a)
Bloom, A.S., Johnson, K.M., Dewey, W.L.: The effects of cannabinoids on body temperature and brain catecholamin synthesis. Res. Commun. Chem. Path. Pharmacol. *20*, 51–57 (1978b)
Borgen, L.A., Davis, W.M.: Vehicle and route of administration as parameters affecting operant behavioral effects of Δ-9-tetrahydrocannabinol. J. Pharmaceut. Sci. *62*, 479–480 (1973)
Borys, H.K., Karler, R.: Cannabidiol and Δ-9-tetrahydrocannabinol metabolism. Biochem. Pharmacol. *28*, 1553–1559 (1979)
Bright, T.P., Farber, M.O., Brown, D.J., Forney, R.B.: Cardiopulmonary toxicity of Δ-9-tetrahydrocannabinol in the anesthetized dog. Toxicol. Appl. Pharmacol. *31*, 100–106 (1975)
Burstein, S., Hunter, S.A.: Prostaglandins and cannabis. VI. Release of arachidonic acid from HeLa cells by Δ-9-tetrahydrocannabinol and other cannabinoids. Biochem. Pharmacol. *27*, 1275–1280 (1978)
Burstein, S., Levin, F., Varanelli, C.: Prostaglandins and cannabis. II. Inhibition of biosynthesis by the naturally occuring cannabinoids. Biochem. Pharmacol. *22*, 2905–2910 (1973)

Burstein, S., Hunter, S.A., Shoupe, T., Taylor, P.: Cannabinoid inhibition of testosterone synthesis by mouse Leydig cells. Res. Commun. Chem. Path. Pharmacol. *19*, 557–560 (1978)

Burstein, S., Hunter, S.A., Shoupe, T.S.: Site of inhibition of Leyding cell testosterone synthesis by Δ-1-tetrahydrocannabinol. Mol. Pharmacol. *15*, 633–640 (1979a)

Burstein, S., Hunter, S.A., Shoupe, T.: Cannabinoid inhibition of rat luteal cell progesterone synthesis. Res. Commum. Chem. Path. Pharmacol. *24*, 413–416 (1979b)

Carchman, R.A., Harris, L.S., Munson, A.E.: The inhibition of DNA synthesis by cannabinoids. Cancer Res. *36*, 95–100 (1976)

Cavero, I., Buckley, J.P., Jandhyala, B.S.: Parasympatholytic activity of (–)-Δ-9-trans-tetrahydrocannabinol in mongrel dogs. Eur. J. Pharmacol. *19*, 301–304 (1972)

Cavero, I., Buckley, J.P., Janhyala, B.S.: Hemodynamic and myocardial effects of (–)-Δ-9-trans-tetrahydrocannabinol in anesthetized dogs. Europ. J. Pharmacol. *24*, 243–251 (1973)

Chan, M.Y., Tse, A.: The effect of cannabinoids (Δ-9-THC and Δ-8-THC) on hepatic microsomal metabolism of testosterone in vitro. Biochem. Pharmacol. *27*, 1725–1728 (1978)

Chari-Bitron, A., Bino, T.: Effect of Δ-1-tetrahydrocannabinol on ATPase activity of rat liver mitochondria. Biochem. Pharmacol. *20*, 473–475 (1971)

Chesher, G.B., Franks, H.M., Hensley, V.R., Hensley, W.J., Jackson, D.M., Starmer, G.A., Teo, R.K.C.: The interaction of ethanol and Δ-9-tetrahydrocannabinol in man. Effects on perceptual cognitive and motor functions. Med. J. Aust. *1976/2* 159–163

Chesher, G.B., Franks, H.M., Jackson, D.M., Starmer, G.A., Teo, R.K.C.: Ethanol and Δ-9-tetrahydrocannabinol. Interactive effects on human perceptual, cognitive and motor functions. II. Med. J. Aust. *1977/1*, 478–481

Chesher, G.B., Jackson, D.M., Starmer, G.A.: Interaction of cannabis and general anaesthetic agents in mice. Brit. J. Pharmacol. *50*, 593–599 (1974)

Clark, S.C., Greene, C., Karr, G.W., MacCannell, K.L., Milstein, S.L.: Cardiovascular effects of marihuana in man. Can. J. Physiol. Pharmacol. *52*, 706–719 (1974)

Clopton, P.L., Janowsky, D.S., Clopton, J.M., Judd, L.L., Huey, L.: Marijuana and the perception of affect. Psychopharmacology *61*, 203–206 (1979)

Cohen, S.: The 94-day cannabis study. Ann. N.Y. Acad. Sci. *282*, 211–220 (1976)

Cohen, S.: Marijuana: Does it have a possible therapeutic use? J. Am. Med. Ass. *240*, 1761–1763 (1978)

Cohen, S., Stillman, R.C. (eds.): The Therapeutic Potential of Marihuana. New York: Plenum Press 1976

Colburn, R.W., Ng, L.K.Y., Lemberger, L., Kopin, I.J.: Subcellular distribution of Δ-9-tetrahydrocannabinol in rat brain. Biochem. Pharmacol. *23*, 873–877 (1974)

Collier, H.O., Francis, D.L., Henderson, G., Schneider, C.S.: Quasi-morphine-abstinence syndrome. Nature *249*, 471–473 (1974)

Collu, R., Letarte, J., Leboeuf, G., Ducharme, J.R.: Endocrine effects of chronic administration of psychoactive drugs to prepuberal male rats. I.: Δ-9-tetrahydrocannabinol. Life Sci. *16*, 533–542 (1975)

Consroe, P.F., Jones, B.C., Akins, F.: Δ-9-tetrahydrocannabinol-methamphetamine interaction in the rabbit. Neuropharmacology *14*, 377–383 (1975)

Consroe, P., Jones, B.C., Laird, H.: Interactions of Δ-9-tetrahydrocannabinol with other pharmacological agents. Ann. N.Y. Acad. Sci. *281*, 198–211 (1976a).

Consroe, P., Jones, B., Laird, H.: EEG and behavioral effects of Δ-9-tetrahydrocannabinol in combination with stimulant drugs in rabbits. Psychopharmacology *50*, 47–52 (1976b)

Consroe, P., Jones, B., Laird, H., Reinking, J.: Anticonvulsant-convulsant effects of tetrahydrocannabinol. In: The therapeutic potential of Marijuana. Cohen, S.., Stillman, R. (eds.), pp. 363–382. New York: Plenum Press (1976c)

Consroe, P., Martin, P., Eisenstein, D.: Anticonvulsant drug antagonism of Δ-9-tetrahydrocannabinol-induced seizures in rabbits. Res. Commun. Chem. Path. Pharmacol. *16*, 1–13 (1977)

Consroe, P., Wolkin, A.: Cannabidiol-antiepileptic drug comparisons and interactions in experimentally induced seizures in rats. J. Pharmacol. Exp. Ther. *201*, 26–32 (1977)

Coper, H.: Wechselwirkungen von Psychopharmaka mit anderen Medikamenten. Nervenarzt *50*, 485–490 (1979)

Coper, H., Fernandes, M., Honecker, H., Kluwe, S.: The influence of solvent agents on the effects of cannabis. Acta Pharmacol. Toxicol. *29*, Suppl. 4, 89 (1971)

Corcoran, M.E., McCaughran, J.A.jr., Wada, J.A.: Acute antiepileptic effects of Δ-9-tetrahydrocannabinol in rats with kindled seizures. Exp. Neurol. *40*, 471–483 (1973)
Dalterio, S., Bartke, A., Burstein, S.: Cannabinoids inhibit testosterone secretion by mouse testes in vitro. Science *196*, 1472–1473 (1977)
Darley, C.F., Trinklenberg, J.R., Hollister, T.E., Atkinson, R.C.: Marihuana and retrieval from short-term memory. Psychopharmacologia *29*, 231–238 (1973)
Davies, B.H., Radcliffe, S., Seaton, A., Graham, J.D.P.: A trial of oral Δ-1-(trans)-tetrahydrocannabinol in reversible airways obstruction. Thorax *30*, 80–85 (1975)
Dewey, W.L., Johnson, K.M., Bloom, A.S., Interactions of active constituents of marihuana with other drugs in the neuron. Ann. N. Y. Acad. Sci. *281*, 190–197 (1976)
Dixit, V.P., Sharma, V.N., Lohiya, N.K.: The effect of chronically administered cannabis extract on the testicular function of mice. Eur. J. Pharmacol. *26*, 111–114 (1974)
Dolby, T.W., Kleinsmith, L.J.: Effects of Δ-9-tetrahydrocannabinol on the levels of cyclic adenosine 3′,5′-monophosphate in mouse brain. Biochem. Pharmacol. *23*, 1817–1825 (1974)
Dornbush, R.L., Fink, M., Freedman, A.M.: Marijuana, memory and perception. Am. J. Psychiat. *128*, 194–197 (1971)
Drewnowski, A., Grinker, J.A.: Food and water intake, meal patterns and activity of obese and lean Zucker rats following chronic and acute treatment with Δ-9-tetrahydrocannabinol. Pharmacol. Biochem. Behav. *9*, 619–630 (1978)
Estevez, V.S., Englert, L.F., Ho, B.T.: Effect of SKF-525-A on the metabolism of (–)-delta^9-tetrahydrocannabinol in the rat brain and liver. Res. Commun. Path. Pharmacol. *8*, 389–392 (1974)
Evans, M.A., Harbison, R.D., Brown, D.J., Forney, R.B.: Stimulant actions of Δ-tetrahydrocannabinol in mice. Psychopharmacology *50*, 245–250 (1976a)
Evans, M.A., Martz, R., Rodda, B.E., Lemberger, L., Forney, R.B.: Effects of marihuana-dextroamphetamine combination. Clin. Pharmacol. Ther. *20*, 350–358 (1976)
Fernandes, M., Coper, H.: The role of vehicles in cannabis application and interaction between cannabis and central active drugs. Acta Pharmaceut. Suecica *8*, 692–693 (1971)
Fernandes, M., Warning, N., Christ, W., Hill, R.: Interactions of several cannabinoids with the hepatic drug metabolizing system. Biochem. Pharmacol. *22*, 2981–2987 (1973)
Fernandes, M., Schabarek, A., Coper, H., Hill, R.: Modification of Δ-9-THC-actions by cannabinol and cannabidiol in the rat. Psychopharmacology *38*, 329–338 (1974)
Fink, M.: Effects of acute and chronic inhalation of hashish, marijuana, and Δ-9-tetrahydrocannabinol on brain electrical activity in man: Evidence for tissue tolerance. Ann. N.Y. Acad. Sci. *282*, 387–398 (1976)
Fleischman, R.W., Baker, J.R., Rosenkrantz, H.: Pulmonary pathologic changes in rats exposed ot marihuana smoke for one year. Toxicol. appl. Pharmacol. *47*, 557–566 (1979)
Fleischman, R.W., Hayden, D.W., Rosenkrantz, H., Brande, M.C.: Teratologic evaluation of Δ^9-tetrahydrocannabinol in mice, including a review of the literature. Teratology *12*, 47–50 (1975)
Fried, P.A., McIntyre, D.C.: Electrical and behavioral attenuation of the anti-convulsant properties of Δ-9-THC following chronic administrations. Psychopharmacology *31*, 215–227 (1973)
Friedman, M.A.: Inhibition of arylhydrocarbon hydroxylase induction in BALB/C mouse liver by Δ-9-tetrahydrocannabinol. Res. Commun. Chem. Path. Pharmacol. *15*, 541–552 (1976)
Frizza, J., Chesher, G.B., Jackson, D.M., Malor, R., Stramer, G.A.: The effect of Δ-9-tetrahydrocannabinol, cannabidiol, and cannabinol on the anaesthesia induced by various anaesthetic agents in mice. Psychopharmacology *55*, 103–107 (1977)
Fujiwara, M., Ueki, S.: Muricide induced by single injection of Δ-9-tetrahydrocannabinol. Physiol. Behav. *21*, 581–585 (1978)
Gaul, Ch. C., Mellors, A.: Δ-9-tetrahydrocannabinol and decreased macrophage migration inhibition. Res. Commum. Chem. Path. Pharmacol. *10*, 559–564 (1975)
Gibbins, R.J., McDougall, J., Miles, C.G., Marshman, J.A.: Tolerance to marijuana-induced tachycardia in man. Acta Pharmacol. Toxicol. *39*, 65–76 (1976)
Gill, E.W., The effects of cannabinoids and other CNS depressants on cell membrane models. Ann. N. Y. Acad. Sci. *281*, 151–161 (1976)

Gottschalk, L.A., Aronow, W.S., Prakash, R.: Effect of marijuana and placebo-marijuana smoking on psychophysiological cardiovascular functioning in anginal patients. Biol. Psychiat. *12*, 255–266 (1977)

Gough, A.L., Olley, J.E.: Catalepsy induced by intrastriatal injections of Δ-9-THC and 11-OH-Δ-9-THC in the rat. Neuropharmacology *17*, 137–144 (1978)

Graham, J.D.P., Lewis, M.J., Li, D.M.F.: The effect of Δ-1-tetrahydrocannabinol on the uptake of (^{3}H)-(–)noradrenaline by the isolated perfused heart of the rat. Brit. J. Pharmacol. *51*, 465–466 (1974)

Green, K.: Marihuana and the eye. Invest. Opthalmol. *14*, 261–263 (1975)

Green, K., Bigger, J.F., Kim, K., Bowman, K.: Cannabinoid penetration and chronic effects in the eye. Exp. Eye Res. *24*, 197–205 (1977)

Greenberg, J.H., Mellors, A., McGowan, J.C.: Molar volume relationships and the specific inhibition of a synaptosomal enzyme by psychoactive cannabinoids. J. Med. Chem. *21*, 1208–1212 (1978)

Haavik, C.O., Hardman, H.F.: Evaluation of the hypothermic action of tetrahydrocannabinols in mice and squirrel monkeys. J. Pharmacol. Exp. Ther. *187*, 568–574 (1973a)

Haavik, C.O., Hardman, H.F.: Hypothermic action of Δ^9-tetrahydrocannabinol, 11-hydroxy-Δ^9-tetrahydrocannabinol and 11-hydroxy-Δ^8-tetrahydrocannabinol in mice. Life Sci. *13*, 1771–1778 (1973b)

Haavik, C.O., Hardman, H.F.: Cannabis and thermoregulation. In: Modern Pharmacology and Toxicology Series, Body Temperature, Regulation, Drug Effects and Therapeutic Implication. Lomax, P., Schönbaum, E. (eds.), Vol. 16. New York: Marcel Dekker 1979

Hansteen, R.W., Miller, R.D., Lonero, L., Reid, L.D., Jones, B.: Effects of cannabis and alcohol on automobile driving and psychomotor tracking. Ann. N.Y. Acad. Sci. *282*, 240–256 (1976)

Harris, L.S., Munson, A.E., Carchman, R.A.: Antitumor properties of cannabinoids. In: Pharmacology of Marihuana. Braude, M., Szara, S. (eds.). New York: Raven Press 1976

Harris, L.S., Dewey, W.L., Razdan, R.K.: Cannabis. Its Chemistry, Pharmacology, and Toxicology. In: Handbook of Experimental Pharmacology, Vol. 45/II: Drug Addiction II: Amphetamine, Psychotogen, and Marihuana Dependence. Martin, W.R. (ed.), pp. 371–429. Berlin, Heidelberg, New York: Springer 1977

Harris, L.S., Carchman, R.A., Martin, B.R.: Evidence for the existence of specific cannabinoid binding sites. Life Sci. *22*, 1131–1137 (1978)

Hartley, J.P.R., Nogrady, S.G., Seaton, A., Graham, J.D.P.: Bronchodilator effect of Δ^1-tetrahydrocannabinol. Brit. J. Clin. Pharmacol. *5*, 523–525 (1978)

Hattendorf, Ch., Hattendorf, M., Coper, H., Fernandes, M.: Interaction between Δ^9-tetrahydrocannabinol and d-amphetamine. Psychopharmacology *54*, 177–182 (1977)

Herha, J., Obe, G.: Chromosomal damage in chronical users of cannabis in vivo investigation with two-day leukocyte cultures. Pharmakopsychiatry *7*, 328–337 (1974)

Hershkowitz, M., Goldman, R., Raz, A.: Effect of cannabinoids on neurotransmitter uptake, ATPase activity and morphology of mouse brain synaptosomes. Biochem. Pharmacol. *26*, 1327–1331 (1977)

Hill, S.Y., Goodwin, D.W., Schwin, R., Powell, B.: Marijuana: CNS depressant or excitant? Am. J. Psychiat. *131*, 313–315 (1974)

Ho, B.T., Estevez, V.S., Englert, L.F.: Effect of repeated administration on the metabolism of (–)-Δ^9-tetrahydrocannabinols in rats. Res. Commun. Chem. Path. Pharmacol. *5*, 215–218 (1973)

Hollister, L.E., Gillespie, H.K.: Delta-8- and delta-9-tetrahydrocannabinol. Comparison in man by oral and intravenous administration. Clin. Pharmacol. Ther. *14*, 353–357 (1973)

Hollister, L.E., Gillespie, H.: Interactions in man of delta-9-tetrahydrocannabinol. II. Cannabinol and cannabidiol. Clin. Pharmacol. Ther. *18*, 80–83 (1975)

Jackson, D.M., Malor, R., Chesher, G.B., Starmer, G.A., Welburn, P.J., Bailey, R.: The interaction between prostaglandin E_1 and Δ^9-tetrahydrocannabinol on intestinal motility and on the abdominal constriction response in the mouse. Psychopharmacology *47*, 187–193 (1976)

Jacobs, J.A., Dellarco, A.J., Manfredi, R.A., Harclerode, J.: The effects of Δ^9-tetrahydrocannabinol, cannabidiol, and shock on plasma corticosterone concentrations in rats. J. Pharm. Pharmacol. *31*, 341–342 (1979)

Järbe, T.U.C.: Δ^9-tetrahydrocannabinol: Tolerance after noncontingent exposure in rats. Arch. Int. Pharmacodyn. Ther. *231*, 49–56 (1978)
Jain, M.L., Curtis, B.M., Bakutis, E.V.: In vivo effect of LSD, morphine, ethanol, and delta^9-tetrahydrocannabinol on mouse brain adenosine triphosphatase activity. Res. Commun. Chem. Path. Pharmacol. *7*, 229–232 (1974)
Johansson, J.O., Järbe, T.U.C., Henriksson, B.G.: Acute and subchronic influences of tetrahydrocannabinols on water and food intake, body weight, and temperature in rats. T.-I.-T.J. Life Sci. *5*, 17–28 (1975)
Johansson, J.O., Järbe, T.U.C., Henriksson, B.G.: Physostigmine attenuation of delta^9-tetrahydrocannabinol induced hyperthermia in rats. Experientia *30*, 779–780 (1974)
Johnson, S., Domino, E.F.: Some cardiovascular effects of marihuana smoking in normal volunteers. Clin. Pharmacol. Ther. *12*, 762–768 (1971)
Jones, G., Pertwee, R.G.: A metabolic interaction in vivo between cannabidiol and delta^1-tetrahydrocannabinol. Brit. J. Pharmacol. *45*, 375–377 (1972)
Jones, R.T., Benowitz, N., Bachman, J.: Clinical studies of cannabis tolerance and dependence. Ann. N.Y. Acad. Sci. *282*, 221–239 (1976)
Jusko, W.J., Schentag, J.J., Clark, J.H., Gardner, M., Yurchak, A.M.: Enhanced biotransformation of theophylline in marihuana and tobacco smokers. Clin. Pharmacol. Ther. *24*, 406–410 (1978)
Kalant, H., LeBlanc, A., Gibbins, R.J.: Tolerance to, and dependence on some non-opiate psychotropic drugs. Pharmacol. Rev. *23*, 135–191 (1971)
Kalofoutis, A., Koutselinis, A., Dionyssiou-Asteriou, A., Miras, C.: The significance of lymphocyte lipid changes after smoking hashish. Acta Pharmacol. Toxicol. *43*, 81–85 (1978)
Kanakis, Ch. jr., Pouget, J.M., Rosen, K.M: The effects of delta^9-tetrahydrocannabinol (cannabis) on cardiac performance with and without beta blockade. Circulation *53*, 703–707 (1976)
Kaymakçalan, S., Sivil, S.: Lack of tolerance to the bradycardic effect of delta^9-trans-tetrahydrocannabinol in rats. Pharmacology *12*, 290–295 (1974)
Kaymakçalan, S., Ercan, Z.S., Türker, R.K.: The evidence of the release of prostaglandin-like material from rabbit kidney and guinea pig lung by (−)-trans-delta^9-tetrahydrocannabinol. J. Pharm. Pharmacol. *27*, 564–568 (1975)
Kelly, L.A., Butcher, R.W.: Effects of delta^1-tetrahydrocannabinol (THC) on cyclic AMP metabolism in cultured human fibroblasts. In: Membrane Mechanisms of Drugs of Abuse. Sharp, Ch.W., Abood, L.G. (eds.), pp. 227–236. New York: Alan R. Liss Inc. 1979
Kilbey, M.M., Moore, J.W.jr., Hall, M.: Delta^9-tetrahydrocannabinol induced inhibition of predatory aggression in the rat. Psychopharmacology *31*, 157–166 (1973)
Klausner, H.A., Dingell, J.V.: The metabolism and excretion of delta^9-tetrahydrocannabinol in the rat. Life Sci. *10/I*, 49–59 (1971)
Kokka, N., Garcia, J.F.: Effects of delta^9-THC on growth hormone and ACTH secretion in rats. Life Sci. *15*, 329–338 (1974)
Kolodny, R.C., Masters, W.H., Kolodner, R.M., Toro, G.: Depression of plasma testosterone levels after chronic intensive marihuana use. N. Engl. J. Med. *290*, 872–874 (1974)
Kolodny, R.C., Lessin, P., Toro, G., Masters, W.H., Cohen, S.: Depression of plasma testosterone with acute marijuana administration. In: The Pharmacology of Marihuana. Braude, M.C., Szara, S. (eds.), pp. 217–225. New York: Raven Press 1976
Koukkou, M., Lehmann, D.: Correlations between cannabis-induced psychopathology and EEG before and after drug ingestion. Pharmakopsychiatry. *11*, 220–227 (1978)
Kubena, R.K., Barry, H. III.: Interactions of delta^1-tetrahydrocannabinol with barbiturates and methamphetamines. J. Pharmacol. Exp. Ther. *173*, 94–100 (1970)
Kubena, R.K., Perhach, J.L., Jr., Barry, H., III: Corticosterone elevation mediated centrally by Δ^1-tetrahydrocannabinol in rats. Eur. J. Pharmacol. *14*, 89–92 (1971)
Kupfer, D., Levin, E., Burstein, S.H.: Studies on the effects of delta^1-tetrahydrocannabinol (delta^1-THC) and DDT on the hepatic microsomal metabolism of delta^1-THC and other compounds in the rat. Chem.-Biol. Interactions *6*, 59–66 (1973)
Larsen, F.F., Pryor, G.T.: Factors influencing tolerance to the effects of delta^9-THC on a conditioned avoidance response. Pharmacol. Biochem. Behav. *7*, 323–329 (1977)
Law, F.C.P.: Metabolism and disposition of delta^1-tetrahydrocannabinol by the isolated perfused rabbit lung. Drug Metab. Disposition *6*, 154–163 (1978)

Lawrence, D.K., Gill, E.W.: The effects of delta^1-tetrahydrocannabinol and other cannabinoids on spin-labeled liposomes and their relationship to mechanisms of general anesthesia. Molec. Pharmacol. *11*, 595–602 (1975)

Lefkowitz, S.S., Klager, K.: Effect of delta^9-tetrahydrocannabinol on in vitro sensitization of mouse splenic lymphocytes. Immun. Commun. *7*, 557–566 (1978)

Lemberger, L., Rubin, A.: Cannabis: The role of metabolism in the development of tolerance. Drug. Metabol. Rev. *8*, 59–68 (1978)

Levy, G.: Pharmacokinetic approaches to the study of drug interactions. Ann. N.Y. Acad. Sci. *281*, 24–39 (1976)

Liakos, A., Boulougouris, J.C., Stefanis, C.: Psychophysiologic effects of acute cannabis smoking in long-term users. Ann. N.Y. Acad. Sci. *282*, 375–386 (1976)

Loewe, S., Goodman, L.S.: Anticonvulsant action of marihuana-active substances. Fed. Proc. *6*, 352 (1947)

Lokhandwala, M.F., Parianai, H.K., Buckley, J.P., Jandhyala, B.S.: Involvement of central alpha-adrenoceptors in the hypotensive and bradycardic effects of (−)-delta^9-trans-tetrahydrocannabinol. Eur. J. Pharmacol. *42*, 107–112 (1977)

Magour, S., Coper, H., Fähndrich, Ch., Hill, R.: Relationship between the subcellular distribution of delta^9-tetrahydrocannabinol and its metabolites in rat brain and the duration of the effect on motor activity. Life Sci. *18*, 575–584 (1976)

Magour, S., Coper, H., Fähndrich, Ch.: Is tolerance to delta^9-THC cellular or metabolic? The subcellular distribution of delta^9-tetrahydrocannabinol and its metabolites in brains of tolerant and non-tolerant rats. Psychopharmacology *51*, 141–145 (1977)

Malor, R., Jackson, D.M., Chesher, G.B.: Possible central dopaminergic modulation of the rise in plasma concentration of non-esterified fatty acids produced in the mouse by (−)-trans-delta^9-tetrahydrocannabinol. Biochem. Pharmacol. *27*, 407–413 (1978)

Manning, F.J.: Chronic delta^9-tetrahydrocannabinol. Transient and lasting effects on avoidance behavior. Pharmacol. Biochem. Behav. *4*, 17–21 (1976)

Mantilla-Plata, B., Harbiso, R.D.: Distribution studies of (^{14}C)-delta^9-tetrahydrocannabinol in mice: Effect of vehicle, route of administration, and duration of treatment. Toxicol. Appl. Pharmacol. *34*, 292–300 (1975)

Marcotte, J., Witschi, H.P.: Induction of pulmonary aryl hydrocarbon hydroxylase by marijuana. Res. Commun. Chem. Path. Pharmacol. *4*, 561–568 (1972)

Martin, B.R., Dewey, W.L., Harris, L.S., Beckner, J.S.: ^{3}H-delta^9-tetrahydrocannabinol tissue and subcellular distribution in the central nervous system and tissue distribution in peripheral organs of tolerant and nontolerant dogs. J. Pharmacol. exp. Ther. *196*, 128–144 (1976)

Martin, B., Agurell, St., Krieglstein, J., Rieger, H.: Perfusion of the isolated rat brain with (^{14}-C)-delta^1-tetrahydrocannabinol. Biochem. Pharmacol. *26*, 2307–2309 (1977)

Martz, R., Brown, D.J., Forney, R.B., Bright, T.P., Kiplinger, G.F., Rodda, B.E.: Propranolol antagonism of marihuana induced tachycardia. Life Sci. *11/1*, 999–1005 (1972)

McCallum, N.K., Eastwood, M.E.E.: In vivo binding of delta^1-tetrahydrocannabinol and cannabinol to rat serum proteins. J. Pharm. Pharmacol. *30*, 384–386 (1978)

McConnell, W.R., Dewey, W.L., Harris, L.S., Borzelleca, J.F.: A study of the effect of delta^9-tetrahydrocannabinol (delta^9-THC) on mammalian salivary flow. J. Pharmacol. Exp. Ther. *206*, 567–573 (1978)

McDonoguh, J.H., jr., Manning, F.J., Elsmore, T.F.: Reduction of predatory aggression of rats following administration of delta^9-tetrahydrocannabinol. Life Sci. *11/1*, 103–111 (1972)

McLendon, D.M., Harris, R.T., Maule, W.F.: Suppression of the cardiac conditioned response by delta^9-tetrahydrocannabinol: A comparison with other drugs. Psychopharmacology *50*, 159–163 (1976)

Mechoulam, R.: Cannabinoid Chemistry. In: Psychotropic Agents. Hoffmeister, F. (ed.), Part 2. Berlin-Heidelberg-New York: Springer 1980

Mendelson, J.H., Babor, T.F., Kuehnle, J.C. Rossi, A.M., Bernstein, J.G., Mello, N.K., Greenberg, J.: Behavioral and biologic aspects of marijuana use. Ann. N.Y. Acad. Sci. *282*, 186–210 (1976)

Mendelson, J.H., Ellingboe, J., Kuehnle, J.C., Mello, N.K.: Effects of chronic marihuana use on integrated plasma testosterone and luteinizing hormone levels. J. Pharmacol. Exp. Ther. *207*, 611–617 (1978)

Miczek, K.A.: Does THC induce aggression? Suppression and induction of aggressive reactions by chronic and acute delta^9-tetrahydrocannabinol treatment in laboratory rats. In: The Pharmacology of Marihuana. Braude, M.C., Szara, S. (eds.), pp. 499–514. New York: Raven Press 1976a
Miczek, K.A.: Mouse-killing and motor activity: Effects of chronic delta^9-tetrahydrocannabinol and pilocarpine. Psychopharmacology *47*, 59–64 (1976b)
Miczek, K.A.: Delta^9-tetrahydrocannabinol: Antiaggressive effects in mice, rats, and squirrel monkeys. Science *199*, 1459–1461 (1978)
Miczek, K.A.: Chronic delta^9-tetrahydrocannabinol in rats: Effect on social interactions, mouse killing, motor activity, consummatory behavior, and body temperature. Psychopharmacology *60*, 137–146 (1979)
Miller, L.L., Drew, W.G.: Cannabis. Review of behavioral effects in animals. Psychol. Bull. *81*, 410–417 (1974)
Milstein, S., McCannel, K.L., Karr, G.W., Clark, S.C.: Marijuana produced changes in pain tolerance: Experienced and naive subjects. J. Pharmacol. (Paris) *5*, suppl. 2: 67–68 (1974)
Mitchell, C.L.: The design and analysis of experiments for the assessment of drug interactions. Ann. N. Y. Acad. Sci. *281*, 118–135 (1976)
Mon, M.J., Jansing, R.L., Doggett, S., Stein, J.L., Stein, G.S.: Influence of delta^9-tetrahydrocannabinol on cell proliferation and macromolecular biosynthesis in human cells. Biochem. Pharmacol. *27*, 1759–1765 (1978)
Munson, A.E., Harris, L.S., Friedman, M.A., Dewey, W.L., Carchman, R.A.: Antineoplastic activity of cannabinoids. J. Natl. Cancer Inst. *55*, 597–602 (1975)
Nowlan, R., Cohen, S.: Tolerance to marijuana: Heart rate and subjective "high". Clin. Pharmacol. Ther. *22*, 550–556 (1977)
Noyes, R., jr., Brunk, S.F., Avery, D.H., Canter, A.: The analgesic properties of delta^9-tetrahydrocannabinol and codeine. Clin. Pharmacol. Ther. *18*, 84–89 (1975)
Parker, J.M., Dubas, T.C.: Automatic determination of the pain threshold to electroshock and the effects of delta^9-THC. Int. J. Clin. Pharmacol. *7*, 75–81 (1973)
Paton, W.D.M., Pertwee, R.G.: Effect of cannabis and certain of its constituents on pentobarbitone sleeping time and phenazone metabolism. Brit. J. Pharmacol. *44*, 250–261 (1972)
Peres-Reyes, M., Lipton, M.A., Timmons, M.C., Wall, M.E., Brine, D.R., Davis, K.H.: Pharmacology of orally administered delta^9-tetrahydrocannabinol. Clin. Pharmacol. Ther. *14*, 48–55 (1973)
Perez-Reyes, M., Timmons, M.C., Wall, M.E.: Long-term use of marihuana and the development of tolerance or sensitivity to delta^9-tetrahydrocannabinol. Arch. Gen. Psychiat. *31*, 89–91 (1974)
Peres-Reyes, M., Brine, D., Wall, M.E.: Clinical study of frequent marijuana use: Adrenal cortical reserve metabolism of a contraceptive agent and development of tolerance. Ann. N. Y. Acad. Sci. *282*, 173–179 (1976)
Pirch, J.H., Cohn, R.A., Osterholm, K.C., Barratt, E.S.: Antagonism of amphetamine locomotor stimulation in rats by single doses of marijuana extract administrated orally. Neuropharmacology *12*, 485–493 (1973)
Prakash, R., Aronow, W.S., Warren, M., Laverty, W., Gottschalk, L.A.: Effects of marihuana and placebo marihuana smoking of hemodynamics in coronary disease. Clin. Pharmacol. Ther. *18*, 90–95 (1975)
Pryor, G.T., Husain, S., Mitoma, C., Braude, M.C.: Acute and subacute interactions between delta^9-tetrahydrocannabinol and other drugs in the rat. Ann. N.Y. Acad. Sci. *281*, 171–189 (1976)
Pryor, G.T., Larsen, F.F., Husain, S., Braude, M.C.: Interactions of delta^9-tetrahydrocannabinol with d-amphetamine, cocaine, and nicotine in rats. Pharmacol. Biochem. Behav. *8*, 295–318 (1978)
Renault, P.F., Schuster, C.R., Freedman, D.X., Sikic, B., Nebel de Mello, D., Halaris, A.: Repeat administration of marihuana smoke to humans. Arch. Gen. Psychiat. *31*, 95–102 (1974)
Revuelta, A.V., Cheney, D.L., Wood, P.L., Costa, E.: GABA-ergic mediation in the inhibition of hippocampal acetylcholine turnover rate elicited by delta^9-tetrahydrocannabinol. Neuropharmacology *18*, 525–530 (1979)

Roth, S.H.: Stereospecific presynaptic inhibitory effect of delta^9-tetrahydrocannabinol on cholinergic transmission in the myenteric plexus of the guinea pig. Can. J. Physiol. Pharmacol. *56*, 968–975 (1978)
Roth, S.H., Williams, P.J.: The non-specific membrane binding properties of delta^9-tetrahydrocannabinol and the effects of various solubilizers. J. Pharm. Pharmacol. *31*, 224–230 (1979)
Sanders, J., Jackson, D.M., Starmer, G.A.: Interactions among the cannabinoids in the antagonism of the abdominal constriction response in the mouse. Psychopharmacology *61*, 281–285 (1979)
Schurr, A., Porath, O., Krup, M., Livne, A.: The effects of hashish components and their mode of action on monoamine oxidase from the brain. Biochem. Pharmacol. *27*, 2513–2517 1978)
Seevers, M.H., Deneau, G.A.: Physiological aspects of tolerance and physical dependence. In: Physiological Pharmacology. A Comprehensive Treatise. Vol. I: Nervous System – Part A: Central Nervous System Drugs. Root, W.S., Hofman, F.G. (eds.), pp. 565–640. New York, London: Academic Press Inc. 1963
Shapiro, B.J., Tashkin, D.P.: Effects of β-adrenergic blockade and muscarinic stimulation on cannabis broncho dilation. In: The Pharmacology of Marihuana. Braude, M.C., Szara, S. (eds.), pp. 277–286. New York: Raven Press 1976
Shapiro, B.J., Tashkin, D.P., Frank, I.M.: Mechanism of increased specific airways conductance with marijuana smoking in healthy young men. Ann. Intern. Med. *78*, 832–833 (1973)
Siemens, A.J., Doyle, O.L.: Cross-tolerance between delta^9-tetrahydrocannabinol and ethanol: The role of drug disposition. Pharmacol. Biochem. Behav. *10*, 49–55 (1979)
Siemens, A.J., Khanna, J.M.: Acute metabolic interactions between ethanol and cannabis. Alcoholism. Clin. Exp. Res. *1*, 343–348 (1977)
Siemens, A.J., DeNie, L.C., Kalant, H., Khanna, J.M.: Effects of various psychoactive drugs on the metabolism of delta^1-tetrahydrocannabinol by rats in vitro and in vivo. Eur. J. Pharmacol. *31*, 136–147 (1975)
Smith, S.H., Harris, L.S., Uwaydah, I.M., Munson, A.E.: Structure-activity relationships of natural and synthetic cannabinoids in suppression of humoral and cell-mediated immunity. J. Pharmacol. Exp. Ther. *207*, 165–170 (1978)
Smith, C.G., Besch, N.F., Smith, R.G., Besch, P.K.: Effect of tetrahydrocannabinol on the hypothalamic-pituitary axis in the ovariectomized rhesus monkey. Fertility Sterility *31*, 335–339 (1979)
Sofia, R.D., Kubena, R.K., Barry, H. III: Comparison among four vehicles and four routes for administering delta^9-tetrahydrocannabinol. J. Pharmaceut. Sci. *63*, 939–941 (1974)
Sofia, R.D., Vassar, H.B., Knobloch, L.C.: Comparative analgesic activity of various naturally occurring cannabinoids in mice and rats. Psychopharmacology *40*, 285–295 (1975)
Sofia, R.D., Strasbaugh, J.E., Banerjee, B.N.: Teratologic evaluation of synthetic delta^9-tetrahydrocannabinol in rabbits. Teratology *19*, 361–366 (1979)
Sprague, G.L., Craigmill, A.L.: Ethanol and delta^9-tetrahydrocannabinol: Mechanism for cross-tolerance in mice. Pharmacol. Biochem. Behav. *5*, 409–415 (1976)
Stenchever, M.A., Allen, M.: The effect of delta^9-tetrahydrocannabinol on the chromosomes of human lymphocytes in vitro. Am. J. Obstet. Gynecol. *114*, 819–821 (1972)
Stillman, R.C., Wyatt, R.J., Murphy, D.L., Rauscher, F.P.: Low platelet monoamine oxidase activity and chronic marijuana use. Life Sci. *23*, 1577–1582 (1978)
Sulkowski, A., Vachon, L., Rich, E.S. jr.: Propranolol effects on acute marihuana intoxication in man. Psychopharmacology *52*, 47–53 (1977)
Takahashi, R.N., Karniol, I.G.: Pharmacological interaction between cannabinol and delta^9-tetrahydrocannabinol. Psychopharmacology *41*, 277–284 (1975)
Tashkin, D.P., Shapiro, B.J., Frank, I.M.: Acute pulmonary physiologic effects of smoked marijuana and oral delta^9-tetrahydrocannabinol in healthy young men. N. Engl. J. Med. *289*, 336–341 (1973)
Tashkin, D.P., Soares, J.R., Hepler, R.S., Shapiro, B.J., Rachelefsky, G.S.: Cannabis, 1977. Ann. Intern. Med. *89*, 539–549 (1978)
Taylor, D.A., Fennessy, M.R.: Biphasic nature of the effects of delta^9-tetrahydrocannabinol on body temperature and brain amines of the rat. Eur. J. Pharmacol. *46*, 93–99 (1977)
Ten Ham, M., DeJong, Y.: Tolerance to the hypothermic and aggression-attenuating effect of delta^8- and delta^9-tetrahydrocannabinol in mice. Eur. J. Pharmacol. *28*, 144–148 (1974)

Vachon, L.: The smoke in marihuana-smoking. N. Engl. J. Med. *294*, 160–161 (1976)
Vachon, L., Fitzgerald, M.X., Soliday, N.H., Gould, I.A., Gaensler, E.A.: Single-dose effect of marihuana-smoke. Bronchial dynamics and respiratory-center sensitivity in normal subjects. N. Engl. J. Med. *288*, 985–989 (1973)
VanWent, G.F.: Mutagenicity testing of 3 hallucinogens: LSD, psilocybin, and delta^9-THC, using the micronucleus test. Experientia *34*, 324–325 (1978)
Varma, D.R., Goldbaum, D.: Effect of delta^9-tetrahydrocannabinol on experimental hypertension in rats. J. Pharm. Pharmacol. *27*, 790–791 (1975)
Webster, C.D., LeBlanc, A.E., Marshman, J.A., Beaton, J.M.: Acquisition and loss of tolerance to 1-delta^9-trans-tetrahydrocannabinol in rats on an avoidance schedule. Psychopharmacology *30*, 217–226 (1973)
Weiss, J.L., Watanabe, A.M., Lemberger, L., Tamarkin, N.R., Cardon, Ph.V.: Cardiovascular effects of delta^9-tetrahydrocannabinol in man. Clin. Pharmacol. Ther. *13*, 671–684 (1972)
Welburn, P.J., Starmer, G.S., Chesher, G.B., Jackson, D.M.: Effect of cannabinoids on the abdominal constriction response in mice: Within cannabinoid interactions. Psychopharmacology *46*, 83–85 (1976)
Widman, M., Nordqvist, M., Dollery, C.T., Briant, R.H.: Metabolism of delta^1-tetrahydrocannabinol by the isolated perfused dog lung. Comparison with in vitro liver metabolism. J. Pharm. Pharmacol. *27*, 842–848 (1975)
Wikler, A.: Aspects of tolerance to and dependence on cannabis. Ann. N.Y. Acad. Sci. *282*, 126–147 (1976)
Wikler, A., Lloyd, B.J.: Effect of smoking marijuanacigarettes on cortical electrical activity. Fed. Proc. *4*, 141–142 (1945)
Willinsky, M.D., Kalant, H., Meresz, O., Endrenyi, L., Woo, N.: Distribution and metabolism in vivo of ^{14}C-tetrahydrocannabinol in the rat. Eur. J. Pharmacol. *27*, 106–119 (1974)
Wilson, R.S., May, E.L.: Analgesic properties of the tetrahydrocannabinols, their metabolites, and analogs. J. Med. Chem. *18*, 700–703 (1975)
Wing, D.R., Paton, W.D.M.: An effect of cannabis treatment in vivo on noradrenaline-stimulated lipolysis in rat adipocytes. J. Pharm. Pharmacol. *30*, 802–803 (1978)
Witschi, H., Saint-Francois, B.: Enhanced activity of benzpyrene hydroxylase in rat liver and lung after acute cannabis administration. Toxicol. Appl. Pharmacol. *23*, 165–168 (1972)
Wrenn, J.M., Friedman, M.A.: Evidence for highly specific interactions between delta^8- and delta^9-tetrahydrocannabinol and hydrocortisone in the rodent tyrosine aminotransferase system. Toxicol. Appl. Pharmacol. *43*, 569–576 (1978)
Zalcman, St., Liskow, B., Cadoret, R., Goodwin, D.: Marijuana and amphetamine: The question of interaction. Am. J. Psychiat. *130*, 707–708 (1973)
Zaluzny, S.G., Chesher, G.B., Jackson, D.M., Malor, R.: The attenuation by delta^9-tetrahydrocannabinol and morphine of the quasi-morphine withdrawal syndrome in rats. Psychopharmacology *61*, 207–216 (1979)
Zwillich, C.W., Doekel, R., Hammill, St., Weil, J.V.: The effects of smoked marijuana on metabolism and respiratory control. Am. Rev. Respir. Dis. *118*, 885–891 (1978)

Alcohol

CHAPTER 9

General Pharmacology and Toxicology of Alcohol

T. L. CHRUŚCIEL

A. Introduction

Ethyl alcohol (Alcohol aethylicus, C_2H_5OH) has been used since the dawn of history in various beverages and, much later in the history of mankind, as a pure fluid substance, for nonmedical, pseudomedical, and medical purposes. At one time it was considered an important remedy for all diseases: the word "whisky" is believed to have its roots in the Gaelic *usquebough*, meaning "water of life" (RITCHIE, 1977). It is now recognized that the therapeutic value of alcohol is limited to its local external use; however, the social use of alcoholic beverages leading eventually to alcohol dependence and concurrent chronic intoxication, as well as frequently occurring cases of acute intoxication, calls for detailed knowledge of its pharmacology and toxicology.

Ethyl alcohol is an inflammable, volatile fluid resulting from carbohydrates fermentation by various species of the genus *Saccharomyces*. It ist also biosynthesized as a byproduct in the process of hexoses oxidation in plant and animal cells. Therefore, small amounts of ethyl alcohol constitute a normal element of animal tissues. In man the blood contains 0.027 mg-%, the liver tissue 0.227 mg-%, and the brain tissue 0.187 mg-% (SUPNIEWSKI, 1965).

B. General Pharmacology

The main effects of ethanol are on the central nervous system. The well-known signs and symptoms, during and following periods of intoxication, from mild inebriation on through drunkenness and the following hangover and to deep coma, illustrate that ethanol has typical and significant effects upon man. The earliest changes are upon the emotional and autonomic functions; a number of intellectual phenomena are adversely affected as intoxication progresses. It should be borne in mind that from the very beginning of its action in man ethanol is always a depressant.

I. Absorption

Alcohol is rapidly absorbed from the stomach, small intestine, and colon. The rate of absorption is variable among individuals and in the same subject at different times. Numerous factors modify the absorption of alcohol from the stomach: the volume, character, and concentration of the alcoholic beverage; the presence in the stomach of food and its characteristics (HAGGARD et al., 1941; LIN et al., 1976); the time sequence of eating and drinking (LIN et al., 1976); the rapidity of ingestion; delayed stomach emptying time; the occurrence of pylorospasmus due to high concentration

of alcohol. All these factors may influence considerably the absorption time. Alcohol itself can inhibit gastric emptying (Haggard et al., 1941; Nimmo, 1976). Food (particularly milk) delays alcohol absorption. An high-carbohydrate meal may have a greater inhibitory effect on alcohol absorption than one rich in fat (Welling et al., 1977). Fasting will bring about an increase in the rate of absorption.
Absorption from the small intestine is extremely rapid and complete: the presence of food does not interfere. Alcohol increases gastric and intestinal perfusion (Magnussen, 1968). The time of gastric emptying may well be the main factor determining the wide individual variation of absorption of alcohol (2–6 h or more).

II. Distribution

Alcohol is fairly uniformly distributed throughout all tissues and body fluids. It passes through placenta and has free access to the fetus. It is soluble and mixes well with water in all proportions. It dissolves lipids, and its water-lipid dissolution coefficient is relatively high. According to Overton-Meyerś theory on the role of lipid-water dissolution coefficient in narcotic action of lipid soluble substances, ethanol has no significant surgical anesthesia potential. In the brain the alcohol concentration quickly approaches that of the blood. The lethal concentration of alcohol in the brain was found to be 270–510 mg-% (Isselbacher, 1977).

III. Metabolism

Up to 98% of the alcohol that is ingested is completely metabolized yielding slightly over 7 calories per gram. The metabolic clearance of alcohol obeys the kinetics of Michaelis-Menten (Lundquist and Wolthers, 1958; Wagner and Patel, 1972; Wagner et al., 1976). The rate of alcohol oxidation is constant with time (zero-order pharmacokinetics). The amount of alcohol oxidized is proportional to body weight. The average rate of oxidation is 85 and 100 mg/kg body wt. per hour in women and men, respectively. The constant rate of metabolizing results in risk of accumulation after ingestion of higher doses. An adult man can metabolize 3–4 g/kg body wt. per day. Kalant (Rotschild et al., 1975) determined the daily maximal metabolism of alcohol to be about 450 ml. At least 80% of alcohol oxidation proceeds via a two-step pathway in which the initial oxidation takes place in the liver. Alcohol dehydrogenase (ADH, alcohol: NAD oxidoreductase; E.C. 11.1.1) oxidizes ethanol to acetaldehyde. ADH is a zinc-containing metalloproteid that utilizes NAD as the hydrogen acceptor (Rubin and Lieber, 1967). Human alcohol dehydrogenase is an NAD-dependent zinc-metalloenzyme (Vallee and Hoch, 1957). Limited studies suggest that human ADH may be dimeric, and its gross physical characteristics are similar to those of well-studied horse ADH (von Wartburg et al., 1964).

$$CH_3CH_2OH - 2H \rightarrow CH_3COH + O_2 + H_2O \rightarrow$$
$$CH_3COOH(+H_2O_2) - 4H \rightarrow 2CO_2 - 2H_2O$$
$$CH_3CH_2OH + H_2O_2 \rightarrow CH_3COOH + 2H_2O\,.$$

The second step is convertion by NAD-dependent aldehyde dehydrogenase, a molybden containing flavoproteid, of acetaldehyde to acetylcoenzyme A, which is then oxidized through the citric acid cycle or utilized in various lipid synthesis cycles. The oxidation of ethanol increases the NADH: NAD ratio. The blood concentration of acetic aldehyde averages between 20 and 50 μM in humans after consumption of an intoxicating dose of alcohol (MAJCHROWICZ and MENDELSON, 1970). Acetic aldehyde at millemolar levels will inhibit Na^{+}-, K^{+}, and Mg^{++}-activated ATPase (TABAKOFF, 1974) protein synthesis (PERIN et al., 1974), and the release of biogenic amines (SCHNEIDER 1974); yet, at lower, potentially physiological levels it does not affect many biological reactions. Westcott et al. (WESTCOTT et al., 1979) have shown that acetic aldehyde enters the brain of the rat treated with ethanol. It appears that an effective acetic aldehyde-metabolizing system exists in the brain that keeps acetic aldehyde at a low level during ethanol metabolism. This is most likely due to the presence of aldehyde dehydrogenase. The finding that acetic aldehyde is detectable in the extracellular fluid (WESTCOTT et al., 1979) shows that acetic aldehyde can cross the blood-brain barrier and is not totally metabolized in the capillaries. Pyrazole and its derivatives inhibit oxidation of ethanol and its elimination from the blood. THEORELL and YONETANI (1963) noted that pyrazole inhibits the activity of hepatic alcohol dehydrogenase. At high blood ethanol concentrations, only 50% of in vivo alcohol oxidation can be suppressed by the potent ADH inhibitor, pyrazole, or its alkyl derivatives (BURNETT and FELDER, 1980).

More recent studies suggest that microsomal oxidases from the smooth endoplasmic reticulum of the liver cell, a microsomal ethanol-oxidizing enzyme system (MEOS) may play a major role (LIEBER and DECARLI, 1968; ROACH, 1975) Catalase also oxidizes alcohol. LIEBER et al. (KALANT et al. 1971) have found the inhibition of MEOS as well as catalase by pyrazole.

Pyrazole is known to activate succinic dehydrogenase and cytochrome oxidase and inhibit lactid dehydrogenase (BESKID et al. 1978a; BESKID et al., 1978b; CEDERBAUM and RUBIN, 1974; KOELICHEN-SUDZIŁOWSKA et al., 1978; SKŁADZIŃSKI, 1976; SKŁADZINSKI and BESKID, 1978).

Concomitant application of pyrazole with ethanol produces hepatic necrosis (LELBACH, 1971; LIEBER et al., 1970; SKŁADZIŃSKI, 1976; SKŁADZIŃSKI and BESKID, 1978) and cortical lesions (BESKID et al., 1978a; BESKID et al., 1978b; KOELICHEN-SUDZIŁOWSKA et al., 1978). Pyrazole-insensitive ethanol oxidation has been attributed to a peroxidative activity of catalase and/or a microsomal ethanol-oxidizing system which bears some relation to the microsomal drug-metabolizing system.

Some portion of in vivo alcohol oxidation and in vitro microsomal alcohol oxidation is suppressed by the catalase inhibitors sodium azide and aminotriazole (BURNETT and FELDER, 1980).

The elevation of the ethanol clearance rate in response to chronic ethanol consumption is a well-established phenomenon (KORVULA and LINDROS, 1975; LIEBER and DE CARLI, 1968; TOBON and MEZEY, 1971).

BURNETT and FELDER (1980), using an Adh^{N}/Adh^{N} deer mouse strain from laboratory populations of *Peromyscus maniculatus* which lack liver ADH activity (BURNETT and FELDER, 1978), have found that these animals eliminated ethanol at a significantly slower rate than those of the normal strain. A comparison of the blood ethanol elimination in the Adh^{N}/Adh^{N} and normal strains indicated that, at high blood ethanol concentrations, non-ADH mediated pathways may account for as much as two-thirds of normal elimination in this species (Burnett and Felder, 1980). These results suggest that ethanol consumption may induce an increase only in the ADH pathway of alcohol oxidation. The increases of the blood alcohol elimination rate, following chronic alcohol consumption, are mediated primarily via the ADH pathway.

IV. Excretion

Normally, about 2% of ingested alcohol is excreted unchanged through the lungs, in perspiration, and with the urine. Exceptionally, this value may be as high as 10%. Efforts to hasten the detoxication by the use of diuretics or hyperpnea-inducing drugs are valueless.

V. Mechanism of Action

Ethanol is a protoplasmic poison which seems to act primarily by disrupting cell membranes (Chin and Goldstein, 1977; Seeman, 1972; Seeman, 1974). This action lacks chemical specificity and apparently results simply from a slight reduction in viscosity of the lipid bilayer. Ethanol precipitates proteins and dehydrates tissues; in the concentration of 70% v/v it is a potent bactericidal agent. Some chronic actions (e.g., physical dependence) of various alcohols correlate with lipid solubility. Four to five times more ethanol than t-butanol exposure was required to produce a given withdrawal reaction severity (McComb and Goldstein 1979). This ratio is the same as the relative lipid solubilities of the two alcohols (Leo et al., 1971; Lieber, 1978). McComb and Goldstein (McComb and Goldstein, 1979) have shown that physical dependence accumulates progressively when the two alcohols are given sequentially.

Quite recently, Jeffcoate et al. (Jeffcoate et al., 1979) have shown in double-blind, crossover study of 20 male volunteers that a single intravenous infusion of 0.4 mg naloxone, a typical opiate-receptor blocking agent, prevented the impairment of psychomotor performance induced by low levels of blood alcohol. Naloxone has been used to rouse comatose patients in alcohol intoxication (Mackenzie, 1979; Schenk et al., 1978; Sürenson and Mattison, 1978). The effects of naloxone tend to agree with the hypothesis that alcohol intoxication is mediated, at least in part, by an action on central opiate (endorphins) receptors. In 1970 Davis and Walsh underlined that dependence on alcohol was analogous to morphine-type dependence and suggested that the effects of alcohol may be caused by the generation of endogenous morphinelike alkaloids. Davis and Walsh (1970) noted that acetic aldehyde can condense with noradrenaline or serotonin to form Schiff bases and then undergo spontaneous rearrangement to tetrahydroisoquinolines or tetrahydropapaveroline. Such substances may be dependence producing and this was suggested as an explanation of the dependence-producing properties of alcohol (Rahwan, 1975). Cohen and Collins (Cohen and Collins, 1970) demonstrated the formation of such alkaloids from catecholamines and acetaldehyde in bovine adrenal tissue in vitro. The recent discovery of enkephalins and endorphins, the endogenous opioid peptides, enables one to complement and to rephrase the original Davis and Walsh theory. It is likely that alcohol produces intoxication by causing release of endorphins. Further research along these lines is necessary.

VI. Central Nervous System

Alcohol is a primary and continuing depressant of the central nervous system. The threshold effects appear when the concentration of ethyl alcohol in the blood is 20–30 mg-%; gross intoxication is seen at concentrations of 100 to 150 mg-%. Tolerance developes easily with chronic drinking. The average concentration in fatal cases is about 400 mg-% (Committee on Medico-legal Problems, 1968). Alcohol exerts its action first on the highly organized structures, particularly on the reticular activating system and the cortex, which is thus released from its integrating control (TOBON and MEZEY, 1971). The lack of inhibition produces the behavioral primary stimulation. The affection of mental processes depending on training and previous experience liquidate self-restriction and soberness. Discrimination, memory, concentration, and insight are dulled and then lost (ISSELBACHER, 1977). Changes in mood and behaviour, well described in all textbooks, follow. In general, the effects of alcohol are proportional to its concentration in the blood, and central effects, due to rapid absorption, may be rapidly obtained. They are, however, of relatively short duration (BEGLEITER and PLATZ, 1972).

The EEG responses to alcohol differ greatly between individuals – even between fraternal twins. Monozygotic twins show an almost identical reaction of the EEG to alcohol (PROPPING 1977). An average α-EEG in a pair of twins in the resting state and after alcohol loading shows that the extent of the alcohol-induced synchronization is similar (PROPPING, 1978) and seems to depend on the genetically determined nature of the resting EEG. PROPPING (1978) assumed that the variability of the normal human EEG may depend to a large extent on the differential tonic influence of the desynchronizing ascending reticular activating system (ARAS). Alcohol has been shown to diminish the spontaneous activity of the ARAS, thus improving synchronization of cortical discharges (CASPERS, 1957; CASPERS, 1958) i.e., the number of α- and ϑ-waves as well as the amplitudes for all frequency classes increase, whereas β-activity is diminished.

Chronic alcoholics show no consistent pathological changes in rhythm (Committee on Medico-legal Problems, 1968).

There is still no adequate understanding of the effect of ethyl alcohol on the human brain. The phenomenon of tolerance for alcohol has never been fully explained. The psychobiological factors predisposing to alcoholism remain unknown. The reason why certain heavy users do not become dependent are unknown.

Purely biological aspects of the effects of alcohol on the brain require further study (WEST, 1972). Alcohol increases neither mental nor physical abilities. Psychometric tests indicate that efficiency is decreased. Only in some special circumstances, e.g., when release of inhibitions is helpful, may alcohol cause some short-lasting improvement of performance. Like morphine, alcohol also causes euphoria, and it changes the patient's reaction to pain from one of concern to one of relative detachment (RITCHIE, 1977). Alcohol anesthesia lasts much longer than conventional anesthesia, and large doses may easily and dangerously depress respiration. For these reasons alcohol is no longer employed as a general surgical narcotic.

The diagnosis of alcohol intoxication is frequently quite easy; for the courts, particularly because of accidents resulting from driving of motor vehicles by persons who are drunk, the determination of blood alcohol concentration is essential for an assessment of drunkenness, and permits the establishment of the degree of intoxication. In most countries recommendations are similar to those issued in the United States by the National Safety Council and the American Medical Association. These recommendations can be summarized as follows: if the defendant's blood has a concentration of alcohol of 100 mg-% or over, he should be considered as being under the influence of alcohol; if 50 mg-% or under, not under the influence; if between 50 and 100 mg-%, other positive evidence indicating the guilt or innocence of the defendant must be considered. RITCHIE (1977) provides a number of examples of the relation of ingested alcohol beverage dose to blood alcohol concentration: on the average the ingestion of 44 g of alcohol taken as whisky (4 oz) or martini cocktail (5.5 oz) on an empty stomach results in a blood alcohol concentration of 41–79 mg-%. After a mixed meal the concentration would be considerably lower: 30–53 mg-%. The same amount of alcohol ingested on an empty stomach as conventional strength beer (1.2 l) results in a maximal blood concentration of 41–49 mg-%; after a mixed meal, 23–29 mg-%. After absorption is complete, the concentration in the blood at some desired time (e.g., at the time of the accident) can be estimated from the volume of distribution of the alcohol, which is 0.68 of the total body weight in men and 0.55 in women, and the metabolic rate of disappearance from the blood, which is about 10–25 (median 18) mg-%.

VII. Cardiovascular System

In general, the effects, particularly the immediate ones, on the heart and circulatory system are minor. Moderate amounts of alcohol do not significantly change the circulatory functional parameters. The pulse rate may temporarily increase. However, in laboratory animals and in men, a depression of the heart was observed after large doses. In the rat the concentration required (1250 mg-%) is about 30% greater than that which produces respiratory arrest (HAGGARD et al., 1941). The toxic effect on respiratory tract function remains the most important preoccupation in acute inebriation. However, recent studies make it clear that chronic excessive dependent use of alcohol has a harmful effect on the heart (BURCH and GILES, 1974; MYERSON, 1971).

Alcohol in moderate doses causes vasodilatation, especially of the cutaneous vessels, and produces the feeling of warmth and flushed skin. The vasodilatation is central in origin since the direct effect of alcohol on vasculary muscles is negligible. Alcohol in man in doses sufficient to produce facial vasodilatation does not change cerebral blood flow, cerebral metabolism, or cerebral vascular resistance (RITCHIE, 1977). Only large, intoxicating doses increase cerebral blood flow. Alcohol does not significantly dilate the coronary vessels. Its pseudo-nitroglycerinlike action seems to be due to its central depressant action.

VIII. Skeletal Muscles

The total amount of work accomplished by a person under the influence of small doses of alcohol may be increased (MYERSON, 1971; RITCHIE, 1977), mainly due to the central action of alcohol (lessened appreciation of fatigue). Large doses of alcohol decrease the amount of muscular work performed and damage the muscles (SONG and RUBIN, 1972).

Alcohol ingestion can cause rhabdomyopathy in man (LANE and MASTAGLIA, 1978). Alcoholic myopathy can be acute, subacute, or chronic (CURRAN and WETMORE, 1972; EKBOM et al., 1964; KUNKERFUSS et al., 1967; PERKOFF et al., 1967; PITTMAN and DECKER, 1971). Acute (or subacute) myopathy is related to the ingestion of excessive amounts of alcohol and is generally characterized by diffuse or focal tenderness and muscle cramps. The serum creatinine phosphokinase (CPK) activity is elevated, and muscle biopsy specimens frequently show a nonspecific pattern with degeneration and regeneration of muscle fibers (EKBOM et al., 1964; LAFAIR and MYERSON, 1978). Chronic alcohol myopathy is characterized by proximal muscle weakness with minimal, nonspecific changes on muscle biopsy specimens (EKBOM et al., 1964; PERKOFF et al., 1967; PITTMAN and DECKER, 1971). An alcohol challenge may be a useful diagnostic test in adult patients with unexplained myopathy or elevation in the serum CPK activity (SPECTOR et al., 1979). Alcoholic patients who drink large amounts or beer while eating little food may develop muscular weakness, dizziness, and confusion associated with hyponatremia, and a low serum and urinary osmolarity (hypoosmolarity syndrome). With a low dietary protein intake urea production is reduced and is insufficient to maintain the minimum urinary osmolarity; sodium is therefore lost in the urine and hyponatremia develops, since beer contains little sodium. Patients usually improve rapidly on a normal diet (HILDEN and SVENDSEN, 1975).

IX. Gastrointestinal Tract

Gastric and salivary secretions are both psychologically and reflexly stimulated by small, individually variable, doses of alcohol. The gastric juice, thus stimulated, is normal in pepsin content and is acidic (RITCHIE, 1977). In addition, alcohol more directly stimulates gastric secretion, probably through indirect stimulation of histamine H_2 receptors. This stimulation cannot be inhibited by therapeutic doses of atropine. Alcohol is, consequently, strongly contraindicated in patients with gastrointestinal diseases, particularly those with peptic ulcers of the stomach and/or duodenum.

Higher doses of alcohol, resulting in the presence of alcohol in the stomach in concentrations of above 20%, produce a stepwise inhibition of gastric secretion and depression of peptic activity. Strong alcoholic beverages (above 40% concentration) irritate the mucosa, cause hyperemia and may provoke inflammation serious enough to lead to erosive gastritis (LEEVY et al., 1971). One of three heavy drinkers suffers from chronic gastritis (RITCHIE, 1977). Very high doses inhibit gastrointestinal motor functions.

Alcohol in moderate amounts has little deleterious effect on intestinal functions. However, in chronic alcohol use a number of abnormalities may occur. Alcohol is an etiological factor in acute and chronic pancreatitis (PIROLA and LIEBER, 1974). Alcoholic liver disease is universal wherever alcoholic beverages are consumed. Alcohol is the major etiological factor in about two-thirds of cases of liver cirrhosis (Editorial, 1978).

Ethanol has a direct toxic effect on the liver and was shown to increase the rate at which isolated liver slices synthesize fat. The enhanced lipid anabolism resulting in deposition of fat in the liver cell occurs because the redox potential of liver is deranged by the constant drain on the coenzyme NAD. The oxidation of ethanol through acetaldehyde to acetic acid results in an increased NADH:NAD ratio. The consequent reduction in fatty acids oxidation results in hepatic fat deposition. The earliest and most common lesion is fatty infiltration, which may develop within 8 days after the start of heavy drinking (Lieber and Jones, 1965). Most patients with fatty liver do not develop cirrhosis, but some progress to alcoholic hepatitis, a precirrhotic lesion prognostic of later cirrhosis (Lieber, 1978). Electron microscopy has shown abnormalities of the subcellular organelles of liver cells. Structurally the changes are most evident in the mitochondria and include swelling and cavitation of the mitochondria, disorientation of their membrane convolutions (cristae) and the appearance of inclusion bodies (Fischer and Rankin, 1977; Svoboda and Manning, 1964). Such abnormal mitochondria have a reduced capacity to metabolize intermediary products of metabolic cycles and to oxidize fatty acids. It is noted, however, that not every mitochondrial function need be depressed and that individual constituents of the liver cell are damaged by alcohol in a varying degree.

Alcohol may also promote the fatty infiltration indirectly, for it causes the mobilization of fat from peripheral tissues (Ritchie, 1977).

In spite of these effects, in acute alcoholic intoxication in man, hepatic function tests do not indicate any great change in hepatic function (Beazell et al., 1942). Duration of drinking is important: most patients with alcoholic hepatitis or cirrhosis have been drinking heavily for many years (Beazell and Ivy, 1940; Wallgren and Barry, 1970).

X. Miscellaneous

Alcohol decreases renal tubular reabsorption of water, and hence it exerts a diuretic effect. It inhibits the secretion of the antidiuretic hormone. The diuretic effect is dose dependent, but repeated doses have an antidiuretic effect (Beard and Knott, 1971).

It is a popular conviction that alcohol is an aphrodisiac. However, the experimental evaluation of the influence of alcohol on sexual reflexes (Ritchie, 1977) support the frequently quoted citation of Shakespeare (Macbeth, act 2, scene 1): Mac Duff: What three things does drink especially provoke? Porter: Marry, Sir, nose-painting, sleep, and urine. Lechery, Sir, it provokes, and it unprovokes; it provokes the desire, but it takes away the performance...

In chronic alcohol use atrophic changes were noted in ovaries and testes; aspermia and infertility were observed.

Fetal alcohol syndrome was first recognized in the United States by Ulleland in 1972 (Government of the USA, 1978). It results in a characteristic pattern of congenital abnormalities including craniofacial and neurological abnormalities and those of the extremities. The syndrome is diagnosed in the United States annually in some 1,400–2,000 newborns, born mostly to alcoholic mothers. Ouellette et al. (1977) found a high percentage of identifiable abnormalities, in children of heavy drinkers. Of 27 women who drank heavily throughout pregnancy, 25 had children with abnormalities including microcephaly, short fissures of the eyelids, midfacial defects, and a flattened elongated vertical groove in the upper lip; abnormal palmar creases; joined, deviated or permanently flexed fingers and toes. In nearly half of reported cases there were cardiac septal defects, genital malformations, and hemangiomas. Prenatal growth retardation, delay in development, and low IQ of affected children, were also observed (Government of the USA, 1978; Jones, et al., 1976).

XI. Tolerance

The repeated use of alcohol results in the development of tolerance. Psychological tolerance is well known: the inexperienced drinker achieves a much greater response to the same dose of alcohol than does the experienced user. Bodily tolerance apparently develops gradually, and the user may become dependent. The degree of tolerance toward various effects of alcohol may differ individually, but in general the degree of tolerance is not as marked as for morphine-like drugs.

C. Interaction of Ethanol and Other Drugs

I. General Remarks

Both acute and chronic ethanol ingestion can alter both the pharmacodynamics and pharmacokinetics of other drugs and/or influence their behavioral effects. Action of ethanol is particularly visible and evident in concomitant use with psychotropic drugs of the depressant type. In general, enhanced effects of all anxiolytics and neuroleptics can be observed after ethanol use, if adequate and sufficiently sensitive measures of drug effects are used. Psychodepressant drug-alcohol interactions are mostly pharmacodynamic in character; potentiation of depressant action of alcohol on the central nervous system is prevalent in the clinical picture. The sedative and hypnotic action of alcohol is increased; the mood and intellectual capacity decreases and depression of respiration may be fatal. The pattern and magnitude of such pharmacodynamic interactions are not easily predicted and are difficult to evaluate because of the unlimited number of possible dose combinations (CARPENTER, 1975, LOEWI, 1953; SELLERS and HOLLOWAY, 1978). A further confusion is due to differences in the pharmacokinetic properties, especially the elimination rate, of each drug. Pharmacokinetic drug-alcohol interactions concern the influence of alcohol on resorption, distribution, metabolism, and elimination of drugs. Alcohol increases resorption from the stomach and intestines, influencing both the vessels and the passage of content in the gastrointestinal tract.

Drugs with long biological half-life, such as benzodiazepines, may potentiate alcohol effects even in cases in which intake of alcohol was 10–11 h preceded by drugs of this group.

Interaction is additionally complicated by changes related to chronic use of alcohol. It leads to tolerance that frequently decreases the pharmacological actions of neuroleptics, anxiolytics and narcotic drugs, if these are given shortly after alcohol is eliminated (KALANT et al., 1971; SELLERS and HOLLOWAY, 1978). This phenomenon, known as cross-tolerance, may in practice prohibit evaluation of interaction, particularly following the use of small doses. SELLERS and HOLLOWAY (1978) emphasize that for psychotropic drugs modification of their action by ethanol is probably much more important than pharmacokinetic interactions. However, our knowledge of the pharmacokinetics of a great number of drugs is as yet incomplete, and studies on pharmacokinetic interactions of alcohol and drugs in man are scarce.

The presence of ethanol in body fluids can alter drug distribution in the brain and other tissues.

There are considerable data indicating the mechanisms by which ethanol might influence drug disposition. It affects not only the central nervous system functions, but also circulation, including tissue blood flow, general metabolism of the body, intermediary metabolism, protein synthesis, and function of cell membranes (ISSELBACHER, 1977; ROTSCHILD et al., 1975; RUBIN and LIEBER, 1967; TOBON and MEZEY, 1971). The resulting changes in organ and tissue function may at least contribute to or modify completely kinetics of other drugs. Again, it is very difficult to foresee the character and direction of changes in effects in view of the complexity of the factors involved. In addition, chronic administration of ethanol stimulates drug metabolism, while acute large doses inhibit action of some enzymes, e.g., oxidase (KALANT et al., 1976; KHANNA et al., 1976; PIROLA, 1977; RUBIN and LIEBER, 1968). Alcohol dehydrogenase catalyzes the oxidation of alcohol to acetic aldehyde with formation of reduced NAD. In chronic users the concentration of NADH in the hepatic cells increases and other dehydrogenases, NAD dependent, decrease their activity. The accumulation of NADH in the liver is hepatotoxic and results in inhibition of glucose catabolism with increase of lactates, compensatory stimulation of lipid synthesis, fatty infiltration, and inhibition of neoglucogenesis (DINNENDAHL, 1980). This complex picture is based only partially on human data, and much additional research is necessary to clarify the issues. SELLERS and HOLLOWAY (1978) note that if ethanol were to substantially modify drug disposition, dosage adjustment might be required for some drugs with narrow margins of safety administered to chronic alcoholics.

II. Interaction of Alcohol with Psychotropic Drugs

LINNOILA and MATTILA (1973) determined that the decrease in driving skill following the intake of 1.2–1.5 g/kg alcohol equalled the decrease resulting when one-third of this dose of alcohol was taken concomitantly with a tranquilizer. WHITEHOUSE et al. (WHITEHOUSE et al., 1977) have found in rats that blood concentrations of methaqualone were statistically significantly higher in rats dosed with ethanol than in controls receiving only methaqualone. Other animal studies with diazepam (PAUL and WHITEHOUSE, 1977), glutethimide, SHETLAND and COURI, 1974) pentobarbital (SEIDEL, 1967), and tetrahydrocannabinol (SIEMENS et al., 1977) have also shown modifications of tissue drug concentrations. In man the plasma elimination half-life of meprobamate, pentobarbital, and tolbutamide is increased by acute ethanol intake (CARULLI and MANENTI, 1971; RUBIN et al., 1970). In the rat ethanol is a less potent inducer of augmentation in drug-metabolizing ability of the microsomes (KHANNA et al., 1972; MISRA et al., 1971; TOBON and MEZEY, 1971). Changes in plasma protein binding of drugs due to ethanol intake, although possible, do not seem to have clinical significance (KOCH-WESER and SELLERS, 1976; SELLERS, 1978). Alcohol pharmacokinetic interactions occur predominantly with uptake-limited binding-sensitive drugs (BLASCHKE, 1977) e.g., benzodiazepines, phenytoin, tolbutamide, warfarin, etc. Less affected are meprobamate, glutethimide, pentobarbital, and phenobarbital, all binding insensitive. Resorption of diazepam (HAYES et al., 1977), barbiturates, meprobamate, and amphetamines is increased. Alcohol increases the toxic gastric side-effects of nonsteroidal antiinflammatory drugs. In general, SELLERS and HOLLOWAY (1978) conclude that for psychoactive drugs cross tolerant with alcohol, the direct additive pharmacological action and the extent of central nervous system tolerance to ethanol will probably be more important than the effects of ethanol on drug metabolism.

III. Interaction of Alcohol with Nonpsychotropic Drugs

Interaction of alcohol with analgesics of the morphine type is particularly dangerous. Fatal cases were described (GREENE et al., 1974; SIMONSES, 1977; SUNDQUIST and PETROVICS, 1977).

Antihypertonics' (methyldopa, guanethidine) orthostatic action is increased by alcohol. β-adrenolytic drugs' central depressant effects are increased.

Antidiabetic biguanides producing lactic acidosis interact with alcohol (BLÖCH and LENHARDT, 1960; CARULLI, et al., 1971; FITZGERALD et al., 1962; KATER et al., 1969; KREISBERG et al., 1972; NELSON, 1962; SHAH et al., 1972; WARDLE and RICHARDSON, 1971) endangering the life of patients.

Since alcohol depresses the activity of NAD-dependent dehydrogenases necessary for steroid synthesis, in chronic use the decrease of the level of sex hormones was recorded, with decrease of libido and symptoms of feminization.

Interactions of alcohol with sulfonylureas, chloramphenicol, griseofulvin, metronidazol, and nitrofurantoin resemble disulfiram-alcohol interactions (FITZGERALD et al., 1962; WARDLE and RICHARDSON, 1971). Bromocryptine decreases alcohol tolerance.

In chronic use MEOS enzymes are involved to a larger extent in alcohol metabolism. Their participation in metabolism rises from approximately 10% to 25%. Drugs susceptible to such enzymes, contained in the endoplasmic reticulum of the liver cell, are not metabolized and their level may be increased, leading to stronger or toxic effects. Therefore, in the presence of alcohol the metabolism of some drugs can be lowered and their effects potentiated, while in the alcohol-free phase in alcoholics such substances are quickly metabolized and their effectiveness diminished.

Enzyme induction in chronic alcoholism results in lower blood level of dicoumarol derivatives, leading to decrease of anticoagulant action. On the contrary, in chronic, high use of alcohol, due to liver damage, inhibition of synthesis of coagulation factors results; the action of dicoumarol is increased and bleeding readiness can occur.

Enzyme induction is also the reason for decrease of blood levels of phenytoin. Even the occasional use of alcohol may lead to the decrease of anticonvulsant properties of this drug.

During concurrent use of strong diuretics (furosemid, thiazide derivatives) and alcohol, an increased frequency of occurrence of acute pancreatitis is noted.

Hepatotoxic effects of some tuberculostatic drugs (rifampicin, isoniazide) are increased by alcohol. Oculotoxic side-effects of ethambutol (retrobulbar neuritis) are increased; the chemotherapeutic activity of p-aminosalicylic acid is decreased.

Table 1. Drugs interacting with alcohol

Amphetamines	Chemotherapeutics
Analgesics, narcotic	Cytostatics
Antidepressants	Diuretics
Antidiabetics	Hormones
Antihistamines	Hypno-sedatives
Antihypertonics	Muscle relaxants
Anticoagulants	Neuroleptics
Anticonvulsants	Tranquilizers

Similarly, in cytostatic therapy with methotrexate or podophyllin and their derivatives the use of alcohol potentiates the frequency and increases the expression of side-effects (Dukes, 1979).

References

Beard, J.O., Knott, D.M.: The effect of alcohol on fluid and electrolyte metabolism. In: The biology of alcoholism. Biochemistry. Kissin, B., Begleiter, H., (eds.), Vol. 1, pp. 353–376. Ney York: Plenum Press 1971

Beazell, J.M. Berman, A.L., Hough, V.H., Ivy, A.C.: The effect of acute alcoholic intoxication on hepatic function. Am J. Dig. Dis. *9*, 82–85 (1942)

Beazell, J.M., Ivy, A.C.: The influence of alcohol in the digestive tract. Q.J. Stud. Alcohol *1*, 45–73 (1940)

Begleiter, H., Platz, A.: The effects of alcohol on the central nervous system in humans. In: The biology of alcoholism. Physiology and behaviour. Kissin, B., Begleiter, H., (eds.), pp. 243–343. New York: Plenum Press 1972

Beskid, M., Koelichen, A., Kwiatkowska, J.: Ultrastrukturalna ocena komórek kory mózgowej szczura w toku skojarzonego stosowania etanolu z pirazolem. Neuropatol. Pol. *16*, 361–373 (1978)

Beskid, M., Składziński, J., Sudziłowska, A., Kwiatkowska, J., Skierkowska, B., Majdecki, T.: Badania morfologiczne i histochemiczne komórek kory mózgowej szczura w toku skojarzonego stosowania etanolu i pirazolu. Probl. Lekarskie *2*, 321–337 (1978)

Blaschke, T.F.: Protein binding and kinetics of drugs in liver disease. Clin. Pharmacokinet. *2*, 32–44 (1977)

Blöch, J., Lenhardt, A.: Vorteile und Nachteile bei der Umstellung von Diabetikern von Rastinon auf Diabinese. Wien. Med. Wochenschr. *110*, 101–105 (1960)

Burch, G.E., Giles, T.D.: Alcoholic cardiomyopathy. In: The biology of alcoholism. Clinical pathology. Kissin, B., Begleiter, H. (eds.), Vol. 3, pp. 435–460. New York: Plenum Press 1974

Burnett, K.G., Felder, M.R.: Ethanol metabolism in Peromyscus genetically deficient in alcohol dehydrogenase. Biochem. Pharmacol. *29*, 125–130 (1980)

Burnett, K.G., Felder, R.N.: Genetic regulation of liver alcohol dehydrogenase in Peromyscus. Biochem. Genet. *16*, 443–454 (1978)

Carpenter, J.A.: Some methodological considerations in research on joint action. In: Clinical pharmacology of psychoactive drugs. Sellers, E.M. (ed.), pp. 147–164. Toronto: Alcoholism and Drug Addiction Research Foundation 1975

Carulli, N., Manenti, F.: Microsomal oxidation of ethanol and the drug metabolizing system. Studies in animals and man. In: Metabolic changes induced by alcohol. Martini, Bode (eds.), pp. 93–100. Berlin, Heidelberg, New York: Springer 1971

Carulli, N., Manenti, F., Gallo, M., Salvioli, G.F.: Alcohol-drugs interaction in man. Alcohol and tolbutamide. Eur. J. Clin. Invest. *1*, 421–424 (1971)

Caspers, H.: Die Beeinflussung der corticalen Krampferregbarkeit durch das aufsteigende Reticulärsystem des Hirnstammes. I. Reizwirkungen. Z. Ges. Exp. Med. *129*, 128–144 (1957)

Caspers, H.: Die Beeinflussung der corticalen Krampferregbarkeit durch das aufsteigende Reticulärsystem des Hirnstammes. II. Narkosewirkungen. Z. Ges. Exp. Med. *129*, 582–600 (1958)

Cederbaum, A.J., Rubin, E.: Effects of pyrazole, 4-bromopyrazole and 4-methylpyrazole on mitochondrial function. Biochem. Pharmacol. *23*, 203–213 (1974)

Chin, J.H., Goldstein, D.B.: Effects of low concentrations of ethanol on the fluidity of spin-labeled erythrocyte and brain membranes. Mol. Pharmacol. *13*, 435–441 (1977)

Cohen, G., Collins, M.: Alkaloids from catecholamines in adrenal tissue: possible role in alcoholism. Sciene *167*, 1749–1751 (1970)

Committee on Medico-legal Problems: Alcohol and the impaired driver: a manual on the medicolegal aspects of chemical tests for intoxication. Chicago: Am. Med. Assoc. 1968

Curran, J.R.,Wetmore, S.J.: Alcoholic myopathy. Dis. Nerv. Syst. *33*, 19–22 (1972)

Davis, V.E., Walsh, M.J.: Alcohol, amines, alkaloids: a possible biochemical basis for alcohol addiction. Science *167*, 1005–1007 (1970)

Dinnendahl, V.: Einfluß von Alkohol auf den Stoffwechsel von Arzneimitteln. Pharm. Z. *125*, 122–126 (1980)
Dukes, M.N.G.: Side effects of drugs. Amsterdam: Excerpta Medica 1979
Editorial. Towards prevention of alcoholic liver disease. Lancet *1978 II*, 353–354
Ekbom, K., Hed, R., Kirstein, L., Astrom, K.E.: Muscular affections in chronic alcoholism. Arch. Neurol. *10*, 449–458 (1964)
Fischer, M.M., Rankin, J.G. (eds.): Alcohol and the liver. New York: Plenum Press 1977
Fitzgerald, M.G., Gaddie, R., Malins, J.M., O'Sullivan, D.J.: Alcohol sensitivity in diabetics receiving chlorpropamide. Diabetes *11*, 40–43 (1962)
Government of the USA: Alcohol and your unborn baby. DHEW Publ. Nr. (ADM) 78–521, Washington, DC: U.S. Government Printing Office 1978
Government of the USA: Third special report of the U.S. Congress on alcohol and health. DHEW Publ. No. (ADM) 78–568. Washington, DC: U.S. Government Printing Office, June 1978
Greene, M.H., Luke, J.L., Dupont, R.L.: Opiate "overdose" death in the District of Columbia. 1. Heroin related fatalities. Med. Ann. D. C. *43*, 175–178 (1974)
Haggard, H.W., Greenberg, L.A., Cohen, L.H., Rakieten, N.: Studies on the absorption, distribution and elimination of alcohol. IX. The concentration of alcohol in the blood causing primary cardiac failure. J. Pharmacol. Exp. Ther. *71*, 358–361 (1941)
Haggard, H.W., Greensberg, L.A., Lolli, G.: The absorption of alcohol with special reference to its influence on the concentration of alcohol appearing in the blood. Q. J. Stud. Alcohol *1*; 684–690 (1941)
Hayes, S.L., Pablo, G., Radomski, T., Palmer, R.F.: Ethanol and oral diazepam absorption. New Engl. J. Med. *296*, 186–189 (1977)
Hetland, L.B., Couri, D.: Effects of ethanol on glutetimide absorption and distribution in relationship to a mechanism for toxicity enhancement. Toxicol. Appl. Pharmacol. *30*, 26–35 (1974)
Hilden, T., Svendsen, T.L.: Electrolyte disturbances in beer drinkers. A specific "hypo"-osmolality syndrome". *Lancet 1975 II*, 245–246
Isselbacher, K.J., Metabolic and hepatic effects of alcohol. New Engl. J. Med. *296*, 612–616 (1977)
Jeffcoate, W.J., Herbert, M., Cullen, M.H., Hastings, A.G., Walder, C.P.: Prevention of effects of alcohol intoxication by naloxone. Lancet *1979 II*, 1157–1159
Jones, K.L., Smith, D.W. Hannson, J.W.: The fetal alcohol syndrome: clinical delineation. Ann. N. Y. Acad. Sci. *273*, 130–139 (1976)
Kalant, H., Khanna, J.M., Lin, G.Y., Ghung, S.: Ethanol – a direct inducer of drug metabolism. Biochem. Pharmacol. *25*, 337–342 (1976)
Kalant, H., Leblanc, A.E., Gibbins, R.J.: Tolerance to and dependence on some non-opiate psychotropic drugs. Pharmacol. Rev. *23*, 135–191 (1971)
Kater, R.M.H., Tobon, F., Iber, F.L.: Increased rate of tolbutamide metabolism in alcoholic patients. J. Am. Med. Assoc. *207*, 363–365 (1969)
Khanna, J.M., Kalant, H., Lin, G.: Significance in vitro of the increase in microsomal ethanol-oxidizing systems after chronic administration of ethanol, phenobarbital and chlorcyclizine. Biochem. Pharmacol. *21*, 2215–2226 (1972)
Khanna, J.M., Kalant, H., Yee, Y., Chung, S., Siemens, A.J.: Effect of chronic ethanol treatment on metabolism of drugs in vitro and in vivo. Biochem. Pharmacol. *25*, 329–335 (1976)
Kunkerfuß, G., Bleisch, V., Dioso, M.M., Perkoff, G.T.: A spectrum of myopathy associated with alcoholism. II. Light and electron microscopic observations. Ann. Intern. Med. *67*, 493–510 (1967)
Koch-Weser, J., Sellers, E.M.: Binding of drugs to serum albumin. New Engl. J. Med. *294*, 526–531 (1976)
Koelichen-Sudziłowska, A., Kwiatkowaska, J., Beskid, M.: Histochemiczna ocena mózgu szczura w toku skojarzonego stosowania etanolu z pirazolem. Neuropatol. Pol. *4*, 519–531 (1978)
Korvula, T., Lindros, K.O.: Effects of long-term ethanol treatment on aldehyde and alcohol dehydrogenase activities in rat liver. Biochem. Pharmacol. *24*, 1937–1942 (1975)
Kreisberg, R.A., Owen, W.C., Siegal, A.M.: Hyperlacticacidemia in man. Ethanol-phenformin synergism. J. Clin. Endocrinol. Metab. *34*, 29–35 (1972)

Lafair, S., Myerson, R.M.: Alcoholic myopathy with special reference to the significance of creatine phosphokinase. Arch. Intern. Med. *122*, 417–422 (1978)
Lane, R.J.M., Mastaglia, F.L.: Drug-induced myopathies in man. *Lancet 1978 II*, 562–566
Leevy, C.M., Tanribilir, A.K., Smith, F.: Biochemistry of gastrointestinal and liver disease in alcoholism. In: The biology of alcoholism. Kissin, B., Begleiter, H. (eds.), vol. I, pp. 307–325. New York: Plenum Press 1971
Lelbach, W.K.: Experimental hepatocellular necrosis induced by ethanol after partial inhibition of liver alcohol dehydrogenase. In: Metabolic changes induced by alcohol, pp. 62–67. Berlin, Heidelberg, New York: Springer 1971
Leo, A., Hansch, C., Elkins,D.: Partition coefficients and their uses. Chem. Rev. *71*, 525–616 (1971)
Lieber, C.S.: Pathogenesis and early diagnosis of alcohol liver injury. New Engl. J. Med. *298*, 888–893 (1978)
Lieber, C.S., DeCarli, L.M.: Ethanol oxidation by hepatic microsomes: adaptive increase after ethanol feeding. Science *162*, 917–918 (1968)
Lieber, C.S., DeCarli, L.M.: Hepatic microsomal ethanoloxidizing system. In vitro characteristics and adaptive properties in vivo. J. Biol. Chem. *245*, 2505–2512 (1970)
Lieber, C.S., Jones, D.P., DeCarli, L.M.: Effects of prolonged ethanol intake: production of fatty liver despite adequate diets. J. Clin. Invest. *44*, 1009–1021 (1965)
Lieber, C.S., Rubin, E., DeCarli, L.M., Misra, P., Gang, H.: Effects of pyrazole on hepatic function and structure. Lab. Invest. *22*, 615–621 (1970)
Lin, Y.J., Weidler, D.J., Garg, D.S., Wagner, J.G.: Effects of solid food on blood levels of alcohol in man. Res. Commun. Chem. Pathol. Pharmacol. *13*, 713–716 (1976)
Linnoila, M., Mattila, M.J.: Drug interaction on driving skills as evaluated by laboratory tests and by a driving simulator. Pharmakopsychiatrie *6*, 127–132 (1973)
Loewi, S.: The problem of synergism and antagonism of combined drugs. Arzneim. Forsch. *3*, 285–290 (1953)
Lundquist, F., Wolthers, H.: The kinetics of alcohol elimination in man. Acta Pharmacol. Toxicol. *14*, 265–269 (1958)
Mackenzie, A.: Naloxone in alcohol intoxication. Lancet *1979 I*, 733–734
Macy, R.: Partition coefficients of fifty compounds between olive oil and water at 20 °. J. Ind. Hyg. Toxicol. *30*, 140–143 (1948)
Magnussen, M.P.: The effect of ethanol on the gastrointestinal absorption of drugs in the rat. Acta Pharmacol. Toxicol. *26*, 130–144 (1968)
Majchrowicz, E., Mendelson, J.H.: Blood concentration of acetaldehyde and ethanol in chronic alcoholics. Science *168*, 1100–1102 (1970)
McComb, J.A., Goldstein, D.G.: Additive physical dependence: evidence for a common mechanism in alcohol dependence. J. Pharmacol. Exp. Ther. *210*, 87–90 (1979)
Misra, P.S., LeFevre, A., Ischii, H., Rubin, E., Lieber, C.S.: Increase of ethanol, meprobamate and pentobarbital metabolism after chronic ethanol administration in man and in rats. Am. J. Med. *51*, 346–351 (1971)
Myerson, R.M.: Effects of alcohol on cardiac and muscular function. In: Biological basis of alcoholism. Israel, Y., Mardones, J. (eds.), pp. 183–208. New York, John Wiley and Sons, 1971
Nelson, E.: Zero-order oxidation of tolbutamide in vivo. Nature *193*, 76–77 (1962)
Nimmo, W.S.: Drugs, diseases and altered gastric emptying. Clin. Pharmacokinetics *1*, 189–203 (1976)
Ouellette, E.M., Rosett, H., Rosman, P., Weiner, L.: Adverse effects on offspring of maternal alcohol abuse during pregnancy. New Engl. J. Med. *297*, 528–530 (1977)
Paul, C.J., Whitehouse, L.W.: Metabolic bases for the supraadditive effect of the ethanol-diazepam combination in mice. Brit. J. Pharmacol. *60*, 83–90 (1977)
Perin,A., Scalabrini, G., Sessa, A., Arnaboldi, A.: In vitro inhibition of protein synthesis in rat liver as a consequence of ethanol metabolism. Biochem. Biophys. Acta *366*, 101–108 (1974)
Perkoff, G.T., Dioso, M.M., Bleisch, V., Klinkerfuss, G.: A spectrum of myopathy associated with alcoholism. I. Clinical and labroatory features. Ann. Intern. Med. *67*, 481–492 (1967)
Pirola, R.C.: Drug metabolism and alcohol. Baltimore: University Park Press 1977
Pirola, R.C., Lieber, C.S.: Acute and chronic pancreatitis. In: The biology of alcoholism. Clinical pathology, vol. 3, pp. 359–402. New York: Plenum Press 1974

Pittman, J.G., Decker, J.W.: Acute and chronic myopathy associated with alcoholism. Neurology *21*, 293–296 (1971)
Propping, P.: Genetic control of ethanol action on the central nervous system.An EEG study in twins. Hum. Genet. *35*, 309–334 (1977)
Propping, P.: Pharmacogenetics. Rev. Physiol. Biochem. *83*, 123–173 (1978)
Rahwan, R.: Toxic effects of ethanol: Possible role of acetaldehyde, tetrahydroisoquinolines and tetrahydro-β-carbolines. Toxicol. Appl. Pharmacol. *34*, 3–27 (1975)
Ritchie, J.M.: The aliphatic alcohols. In: Goodman, L.S., Gilman, A.: The pharmacological basis of therapeutics. 5th ed., pp. 137–151. New York: Mac Millan Publ. Co. Inc. 1977
Roach, M.K.: Microsomal ethanol oxidation: activity in vitro and in vivo. Adv. Exp. Med. Biol. *56*, 33–55 (1975)
Rotschild, M.A., Oratz, M., Schreiber, S.S. (eds.): Alcohol and abnormal protein biosynthesis-biochemical and clinical. Oxford: Pergamon Press Inc. 1975
Rubin, E., Gang, H., Misra, P.S., Lieber, C.S.: Inhibition of drug metabolism by acute ethanol intoxication. A hepatic microsomal mechanism. Am. J. Med. *49*, 801–806 (1970)
Rubin, E., Lieber, C.S.:Early fine structural changes in the human liver induced by alcohol. Gastroenterology *52*, 1–13 (1967)
Rubin, E., Lieber, C.S.: Hepatic microsomal enzymes in man and rat: induction and inhibition by ethanol. Science *162*, 690–691 (1968)
Schenk, G.K., Engelmeier, M.P., Matz, D., Pach, J.: High dosage naloxone treatment in acute alcohol intoxication, p. 386. Proc. CINP Congress, Vienna 1978
Schneider, F.H.: Effects of length of exposure to and concentration of acetaldehyde on the release of catecholamines. Biochem. Pharamcol. *23*, 223–229 (1974)
Seeman, P.: The membrane actions of anesthetics and tranquilizers. Pharmacol. Rev. *24*, 583–655 (1972)
Seeman, P.: The membrane expansion theory of anesthesia: Direct evidence using ethanol and a high-precision density meter. Experientia *30*, 759–760 (1974)
Seidel, G.: Distribution of pentobarbital, barbital and thiopenthal under ethanol. N.S. Arch. Pharmakol. Exp. Pathol. *257*, 221–229 (1967)
Sellers, E.M.: The clinical importance of interactions based on displacement of protein bound drugs. Proc. VIIth Intl Congress of Pharmacol., Paris 1978
Sellers, E.M., Holloway, M.R.: Drug kinetics and alcohol ingestion. Clin. Pharmacokinet. *3*, 440–452 (1978)
Shah, M.N., Clancy, B.A., Iber, F.L.: Comparison of blood clearence of ethanol and tolbutamide and the activity of hepatic ethanol-oxidizing and drug-metabolizing enzymes in chronic alcoholic subjects. Am. J. Clin. Nutr. *25*, 135–139 (1972)
Siemens, A.J., Jatinder, M., Khanna, J.M.: Acute metabolic interactions between ethanol and cannabis. Alcoholism. Clin. Exp. Res. *1*, 343–348 (1977)
Simonses, J.: Accidental fatal drug poisoning with particular reference to dextropropoxyphene. Forens. Sci. *10*, 127–131 (1977)
Składzinski, J.: Morfologiczne, histochemiczne i ultrastrukturalne badania wątroby szczura w toku skojarzonego stosowania pirazolu i etanolu. Zeszyty Naukowe ASW, Suppl. *14*, 1–3 (1976)
Składziński, J., Beskid, M.: Combined action of pyrazole and ethanol on a rat liver: Histochemical and ultrastructural study. Folia Histochem. Cytochem. *16*, 13–18 (1978)
Song, S.K., Rubin, E.: Ethanol produces muscle damage in human volunteers. Science *175*, 327–382 (1972)
Sörensen, S.C., Mattison, K.W.: Naloxone as an antagonist in severe alcohol intoxication. Lancet *1978 II*, 688–689
Spector, R., Choudhury, A., Cancilla, P., Lakin, R.: Alcohol myopathy. Diagnosis by alcohol challenge. J. Am. Med. Assoc. *242*, 1648–1649 (1979)
Sundquist, L., Petrovics, J.: Fatal poisoning with dextropropoxyphene containing analgetics – suicide or not? Acta Med. Scand. *196*, 467–470 (1977)
Supniewski, J.: Farmakologia. Warszawa: PZWL 1965
Svoboda, D.J., Manning,R.T.: Am. J. Pathol. *44*, 645–650 (1964)
Tabakoff, B.: Inhibition of sodium, potassium and magnesium activated ATPases by acetaldehyde and "biogenic" aldehydes. Res. Commun. Chem. Path. Pharmacol. *7*, 621–624 (1974)

Theorell, H., Yonetani, T.: Liver alcohol dehydrogenase-DPN-Pyrazole complex. Biochem. Z. *338*, 537–553 (1963)
Tobon, F., Mezey, E.: Effect of ethanol administration on hepatic ethanol and drug-metabolizing enzymes and on rates of ethanol degradation. J. Lab. Clin. med. *77*, 110–121 (1971)
Vallee, B.L., Hoch, F.L.: Zinc in horse liver alcohol dehydrogenase. J. Biol. Chem. *225*, 185–195 (1957)
Von Wartburg, J.P., Bethune, J.L., Vallee, B.L.: Human liver alcohol dehydrogenase kinetic and physicochemical properties. Biochemistry *3*, 1775–1782 (1964)
Wagner, J.G., Patel, J.A.: Variations in absorbtion and elimination rates of ethyl alcohol in a single subject.Res. Commun. Chem. Path. Pharmacol. *4*, 61–67 (1972)
Wagner, J.G., Wilkinson, P.K., Sedman, A.J., Kay, D.R., Weidler, D.J.: Elimination of alcohol from human blood. J. Pharm. Sci. *65*, 152–158 (1976)
Wallgren, H., Barry, H. III: Actions of alcohol, vols. I and II. New York: Elsevier Publ. Co. Inc. 1970
Wardle, E.N., Richardson, G.O.: Alcohol and glibenclamide. Brit. med. J. *1971 III*, 309–310
Welling, P.G., Lyons, L.L. Elliott, M.S., Amidon, G.L.: Pharmacokinetics of alcohol following single low doses to fasted and nonfasted subjects. J. Clin. Pharmacol. 199–206 (1977)
West, L.J.: Research strategies in alcoholism. Ann. N.Y. Ac. Sci. *197*, 13–15 (1972)
Westcott, J.Y., Weiner, H., Shultz, J., Myers, R.D.: In vivo acetaldehyde in the brain of the rat treated with ethanol. Biochem. Pharmacol. *29*, 411–417 (1979)
Whitehouse, L.W., Peterson, G., Paul, C.J., Thomas, B.H.: Effect of ethanol on the pharmacokinetics of 2-^{14}C-methaqualone in the rat. Life Sci. *20*, 1871–1878 (1977)

CHAPTER 10

Behavioral Pharmacology of Alcohol

N. K. MELLO

A. Introduction

Although alcohol is one of the earliest drugs used by man to change behavior and to modulate subjective states, less is known about its behavioral pharmacology than about many drugs of more recent origin. This is probably due to a complex interweaving of social attitudes and beliefs about alcohol which have evolved from a common familiarity with drinking and the effects of alcohol intoxication. For many years, the assumption that all is known, coupled with denial that alcoholism is a form of drug addiction, and ambivalence about problem drinking, tended to limit experimental interest in the study of alcohol and behavior (MELLO, 1976b, 1978b). Gradually, over the past 15 years, an increasing number of studies have examined the behavioral effects of alcohol in normal social drinkers and in alcohol addicts. The early evidence that alcoholism is a form of addiction (VICTOR and ADAMS, 1953; ISBELL et al., 1955; MENDELSON, 1964) has been consistently reaffirmed (MELLO and MENDELSON, 1977 for review). As more empirical studies have examined the effects of alcohol during intoxication rather than relying on retrospective self-reports, the limitations of commonly shared expectancies about alcohol's effects have become increasingly evident. The disparities between anticipated and observed effects of intoxication illustrate how far we now are from a comprehensive understanding of the behavioral pharmacology of alcohol (MELLO and MENDELSON, 1978a for review).

This review will discuss some methodological issues which continue to affect the interpretation of behavioral data (MELLO, 1968). A selective review of clinical research will focus on the effects of alcohol intoxication on those aspects of behavior and subjective states which are often alleged to account for alcohol abuse. The implications of these findings for understanding the way in which alcohol maintains behavior leading to its administration, i.e., alcohol's reinforcing properties, will also be considered. The clinical aspects of alcoholism, i.e., tolerance and physical dependence, the clinical expression and treatment of the alcohol withdrawal syndrome, and theoretical models which attempt to account for alcohol dependence were described in a previous volume of this handbook (MELLO and MENDELSON, 1977). Consequently, this review will be restricted to the behavioral pharmacology of alcohol in man and animal models.

Alcohol has now been shown to be an effective reinforcer in primate drug self-administration models. The reinforcing properties of alcohol have been demonstrated in preparations which are not physically dependent on alcohol. Systematic analysis of the variables which influence alcohol self-administration has begun quite recently and illustrative studies will be described. Since these data are best understood in the context of the struggle to develop adequate animal models of alcoholism, the current status of models of alcohol dependence will also be summarized. This review will not include studies of the *effects* of alcohol on psychomotor performance or schedule-controlled behavior, since recent descriptions of these data are available elsewhere (ISRAELSTAM and LAMBERT, 1975; MCMILLAN and LEANDER, 1976; MELLO and MENDELSON, 1978a).

B. Issues in Measurement and Interpretation

Clinical studies of the behavioral and subjective effects of alcohol have shown that the consequences of intoxication often are not entirely predictable from the dose of alcohol given or from the blood alcohol level achieved. In addition to physiologic factors which influence the rate of alcohol absorption and the effective dose achieved, a number of nonpharmacologic factors, such as expectancy, experience with alcohol, and motivation to perform accurately, may also modulate the behavioral effects of alcohol. Studies of the behavioral effects of alcohol continue to share a series of methodological problems which often limit the generality of the findings obtained. Some frequent common problems are discussed in this section. Several problems are specific to behavioral studies of alcohol, and others apply equally to behavioral studies of any drug.

I. Methodological Issues Specific to Alcohol Studies

1. Blood Alcohol Level Measurement

Alcohol offers a particular advantage over many other psychoactive drugs for behavioral studies in man. The effective dose of alcohol can be rapidly and efficiently measured, at any point in time, by some variant of a breathalyzer device, which measures the concentration of alcohol in expired air (DUBOWSKI, 1970). Consequently, it is not necessary to rely on estimates of effective dosage on the basis of the amount of alcohol administered; the effective blood alcohol concentration can be quantitatively assessed. Direct measures are important because blood alcohol levels are not constant through time, but rather rise to a peak and then fall at a rate which is influenced by all of the factors which affect absorption, distribution, and metabolism. There are now considerable behavioral data which support Goldberg's (GOLDBERG, 1943) early observation that the greatest impairment in performance occurs during the rising phase of the blood alcohol curve, and there may be no impairment at equivalent blood alcohol levels during the falling phase of the curve (JONES, 1973; JONES and VEGA, 1972). In animals, alcohol concentration in small samples of blood can be measured with a variety of enzymatic and gas chromatographic techniques. It is also possible to measure alcohol concentration in urine.

It is unfortunate that many investigators still neglect to determine the effective alcohol concentration, fail to report blood alcohol levels, and occasionally even fail to specify the alcohol dosage. This perpetuates the inconsistent and ambiguous status of behavioral data on alcohol. Without information about alcohol dose and blood alcohol level it is impossible to compare studies and identify the basis for discrepant findings. Some would argue that since alcohol is metabolized at the rate of about 1 oz per hour, it is possible to estimate changes through time, if the initial dose is known. The difficulties involved in the quantitative analysis of blood levels of many other psy-

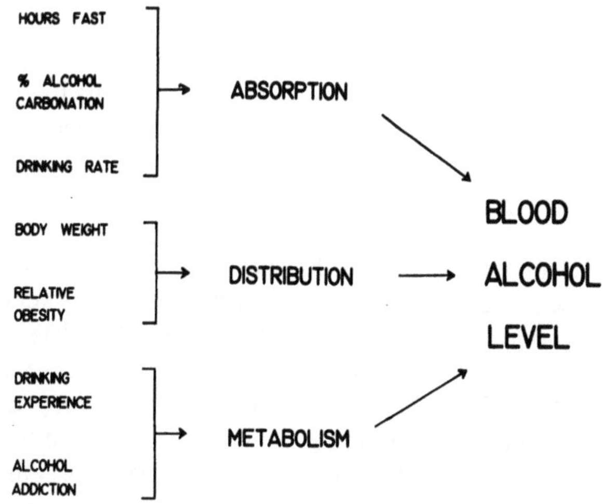

Fig. 1. Factors which Influence Blood Alcohol Levels are shown schematically. These are some variables which can affect alcohol absorption, distribution, and metabolism. A combination of these factors in turn determine the effective blood alcohol level following a standard dose of alcohol

choactive drugs have forced behavioral pharmacologists to rely on this approach. However, in studies of alcohol effects, such extrapolations are extremely hazardous and almost certainly unjustified because blood alcohol levels are influenced by so many factors. Physiologic variables and species differences also affect blood alcohol levels in animals.

Some of the major variables which can affect the concentration of alcohol, following administration of a standard dose, are summarized in Fig. 1. Each contributes to the variability in alcohol absorption or metabolism and to the resulting unpredictability of alcohol effects for the drinker and the investigator alike.

2. Alcohol Absorption

The rate of alcohol absorption determines when peak blood alcohol levels occur. Absorption is influenced by a number of factors, including the presence of food in the stomach, the concentration of alcohol consumed, the carbonation of the alcohol vehicle, and the speed of drinking. It is essential to specify the number of hours of fasting before oral alcohol administration. Since alcohol is absorbed primarily from the small intestine, food in the stomach will delay the gastric emptying with a resultant delay in absorption and peak blood alcohol concentration. Alternatively, if a large amount of alcohol is consumed rapidly on an empty stomach, pylorospasm and vomiting may occur. Since the emptying time of the stomach is estimated at between 3½ and 4 h, a 6–8 h fast prior to the administration of alcohol will insure that absorption rates are not altered by food in the stomach. If alcohol is consumed slowly, normal social drinkers can usually tolerate doses up to 2 mg/100 ml without emesis.

The higher the concentration of beverage alcohol, the more rapid the absorption up to a maximum of about 40% – the alcohol concentration of most distilled spirits. Distilled spirits, e.g., bourbon, scotch, and gin, will be absorbed considerably more rapidly than low concentration alcohol beverages such as beer and wine. Alcohol is absorbed more rapidly in a carbonated vehicle, and for this reason champagne is absorbed more rapidly than still wine. However, distilled spirits have a higher *congener* content than wine or beer, and the rate of alcohol absorption decreases with increasing congener concentrations. Rapid drinking will produce a higher concentration of alcohol in blood than slowly sipping an equivalent amount of alcohol (Moskowitz and Burns, 1975).

However, the common impression that beer and wine are less intoxicating than distilled spirits appears to be incorrect. Kalant and co-workers (1975) examined the effects of a standard dose of alcohol (1.3 g/kg), administered in the form of rye whiskey, beer, and sparkling wine, on sensory-motor tasks and the physiologic variables in normal drinkers. Peak blood alcohol levels ranged between 90 and 120 mg/100 ml. No significant differences between the effects of these three alcoholic beverages on sensory-motor or physiologic measures were observed at any blood alcohol level. The relevant variable influencing performance appeared to be blood alcohol concentration as a function of dose of alcohol ingested, and not the type of beverage consumed (Kalant et al., 1975).

3. Alcohol Distribution

Once alcohol has been absorbed, the effective concentration in the central nervous system (CNS) is influenced by the body weight and the relative obesity of the subject. Following absorption, alcohol is distributed equally throughout body water. Even if two subjects are of equal weight, total body water may be less in an obese subject, because water content of tissues which contain a high concentration of lipid is lower than a similar tissue mass with high protein content (Mendelson, 1968). Consequently, an obese subject would attain a higher blood alcohol level than a nonobese subject after administration of the same alcohol dose, because alcohol would be distributed in a smaller total body water pool. Obtaining equivalent alcohol doses in subjects of different weights is even more difficult. After the same initial dose, a 180-lb man will have a lower blood alcohol level than a 130-lb man, due to the relatively larger body water compartment.

4. Alcohol Metabolism

Once alcohol has been absorbed and distributed, several factors may affect the rate at which it is metabolized. The primary factor is the status of hepatic function. Most alcohol is metabolized by the liver, and impairment of liver function may retard the rate of alcohol metabolism. The presence of other drugs may also interact with alcohol to reduce the rate of metabolism. Malnutrition can also slow the rate of alcohol metabolism (Smith and Newman, 1959; Mendelson, 1970).

Suggestions that certain ethnic groups may metabolize alcohol differently (and therefore the risk of problem drinking is concomitantly enhanced or reduced) have not been substantiated in controlled studies (Bennion and Li, 1976). Differences in blood alcohol levels as a function of age or sex (Dubowski, 1976) do not appear to be related to metabolism per se, but rather reflect the proportional composition of lipid, protein, and water in the body.

In summary, these several factors which may interact to accelerate or retard the rate of alcohol absorption make it impossible to accurately predict blood alcohol concentrations following alcohol ingestion. Different behavioral effects may occur at different points on the blood alcohol curve and interpretation requires specification of the effective alcohol dose through time. There is no substitute for periodic monitoring of blood alcohol levels in both clinical and animal studies. Under optimal conditions, breath–alcohol values correspond closely to serum alcohol determinations carried out with enzymatic or gas chromatographic methods (DUBOWSKI, 1970). However, the accuracy of a breathalyzer can be affected by several variables including smoking, eating, residual alcohol in the mouth of the subject, and incorrect calibration of the instrument.

II. General Problems of Experimental Design

There are many methodological considerations which may affect the interpretation of data from the clinical and animal studies reviewed in Sect. C and D. Often, these are specific and unique to the type of study and the variables measured. However, there are also some general problems in design which transcend the specific ones and seriously limit generalizations from studies so afflicted.

1. Baseline Assessments

It is obvious that evaluation of the effect of alcohol upon any behavioral or biologic variable requires baseline assessment of that variable under conditions of sobriety. Evaluation of normal functioning under nondrug conditions is essential, whether subjects are used as their own control, during successive phases of a sequential study, or whether subjects are compared with a "matched" control group. Unless a behavioral baseline is obtained prior to alcohol intoxication, it is impossible to determine the contribution of alcohol to apparent changes in behavior. If one group of subjects performs less well than a matched control group, it is impossible to ascertain whether this is the effect of alcohol or some preexisting deficit. Although this basic principle of experimental design is so elementary that its elaboration may seem unnecessary, many behavioral studies of alcohol effects have neglected to assess baseline functioning.

2. Sex and Menstrual Cycle Phase

Failure to control for the sex of the subject may present a further complication. There is recent evidence that women develop higher blood alcohol levels than men after an equivalent dose of alcohol (JONES and JONES, 1976a, b; DUBOWSKI, 1976). Women also absorb alcohol faster and reach a peak blood alcohol level sooner than male controls (JONES and JONES, 1976b). These data presumably reflect the fact that alcohol is distributed throughout the total body water, and women have less water per body unit than men. However, there are no significant differences in the rate of alcohol elimination in men and women (DUBOWSKI, 1976).

Moreover, there is suggestive evidence that blood alcohol levels following a standard dose of alcohol tend to vary as a function of the phase of the menstrual cycle in women. Specifically, blood alcohol levels were higher at ovulation and during the premenstruum than at other phases of the menstrual cycle (JONES and JONES, 1976a, b). The extent to which behavioral and subjective effects of alcohol covary with these apparent biologic changes associated with phases of the menstrual cycle remain to be determined, and existing data are inconsistent (MELLO, 1980 for review). In studies unrelated to drug effects, there is considerable evidence that objective performance measures usually fail to show any menstrual cycle-related changes (SOMMER, 1973). However, it does appear that sensory acuity may change as a function of menstrual cycle phases (SOMMER, 1973; WARD et al., 1978).

Although the replicability and generality of reported sex specific and menstrual cycle-related differences in alcohol effects remain to be demonstrated, it is apparent that additional controls may be necessary in studies of alcohol effects in women. In addition to baseline measures under alcohol-free conditions, it may also be important to compare alcohol effects across several phases of the menstrual cycle.

3. Expectancy About Drug Effects

Although it is generally agreed that nonpharmacologic, situational, and social factors influence reactions to psychoactive drugs, the fact that the expectancy of a drug effect can influence behavior even when no drug is given has rarely been considered. The potent effects of expectancy have recently been demonstrated in an elegant series of carefully designed studies of drug effects (MARLATT and ROHSENOW, 1980 for review). It has now been shown that diverse behaviors, such as aggressivity, anxiety, laughter in response to humorous stimuli, and arousal to sexual stimuli, may be enhanced by the expectation of receiving alcohol, even though an alcohol-placebo was given. On tasks involving motor performance, the effects of expectancy were diminished, and variables such as reaction time were consistently affected by alcohol. Moreover, alcohol adversely affected performance of subjects who had expected to receive the placebo, but subjects who had expected to receive alcohol appeared able to compensate for this effect.

MARLATT and ROHSENOW (1980) argue convincingly for the importance of a *balanced placebo design* to control for the effects of expectancy about drug effects on behavior. This design involves two groups of subjects; one group expects to receive drug and the other expects to receive placebo. Within each of these two groups, half of the subjects actually receive drugs and half actually receive placebo. This design permits an independent manipulation of the instructions given to the subject and the actual substance (active drug or placebo) administered.

Studies using the balanced placebo design have shown that a wide range of behaviors are influenced by expectancies about drug effects rather than by the drug itself. MARLATT and ROHSENOW (1980) conclude that if the effects of alcohol are believed to be positive or desirable, then the effects of expectancy may be as potent as the actual effect of alcohol, whereas if subjects believe that drinking may have a negative or undesirable outcome, experimental manipulation of expectancy appears to have less impact.

Since very few of the clinical studies to be reviewed employed a balanced placebo design, and the effectiveness of double-blind manipulations is often open to question, the possible influence of expectancy is still one further qualification to be considered in evaluation of data obtained. In studies of alcoholic individuals, subjects were usually aware that they were receiving alcohol and brought a complex host of expectancies to the drinking situation (McGuire et al., 1966).

4. Motivation to Perform

Most studies of the behavioral effects of alcohol require the subjects cooperation and performance on some task. Unless subjects are motivated to perform as well as possible, any performance decrement during alcohol intoxication could be accounted for by boredom, indifference, or fatigue rather than alcohol. Apparently most investigators assume that their subjects will try to perform as well as possible. Subjects are often paid for their participation in the study. However, this payment is rarely made contingent upon performance accuracy. There is no reason to assume that paid volunteers will consistently perform at the upper limits of their capacity unless they are specifically paid to do so, i.e., unless the accuracy of their performance results in a task-specific reinforcement. The wide diversity of behavioral effects attributed to alcohol may reflect in part a failure to insure optimal performance by the subject.

There is a considerable literature attesting to the powerful behavioral control exerted by contingent reinforcements. Both student volunteers and alcohol addicts might perform better during intoxication if they were reinforced for accurate performance. It is also essential to establish that the reinforcement offered is an adequate reinforcement. Pennies and candy may not be effective reinforcements for college students. Alcohol appears to be the only reinforcer that will consistently maintain accurate performance in alcoholic subjects during intoxication (Mello, 1972; 1973b). Differences in the conditions of reinforcement for accurate performance are probably among the most important factors which account for reported differences in performance on a variety of behavioral tasks during sobriety and during alcohol intoxication.

5. Attention to the Task

Certain types of behavioral tasks are more vulnerable to subject distractibility than others. Most tasks which attempt to assess some aspect of cognitive function before and during alcohol intoxication require the subject to attend to, and perhaps learn, some verbal, visual, or auditory stimulus pattern. The potentially devastating effects of inattention and distractibility can be illustrated in studies of memory function. Although it seems obvious that the subject's attention to the stimuli to be recalled is essential for the evaluation of drug intoxication on subsequent recall, this variable is seldom controlled, and apparent memory failure during or after alcohol intoxication could be a lack of attention to the stimulus to be remembered. Some investigators have attempted to manipulate attention by presenting materials which are presumably interesting to the subject, such as erotic movies (Goodwin et al., 1970).

A more reliable technique for controlling attention, which is independent of stimulus content, is to require an observing response. This is a standard behavioral technique commonly used with both human and animal subjects to insure that the subject does attend to the discriminative stimulus upon which subsequent performance is based (e.g., Mello, 1973b). There are many variations on this procedure, which in essence requires the subject to produce a stimulus by some motor or verbal response. It is assumed that the subject is more likely to attend to a self-produced stimulus than one which is introduced by the investigator (or the programing apparatus).

6. Patterns of Alcohol Administration

Alcohol can be given in fixed doses at specified times (programed administration) or the subject can control the dose and frequency of alcohol intake (spontaneous administration). Each paradigm has limitations and advantages, and the choice ultimately depends upon the type of questions asked.

Spontaneous alcohol self-administration paradigms necessarily involve unpredictable variation in alcohol dose and the interval between successive doses. In some instances, the spontaneous pattern of alcohol self-administration may be the dependent variable of interest in both clinical (Mello and Mendelson, 1978c) and animal studies (Mello, 1976a). It is generally agreed that data obtained under spontaneous alcohol administration conditions are most behaviorally relevant. However, spontaneous administration paradigms are not optimal for study of the effects of alcohol when precise time-dose response curves are essential for interpretation of data obtained.

Programed drinking regimens are traditionally used in experimental pharmacology. There is little question that a programed dosage regimen provides better control over dose and interdose interval than does a spontaneous alcohol administration paradigm. One disadvantage of programed alcohol self-administration is that it bears little resemblance to naturalistic alcohol use and may have different biologic as well as behavioral consequences. For example, a comparison of alcoholic subjects during two successive programed (Q4H) or spontaneous drinking periods indicated that spontaneous drinking resulted in withdrawal signs and symptoms most concordant with real-life drinking patterns (Mello and Mendelson, 1970). These data were interpreted to suggest that given an equivalent volume and duration of exposure to alcohol, the essential determinant of the behavioral and biologic concomitants of alcohol intoxication *and* alcohol withdrawal is the distribution or pattern of drinking through time. Consequently, clinical studies of alcohol withdrawal are probably best conducted using a spontaneous drinking paradigm. Alternatively, in studies with animal models, programed alcohol procedures induce physical dependence most rapidly and reliably (Mello, 1976b, for review).

III. Route of Alcohol Administration

In clinical studies, alcohol is usually consumed in beverage form by cooperative subjects. However, in self-administration studies with animals, the choice of route of alcohol administration can be a critical determinant of data obtained (Mello, 1976b). It has been repeatedly shown that intravenous and intragastric routes of alcohol administration are effective and reliable (Winger and Woods, 1973; Karoly et al., 1978; Altschuler and Talley, 1977). Alcohol is usually reinforcing under these conditions of administration.

Conversely, when alcohol is administerd orally, alcohol is not always reinforcing and appears to be noxious to many animals. Use of an oral administration procedure makes it especially important to monitor blood alcohol levels, to control variables which may effect delay of absorption, and most important, to devise techniques to insure that the animal actually drinks the alcohol presented (MELLO, 1976c, for discussion). Despite the recurrent problems with oral alcohol administration in animals, two approaches appear to yield successful control of drinking behavior. Falk and co-workers have used schedule-induced polydipsia procedures to induce alcohol consumption in rodents and have succeeded in producing physical dependence upon alcohol (FALK et al., 1972; FALK and SAMPSON, 1976). Meisch and co-workers have devised a series of procedures to control alcohol consumption in the monkey, and they conclude that oral alcohol is reinforcing (MEISCH, 1977 for review).

Despite these ingenious efforts to control and maintain oral alcohol intake in animals, intravenous administration offers an important advantage for behavioral studies. Each alcohol infusion is rapidly distributed throughout the circulatory system and produces an immediate effect. The delay in absorption of alcohol taken orally may be 1–3 h (MELLO, 1971). Moreover the delay in absorption may be influenced by all the factors previously discussed. Consequently the animal presumably must learn to associate the initially noxious taste of alcohol with some delayed "reinforcing" effect. Immediate reinforcement is known to be more effective than delayed reinforcement in shaping behavior.

IV. Implications of Behavioral Tolerance

Tolerance to alcohol can develop as a function of prolonged exposure, just as tolerance develops to many psychoactive drugs of abuse. When progressively higher doses of alcohol are required to produce comparable subjective and behavioral effects, tolerance is inferred. The three types of tolerance which are common to alcohol addiction and other forms of drug addiction are: behavioral tolerance, pharmacologic tolerance, and cross tolerance to other potentially addictive drugs (SEEVERS and DENEAU, 1963).

Behavioral tolerance is illustrated by the fact that alcohol may not induce significant impairment in the performance of behavioral tasks even when blood alcohol levels are twice the legal limit of intoxication, i.e., above 200 mg/100 ml (MELLO, 1972; TALLAND, 1966; TALLAND et al., 1964a, b). The dramatic behavioral tolerance for alcohol shown by the alcohol addict cannot be accounted for by a more rapid or effective capacity to metabolize alcohol. Alcoholics can perform very well on difficult tasks at the time when their blood alcohol levels are above 200 mg/100 ml (MELLO, 1973b). Some tolerant alcohol addicts can consume between 4/5 and 1 quart of bourbon per day, often without signs of gross intoxication (MELLO, 1972; MELLO and MENDELSON, 1970, 1972). Behavioral tolerance has been observed in alcohol addicts *and* in moderate drinkers under certain conditions (GOODWIN et al., 1970). The duration of alcohol-induced tolerance in man is unknown.

Most clinical investigators have been insensitive to the possible effects of behavioral tolerance upon a subject's reaction to alcohol. Many attempt to compare normal drinkers with alcoholics, and alcoholics with each other, without indicating the duration of intoxication or sobriety. There is no reason to assume that it is valid to compare an alcoholic who has been sober for 1 day with an alcoholic who has been sober for 3 weeks or with an alcoholic who is intoxicated.

Behavioral tolerance may also influence performance in animal studies. In the rat, behavioral tolerance has been shown to develop within 3 weeks of daily alcohol administration (LEBLANC et al., 1969). Following cessation of alcohol administration, tolerance began to dissipate within 1 week and returned to baseline levels after 3 or 4 weeks. It was subsequently observed that rats given alcohol before training on a circular maze or testing on a moving belt developed tolerance to alcohol more rapidly than animals trained under identical conditions, but given equivalent doses of alcohol after the session (LEBLANC et al., 1973; LEBLANC et al., 1976). In both situations, pre- and postsession alcohol groups reached the same maximum level of tolerance, and upon cessation of alcohol administration, tolerance was lost at the same rate. The investigators have termed this phenomenon "behaviorally augmented tolerance." They conclude that tolerance reflects CNS changes which accompany prolonged exposure to alcohol, since blood alcohol levels were equivalent despite improved performance in the presession alcohol administration groups (LEBLANC et al., 1973).

V. Operational Definitions

The primary subjective effects of alcohol appear to involve changes in perceived mood and self-esteem, social receptivity, aggressivity, sexuality, somnolence, and memory. Each of these descriptive terms encompasses a complex of variables which cannot all be directly measured. Each is a hypothetical construct which is operationally defined by the various measures used for assessment.

Reification of hypothetical constructs and a tendency toward imprecision and inconsistency in operational definitions is not unique to the behavioral literature on alcohol. Given that any single construct, such as mood, may be conceived differently by each discipline, some degree of inconsistency is to be expected and is often valuable. However, when the underlying rationale and assumptions for a particular operational definition are not described with sufficient precision to permit critical evaluation, the research process can deteriorate into a naming exercise. For example, RUSSELL and MEHRABIAN (1975) have criticized studies of the effects of alcohol on emotion because of the ambiguity and inconsistency with which emotional states have been defined. They conclude that the emotional impact of the given dose of alcohol may depend upon the environmental setting, the drinker's prior mood, and the underlying personality. To the extent that most research has neglected examination of all of these variables in relation to alcohol, findings in this area are at best inconclusive (RUSSELL and MEHRABIAN, 1975). CAPPELL (1975) and CAPPELL and HERMAN (1972) have advanced a comparable critique in a review of data relevant to the hypothesis that alcohol consumption can be accounted for by its "tension reduction" effects.

An illustration of the confusion that an imprecise operational definition may cause comes from studies of the effects of alcohol on short-term memory function. It is obvious that the temporal definition of memory span is essential to any assessment of memory function. Nonetheless, short-term memory has been variously defined as 5 s, 5 min, and 30 min. Some investigators use the descriptive term without providing any temporal limits at all.

Admittedly, the study of subjective variables such as mood present many difficulties in measurement as well as definition. It is difficult to devise adequate measures of affect which reflect the mood states presumably tested. Since mood changes can only be subjective reports, the assumption that a subject's verbal behavior has some relationship to actual feeling states cannot be satisfactorily established with reference to any objective criteria. Variables related to the cooperativeness, expectancy, and compliance of the subject may influence answers on a mood assessment inventory as much or more than the presence or absence of alcohol. No satisfactory resolution of this problem appears imminent, and the usual strategy is to use a combination of several apparently sensitive instruments and global clinical impressions.

C. Clinical Studies of Alcohol Effects

Alcohol has many varied, and often inconsistent effects on human behavior (MELLO and MENDELSON, 1978 a, for review). Among the most prominent of these are changes in mood, sociability, sexuality, aggressivity, and relative states of tension or relaxation. Most clinical research has focused upon these variables, in part because it is commonly believed that related changes in subjective feelings and behavior may account for alcohol use and abuse. The belief that alcohol intoxication is consistently associated with an elevation in mood, enhanced sociability and sexuality, and relaxation has only recently been challenged. As direct observations of behavior and assessment of subjective states *during* intoxication have replaced reliance on retrospective self-reports, the limitations of accustomed beliefs and simplistic formulations about the effects of alcohol have become increasingly apparent. Although drinking may be initiated with an intent to achieve the alleged positive effects of intoxication, it now appears that the expected effects often do not occur.

This section will briefly discuss some of the major finding relevant to the alleged subjective and behavioral effects of alcohol intoxication. Many of these studies described suffer from one or more of the methodological problems noted in Sect. B of this review. Nevertheless, a number of concordant findings have emerged despite a diversity of approaches and frequent procedural limitations.

I. Alcohol and Mood

One of the most puzzling findings to emerge from behavioral studies of alcohol addicts is that chronic intoxication may increase rather than alleviate anxiety and depression (MELLO and MENDELSON, 1978 a). Usually, the severity of depression and anxiety tends to increase in alcoholic individuals as heavy drinking continues (ALTERMAN et al., 1975). Yet these aversive consequences of intoxication are seldom recalled during sobriety, and alcoholics usually report that the anticipated positive effects in fact occurred (MCGUIRE et al., 1966; TAMERIN et al., 1970).

An alcohol-related despondency does not occur only in alcoholics; social drinkers also report increased anxiety and depression after consuming 6–8 oz alcohol (WARREN and RAYNES, 1972; WILLIAMS, 1966). An alcohol dose-dependent increase in self-reported anxiety was observed in male and female social drinkers over a range of 0.5–1.2 g/kg (LOGUE et al., 1978). These data are consistent with the clinical impression that the degree of dysphoria and anxiety induced by alcohol appears to be related to the dose of alcohol consumed, both in alcohol addicts and social drinkers. Since the alcohol addict has greater tolerance for alcohol, larger quantities of alcohol may be necessary to produce an increase in depression and anxiety. It is not unusual for an alcohol addict to ingest between 26 and 32 oz of distilled spirits each day (MELLO and MENDELSON, 1972).

Depression and anxiety during intoxication are inconsistent with the commonplace notion that alcohol is an effective euphorigen. Supporting clinical data come from the high concordance between alcohol intoxication and suicidal behavior (GOODWIN, 1973). At low doses, alcohol may have some euphorigenic effects for the social drinker (SMITH et al., 1975) and probably very little effect for the behaviorally tolerant alcohol addict. These reactions are undoubtedly influenced by previous experience with alcohol, the pattern, volume, and duration of drinking, as well as expectancy and social context. It is interesting that even reports of euphoria in social drinkers at moderate blood alcohol levels (67–100 mg/100 ml) were not associated with a diminution of anxiety and depression (SMITH et al., 1975).

II. Alcohol and Aggression

Since alcohol intoxication often increases feelings of despondency and anxiety, perhaps it is not surprising that aggressive behavior is another frequent accompaniment of heavy drinking (TINKLENBERG, 1973; WALLER, 1972; WOLFGANG, 1958; MENDELSON and MELLO, 1974). Clinical studies of alcohol addicts during intoxication have consistently reported aggressive behavior ranging from sarcasm and verbal insults to threats of physical assault, actual assaults, temper tantrums, and occasionally self-destructive behaviors (MENDELSON and MELLO, 1974; TAMERIN and MENDELSON, 1969; NATHAN et al., 1970, 1972; STEINGLASS and WOLIN, 1974). It is possible that some critical number of subjects (four or more) facilitates these gross expressions of aggression, since comparable increases in aggressive behavior were not observed in pairs of alcoholic men given unrestricted access to alcohol, despite increased dysphoria (PERSKY et al., 1977).

Social drinkers also may engage in verbal and physical assaultive behavior during intoxication (SMITH et al., 1975; BOYATZIS, 1974, 1975). Clinical impressions of spontaneous aggression during drinking are consistent with findings from experiments in which aggression is defined by the frequency or intensity of electric shock delivered to another individual (TAYLOR and GAMMON, 1975). However, expectancy about alcohol effects has also been shown to be an important determinant of aggressive behavior in an experimental paradigm (LANG et al., 1975). Subjects who expected to receive alcohol exhibited more aggression, defined as intensity and duration of shock administered to another, than subjects who expected to drink tonic. Subjects who expected to receive tonic and in fact received alcohol were far less aggressive than subjects who expected alcohol and in fact received tonic (LANG et al., 1975). These data are eloquent testimony to the importance of expectancies in influencing the behavioral effects of drugs (MARLATT and ROHSENOW, 1980). The investigators suggest that alcohol may provide a culturally accepted excuse for behavior such as aggression which is normally unacceptable (LANG et al., 1975; MARLATT and ROHSENOW, 1980). It does appear that aggression associated with alcohol intoxication may be facilitated by stereotypes about alcohol effects.

III. Alcohol and Sexuality

Alcoholic men often report diminished heterosexual desire, diminished sexual activity, and impotence. The biologic effects of alcohol which may contribute to these changes in sexuality are discussed elsewhere (MELLO and MENDELSON, 1978a; MENDELSON et al., 1978). A comprehensive review of alcohol and sexual behavior has been prepared by WILSON (1977).

Accumulating evidence that sexual function is compromised by alcohol has now been extended to include nonalcoholic, healthy men and women. It is only recently that clinical impression and anecdotal accounts have been replaced by careful behavioral studies of the effects of alcohol on sexual arousal in response to an erotic or neutral control film (WILSON, 1977 for review). It has been consistently reported that alcohol attenuates sexual responsivity, as defined by measures of penile tumescence in healthy young males (BRIDDELL and WILSON, 1976; FARKAS and ROSEN, 1976; RUBIN and HENSON, 1976; WILSON and LAWSON, 1976a). Relatively low doses of alcohol also decreased sexual responsivity in young women, as measured by photoplethysmographic recordings of vaginal pulse pressure and blood volume (WILSON and LAWSON, 1976b). However, women reported feelings of enhanced sexual arousal with increasing levels of alcohol intoxication. In males, reports of sexual arousal and estimates of penile erection were positively correlated with penile tumescence measures (FARKAS and ROSEN, 1976; RUBIN and HENSON, 1976).

Despite evidence to the contrary, male subjects often continue to believe that alcohol enhances their sexual function. These data illustrate the difficulty in reconciling objective and subjective information about sexual behavior. RUBIN and HENSON (1976) concluded that "an individual whose threshold for penile erection or ejaculation has been raised by the ingestion of alcohol may consider this depressant effect to be an enhancement of sexual abilities because it increases the time available for sexual stimulation of his partner which could well increase the possibility of her being brought to orgasm."

The well-entrenched expectancy about alcohol's effects on sexuality have been shown to effect sexual arousal even in the absence of alcohol. Young men were shown erotic films and arousal was measured by penile tumescence. Those subjects who believed they had consumed alcohol showed greater levels of sexual arousal than subjects who believed they drank only tonic irrespective of whether their drinks in fact contained any alcohol (WILSON and LAWSON, 1976b). These basic findings have recently been replicated in studies of male social drinkers exposed to normal and deviant erotic stimuli. Subjects who believed they had alcohol were significantly more aroused by deviant sexual stimuli than subjects who believed they had a nonalcoholic drink (BRIDDELL et al., 1978).

IV. Alcohol and Tension

Although alcohol intoxication is usually associated with increased relaxation, the effectiveness of alcohol as a tension reducer has also been repeatedly challenged. CAPPELL and HERMAN (1972) critically reviewed the animal and human literature and found that acute alcohol administration did not consistently result in decreased "tension." STEFFAN and co-workers (1974) studied the effects of alcohol on subjective and objective measures of tension in four alcoholic men given free access to bourbon for 12 consecutive days. Electromyographic activity was recorded from the frontalis muscle. It was found that reports of subjective distress were positively correlated with blood alcohol levels, but unrelated to electromyographic activity.

There was a significant negative correlation between muscle tension and blood alcohol levels (STEFFAN et al., 1974).

These data illustrate the problem with an over-inclusive definition of "tension," since muscle tension was not correlated with subjective distress reports, and each subject was affected differently by increasing blood alcohol levels. These data suggest that "tension reduction" probably is not a viable explanatory construct to account for alcohol abuse. This impression is strengthened by studies which have shown that antecedent naturally occurring or experimentally induced "stress" does not necessarily result in increased alcohol consumption by alcoholics or social drinkers (MELLO, 1972; HIGGINS and MARLATT, 1973; MILLER et al., 1974). The previously described studies of aggression, dysphoria, and anxiety as a consequence of drinking would suggest that at sufficiently high doses, alcohol may be a more effective "stressor" than tension reducer.

V. Alcohol and Sociability

Under conditions where both alcohol and socializing are freely accessible, drinking is often associated with an increase in social behavior (GRIFFITHS et al., 1978, for review). However, as is evident from the foregoing descriptions of alcohol-related depression, anxiety, and aggressivity, the quality of the social interaction may not be uniformly pleasant. Social behavior has usually been measured by intermittent observations of whether or not the subject is interacting with another person, and the type of interchange is not always reported. Moreover, many of the existing studies have not used the balanced placebo design which MARLATT and ROHSENOW (1980) argue is essential for controlling for the effects of expectancy. Parametric dose-response studies of the effect of alcohol on socialization in alcoholics and social drinkers are not yet available.

Despite these limitations, the question of whether or not alcohol facilitates social interaction has been asked in a variety of experimental and naturalistic situations in both alcoholics and social drinkers (GRIFFITHS et al., 1978; MELLO, 1972; MELLO and MENDELSON, 1978 a, for review). Under conditions of continuous alcohol availability, intoxication does not uniformly increase or maintain spontaneous social interaction. THORNTON and co-workers (1976) compared social behavior in male alcoholic abstainers and heavy drinkers over a 4-week period of alcoholic availability. The abstainers maintained a relatively constant level of socializing throughout the baseline and alcohol-available periods of the study. The heavy drinkers increased socializing significantly during the first week of alcohol availability. During the final 3 weeks of alcohol availability, the overall level of socializing decreased somewhat and then declined sharply when alcohol was no longer available. Subjects within the abstaining and heavy drinking group were characterized as extroverted or introverted on the Eysenck Personality Inventory (Form A) and this categorization was confirmed by observations of actual social behavior. However, alcohol did not appear to affect the socialization behavior of introverted alcoholics more than that of extroverted alcoholics. The socialization rates of extroverts were higher than introverts in both the abstinent and alcohol drinking group, across all phases of the study (THORNTON et al., 1976). In studies where alcohol was available intermittently, spontaneous rates of social interaction increased in alcoholic subjects (GRIFFITHS et al., 1974).

In an effort to further analyze the apparent relationship between alcohol intoxication and social interaction, NATHAN and co-workers (1970, 1971, and 1972) examined the effect of experimentally controlled social isolation on drinking. In the initial studies, 3 days of unrestricted socialization were alternated with 3-day periods of complete isolation. Subjects worked at a simple operant task for points which could be exchanged for alcohol (20 ml bourbon) or for socialization (15 min out of isolation). Given a choice between buying alcohol and buying social interaction, these alcoholics preferred to spend their resources on alcohol. Most subjects drank about the same amount of alcohol during periods of socialization and isolation. When alcoholic subjects were given a choice every 20 min of some money (10–35 cents) and no social interaction *or* no money and 20 min of social interaction, subjects chose socialization over money on days when they were consuming alcohol (GRIFFITHS et al., 1975).

GRIFFITHS and co-workers have also given alcoholic subjects a choice between: (a) alcohol and a brief period (10–15 min) of isolation (BIGELOW et al., 1974); (b) alcohol and 40 min of isolation; and (c) alcohol and a time-out from other activities (GRIFFITHS et al., 1978). In each situation, the period of isolation was contingent upon alcohol consumption. This contingent choice procedure differs from that used by NATHAN in which points could be exchanged for alcohol, socialization, or both. Several other procedural differences also limit comparisons between studies of NATHAN and co-workers and studies by GRIFFITHS and co-workers. For example, GRIFFITHS' alcoholic subjects were studied sequentially, rather than together, and their interaction opportunities were with other psychiatric patients or subjects involved in other drug-related experiments. In most other studies of social interaction, groups of three or more alcoholics have been studied together. Also, whereas NATHAN's subjects were completely isolated from social interaction in individual bedrooms, GRIFFITHS' subjects were usually isolated on the research ward where they could still see, hear, and be close to other individuals.

Although the degree of social isolation was less stringent, alcohol-contingent social isolation effectively suppressed drinking in comparison to baseline conditions (GRIFFITHS et al., 1978, for review). Alcohol-contingent restriction of activities produced a somewhat greater suppression of alcohol intake (36% of baseline) than the alcohol-contingent time-out from socialization (71% of baseline). When an alcohol-contingent time-out from activity was combined with an alcoholic-contingent time-out from socialization, alcohol intake was further decreased to an average of 24% of baseline. Comparable results were obtained whether the contingent time-out procedures were in effect continuously over several days, or intermittently on occasional days. Extensions of the contingent relationship between alcohol and drinking to external socialization conditions produced similar results in two subjects. Subjects could earn prearranged social privileges outside the ward by drinking five or fewer drinks each day for a specified number of days. These social contingencies were effective in controlling the drinking behavior (GRIFFITHS et al., 1978).

It is evident from the foregoing that drinking behavior can be manipulated by contingent socialization or isolation under some conditions, and that spontaneous socialization may increase as a function of alcohol intoxication. GRIFFITHS et al. (1978) conclude that "...it is clear that social access is a reinforcer for which alcoholics will modify their drinking. However, it is not clear whether ethanol-induced socializing acts as a reinforcer to maintain alcoholics drinking. The fact that alcoholics will continue to drink heavily under conditions of social impoverishment and isolation certainly demonstrates that facilitation of social behavior is not a necessary element for the maintenance of drinking" (p. 372).

VI. Implications for Analysis of the Reinforcing Properties of Alcohol

It now appears that alcohol does not reliably provide the euphoria, relaxation, or relief from anxiety and tension usually anticipated. Although social interaction may increase during intoxication, verbal and physical aggression may be an important component of the social interchange. These data are not consistent with the hypothesis that alcohol abuse is maintained by its immediate "positive" effects, usually alleged to outweigh the delayed adverse social, legal, and medical consequences of alcoholism. Although alcohol abuse is often assumed to magnify and extend the several satisfactions of social drinking, it may in fact distort the simplest pleasures and transform the expected rewards of intoxication into their antithesis. Despite the powerful influence of expectancy, it is not clear why the seeming adverse consequences of alcohol abuse which occur during intoxication have so little effect on drinking behavior. Recall is somewhat selective, and alcoholics interviewed before, during, and after an episode of intoxication tended to remember predrinking expectancies, even when these were completely at variance with the actual effects of intoxication (McGUIRE et al., 1966).

Dysphoric effects during intoxication are not unique to alcohol, and many abused drugs have now been shown to increase anxiety and depression (MIRIN et al., 1976; MELLO, 1978 a; MELLO and MENDELSON, 1978 b; MEYER and MIRIN, 1979). These clinical findings appear somewhat paradoxical, and present many problems for reward-related constructs often advanced to account for alcoholism and drug abuse. Since drug self-administration is presumably controlled or maintained by its consequences, it may be that these "aversive" consequences are an important aspect of the reinforcement for drinking (MELLO, 1977, 1978 a for review).

In this context, it is of interest to recall that an initial drug experience often has a variety of aversive emotional and somatic consequences for the naive user. For example, alcohol addicts tend to have a clear recollection of their first drink (KUEHNLE et al., 1974), which was often associated with despondency, nausea, and vomiting rather than with relaxation and euphoria. The process by which an aversive initial drug experience becomes translated into a repetitive drug use pattern is not understood, and the contribution of drug tolerance is unclear. It is tempting to postulate that the aversive consequences associated with the initial alcohol intoxication event may remain an integral part of the reinforcing complex for subsequent alcohol abuse.

There is considerable evidence that aversive events may control behavior leading to their self-administration in animal models (MORSE et al., 1977; MORSE and KELLEHER, 1970, for review). One example is the repetitive self-administration of an electric shock. Although the aversive properties of electric shock have been amply documented, it has been consistently observed that the same electric shock that can maintain escape and avoidance behavior, may under certain conditions, be self-administered by the same monkey. A second example of the aversive control of behavior, is the self-administration of narcotic antagonist drugs by opiate-dependent monkeys despite the occurrence of opiate withdrawal signs (WOODS et al., 1975; GOLDBERG et al., 1972). It is now evident that many forms of drug abuse continue despite the recurrence of seemingly aversive consequences during intoxication (MELLO, 1978a).

Since the positive effects of alcohol appear to be so ephemeral and somewhat less predictable than both the immediate and delayed aversive consequences, more careful attention to the possible role of aversive consequences in maintaining human drug self-administration seems indicated.

Analysis of the reinforcing properties of alcohol abuse clearly requires examination of the actual consequences of drinking. The term reinforcement does not imply anything about the nature of the reinforcing event, but rather describes a functional relationship between events and behavior. MORSE and KELLEHER (1977) have criticized the common tendency to think about reinforcers in terms of the alleged properties of events. It is important to recognize that the same event, alcohol intoxication, may have either reinforcing or punishing consequences (i.e., may increase or decrease behavior leading to its presentation), depending upon the conditions under which it is presented. The dose-response function for subjective effects of alcohol remains to be accurately characterized. The critical alcohol dose necessary for a transient feeling of well-being at the beginning of a drinking episode has not been determined and the influence of alcohol tolerance and expectancy remain to be clarified (MELLO and MENDELSON, 1978a).

At present there are no satisfactory explanations for the repetition of excessive drinking and alcohol withdrawal episodes which define the clinical expression of alcoholism (MENDELSON and MELLO, 1979). Further study of the behavioral consequences of alcohol intoxication, under controlled conditions, should eventually contribute to an improved understanding of this complex behavior disorder.

D. Behavioral Studies of Alcohol in Animal Models

Over the past decade there has been a concerted effort to develop animal models of alcoholism. This goal has recently been accomplished in several species with a variety of techniques. The technological advances necessary for the development of animal models of alcohol addiction have also permitted examination of the behavioral pharmacology of alcohol. Although the primary focus remains on alcohol-dependent models to examine biologic effects of alcohol intoxication and withdrawal, it is now possible to study a number of behavioral questions which have already been addressed for many other drugs of abuse (SCHUSTER and JOHANSON, 1974; JOHANSON, 1978; GRIFFITHS et al., 1980).

I. Animal Models of Alcohol Addiction

Since the development of animal models of alcohol addiction has been one of the most significant recent advances in research on alcoholism, it is important to briefly review some of the relevant conceptual and methodological issues. A number of comprehensive critical reviews of animal models of alcohol addiction are currently available (CICERO, 1979; FALK and TANG, 1977; GOLDSTEIN, 1978; MELLO, 1973a, 1976b, 1979b; WOODS and WINGER, 1971, 1974).

Models are now available which fulfill the pharmacologic criteria of alcohol addiction, i.e., tolerance for and physical dependence upon alcohol. These criteria are distinct from, and do not necessarily include, oral preference for alcohol. It is somewhat surprising that animal models of alcoholism have only been developed within the past 10 years, since opiate addiction models have been available for decades (SCHUSTER and JOHANSON, 1974). This delay appears to reflect an anthropomorphic tendency to restrict animal models of alcoholism to oral preference for alcohol, since this is the way alcohol is consumed by man. Advocates of preference criteria argue that voluntary ingestion of alcohol to the point of sustained intoxication, in preference to other fluids, is essential for any analog of human alcoholism (LESTER and FREED, 1973). Unfortunately, most animals do not prefer alcohol, and actively avoid alcohol solutions in sufficient concentration to produce any discernible pharmacologic effects (MELLO, 1976b, c). Although a transient preference for alcohol can be induced by a variety of techniques, once the controlling variables are removed there is usually a precipitous decrease in alcohol preference (MYERS and VEALE, 1972). Moreover, oral alcohol preference has rarely been associated with tolerance and physical dependence upon alcohol. One exception to this general finding is the miniature pig (PRESTON et al., 1972; PRESTON et al., 1973).

Empirical progress with animal alcoholism models which do not involve a voluntary preference component would tend to refute the argument that unless an animal exhibits spontaneous alcohol selection (LESTER and FREED, 1973) it is not analogous or relevant to the condition of human alcoholism. One of the most important findings using animal models involved the development of an animal model of cirrhosis in which preference for alcohol did not play an important role (LIEBER et al., 1975). The issue is rather one of selecting the most appropriate model for the biochemical, pharmacologic, toxicologic, or behavioral questions asked.

Animal models of alcoholism can be categorized as either pharmacologic or behavioral on the basis of the technique used to induce alcohol dependence. In a *pharmacologic* or forced administration model, alcohol is administered to the experimental animals in sufficient doses over sufficient time to induce physical dependence. In a *behavioral* or self-administration model, the animal works at a task to obtain alcohol or freely ingests alcohol solutions, usually in the context of working for food (MELLO, 1976a).

Pharmacologic and behavioral models of alcohol addiction involve a variety of procedures which can be further subdivided according to the route of alcohol administration. The route of administration determines the rate at which a pharmacologically effective dose of alcohol is reached, as well as the direction and stability of the drug effect. Among the routes of administration that have proven effective in inducing alcohol dependence are: oral, intragastric, nasogastric, intravenous, subcutaneous (ERICKSON et al., 1978), and the inhalation of alcohol vapors (GOLDSTEIN, 1972). A detailed description and evaluation of the several procedures has appeared in previous reviews (MELLO, 1973a, 1976b; CICERO, 1979; GOLDSTEIN, 1978) and will not be detailed here. Some problems with oral alcohol administration were described in Sect. B of this review (MELLO, 1976c).

The dose and duration of alcohol exposure required to produce physical dependence varies as a function of the species and the technique used to induce addiction. Usually, physical dependence develops much more rapidly than has been reported in man (MELLO and MENDELSON, 1977). For example, mice may develop withdrawal signs after 36–48 h of alcohol exposure to an alcohol vapor (GOLDSTEIN, 1972). Rhesus monkeys given intravenous infusions of alcohol every 8 h until the eye blink reflex was lost, may develop withdrawal tremors within 8 days, and severe withdrawal signs within 16 days of chronic infusion (TARIKA and WINGER, 1979). A comparable time course of physical dependence development was observed in rhesus monkeys given alcohol nasogastrically (ELLIS and PICK, 1970). The time course and expression of the alcohol withdrawal syndrome in some rodent and primate models is comparable to that in man.

The relative value of pharmacologic versus behavioral models is entirely dependent upon the types of questions that are subsequently asked. One advantage of a pharmacologic (forced administration) model is that the induction of physical dependence upon alcohol has been consistently more rapid and reliable than with behavioral (self-administration) techniques. The rapid induction of physical dependence provides an extremely important tool for assessing the end product of addiction, alcohol withdrawal. It is probably the most practical and efficient way to induce alcohol dependence in order to examine neural, endocrine, and metabolic correlates of alcohol withdrawal and to assess the effects of various pharmacologic agents or other forms of intervention on the alcohol abstinence syndrome. In studies which require chronic long-term exposure to alcohol, a pharmacologic forced administration procedure provides stable and reliable alcohol doses.

The major disadvantage of a pharmacologic model of alcoholism is that there are few meaningful behavioral questions about the addictive process that can be examined with these procedures. Pharmacologic models are limited to studies of the *effects* of alcohol on various aspects of behavior. Behavioral pharmacologists are primarily interested in the identification and analysis of the processes involved in drug-related reinforcement (KELLEHER et al., 1976). Since drug self-administration behavior presumably is maintained by its consequences, analysis of the variables which maintain drug use and abuse are of critical importance. This is why an adequate behavioral model of alcohol addiction must show that alcohol functions as a reinforcement, in addition to fulfilling the pharmacologic criteria of tolerance and physical dependence (WOODS and WINGER, 1974). Behavioral (self-administration) models facilitate the examination of factors which contribute to the development of the addictive process as a function of time. Eventually, behavioral models should permit the identification and subsequent manipulation of environmental determinants which affect the acquisition and maintenance of addictive drinking (MEISCH, 1977).

II. Behavioral Studies of Alcohol Reinforcement

WINGER, WOODS, and co-workers have systematically analyzed the reinforcing properties of alcohol using a monkey intravenous self-administration model (WOODS and WINGER, 1971; WOODS et al., 1971; WINGER and WOODS, 1973; KAROLY et al., 1978) and have compared alcohol to other reinforcing drugs such as codeine (CARNEY et al., 1976). Their major findings concerning the effects of alcohol dose per injection, alcohol pretreatment, and duration of access on intravenous alcohol self-administration are described in the remainder of this section. Alcohol also has been shown to maintain behavior leading to its administration when presented nasogastrically

(YANAGITA, 1968; 1970), intragastrically (ALTSHULER and TALLEY, 1977), and orally (MEISCH, 1977). However, the intravenous model will be the focus of this review, since the widest range of behavioral pharmacologic studies have been conducted with that preparation.

There is considerable variation in the initial reaction to drugs among naive monkeys and across drug types. Systematic comparisons of the development of drug self-administration behavior in large groups of naive monkeys given access to a variety of drugs under identical conditions have not been published. Moreover, the difficulties in studying acquisition make it unlikely that such a compendium will become available. Lacking such information, it is difficult to assess the significance of the fact that only 6 of 14 naive monkeys initiated intravenous alcohol self-administration within 10 days of continuous access to alcohol (0.1 g/kg/inf) on a continuous reinforcement schedule (CRF) (WINGER and WOODS, 1973). Moreover, only 8 of 12 naive monkeys initiated intragastric alcohol self-administration (100 mg/kg/inf) on a CRF schedule under continuous access conditions (ALTSHULER and TALLEY, 1977). WINGER and WOODS' recalcitrant monkeys were later exposed to cocaine (0.5 mg/kg/inf) or sodium methohexital (0.5 mg/kg/inf) under the same schedule conditions. Ethanol was then substituted for cocaine or sodium methohexital after monkeys were responding for these drugs. Each animal continued to self-administer alcohol, and differences in patterns and amount of alcohol intake between monkeys with different drug initiation histories were unremarkable. WINGER and WOODS (1973) emphasize that alcohol dose and access time were more important determinants of alcohol self-administration than the initiating conditions. The observation that higher alcohol doses (0.2 vs 0.1 g/kg/inj) increased alcohol self-administration in some monkeys, led WINGER and WOODS to suggest that there may be a dose-time threshold for alcohol reinforcement. If too few injections occur over long interinjection intervals, the reinforcing property of the drug may not be established (WINGER and WOODS, 1973).

1. Effects of Alcohol Dose Per Injection on Alcohol Self-Administration Patterns

Recent studies have shown that intravenous alcohol is an effective reinforcer over a wide range of doses (KAROLY et al., 1978). After 20 or more sessions at an alcohol dose of 0.1 g/kg/inj, monkeys were exposed to each of four other doses (0.05, 0.075, 0.15, or 0.2 g/kg/inj) for at least five 3-h sessions. The alternative doses were presented in an irregular sequence. Each dose change was followed by five or more sessions at the accustomed alcohol dose (0.1 g/kg/inj). It was found that the number of alcohol injections during each 3-h session were inversely related to the dose per injection over an eightfold range. Moreover, there was a slight, nonsignificant tendency for total alcohol intake per session to increase with increasing doses per injection. Monkeys usually adjusted their self-administration behavior to the dose per injection within the first 3-h session of exposure. However, responding maintained by the accustomed dose of alcohol (0.1 g/kg) was stable over the course of the study.

A similar pattern of responding occurred at each alcohol dose, i.e., more injections at the beginning of the session and fewer as the session continued. The decrease in the rate of alcohol injections occurred soonest at the highest dose per injection (0.2 g/kg/inj). Figure 2 shows patterns of alcohol injections cumulated over 15-min segments and averaged over five consecutive 3-h sessions for each of three monkeys. The dose of alcohol per injection is shown above each cumulative curve.

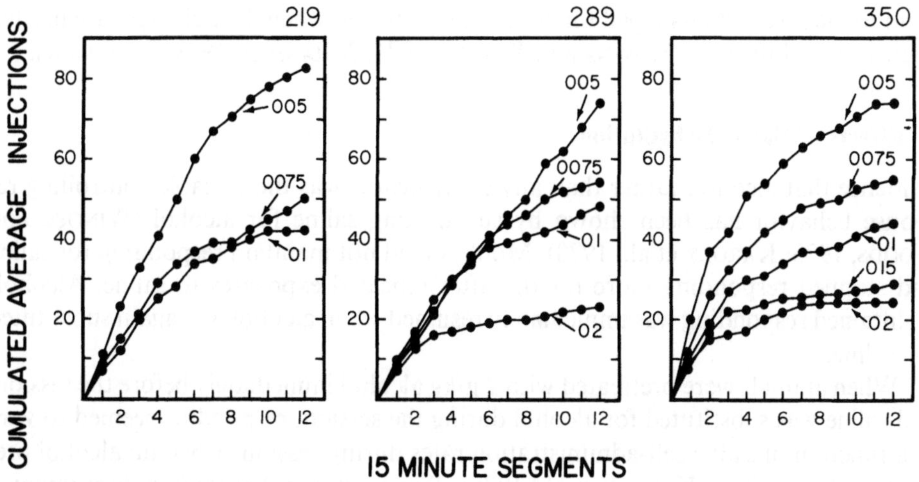

Fig. 2. The effects of Alcohol Dose on Alcohol Self-Administration are illustrated. The effects of varying the injection dose of ethanol on patterns of intrasession alcohol injections for three monkeys (219, 289, and 350). *Abscissa*, each number designates the number of 15-min segments in a 3-h alcohol self-administration session. *Ordinate*, the cumulative number of alcohol injections received. Injections were cumulated in 15-min segments over a 3-h session and averaged over five consecutive sessions. When more than five sessions were available at a given dose, those used in the figure were randomly selected from those available. The numbers associated with the *arrows* indicate the ethanol dose (g/kg) that was administered following each lever response. KAROLY et al. (1978), reprinted with permission

In contrast to these findings in monkey, increases in alcohol dose per ingestion from 1.86 to 11.14 g in human drug abusers resulted in an increase in the number of drinks per session (GRIFFITHS et al., 1976). Increases in the dose per ingestion of diazepam and pentobarbital produced similar results. Although species and procedural differences limit comparisons between these studies, the overall range of doses studied is probably the critical determinant of effects on self-administration behavior. In procedures in which the rate-decreasing effects of successive drug injections cannot confound evaluation of relative dose preference, higher doses are usually preferred to lower doses, up to some critical dose level (JOHANSON, 1978 for discussion).

When the reinforcing properties of intravenous ethanol and codeine were compared, it was found that ethanol maintained behavior leading to its administration as effectively as codeine (CARNEY et al., 1976). Three naive monkeys were trained to self-administer codeine (0.1 mg/kg/inj) and two naive monkeys were trained to self-administer ethanol (100 mg/kg/inj) on ascending values of a variable interval schedule. The effects of a range of doses of codeine (0.003–1.0 mg/kg/inf) and ethanol (32.0–560 mg/kg/inf) were examined in 1-h sessions, under a final schedule of VI 2 min. Response rates were highest at a codeine dose of 0.01 mg/kg/inj and an ethanol dose of 180 mg/kg/inj. Higher and lower doses of each drug resulted in lower rates of responding. Patterns of responding for ethanol and codeine were negatively accelerated within a session. Although codeine produced minimal signs of intoxication at the doses studied, alcohol doses of 180 mg/kg/inj and above resulted in ataxia and impaired corneal reflexes. Blood alcohol levels were not reported (CARNEY et al., 1976). These data conform to the inverted U-shaped function often reported when dose changes are plotted against drug infusions (DOWNS and WOODS, 1974; JOHANSON, 1978, for review).

2. Effects of Saline Substitution

Evidence that alcohol, rather than any other factor, was the variable controlling response behavior has been shown by substituting saline for alcohol (WINGER and WOODS, 1973; KAROLY et al., 1978). Monkeys did not maintain responding for saline and stopped responding more rapidly after repeated exposures to saline. Alcohol-maintained responding was immediately resumed when alcohol was again substituted for saline.

When animals were pretreated with 2 g/kg alcohol immediately before the session, and saline was substituted for alcohol during the session, responding seemed to vary as a function of saline self-administration rates during sessions when no alcohol pretreatment was given (KAROLY et al., 1978). Two monkeys that rapidly discriminated saline from alcohol under the no pretreatment condition, increased the number of saline self-injections following alcohol pretreatment. Monkeys that self-administered saline at a rate approximately equivalent to previous rates of alcohol self-administration did not show a concomitant increase following alcohol pretreatment.

Subsequently, monkeys were given only saline during 3-h sessions over 17 days and were pretreated with alcohol (2 g/kg) on alternate days. Alcohol pretreatment consistently increased the number of saline injections in comparison to the previous session, but this effect gradually diminished over the period of saline exposure. However, when saline sessions were alternated with ethanol sessions, and each saline session was preceded by pretreatment with alcohol, more saline injections were administered than in the absence of alcohol pretreatment (KAROLY et al., 1978). The investigators suggest that the discriminative stimulus potency of ethanol may decrease under conditions when ethanol is no longer available as a reinforcer (KAROLY et al., 1978). Alternatively, it may be that pretreatment with ethanol impaired the monkeys capacity to discriminate alcohol from saline and therefore tended to maintain saline-contingent responding.

3. Effects of Alcohol Pretreatment on Alcohol Self-Administration Patterns

After monkeys had self-administered alcohol (0.1 g/kg/inj) on a continuous reinforcement schedule during 3-h access conditions for at least 15 sessions, the effects of alcohol or saline pretreatment on alcohol self-administration patterns was examined (KAROLY et al., 1978). Each of three doses of alcohol (1.0, 2.0, or 3.0 g/kg) was infused through the intravenous catheter immediately before a daily 3-h session. Each pretreatment dose was separated by a 1-week interval. It was found that alcohol intake was reduced by exactly the dose of alcohol given prior to the self-administration session. These data confirm and extend previous reports of the effects of ethanol pretreatment on intravenous alcohol self-administration (WOODS et al., 1971). The effect of alcohol pretreatment on alcohol intake by three monkeys is shown on the left of Fig. 3.

Despite the consistent dose-related decrease in total alcohol intake, the temporal pattern of alcohol self-injection *within* a session was similar across pretreatment doses.

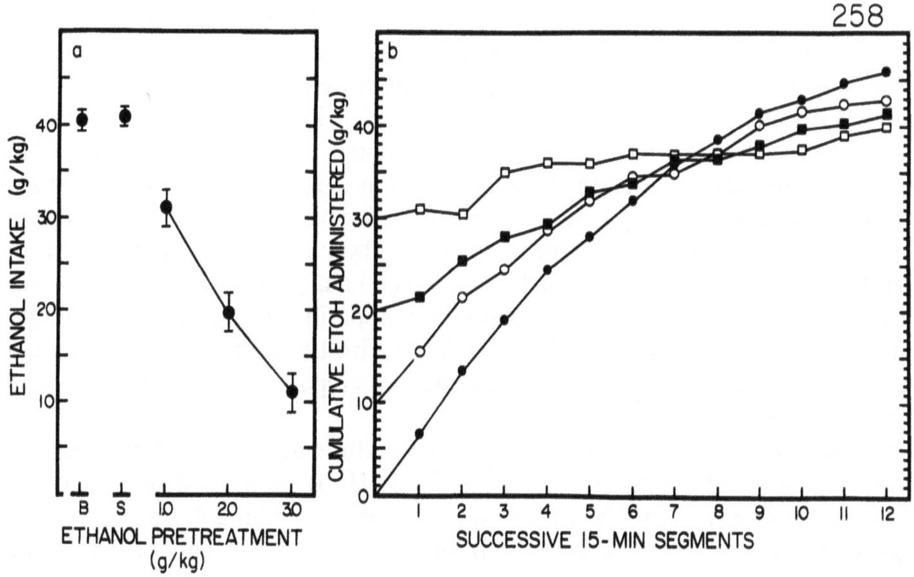

Fig. 3 a, b. The Effects of Alcohol Pre-Treatment on Alcohol Self-Administration are illustrated. **a** The effects of various ethanol pretreatment doses on ethanol intake in three monkeys. *Abscissa*, dose of alcohol in g/kg given immediately before a 3-h session in which each response on the lever resulted in injection of 0.1 g/kg ethanol. *S*, saline, average ethanol intake following saline injections; *B*, baseline, average ethanol intake without pretreatment. Each point is the mean of at least four observations at the designated condition ± 1 sem. **b** The pattern of ethanol intake in daily 3-h sessions for one monkey (258). *Abscissa*, successive 15-min segments in a 3-h session. *Ordinate*, cumulative ethanol administered (g/kg), i.e., the intake incremented by amount given before the session. The pattern of self-injection of ethanol was averaged over at least three sessions at each pretreatment dose and cumulated in 15-min sements over a 3-h session. Although data for this monkey (258) suggest an inverse relation between the alcohol pretreatment dose and total alcohol intake after 3-h, this was not true of other monkeys. KAROLY et al. (1978), reprinted with permission

The pattern of alcohol intake during each 15-min segment of daily 3-h sessions following pretreatment with saline (●) or ethanol at doses of 1.0 g/kg (○), 2.0 g/kg (■), and 3.0 g/kg (□) is shown at the right of Fig. 3.

Although it is not surprising that alcohol pretreatment reduced the level of alcohol self-administration since comparable effects have been seen on opiate self-administration following pretreatment with opiates (JOHANSON, 1978), the effect of alcohol pretreatment has been an issue of acrimonious debate in the clinical literature. One persistent myth about the effects of small doses of alcohol on subsequent drinking by alcoholics is that one drink is sufficient to unleash an episode of uncontrolled drinking. Despite the considerable evidence contrary to this belief (MELLO, 1975 for review), the notion that alcohol exposure can induce alcohol "craving" and uncontrolled drinking continues to influence treatment strategies for alcohol problems. This belief is central to treatment approaches which require total abstinence (PATTISON, 1976).

Clinical studies of drinking behavior following pretreatment with alcohol have yielded inconsistent results. BIGELOW et al. (1977) report that four alcoholic men increased the number of drinks per session from approximately two to more than eight drinks after pretreatment with 33.3 and 77.7 g ethanol. Pretreatment with 11.1 g alcohol did not produce a change in drinking in comparison to the baseline. Conversely, 20 casual and 14 heavy social drinkers did not increase alcohol consumption during a 6-h period following a "happy hour" (BABOR et al., 1978). Alcohol was available at one-half the usual price for 3 h each day during a 20-day period of alcohol access. Subjects drank significantly more during the happy hour. However, there were no significant differences in drinking between subjects participating in the happy hour and controls during the 6 h following the happy hour. BABOR and co-workers (1978) conclude that the happy hour condition did not exert a kindling or priming effect on subsequent alcohol consumption. Further studies comparing the effects of alcohol pretreatment on drinking by alcoholics and heavy drinkers, under comparable conditions, would be necessary to determine if these discrepant findings primarily reflect differences in subject variables.

Expectancy has also been shown to be a powerful determinant of drinking after alcohol pretreatment. MARLATT and co-workers (1973) found that both alcoholics and social drinkers who believed that they were drinking alcohol drank more than subjects who believed they were receiving placebo, regardless of the actual alcohol content of the beverage.

In a recent review of the effects of preloading with alcohol, opiates, and stimulants in man and animal models, GRIFFITHS et al., (1980) conclude that the previous drug baseline is a critical controlling factor. In general, a preload superimposed on a low drug self-administration baseline tends to increase drug intake, whereas a preload superimposed on a high drug self-administration baseline is unlikely to result in a further increase and may in fact decrease subsequent drug self-administration. This appears to be a parsimonious interpretation of an otherwise conflicting literature.

4. Effects of Duration of Alcohol Access on Alcohol Self-Administration

We have seen that patterns of responding within a session are controlled by the dose of alcohol per infusion and the presence or absence of alcohol pretreatment (WINGER and WOODS, 1973; KAROLY et al., 1978). The effects of the schedule of reinforcement on alcohol-maintained responding have not been systematically studied and with only occasional exceptions (CARNEY et al., 1976) investigators have used a CRF.

However, day-to-day patterns of alcohol self-administration appear to be controlled by the number of hours of alcohol access. Under conditions of unrestricted, 24-h access to alcohol, a recurrent alternation of periods of sustained intoxication with periods of self-imposed abstinence has been observed in the intravenous monkey model (DENEAU et al., 1969; WOODS et al., 1971), the intragastric monkey model (ALTSHULER and TALLEY, 1977), and in alcoholic men (NATHAN et al., 1970; MELLO and MENDELSON, 1972). The similarity between alcohol self-administration patterns in men and monkey models is striking.

Under conditions of continuous access, a number of other drugs are also self-administered in a cyclic pattern in both the intravenous and intragastric model. For example, daily self-administration of morphine, cocaine, pentobarbital, and caffeine showed episodic increases and decreases in an intravenous monkey model (DENEAU et al., 1969). Cyclic patterns of intragastric self-administration of pentobarbital, methaqualone, methadone, d-amphetamine, and cocaine have also been observed

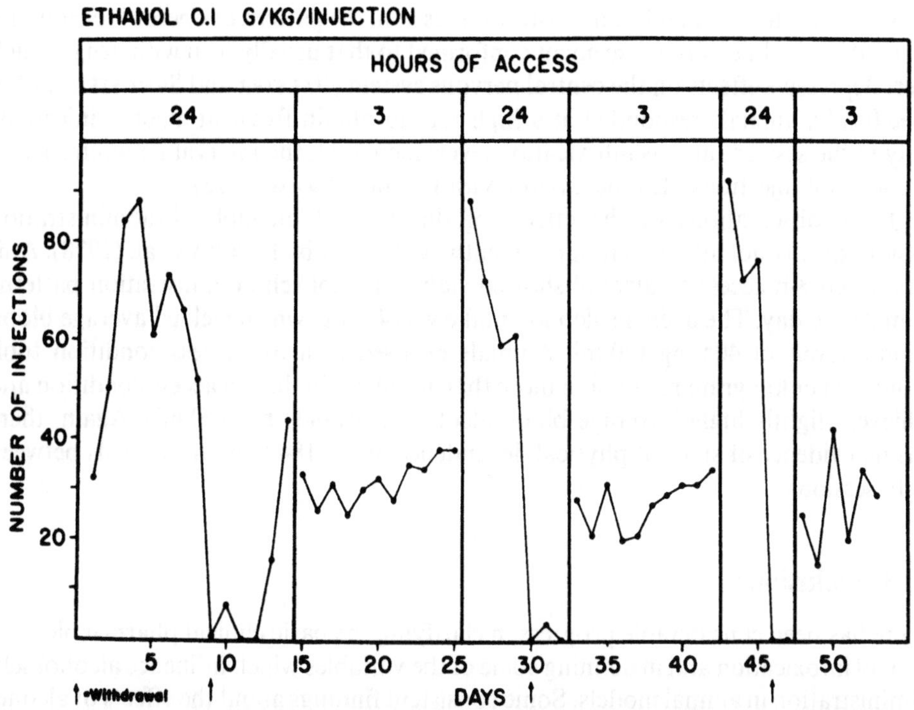

Fig. 4. Effect of hours of access on alcohol self-administration. Periods of 24-h access were alternated with periods of 3-h access to alcohol. This monkey was given 24-h access to 0.1 g/kg/inj ethanol until responding terminated and withdrawal ensued. When responding increased again, the access was limited to 3-h per day for approximately 10 days, and then the 24-h access condition was reinitiated. Occurrences of withdrawal signs are indicated by *arrows*. WINGER and WOODS (1973), reprinted with permission

(ALTSHULER et al., 1975; ALTSHULER and PHILLIPS, 1978). Over the course of many episodes of several days of high drug intake, alternating with several days of low drug intake, animals increase the amount of drug taken during each successive epoch. Total drug intake therefore tends to increase over time (ALTSHULER and PHILLIPS, 1978).

WINGER and WOODS (1973) have compared the effects of unrestricted, 24-h access and limited, 3-h access on patterns of intravenous alcohol administration in seven rhesus monkeys. Alcohol (1.0 or 0.2 g/kg/inj) was available on a continuous reinforcement schedule (CRF). Unrestricted access conditions were associated with episodic intoxication and abstinence as was previously observed. Monkeys took relatively high doses of alcohol (8 g/kg/24 h) and showed signs of physical dependence upon cessation of alcohol-maintained responding. Blood alcohol levels were not reported.

However, when alcohol access was limited to only 3 h each day, and all other conditions were identical, a very different pattern of alcohol self-administration was observed. Animals self-administered less alcohol although in a relatively stable pattern. During the limited access condition, animals averaged between 3 and 5 g/kg per 3-h session. The contrast between the stable daily alcohol intake under 3-h access conditions and the variable self-administration patterns under the 24-h access conditions is clearly illustrated in Fig. 4.

Within each alcohol self-administration session, the pattern of operant responding on a CRF schedule of reinforcement conformed to that usually seen with drugs which exert depressive effects on the central nervous system (Balster and Schuster, 1973). Specifically, animals responded at a high rate to obtain frequent alcohol injections early in the session, and as intoxication levels increased, the interval between successive alcohol injections also increased (Winger and Woods, 1973).

These observations of the effects of duration of alcohol self-administration sessions on alcohol intake were subsequently reaffirmed by Karoly et al. (1978). Animals given 3-h access to alcohol showed stable alcohol self-administration patterns from day to day. The average alcohol intake was 4 g/kg, which yielded average blood alcohol levels of 405 mg/100 ml. Animals exposed to a 6-h access condition took about 1 g per kilogram per session more than monkeys in the 3-h access condition and achieved slightly higher average blood alcohol levels (431 mg/100 ml). Again, there was no evidence of signs of physical dependence in the 18–21 hour intervals between daily sessions.

E. Conclusions

There has been considerable progress in clarifying the basic clinical pharmacology of alcohol intoxication and in defining some of the variables which influence alcohol self-administration in animal models. Some consistent findings about the effects of alcohol on behavior have emerged, despite the pervasive methodological problems which continue to plague studies of the behavioral pharmacology of alcohol. Although a clearer characterization of the dose-response relationships which determine the behavioral and subjective effects of alcohol is urgently needed, it does appear that alcohol intoxication is often less benign and pleasurable than was once believed. These data illustrate how little is known about the reinforcing properties of alcohol and the determinants of the way in which alcohol maintains behavior leading to its self-administration. A focused behavioral analysis of the actual consequences of alcohol intoxication should eventually lead to a clearer understanding of the variables which maintain alcohol use and abuse.

Traditionally, alcohol and alcoholism have been studied separately, and there has been relatively little interest in examining the similarities and differences between the acute and chronic effects of alcohol and other drugs. A comparative analysis of the behavioral pharmacology of many drugs, including alcohol, is one important area for future studies. Although alcohol is frequently used in combination with other drugs, little is known about the behavioral consequences of various polydrug combinations involving alcohol. It is evident that the list of unanswered questions far exceeds the current reservoir of information about the behavioral pharmacology of alcohol.

Acknowledgment. Preparation of this review was supported in part by Grant No. DA-02519 from the National Institute of Drug Abuse and Grant No. AA-04368 from the National Institute on Alcohol Abuse and Alcoholism, ADAMHA. I thank Marjorie Donohoe for excellent editorial assistance in the preparation of this manuscript.

References

Alterman, A.I., Gottheil, E., Crawford, H.D.: Mood changes in an alcoholism treatment program based on drinking decisions. Am. J. Psychiatry *132*, 1032–1037 (1975)

Altshuler, H.L., Phillips, P.E.: Intragastric self-administration of drugs by the primate. In: Drug discrimination and state dependent learning. Ho, B., Chute, D., Richards, D. (eds.), pp. 263–280. New York: Academic Press 1978

Altshuler, H.L., Talley, L.: Intragastric self-administration of ethanol by the rhesus monkey: An animal model of alcoholism. In: Currents in alcoholism. Seixas, F. (ed.), pp. 243–253. New York: Grune & Stratton 1977

Altshuler, H.L., Weaver, S.S., Phillips, P.E., Burch, N.R.: Gastric self-administration in monkeys: Neurophysiological correlates and recent developments. Proc. West. Pharmacol. Soc. *18*, 58–61 (1975)

Babor, T.F., Mendelson, J.H., Greenberg, I., Kuehnle, J.C.: Experimental analysis of the "happy hour": Effects of purchase price on alcohol consumption. Psychopharmacology *58*, 35–41 (1978)

Balster, R.L., Schuster, C.R.: Fixed-interval schedule of cocaine reinforcement: Effect of dose and infusion duration. J. Exp. Anal. Behav. *20*, 119–129 (1973)

Bennion, L.J., Li, T-K.: Alcohol metabolism in American indians and whites: Lack of racial differences in metabolic rate and liver alcohol dehydrogenase. N. Engl. J. Med. *294* (1), 9–13 (1976)

Bigelow, G., Griffiths, R.R., Liebson, I.: Pharmacological influences upon human ethanol self-administration. In: Alcohol intoxication and withdrawal: experimental studies III. Gross, M. (ed.), pp. 523–536. New York: Plenum 1977

Bigelow, G., Liebson, I., Griffiths, R.: Alcoholic drinking: Suppression by a brief time-out procedure. Behav. Res. Ther. *12*, 107–115 (1974)

Boyatzis, R.E.: The effect of alcohol consumption on the aggressive behavior of men. J. Stud. Alcohol *35*, 959–972 (1974)

Boyatzis, R.E.: The predisposition toward alcohol-related interpersonal aggression in men. J. Stud. Alcohol *36*, 1196–1207 (1975)

Briddell, D.W., Wilson, G.T.: Effects of alcohol and expectancy set on male sexual arousal. J. Abnorm. Psychol. *85* (2), 225–234 (1976)

Briddell, D.W., Rimm, D.C., Caddy, G.R., Krawitz, G., Sholis, D., Wunderlin, R.J.: The effects of alcohol and cognitive set on sexual arousal to deviant stimuli. J. Abnorm. Psychol. *87*, 418–430 (1978)

Cappell, H.: An evaluation of tension models of alcohol consumption. In: Research advances in alcohol and drug problems. Gibbins, R., et al. (eds.), Vol. 2., pp. 177–209. New York: Wiley & Sons 1975

Cappell, H., Herman, P.C.: Alcohol and tension reduction: A review. J. Stud. Alcohol *33*, 33–64 (1972)

Carney, J.M., Llewellyn, M.E., Woods, J.H.: Variable interval responding maintained by intravenous codeine and ethanol injections in the rhesus monkey. Pharmacol. Biochem. Behav. *5*, 577–582 (1976)

Cicero, T.J.: A critique of animal models of alcohol self-administration, preference, tolerance and physical dependence. In: The pharmacology of ethanol. Majchrowicz, E. (ed.), pp. 533–560. New York: Plenum 1979

Deneau, G., Yanagita, T., Seevers, M.H.: Self-administration of psychoactive substances by the monkey. Psychopharmacology *16*, 30–48 (1969)

Downs, D.A., Woods, J.H.: Codeine- and cocaine-reinforced responding in rhesus monkeys: Effects of dose on response rates under a fixed ratio schedule. J. Pharmacol. Exp. Ther. *191* (1), 179–188 (1974)

Dubowski, K.M.: Measurement of ethyl alcohol in breath. In: Laboratory Diagnosis of Disease Caused by Toxic Agents. Sunderman, F.J., Sunderman, F.J., jr. (ed.), pp. 316–342. St. Louis: Warren H. Green 1970

Dubowski, K.M.: Human pharmacokinetics of ethanol. 1. Peak blood concentrations and elimination in male and female subjects. Alcohol Tech. Rep. *5* (4), 55–72 (1976)

Ellis, F.W., Pick, J.R.: Experimentally induced ethanol dependence in rhesus monkeys. J. Pharmacol. Exp. Ther. *175*, 88–93 (1970)
Erickson, C.K., Koch, K.I., Mehta, C.S.: Sustained release of alcohol: Subcutaneous silastic implants in mice. Science *199*, 1457–1458 (1978)
Falk, J.L., Samson, H.H.: Schedule-induced dependence on ethanol. In: Control of drug taking behavior by schedules of reinforcement. Kelleher, R.T., Goldberg, S.R., Krasnegor, N. (eds.), pp. 449–464. Baltimore: Williams & Wilkins 1976
Falk, J.L., Tang, M.: Animal model of alcoholism: Critique and progress. In: Alcohol intoxication and withdrawal: experimental studies, III. Gross, M.M. (ed.), pp. 465–493. New York: Plenum 1977
Falk, J.L., Samson, H.H., Winger, G.: Behavioral maintenance of high concentrations of blood ethanol and physical dependence in the rat. Science *177*, 811–813 (1972)
Farkas, G.M., Rosen, R.C.: Effect of alcohol on elicited male sexual response. J. Stud. Alcohol *37*(3), 265–272 (1976)
Goldberg, L.: Quantitative studies on alcohol tolerance in man. The influence of ethyl alcohol on sensory, motor and psychological functions referred to blood alcohol in normal and habituated individuals. Acta Physiol. Scand. [Suppl. 16] *5*, 1–128 (1943)
Goldberg, S.R., Hoffmeister, F., Schlichting, U.U.: Morphine antagonists: Modification of behavioral effects by morphine dependence. In: Drug addiction. I. experimental pharmacology. Singh, J.M., Miller, L., Lal, H. (eds.), pp. 31–48. Mt. Kisco: Futura 1972
Goldstein, D.B.: An animal model for testing effects of drugs on alcohol withdrawal reactions. J. Pharmacol. Exp. Ther. *183*(1), 14–22 (1972)
Goldstein, D.B.: Animal studies of alcohol withdrawal reactions. In: Research advances in alcohol and drug problems. Israel, Y., Glaser, F., Kalant, H., Popham, R.E., Schmidt, W., Smart, R.G. (eds.), Vol. 4, pp. 77–109. New York: Plenum 1978
Goodwin, D.W.: Alcohol in suicide and homicide. J. Stud. Alcohol *34*(1), 144–156 (1973)
Goodwin, D.W., Othmer, E., Halikas, J.A., Freemon, F.: Loss of shortterm memory as a predictor of the alcoholic "blackout". Nature *227*, 201 (1970)
Griffiths, R.R., Bigelow, G., Henningfield, J.E.: Similarities in animal and human drug taking behavior. In: Advances in substance abuse, behavioral and biological research. Mello, N.K. (ed.), Vol. 1, pp. 1–90. Greenwich: JAI 1980
Griffiths, R.R., Bigelow, G., Liebson, I.: Suppression of ethanol self-administration in alcoholics by contingent time-out from social interactions. Behav. Res. Ther. *12*, 327–334 (1974)
Griffiths, R.R., Bigelow, G., Liebson, I.: Effect of ethanol self-administration on choice behavior: Money vs. socializing. Pharmacol. Biochem. Behav. *3*, 443–446 (1975)
Griffiths, R.R., Bigelow, G.E., Liebson, I.: Relationship of social factors to ethanol self-administration in alcoholics. In: Alcoholism: new directions in behavioral research and treatment. Nathan, P.E., Marlatt, G.A., Loberg, T. (eds.), pp. 351–359. New York: Plenum 1978
Griffiths, R.R., Wurster, R.N., Brady, J.V.: Discrete trial choice procedure: Effects of naloxone and methadone on choice between food and heroin. In: Control of drug taking behavior by schedules of reinforcement. Kelleher, R.T., Goldberg, S.R., Krasnegor, N.A. (eds.), pp. 357–365. Baltimore: Williams & Wilkins 1976
Higgins, R.L., Marlatt, G.A.: Effects of anxiety arousal on the consumption of alcohol by alcoholics and social drinkers. J. Consult. Clin. Psychol. *41 (3)*, 426–433 (1973)
Isbell, H., Fraser, H., Wikler, A., Belleville, R., Eisenman, A.: An experimental study of the etiology of rum fits and delirium tremens. Q. J. Stud. Alcohol. *16*, 1–33 (1955)
Israelstam, S., Lambert, S. (eds.): Alcohol, drugs and traffic safety. Proceedings, Sixth International Conference on alcohol, drugs and traffic safety, Toronto, September 8–13, 1974, pp. 939. Toronto: Addiction Research Foundation of Ontario 1975
Johanson, C.E.: Drugs as reinforcers. In: Contemporary research in behavioral pharmacology. Blackman, D.E., Sanger, D.J. (eds.), pp. 325–390. New York: Plenum 1978
Jones, B.M.: Memory impairment on the ascending and descending limbs of the blood alcohol curve. J. Abnorm. Psychol. *82*, 24–32 (1973)
Jones, B.M., Jones, M.K.: Alcohol effects in women during the menstrual cycle. Ann. NY Acad. Sci. *273*, 567–587 (1976a)
Jones, B.M., Jones, M.K.: Women and alcohol: Intoxication, metabolism, and the menstrual cycle. In: Alcoholism problems in women and children. Greenblatt, M., Schuckit, M.A. (eds.), pp. 103–136. New York: Grune & Stratton 1976b

Jones, B.M., Vega, A.: Cognitive performance measured on the ascending and descending limb of the blood alcohol curve. Psychopharmacologia *23*, 99–114 (1972)

Kalant, H., Leblanc, A.E., Wilson, A., Homatidis, S.: Sensorimotor and physiological effects of various alcoholic beverages. In: Alcohol, drugs and traffic safety. Israelstam, S., Lambert, S. (eds.), pp. 371–380. Toronto: Addiction Research Foundation 1975

Karoly, A.J., Winger, G., Ikomi, F., Woods, J.H.: The reinforcing property of ethanol in the rhesus monkey. Psychopharmacology *58*, 19–25 (1978)

Kelleher, R.T., Goldberg, S.R., Krasnegor, N. (eds.): Control of drug taking behavior by schedules of reinforcement, pp. 555. Baltimore: Williams&Wilkins 1976

Kuehnle, J.C., Anderson, W.H., Chandler, E.: Report on first drinking experience in addictive and nonaddictive drinkers. Arch. Gen. Psychiatry *31*, 521–523 (1974)

Lang, A.R., Goeckner, D.J., Adesso, V.J., Marlatt, G.A.: Effects of alcohol on aggression in male social drinkers. J. Abnorm. Psychol. *84*(5), 508–518 (1975)

Leblanc, A.E., Gibbins, R.J., Kalant, H.: Behavioral augmentation of tolerance to ethanol in rat. Psychopharmacologia *30*, 117–122 (1973)

Leblanc, A.E., Kalant, H., Gibbins, R.J.: Acquisition and loss of behaviorally augmented tolerance to ethanol in the rat. Psychopharmacology *48*, 153–158 (1976)

Leblanc, A.E., Kalant, H., Gibbins, R.J., Berman, N.D.: Acquisition and loss of tolerance to ethanol by the rat. J. Pharmacol. Exp. Ther. *168*, 244–250 (1969)

Lester, D., Freed, E.X.: Criteria for an animal model of alcoholism. Pharmacol. Biochem. Behav. *1*, 103–107 (1973)

Lieber, C.S., Decarli, L.M., Rubin, E.: Sequential production of fatty liver, hepatitis, and cirrhosis in sub-human primates fed ethanol with adequate diets. Proc. Natl. Acad. Sci. USA *72*(2), 437–441 (1975)

Logue, P.E., Gentry, W.D., Linnoila, M., Erwin, C.W.: Effect of alcohol consumption on state anxiety changes in male and female nonalcoholics. Am. J. Psychiatry *135*(9), 1079–1081 (1978)

Marlatt, G.A., Rohsenow, D.J.: Cognitive processes in alcohol use: Expectancy and the balanced placebo design. In: Advances in substance abuse: Behavioral and biological research. Mello, N.K. (ed.), Vol. 1, pp. 159–199. Greenwich: JAI 1980

Marlatt, G.A., Demming, B., Reid, J.B.: Loss of control drinking in alcoholics: An experimental analogue. J. Abnorm. Psychol. *81*(3), 233–241 (1973)

McGuire, M.T., Mendelson, J.H., Stein, S.: Comparative psychosocial studies of alcoholic and non-alcoholic subjects under going experimentally induced ethanol intoxication. Psychosom. Med. *28*, 13–25 (1966)

McMillan, D.E., Leander, J.D.: Effects of drugs on schedule-controlled behavior. In: Behavioral pharmacology. Glick, S.D., Goldfarb, J. (eds.), pp. 85–139. St. Louis: Mosby 1976

Meisch, R.A.: Ethanol self-administration: Infrahuman studies. In: Advances in behavioral pharmacology. Thompson, T., Dews, P.B. (eds.), Vol. 1, pp. 35–84. New York: Academic Press 1977

Mello, N.K.: Some aspects of the behavioral pharmacology of alcohol. In: Psychopharmacology. A review of progress 1957–1967. Efron, D.H. (ed.), pp. 787–809. PHS Publ. No. 1863, Washington: U.S. Gov Printing Office 1968

Mello, N.K.: Alcohol effects on delayed matching to sample performance by rhesus monkey. Physiol. Behav. *7*, 77–101 (1971)

Mello, N.K.: Behavioral studies of alcoholism. In: The biology of alcoholism: Physiology and behavior. Kissin, B., Begleiter, H. (eds.), Vol. II, pp. 219–291. New York: Plenum 1972

Mello, N.K.: A review of methods to induce alcohol addiction in animals. Pharmacol. Biochem. Behav. *1*, 89–101 (1973a)

Mello, N.K.: Short-term memory function in alcohol addicts during intoxication. In: Alcohol intoxication and withdrawal: experimental studies. Gross, M.M. (ed.), Proc. 30th internat. congress on alcoholism and drug dependence, pp. 333–344. New York: Plenum 1973b

Mello, N.K.: A semantic aspect of alcoholism. In: Biological and behavioral approaches to drug dependence. Cappell, H.D., LeBlanc, A.E. (eds.), pp. 73–87. Toronto: Addiction Research Foundation of Ontario 1975

Mello, N.K.: Animal models for the study of alcohol addiction. Psychoneuroendocrinology *1*, 347–357 (1976a)

Mello, N.K.: Some issues in research on the biology of alcoholism. In: Alcohol and alcohol problems: New thinking and new directions. Filstead, W.J., Rossi, J.J., Keller, M. (eds.), pp. 167–191. Cambridge: Ballinger 1976b

Mello, N.K.: Schedule-induced polydipsia and oral drug intake. In: Control of drug taking behavior by schedules of reinforcement. Kelleher, R.T., Goldberg, S.R., Krasnegor, N. (eds.), pp. 489–498. Baltimore: Williams & Wilkins 1976c

Mello, N.K.: Stimulus self-administration: Some implications for the prediction of drug abuse liability. In: Predicting dependence liability of stimulant and depressant drugs. Thompson, T., Unna, K.R. (eds.), pp. 243–260. Baltimore: University Park Press 1977

Mello, N.K.: Control of drug self-administration: The role of aversive consequences. In: Phencyclidine abuse: An appraisal. Peterson, R.C., Stillman, R.C. (ed.), pp. 289–308. Washington: U.S. Gov Printing Office 1978a

Mello, N.K.: Alcoholism and the behavioral pharmacology of alcohol: 1967–1977. In: Psychopharmacology. A generation of progress. Lipton, M.A., DiMascio, A., Killam, K.F. (eds.), pp. 1619–1637. New York: Raven 1978b

Mello, N.K.: Animal models of alcoholism: Progress and prospects. In: Modification of pathological behavior, experimental analysis of etiology and therapy. Davidson, R.S. (ed.), pp. 273–333. New York: Gardner 1979

Mello, N.K.: Behavioral and biological aspects of alcohol problems in women. In: Research advances in alcohol and drug problems. Alcohol and drug problems in women. Kalant, O. (ed.), Vol. V, pp. 263–298. New York: Plenum 1980

Mello, N.K., Mendelson, J.H.: Experimentally induced intoxication in alcoholics: A comparison between programmed and spontaneous drinking. J. Pharmacol. Exp. Ther. *173*, 101–116 (1970)

Mello, N.K., Mendelson, J.H.: Drinking patterns during work-contingent and non-contingent alcohol acquisition. Psychosom. Med. *34 (2)*, 139–164 (1972)

Mello, N.K., Mendelson, J.H.: Clinical aspects of alcohol dependence. In: Handbook of experimental pharmacology. Martin, W. (ed.), pp. 613–666. Berlin, Heidelberg, New York: Springer 1977

Mello, N.K., Mendelson, J.H.: Alcohol and human behavior. In: Handbook of psychopharmacology. Vol. 12 Drugs of Abuse. Iversen, L.L., Iversen, S.D., Snyder, S.H. (eds.), pp. 235–317. New York: Plenum 1978a

Mello, N.K., Mendelson, J.H.: Behavioral pharmacology of human alcohol, heroin and marihuana use. In: The bases of addiction. Fishman, J. (ed.), pp. 133–158. Berlin: Dahlem Konferenzen 1978b

Mello, N.K., Mendelson, J.H.: Marihuana, alcohol, and polydrug use: Human self-administration studies. In: Self-administration of abused substances: Methods for study. Krasnegor, N. (ed.), pp. 93–127. Washington: U.S. Gov Printing Office 1978c

Mendelson, J.H.: Experimentally induced chronic intoxication and withdrawal in alcoholics. J. Stud. Alcohol [Suppl.] *2*, pp. 108–116 (1964)

Mendelson, J.H.: Ethanol-1-C^{14} metabolism in alcoholics and non-alcoholics. Science *159*, 319–320 (1968)

Mendelson, J.H.: Biological concomitants of alcoholism. N. Engl. J. Med. *283*, 24–32 and 71–81 (1970)

Mendelson, J.H., Mello, N.K.: Alcohol, aggression and androgens. In: Aggression, proceedings A.R.N.M.D. Frazier, S.H. (ed.), pp. 225–247. Baltimore: Williams & Wilkins 1974

Mendelson, J.H., Mello, N.K.: The diagnosis of alcoholism. In: Diagnosis and treatment of alcoholism. Mendelson, J.H., Mello, N.K. (eds.), pp. 1–18. New York: McGraw-Hill 1979

Mendelson, J.H., Mello, N.K., Ellingboe, J.: Effects of alcohol on pituitary-gonadal hormones, sexual function and aggression in human males. In: Psychopharmacology, a generation of progress. Lipton, M.A., DiMascio, A., Killiam, K.F. (eds.), pp. 1677–1691. New York: Raven 1978

Meyer, R.E., Mirin, S.M.: The heroin stimulus. pp. 254. New York: Plenum 1979

Miller, P.M., Hersen, M., Eisler, R.M., Hilsman, G.: Effects of social stress on operant drinking of alcoholics and social drinkers. Behav. Res. Ther. *12*, 67–72 (1974)

Mirin, S.M., McNamee, H.B., Meyer, R.E.: Psychopathology, craving and mood during heroin acquisition: An experimental study. Int. J. Addict. *11 (3)*, 525–543 (1976)

Morse, W.H., Kelleher, R.T.: Schedules as fundamental determinants of behavior. In: The theory of reinforcement schedules: Schoenfeld, W.N. (ed.), pp. 139–185. New York: Appleton-Century-Crofts 1970
Morse, W.H., Kelleher, R.T.: Determinants of reinforcement and punishment. In: Operant behavior. Honig, W.K., Staddon, J.E.R. (eds.), Vol. 2, pp. 174–200. Englewood Cliffs: Prentice Hall 1977
Morse, W.H., McKearney, J.W., Kelleher, R.T.: Control of behavior by noxious stimuli. In: Handbook of psychopharmacology. Iversen, L.L., Iversen, S.D., Snyder, S.H. (eds.), Vol. 7, pp. 151–180. New York: Plenum 1977
Moskowitz, H., Burns, M.: Effects of rate of drinking on human performance. J. Stud. Alcohol *37 (5)*, 598–605 (1975)
Myers, R.D., Veale, W.L.: The determinants of alcohol preference in animals. In: Biology of alcoholism: Physiology and behavior. Kissin, B., Begleiter, H. (eds.), Vol. II, pp. 131–168. New York: Plenum 1972
Nathan, P.E., O'Brien, J.S.: An experimental analysis of behavior of alcoholics and nonalcoholics during prolonged experimental drinking: A necessary precursor of behavior therapy? Behav. Ther. *2 (4)*, 455–476 (1971)
Nathan, P.E., O'Brien, J.S., Norton, D.: Comparative studies of the inter-personal and affective behavior of alcoholics and non-alcoholics during prolonged experimental drinking. In: Recent advances in studies of alcoholism. Mello, N.K., Mendelson, J.H. (eds.), pp. 619–646. Washington: U.S. Gov Printing Office 1971 a
Nathan, P.E., O'Brien, J.S., Lowenstein, L.M.: Operant studies of chronic alcoholism: Interaction of alcohol and alcoholics. In: Biological aspects of alcohol. Roach, M.K., McIsaac, W.M., Creaven, P.J. (eds.), pp. 341–370. Austin: University of Texas 1971 b
Nathan, P.E., Goldman, M.S., Lisman, S.A., Taylor, H.A.: Alcohol and alcoholics: A behavioral approach. Trans. N. Y. Acad. Sci. *34*, 602–627 (1972)
Nathan, P.E., Titler, N.A., Lowenstein, L.M., Solomon, P., Rossi, A.M.: Behavioral analysis of chronic alcoholism: Interaction of alcohol and human contact. Arch. Gen. Psychiatry *22*, 419–430 (1970)
Pattison, E.M.: Nonabstinent drinking goals in the treatment of alcoholics. In: Research advances in alcohol and drug problems. Gibbins, R.V., Israel, Y., Kalant, H., Popham, R.E., Schmidt, W., Smart, R.G. (eds.), Vol. 3, pp. 401–455. New York: Wiley & Sons 1976
Persky, H., O'Brien, C.P., Fine, E., Howard, W.J., Khan, M.A., Beck, R.W.: The effect of alcohol and smoking on testosterone function and aggression in chronic alcoholics. Am. J. Psychiatry *134 (6)*, 621–625 (1977)
Preston, A.M., Tumbleson, M.E., Hutcheson, D.P., Middleton, C.C.: Alcohol consumption and vehicle preference in young sinclair (S-1) miniature swine fed two levels of dietary protein (36828). Proc. Soc. Exp. Biol. Med. *141*, 585–589 (1972)
Preston, A.M., Tumbleson, M.E., Hutcheson, D.P.: Ethanol consumption and enzyme activities in sinclair miniature pigs. J. Stud. Alcohol *34*, 1293–1302 (1973)
Rubin, H.B., Henson, D.E.: Effects of alcohol on male sexual responding. Psychopharmacology *47 (2)*, 1323–1324 (1976)
Russell, J.A., Mehrabian, A.: The mediating role of emotions in alcohol use. J. Stud. Alcohol *36 (11)*, 1508–1536 (1975)
Schuster, C.R., Johanson, C.E.: The use of animal models for the study of drug abuse. In: Research advances in alcohol and drug problems. Gibbons, R.J., Israel, Y., Kalant, H., Popham, R.E., Schmidt, W., Smart, R.G. (eds.), Vol. 1, pp. 1–31. New York: Wiley & Sons 1974
Seevers, M.H., Deneau, G.A.: A critique of the dual action hypothesis of morphine physical dependence. Arch. Int. Pharmacodyn. Ther. *140*, 514–520 (1963)
Smith, M.E., Newman, H.W.: The rate of ethanol metabolism in fed and fasting animals. J. Biol. Chem. *234*, 1544 (1959)
Smith, R.C., Parker, E., Noble, E.P.: Alcohol and affect in dyadic social interaction. Psychosom. Med. *37*, 25–40 (1975)
Sommer, B.: The effect of menstruation on cognitive and perceptual-motor behavior: A review. Psychosom. Med. *35*, 515–534 (1973)
Steffan, J.J., Nathan, P.E., Taylor, H.A.: Tension-reducing effects of alcohol: Further evidence and some methodological considerations. J. Abnorm. Psychol. *83 (5)*, 542–547 (1974)

Steinglass, P., Wolin, S.: Explorations of a systems approach to alcoholism: Clinical observations of a simulated drinking gang. Arch. Gen. Psychiatry *31*, 527–532 (1974)
Talland, G.A.: Effects of alcohol on performance in continuous attention in tasks. Psychosom. Med. *28 (II)*, 596–604 (1966)
Talland, G.A., Mendelson, J.H., Ryack, P.: Experimentally induced chronic intoxication and withdrawal in alcoholics. Pt. 4, tests of motor skills. Q. J. Stud. Alcohol [Suppl.] 2, 53–73 (1964a)
Talland, G.A., Mendelson, J.H., Ryack, P.: Experimentally induced chronic intoxication and withdrawal in alcoholics. Pt. 5, tests of attention. Q. J. Stud. Alcohol [Suppl.] 2, 74–86 (1964b)
Tamerin, J.S., Mendelson, J.H.: The psychodynamics of chronic inebriation: Observations of alcoholics during the process of drinking in an experimental group setting. Am. J. Psychiatry *125*, 886–899 (1969)
Tamerin, J.S., Weiner, S., Mendelson, J.H.: Alcoholics' expectancies and recall of experiences during intoxication. Am. J. Psychiatry *126*, 1697–1704 (1970)
Tarika, J.S., Winger, S.: The effects of ethanol, phenobarbital, and baclofen on alcohol withdrawal in the rhesus monkey. Personal Communication (1979)
Taylor, S.P., Gammon, C.B.: Effects of type and dose of alcohol on human physical aggression. J. Pers. Soc. Psychol. *32 (1)*, 169–175 (1975)
Thornton, C.C., Alterman, A.I., Skoloda, T.E., Gottheil, E.: Drinking and socializing in "introverted" and "extroverted" alcoholics. Ann. NY Acad. Sci. *273*, 481–487 (1976)
Tinklenberg, J.R.: Alcohol and violence. In: Alcoholism: Progress in research and treatment. Bourne, P., Fox, R. (eds.), pp. 195–210. New York: Academic Press 1973
Victor, M., Adams, R.D.: The effect of alcohol on the nervous system. Res. Publ. Assoc. Res. Nerv. Ment. Dis. *32*, 526–573 (1953)
Waller, J.A.: The roles of alcohol and problem drinking, drugs and medical impairment. Report to the Department of Health Education and Welfare, Environmental Control Administration (1972)
Ward, M.M., Stone, S.C., Sandman, C.A.: Visual perception in women during the menstrual cycle. Physiol. Behav. *20*, 239–243 (1978)
Warren, G.H., Raynes, A.E.: Mood changes during three conditions of alcohol intake. J. Stud. Alcohol *33*, 979–989 (1972)
Williams, A.F.: Social drinking, anxiety and depression. J. Pers. Soc. Psychol. *3*, 689–693 (1966)
Wilson, G.T.: Alcohol and human sexual behavior. Behav. Res. Ther. *15*, 239–252 (1977)
Wilson, G.T., Lawson, D.M.: Expectancies, alcohol and sexual arousal in male social drinkers. J. Abnorm. Psychol. *85*, 587–594 (1976a)
Wilson, G.T., Lawson, D.M.: Effects of alcohol on sexual arousal in women. J. Abnorm. Psychol. *85 (5)*, 489–497 (1976b)
Winger, G.D., Woods, J.H.: The reinforcing property of ethanol in the rhesus monkey: I. Initiation, maintenance and termination of intravenous ethanol-reinforced responding. Ann. NY Acad. Sci. *215*, 162–175 (1973)
Wolfgang, M.E.: Patterns in criminal homicide. Philadelphia: University of Pennsylvania Press 1958
Woods, J.H., Winger, G.: A critique of methods for inducing ethanol self-intoxication in animals. In: Recent advances in studies of alcoholism. Mello, N.K., Mendelson, J.H. (eds.), pp. 413–436. Washington: U.S. Gov Printing Office 1971
Woods, J.H., Ikomi, F., Winger, G.: The reinforcing property of ethanol. In: Biological Aspects of Alcohol. Roach, M.K., McIsaac, W.M, Creaven, P.J. (eds.), pp. 371–388. Austin: Univ. of Texas Press 1971
Woods, J.H., Winger, G.D.: Alcoholism and animals. Prev. Med. *3*, 49–60 (1974)
Woods, J.H., Downs, D.A., Carney, J.: Behavioral functions of narcotic antagonists: Response-drug contingencies. Fed. Proc. *34 (9)*, 1777–1784 (1975)
Yanagita, T.: A technique for self-administration of water-insoluble drugs to monkeys by means of chronically implanted stomach catheters. Bull. Comm. Prob. Drug Depend. *30*, 5631 (1968)
Yanagita, T.: Self-administration studies on various dependence producing agents in monkeys. Univ. Mich. Med. Cent. J. *36 (4)*, 216–224 (1970)

CHAPTER 11

Biochemical Pharmacology of Alcohol

J. Ellingboe and J. H. Mendelson

A. Introduction

During recent years, a large amount of data has been obtained describing the diversity of alcohol actions on biologic systems. While the study of opiate drugs has led to the discovery of endogenous opioid peptides and specific receptors mediating their actions, investigations of alcohol have revealed increasingly complex primary effects and a multitude of secondary biologic consequences. In contrast to opiate alkaloids and endogenous peptides, ethanol is lacking in informational content. Its much simpler molecular structure is less likely to be able to interact specifically with a particular putative receptor. Because of its physical and chemical properties, ethanol can be considered to have dual actions on biologic systems. Like other nonspecific anesthetics, it produces some of its effects because of its particular balance of polar and nonpolar interactions with biologic membranes. The other important property of ethanol is that of an oxidizable substrate, with multiple consequences that include perturbation of normal metabolism and the production of the highly reactive and potentially toxic agent, acetaldehyde.

In a preceding volume of this series, Smith (1977) has already provided an exhaustive survey and discussion of sites and mechanisms of action of sedative-hypnotics, anesthetics, and alcohol. We have also chosen to review effects of alcohol on the central nervous system, however, only selected topics related to biochemical mechanisms will be presented. We will focus particularly on the effects of ethanol on brain metabolism, neurotransmitters, and membrane function. Because of space limitations, certain areas of current research on alcohol, such as those related to genetics, the effects on neuroendocrine systems, alcohol preference, and behavior, are not considered in our discussion. Tolerance, dependence, and withdrawal are discussed with respect to particular biochemical effects of ethanol.

B. Physical and Chemical Properties of Ethanol

Many of the biologic effects of lower aliphatic alcohols appear to be correlated with their physical and chemical properties. Like water, these alcohols have high dielectric constants, an indication of strong hydrogen bonding due to polar hydroxyl groups. Such properties result in a relatively high boiling point for ethanol compared to its corresponding hydrocarbon, ethane. With the addition of methylene units, lengthening the hydrocarbon chain, hydrophilicity of the lower alcohols does not decrease greatly, but rapidly increasing van der Waals/London interactions between hydrocarbons result in enhanced lipophilicity. Nevertheless, the affinity of ethanol toward a strongly lipophilic phase is small compared with that of the higher alcohols. The triolein-water partition coefficient for ethanol is only 0.035, compared to 59.0 for *N*-octanol (25 °C).

The partitioning of alcohols between biologic membranes and physiologic buffer solutions parallels the affinity for extremely lipophilic (oil) phases. For methanol and ethanol, the stronger intramolecular forces between hydroxyl groups predominate. These alcohols are infinitely soluble in water and appear to move freely across biologic membranes, primarily as a function of the concentration gradient. Studies with synthetic and natural biologic membranes indicate that ethanol does not penetrate deeply into the hydrophobic regions of the membrane. Because ethanol cannot easily move through the membrane lipid bilayer, it must diffuse into cells through the channels that regulate entry of cations and certain organic molecules. Unlike water, however, ethanol is potentially oxidizable, with a caloric value of 7.1 cal/g. The extent of oxidation depends upon the oxidative capacity of each particular cell type.

C. Peripheral Actions of Ethanol Having Indirect Effects in the Brain

Before discussing the direct action of alcohol on the brain, we should not neglect the possibility that ethanol might affect the central nervous system indirectly, as a consequence of its peripheral metabolism. Quantitative and qualitative changes in blood-borne substances that normally pass the blood-brain barrier, or that might affect the transport of other compounds into the brain, can alter central nervous system function. Among such substances are acetaldehyde, steroid hormones, glucose, amino acids, and lipids.

The major site of acetaldehyde production from ethanol is the liver, where 90%–95% of ethanol metabolism occurs. The most important route of ethanol oxidation in the liver is through catalysis by alcohol dehydrogenase (alcohol NAD oxidoreductase; EC 1.1.1.1.), a zinc-containing cytoplasmic enzyme of low substrate specificity that requires nicotinamide adenine dinucleotide (NAD) as a cofactor. Other liver enzymes such as catalase and the microsomal ethanol oxidizing system (MEOS) are quantitatively less important in the normal metabolism of ethanol, although there is now considerable evidence to support early reports of an adaptive increase in MEOS activity during long-term ethanol consumption (LIEBER and DECARLI, 1968). Another NAD-requiring enzyme, aldehyde dehydrogenase (aldehyde NAD oxidoreductase; EC 1.2.1.3.), located primarily in mitochondria, catalyzes the oxidation of acetaldehyde to acetate. Acetate is the main product of ethanol metabolism, entering the general circulation and acting as a substrate in the Krebs cycle.

Acetaldehyde is also produced and released into the blood during ethanol oxidation. For technical reasons, the extent of acetaldehyde transport into the brain, and the levels of acetaldehyde in brain tissue, have been difficult to assess until recently. Some earlier studies had indicated that ethanol caused large increases in brain acetaldehyde, but with the use of more modern procedures, which avoid nonenzymatic acetaldehyde formation from ethanol, SIPPEL (1974) and others (SIPPEL and ERIKSSON, 1975; TABAKOFF et al., 1976) have found very little acetaldehyde in the brain following ethanol administration. Nevertheless, acetaldehyde inhalation experiments do increase the acetaldehyde level in brain tissue and cause physical dependence on acetaldehyde and cross-tolerance to ethanol (ORTIZ et al., 1974). Furthermore, a role for acetaldehyde in alcohol dependence is indicated by findings that an acetaldehyde dehydrogenase inhibitor (cyanamide), with or without acetaldehyde administration, was effective in decreasing the symptoms of ethanol withdrawal (DEITRICH and ERWIN, 1975). Some investigators now believe that acetaldehyde, from both central and peripheral sources, may play a role in the neuronal effects of alcohol by condensing with biogenic amines to form pharmacologically active alkaloids (see Sect. D.V.).

On the other hand, the results of many studies suggest that alcohol itself is the important pharmacologic agent in the development of ethanol dependence. An alcohol dehydrogenase inhibitor (pyrazole) has been used to facilitate the development of physical dependence on ethanol (GOLDSTEIN, 1975). Pyrazole potentiates both the acute and chronic effects of ethanol (GOLDSTEIN and PAL, 1971). Considering these and other experimental findings, one is forced to conclude that ethanol and acetaldehyde can both act pharmacologically on the central nervous system. Only at high ethanol doses, however, is acetaldehyde likely to play a significant role. Although cross-tolerance can be demonstrated to many effects of these agents, one should also expect to find dose-related differences in their specific central effects.

Formaldehyde has also been implicated as an agent that could affect the central nervous system during ethanol withdrawal. Apparently a small endogenous production of methanol can normally be handled by the liver, but during ethanol metabolism, methanol oxidation may be delayed until blood ethanol levels drop, during withdrawal. MAJCHROWICZ (1975) has found that a rapid increase in formaldehyde formation occurs when blood ethanol levels are declining, raising the possibility that the well-known toxicitiy of formaldehyde might contribute to the severity of the withdrawal syndrome.

Ethanol metabolism interferes with normal oxidative processes in the liver. As much as three-quarters of the oxidative capacity of the liver may be preempted for the metabolism of ethanol. Oxygen consumption, carbon dioxide production, the respiratory quotient and the ratio of oxidized to reduced nicotinamide adenine dinucleotide (NAD/NADH) are all decreased during ethanol metabolism (LUNDSGAARD, 1938; LELOIR and MUÑOZ, 1938; BÜTTNER et al., 1961; LUNDQUIST et al., 1962; FORSANDER, 1966).

Such dramatic shifts in liver function may have important indirect effects on the brain. Endogenous compounds having functional roles in the brain may be altered by the metabolism of alcohol. For example, steroid hormone metabolism in the liver appears to be affected by the NAD/NADH balance, as the ratio of keto steroids to hydroxy steroids increases during ethanol oxidation, probably because of the reduced availability of the oxidized cofactor NAD. Gonadal steroid biosynthesis, as well as adrenocorticosteroid production, may also be affected because of ethanol metabolism, although effects in vivo may be difficult to interpret because of concomitant direct central effects and compensatory central neuroendocrine mechanisms. Recent experiments indicate that the production of testosterone in Leydig cells from rats testis may be inhibited by limiting amounts of NAD in the presence of ethanol (ELLINGBOE and VARANELLI, 1979). In the brain, especially in the limbic system where specific sex steroid hormone binding sites are localized, changes in the concentrations of androgens, estrogens, and other steroids can have important consequences for neuroendocrine regulation, reproductive function, sexual behavior, and perhaps mood.

Compounding the acute inhibitory effect of ethanol on testicular testosterone synthesis is an increase in testosterone catabolism that occurs in the liver during chronic alcoholism (Rubin et al., 1976). This effect is probably explained by ethanol induction of microsomal oxidizing systems. Alcoholics have long been known to have a greater resistance to certain anesthetic drugs, such as barbiturates, which are catabolized by this detoxification system of the liver.

Among other metabolic effects of ethanol in the periphery is inhibition of gluconeogenesis, which in the absence of other nutritional sources can cause hypoglycemia, with obvious cerebral consequences. Gluconeogenesis is depressed because the lower NAD/NADH ratio of liver cells decreases the availability of pyruvate, which results in reduced decarboxylation of pyruvate to oxaloacetate, and increased lactate production (Krebs et al., 1969). Uridine diphosphate glucose isomerase is similarly inhibited by the change in redox potential, causing suppression of galactose oxidation.

Amino acid metabolism and protein production are also affected by ethanol in liver cells. Free amino acids accumulate during ethanol exposure in the perfused liver (Krebs et al., 1973) and following acute doses of ethanol in the intact rat (Pohorecky and Newman, 1978). Because cerebral serotonin levels are determined in part by the rate of tryptophan transport into brain, and because this depends upon the relative concentration of tryptophan in plasma (Fernstrom and Wurtman, 1971), experiments have been carried out to learn if ethanol-induced changes in plasma tryptophan might alter brain serotonin. Although decreased plasma levels of tryptophan were found following ethanol administration, similar changes were observed for phenylalanine and tyrosine (amino acids that compete with tryptophan for transport into brain), and brain serotonin levels were found to be decreased (Pohorecky and Newman, 1978).

The predominant effect of acute ethanol treatment upon hepatic protein synthesis is inhibition (Rothschild et al., 1971; Jeejeebhoy et al., 1972; Kirsch et al., 1973), while chronic ethanol consumption enhances liver protein synthesis and causes intrahepatic accumulation of proteins that are normally secreted (Baraona and Lieber, 1977). Because ethanol affects the synthesis of "exported" protein such as albumin, a carrier for tryptophan, fatty acids, and other compounds in the peripheral circulation, it is conceivable that the ratio of free to bound plasma metabolites might be altered as a consequence of changing plasma albumin levels. Ethanol-induced alteration in plasma pH or free fatty acids (Lieber et al., 1962; Abramson and Arky, 1968) might also change the proportion of free to bound tryptophan (Curzon et al., 1973), which has been reported to affect its transport into brain (Knott and Curzon, 1972), although there are contradictory data on this point (Madras et al., 1974).

Other peripheral effects of acute and chronic ethanol ingestion include increased oxygen consumption, depleted serum magnesium, calcium and phosphate, alcoholic ketoacidosis, decreased citric acid cycle activity, increased lactate production, increased δ-aminolevulinic acid and porphobilinogen synthesis, increased plasma triglyceride levels, and altered secretory activity in the pancreas and gut. These and other effects of ethanol depend greatly upon the dose, the time course, and the degree of intoxication, dependence, and withdrawal, as well as nutritional factors. At present it is uncertain to what degree such ethanol-induced changes in peripheral biochemistry might affect brain function. Nevertheless, the possibility of such indirect effects should not be dismissed. More holistic research approaches may reveal unforeseen interactions between the peripheral and central effects of ethanol.

D. Pharmacologic Effects and Mechanisms of Ethanol Action in the Brain

I. Effects on Oxidative Metabolism

Although the brain can oxidize some ethanol (HIMWICH et al., 1933), the extent of ethanol metabolism in cerebral tissue is clearly inadequate to supply significant amounts of energy (GOLDFARB and WORTIS, 1940). The capacity of the brain to metabolize ethanol is significantly lower than that of the liver. Brain has only about 1/5000 as much alcohol dehydrogenase activity, based on tissue wet weight, as liver (RASKIN and SOKOLOFF, 1972). Because of the lower ethanol oxidizing capacity of the brain, it is less likely that ethanol would cause a change in the NAD/NADH ratio of brain tissue, as it does in liver. Some investigators have reported that there are small but significant reductions in the brain NAD/NADH ratio during alcohol treatment in vivo (RAWAT et al., 1973); however, others detected no change in the ratio of these cofactors (VELOSO et al., 1972; GUYNN, 1976). Because of low brain alcohol dehydrogenase activity, it is more likely that the enzyme, rather than NAD, might become rate limiting for normal cell function in the presence of ethanol.

Alcohol can affect cerebral oxygen consumption in a number of ways. The vasodilatory effects of ethanol, which result in increased brain blood flow, have been known for some time (THOMAS, 1937). Low doses of ethanol can cause relaxation of vascular smooth muscle and inhibit the actions of vasoconstrictive agonists on small blood vessels, but acetaldehyde is even more potent in this respect in vitro (ALTURA et al., 1978). While net cerebral blood flow increases following acute ethanol administration, dose-related agglutination of red blood cells ("sludging") has been reported to cause reductions in the blood flow of small vessels (MOSKOW et al., 1968). Such mechanical effects can interfere with local oxygen supply and furthermore increase the toxic effects of tissue metabolites for lack of adequate removal. Large doses of ethanol in human subjects can cause a significant decrease (25%–20%) in oxygen uptake from cerebral blood (LOMAN and MYERSON, 1942; BATTEY et al., 1953). Respiratory acidosis has also been shown to occur during heavy intoxication (BATTEY et al., 1953). To a certain degree such acidosis may actually protect against regional hypoxia through centrally mediated increases in brain blood flow and enhanced oxygen delivery (METZGER et al., 1971). At the same time, hypercapnic acidosis inhibits brain glucose utilization (MILLER et al., 1975).

Under normal circumstances the brain is critically dependent upon glucose as its sole energy source (KETY and SCHMIDT, 1948; HAWKINS et al., 1971). There is some evidence that ethanol depresses brain metabolism (GOLDFARB et al., 1940). Nevertheless, it has not been until recently that more rigorous studies have supported the earlier reports of reduced cerebral oxygen consumption in humans by demonstrating depressed glucose uptake and utilization (25% maximum decrease 60 min after ethanol administration) in the brains of heavily intoxicated rats (NIELSEN et al., 1975). Although ethanol has little effect on unstimulated respiration in brain tissue in vitro (BEER and QUASTEL, 1958; WALLGREN and KULONEN, 1960), electric or potassium-stimulated respiration is slightly but significantly decreased by pharmacologic concentrations of ethanol (MAJCHROWICZ, 1965). The time course of respiratory inhibition relative to ethanol-induced narcosis suggests that the inhibitory effect on cerebral energy metabolism is secondary to central depressant effects of ethanol (NIELSEN et al., 1975). The latter effects are believed to be caused primarily by inhibition of sodium and potassium-dependent adenosine triphosphatase (ATPase) activity (JÄRNEFELT, 1961c) (see Sect. D. IV. 3). This would cause a decreased cerebral adenosine triphosphate (ATP) requirement, resulting in an increased [ATP]/[ADP] × [HPO_4^{2-}] ratio (WILSON et al., 1974), increased levels of reduced cytochrome a,a_3 (LAMANNA et al., 1977), and decreased oxygen consumption.

Acetaldehyde has a greater inhibitory effect on mitochondrial respiration than ethanol in homogenates or subcellular fractions of brain tissue (BEER und QUASTEL, 1958; MAJCHROWICZ, 1965). This effect is probably due to interference with the Krebs cycle. Using ^{14}C-labeled substrates such as palmitate and pyruvate, ^{14}C-carbon dioxide production is inhibited only in the absence of the alcohol dehydrogenase inhibitor pyrazole (RAWAT et al., 1973). Although the mechanisms underlying alcohol (or acetaldehyde) inhibition of the Krebs cycle have not yet been clearly delineated in brain, RAWAT and KURIYAMA (1972) and RAWAT et al., (1973) have suggested that it may be due to a shift in the NAD/NADH ratio, while AMMON et al. (1969) proposed that acetaldehyde might prevent entry of acetate into the Krebs cycle by reacting with the sulfhydryl group of coenzyme A (CoA). The latter interpretation may not explain suppression of the Krebs cycle in the intact animal, as brain concentrations of acetaldehyde in vivo are unlikely to reach the level required for inhibition of transacetylation reactions (SIPPEL and ERIKSSON, 1975; TABAKOFF et al., 1976). Furthermore, there is no evidence for ethanol-induced alterations in brain CoA or acetyl CoA levels (GUYNN, 1976).

Chronic ethanol treatment reduces steady-state levels of ATP and creatine phosphate in the quick-frozen rat brain, while adenosine diphosphate (ADP) and adenosine monophosphate (AMP) levels are reported to increase (RAWAT et al., 1973). Such changes in the concentrations of the energy-rich phosphates do not appear to be caused by acute ethanol administration in vivo (RAWAT and KURIYAMA, 1972; VELOSO et al., 1972; RAWAT et al., 1973). These observations may be related to increased membrane ATPase activity during tolerance development (ISRAEL and KURIYAMA, 1971).

II. Effects on Ribonucleic Acid and Protein Synthesis

Cerebral protein synthesis has been found by several groups to be suppressed by long-term ethanol administration to apparently well-nourished experimental animals (TEWARI and NOBLE, 1971; KURIYAMA et al., 1971a; JARLSTEDT, 1972; JARLSTEDT and HAMBERGER, 1972; KHAWAJA et al., 1978). These and other studies have examined the incorporation of radioactively labeled amino acids into protein in vivo and in vitro. Analogous experiments have been carried out to determine the effect of ethanol on ribonucleic acid (RNA) biosynthesis, because interference with RNA metabolism could explain perturbed protein production. The synthesis of RNA was also found to be inhibited by chronic alcohol administration, and several reports have described details of this effect (NOBLE and TEWARI, 1973; FLEMING et al., 1975; TEWARI and NOBLE, 1975). Recent data from TEWARI's laboratory (TEWARI and NOBLE, 1977) demonstrate that long-term ethanol ingestion decreases the synthesis and transport of a rapidly labeled nuclear RNA fraction associated with ribosomes. These data suggested that an essential enzymatic activity such as ATP polymerase, or the availability of polyadenylic acid, might be adversely affected by long-term ethanol treatment (TE-

WARI and NOBLE, 1977). KHAWAJA et al. (1978) also reported that chronic ethanol treatment of weanling rats causes a decrease in labeling of bound ribosomal RNA in vitro, but that amino acid incorporation into free ribosomal RNA is actually increased in preparations from the brains of chronically treated rats.

The significance of these findings and their underlying mechanisms are unclear. It would be of great interest if further studies were to reveal specific effects on proteins that have critical importance to central nervous system function, particularly if such effects relate to adaptive responses underlying the development of tolerance and physical dependence. A cautious approach should be taken in evaluating these and other results from experiments with long-term ethanol-treated experimental animals. Recent studies by JARLSTEDT (1977) reveal no measurable differences in amino acid incorporation or tissue amino acid pools in equally well-nourished rats. The only difference found in the well-nourished animals was greater incorporation of amino acids into liver protein, an observation that is consistent with the known proliferation of smooth endoplasmic reticulum and induction of drug metabolizing enzymes found during chronic alcohol consumption. By varying the nature of the experimental diet, JARLSTEDT obtained no evidence for an effect of ethanol per se, in the absence of dietary deficiencies, on brain protein biosynthesis.

III. Effects on Neurotransmitters

Recognizing the importance of intraneuronal communication for brain function, many investigators have attempted to delineate the effects of alcohol on central neurotransmitters. A large number of publications in this area serve mainly to illustrate the difficulty in drawing general conclusions from highly complex, incomplete, and apparently contradictory reports. In comparing the many published results, it should be apparent that most studies are not directly comparable. Usually, difficulties of interpretation arise because of differences in the ethanol dosage, route and duration of administration, the degree of stress, dependence development or withdrawal, the region of the brain examined, the nutritional status, and biologic differences between species or strains. Often it must be acknowledged that the experimental methodology has been inadequate to measure true steady-state levels of a neurotransmitter or its metabolites at the time of sacrifice. Interpretation of even the best steady-state data may be difficult without further information on the dynamics of synthesis, release, reuptake, catabolism, transport, and the responsiveness of specific receptors. Despite these problems, an attempt will be made to summarize highlights in this field, emphasizing findings that have been confirmed in several laboratories.

1. Biogenic Amines

In early studies of the effect of alcohol on putative neurotransmitters, investigators examined the patterns of urinary metabolites, which reflect peripheral as well as central action of alcohol. Several groups described a shift from the predominant oxidative metabolism of epinephrine, norepinephrine, and serotonin to a reductive pathway during ethanol oxidation (KLINGMAN and GOODALL, 1957; ROSENFELD, 1960; MURPHY et al., 1962; DAVIS et al., 1967a, b; FELDSTEIN et al., 1967; OGATA et al., 1971). Such effects are consistent with the consequence of ethanol metabolism on the redox potential (NAD/NADH ratio) in the liver, but could also be explained by competition between acetaldehyde and biogenic aldehyde (derived from biogenic amines) for rate-limiting levels of aldehyde dehydrogenase activity in the liver. Other investigations have provided evidence supporting the latter explanation as a way of diverting biogenic aldehyde catabolism toward the formation of alcohol derivatives rather than the carboxylic acid products which normally predominate. WALSH and TRUITT (1970) showed that acetaldehyde caused a reductive shift in the metabolism of labeled norepinephrine in vivo, but that ethanol was effective only when administered with an aldehyde dehydrogenase inhibitor. Studies with liver homogenates also demonstrated that the reductive pathway of serotonin metabolism was increased by acetaldehyde, but not by an increase in the NAD concentration (LAHTI and MAJCHROWICZ, 1967, 1969).

In contrast to the ethanol-induced shift from a predominantly oxidative to reductive route of biogenic amine metabolism in the periphery, there is little evidence to support such a change in the brain. Although acetaldehyde can compete strongly for brain aldehyde dehydrogenase and redirect biogenic amine metabolism toward the formation of reduced metabolites in vitro (LAHTI and MAJCHROWICZ, 1969) and in vivo (WALSH and TRUITT, 1970), ethanol itself does not alter the metabolism of serotonin, either in vitro (ECCLESTON et al., 1969) or in vivo (TYTELL and MYERS, 1973), nor does it shift the metabolism of norepinephrine or dopamine (WALSH and TRUITT, 1970; POHORECKY, 1974; KAROUM et al., 1976).

Acute and chronic administrations of ethanol do appear, however, to change the turnover of central catecholamines (POHORECKY, 1974; HUNT and MAJCHROWICZ, 1974; KAROUM et al., 1976; GITLOW et al., 1976), although the specific effects observed are complex and difficult to interpret. When catecholamine synthesis was inhibited using α-methyl-p-tyrosine, acute ethanol administration to rats caused an initial increase in norepinephrine turnover and no effect on dopamine; after several hours the turnover of both catecholamines was reduced. In dependent animals, during both intoxication and withdrawal, norepinephrine turnover was increased while dopamine turnover was lower than normal (HUNT and MAJCHROWICZ, 1974). Other data also suggest that there is an increased turnover of norepinephrine during withdrawal, but either decreased or unaltered dopamine turnover (POHORECKY, 1974; GRIFFITHS et al., 1974; AHTEE and SVARTSTRÖM-FRASER, 1975; DARDEN and HUNT, 1977). Several studies had suggested that acute administration of ethanol increased synthesis and/or release of dopamine (CARLSSON and LINDQVIST, 1973; CARLSSON et al., 1973; SEEMAN and LEE, 1974), but reports from other laboratories did not confirm these findings, indicating instead that dopamine turnover is decreased both in vivo and in vitro following a single dose of ethanol (BUSTOS and ROTH, 1976; DARDEN and HUNT, 1977; GYSLING et al., 1976; POHORECKY and NEWMAN, 1977).

The concept of relative noradrenergic deprivation during withdrawal is reinforced by the effects of certain drugs. Catecholamine agonists and agents that promote endogenous catecholamine production tend to alleviate withdrawal symptoms, while inhibitors of catecholamine synthesis and certain catecholamine antagonists appear to accentuate withdrawal signs (GOLDSTEIN, 1973; GRIFFITHS et al., 1974; BLUM and WALLACE, 1974; COLLIER et al., 1976; BLUM et al., 1976). Such findings are also consistent with the development of noradrenergic receptor subsensitivity during long-term ethanol administration, and supersensitivity of norepinephrine-stimulated adenylate cyclase during late withdrawal (FRENCH et al., 1975, 1977).Evidence for changes in dopamine receptor sensitivity is contradictory, with data supporting the development of dopamine receptor subsensitivity in mice during long-term ethanol treatment and supersensitivity during withdrawal (HOFFMAN and TABAKOFF, 1977; TABAKOFF et al., 1978), and a report that withdrawal in rats is not necessarily associated with postjunctional dopamine receptor supersensitivity (SEEBER and KUSCHINSKY, 1976).

Interest in the effect of ethanol on brain serotonin has been particularly great because of the involvement of both of these pharmacologically active agents in respiratory depression, analgesia, sleep, and hypothermia. Interest has also been stimulated by reports that *p*-chlorophenylalanine (a depletor of central serotonin) reduced ethanol consumption by experimental animals (MYERS and VEALE, 1968). Furthermore, increased brain serotonin levels have been reported during ethanol consumption in ethanol-preferring rats, but not in their water-preferring controls (AHTEE and ERIKSSON, 1972). Because of the demonstration that alcohol intake was not affected by depleting serotonin using means other than *p*-chlorophenylalanine, brain serotonin levels per se may not be involved in ethanol choice (KIIANMAA, 1976). It may also be fortuitous that brain serotonin levels are higher in ethanol-preferring rats, as the genetic selection pressure was not exclusively for ethanol choice.

Studies of ethanol effects on serotonin levels and turnover have also been especially difficult to evaluate. Many reports are contradictory, indicating that ethanol enhances, reduces, or does not change brain serotonin levels. Strain differences (as suggested above), as well as methodological problems, may contribute to the confusing literature on this subject. Most turnover studies, for example, suffer from the nonspecificity of pargyline, the monoamine oxidase inhibitor used to prevent serotonin catabolism, since pargyline acts also as an aldehyde dehydrogenase inhibitor (DEMBIEC et al., 1976).

The more consistent finding regarding serotonin is that brain serotonin levels are not significantly affected by acute ethanol administration, but its major metabolic product, 5-hydroxyindoleacetic acid (5-HIAA), is increased (KURIYAMA et al., 1971b; TABAKOFF and BOGGAN, 1974; POHORECKY and NEWMAN, 1978). Brain tryptophan, the amino acid precursor of serotonin, has also been reported to be elevated modestly after ethanol, but serum tryptophan was reduced (POHORECKY and NEWMAN, 1978). Ethanol might cause an increase in central serotonin turnover, as these results suggest, but impaired removal of 5-HIAA from the brain could also explain increases in this metabolite following ethanol administration (TABAKOFF et al., 1975). Direct inhibition of tryptophan hydroxylase by ethanol (ROGAWSKI et al., 1974), and indirect inhibition of this enzyme through ethanol stimulation of corticosteroid release (ELLIS, 1966; AZMITIA and MCEWEN, 1969; SZE and NECKERS, 1974), have also been suggested as mechanisms to explain apparent ethanol-induced increases in serotonin turnover.

2. Acetylcholine

Some of the complexity and inconsistency of reported ethanol action on catecholaminergic and serotonergic systems may be the consequence of multiple indirect effects from other neurotransmitter systems such as cholinergic neurons, which synapse upon dopamine neurons in the nigrostriatum and affect dopamine turnover. Ethanol probably acts more directly upon acetylcholine release, as is indicated by more consistent experimental findings from studies on this neurotransmitter. Acetylcholine release is decreased by ethanol in brain tissues in vivo (ERICKSON and GRAHAM, 1973) and in cortical slices (CARMICHAEL and ISRAEL, 1975; KALANT and GROSE, 1967). After a single dose of ethanol, brain concentrations of acetylcholine were reported to increase, followed by a later decrease (HUNT and DALTON, 1976). This biphasic effect appears to parallel the rise and fall in blood ethanol levels and is not unlike the effect of ethanol on catecholamine turnover (HUNT and MAJCHROWICZ, 1974). Both acetylcholine and dopamine were reported to rise again after low blood ethanol levels had been reached. In studies of chronic ethanol administration, KALANT and GROSE (1967) found that slices of brain cortex from dependent rats and guinea pigs were refractory to the inhibitory effect of ethanol on acetylcholine release in vitro. Other investigators have shown, however, that cholinergic systems may not be involved directly in ethanol withdrawal (GOLDSTEIN, 1973) or in behavioral intoxication (KLEMM, 1974).

3. Amino Acids

Among the putative amino acid neurotransmitters, γ-aminobutyric acid (GABA) has been more widely studied with respect to alcohol effects. Work done with the whole brain (or brain regions) following administration of ethanol in vivo has yielded conflicting results, some reports describing an increase in steady-state levels of GABA (HÄKKINEN and KULONEN, 1959, 1961; RAWAT, 1974; CHAN, 1976) after a single dose of ethanol, while others have found marked decreases in GABA concentrations (FERRARI and ARNOLD, 1961; HIGGINS, 1962; GORDON, 1967). The action of ethanol in vitro on brain slices has also been examined; a small but significant inhibition of GABA release was found in cortex slices under resting conditions, but not during potassium stimulation (LIN and SUTHERLAND, 1974).

Chronic ethanol intoxication is reported to produce decreases in whole brain or regional GABA levels (PATEL and LAL, 1973; RAWAT, 1974; GRIFFITHS and LITTLETON, 1977). CHOPDE and his colleagues (1977), however, while finding GABA decrements during intoxication, observed increased GABA levels in the brain during withdrawal.

VOLICER et al. (1977) have also found regional differences in the ethanol effect on GABA, levels being reduced only in the cerebellum, subcortex, and pons-medulla oblongata. Subsequent experiments revealed that ethanol lowered GABA only in the brains of animals that had been stressed before being killed (VOLICER et al., 1979). Such results suggest that the contradictory reports found in the literature might be due to different degrees of stress experienced by the animals prior to being killed. The association between ethanol, stress, and GABA may be important to expression of the withdrawal syndrome, as GOLDSTEIN (1973) has found that GABA (also catecholamines) can relieve withdrawal convulsions in mice. Studies of synaptosomal glutamate (an excitatory neurotransmitter) binding are consistent with GOLDSTEIN's observations, as glutamate binding changes in the opposite direction of the presumed decrease in GABA (an inhibitory neurotransmitter) during withdrawal (MICHAELIS et al., 1978). In the latter report, ethanol intake was found to cause a time-dependent increase in glutamate binding in ethanol-tolerant rats.

IV. Effects on Membranes

1. Fluidity

Early hypotheses for the mechanism of action of general anesthetics were based largely upon studies with a homologous series of alcohols. OVERTON (1901) and MEYER (1901) determined that anesthetic potency was related directly to lipid solubility and suggested that the degree of narcosis produced by an anesthetic was proportional to its concentration in the lipid phase of the biologic system affected. Ethanol has therefore been thought to exert its central narcotic effect because of a limited degree of solubility in the lipid regions of neuronal membranes.

Some of the electrophysiologic effects of ethanol may indeed be similar to those of higher alcohols and general anesthetics, attributable to actions that have been called "membrane-fluidization," "membrane-expansion," and "lateral phase separation" (HUBBELL and MCCONNELL, 1968; PATERSON et al., 1972; SEEMAN, 1972; TRUDELL, 1977). Ethanol and some other polar, less potent anesthetics are somewhat different from longer-chain alcohols and the classic general anesthetics in that they appear to be as effective in depressing axonal conductance as in depressing postsynaptic excitation (BARKER, 1974).

Because of its low oil–water partition coefficient, ethanol might not be expected to enter into the hydrophobic core of membrane bilayers as readily as the more lipophilic anesthetics. Using fluorescent probes that penetrate deeply into the membrane, it has been found that the concentration of ethanol must be two orders of magnitude greater than that of general anesthetics to lower the phase transition of synthetic membranes by 2 °C (VANDERKOOI et al., 1977). The actual concentration of ethanol probably required for any significant deep membrane effects is therefore unlikely to be pharmacologically meaningful. On the other hand, using a less hydrophobic probe, aminopyrene, effects of ethanol at the membrane–water interface have been clearly demonstrated at concentrations that can be achieved in vivo (VANDERKOOI, 1979). Studies by GRENELL (1975), utilizing the technique of microwave absorption to measure changes in free and membrane-bound water, suggest that ethanol fluidizes and displaces water associated with outer membrane surfaces.

In GOLDSTEIN's laboratory, paramagnetic resonance has been used to study the effect of ethanol on nerve cell membranes prepared from mice (DBA strain). The particular spin-labeled probe used in these studies, 5-doxylstearic acid, is believed to reflect alterations in the order of the outer membrane, closer to the water interface. In moderate concentrations (1–4 mg/ml) in vitro, ethanol produced a concentration-dependent increase in the fluidity of synaptosomal, erythrocyte, and mitochondrial membranes (CHIN and GOLDSTEIN, 1977a). Fluidity was also increased in cell membranes prepared from mice that had been treated acutely with a single intoxicating dose of ethanol. When the mice were fed ethanol for 8 days, synaptosomal and erythrocyte membranes became more resistant to the disordering effect of ethanol (CHIN and GOLDSTEIN, 1977b). Only when ethanol was present in vitro, however, could differences in membrane fluidity be detected between the control and ethanol-fed mice.

CURRAN and SEEMAN (1977) have also reported the development of tolerance to membrane-fluidizing effects of ethanol. They found that phrenic nerve terminals from ethanol-tolerant rats were more resistant than those from control rats to the acute effect of ethanol in increasing the frequency of miniature end-plate potentials. This particular electrophysiologic measure is believed to reflect spontaneous acetylcholine release (QUASTEL et al., 1971), which is thought to be enhanced by increased membrane fluidity and membrane expansion effects of alcohols and anesthetics (SEEMAN, 1972). Only upon the application of ethanol in vitro was it possible to demonstrate a significant difference between control and ethanol-fed rats. As has been the case with many studies, relatively high levels of ethanol were employed in vitro, with the assumption that measurements at high ethanol concentrations reflect less detectable, but nevertheless meaningful effects at more physiologic concentrations. In this particular report, the investigators demonstrated a linear dose-response relationship from reasonable pharmacologic amounts of ethanol to the higher doses used for most of their experiments.

Because cell membrane fluidity is correlated with temperature (CHAPMAN, 1975), temperature effects on electrophysiologic measures of presynaptic function have been used to indicate degree of dependence upon membrane fluidity. As temperature is lowered, there is a slower decay of posttetanic potentiation of synaptic transmission in model systems such as the abdominal ganglion of *Aplysia californica* (SCHLAPFER et al., 1975). Ethanol accelerates decay of posttetanic potentiation, suggesting that it increases membrane fluidity (WOODSON et al., 1976). After prolonged exposure to ethanol or to lowered temperature, the electrophysiologic response returns to normal (TRAYNOR et al., 1976; SCHLAPFER et al., 1975). In other words, the preparation had developed tolerance to ethanol and had adapted to a colder temperature. Unexpected, however, was the observation that cold-adapted preparations had a normal, preadaptation rate of decay of posttetanic potentiation when tested at the control temperature. Ethanol-tolerant preparations were also normal under control conditions. Temperature-adapted preparations behaved as though they were ethanol-tolerant, and ethanol-tolerant preparations exhibited adaptation to temperature effects, i. e., there was cross tolerance between the effects of temperature and ethanol (TRAYNOR et al., 1979). These observations are difficult to interpret in relation to proposed models for both ethanol tolerance (HILL and BANGHAM, 1975) and temperature adaptation (SINENSKY, 1971) that suggest compensatory changes in lipid composition of the membrane. However, TRAYNOR et al. (1979) point out that there are other examples of bidirectional adaptation that protects organisms against both heat and cold following cold adaptation.

2. Lipids

In an attempt to determine the molecular basis for the apparent development of tolerance to ethanol-induced membrane fluidization, CHIN and her co-workers (1978) examined the membrane lipid composition of synaptosomes and erythrocytes from mice treated chronically with ethanol. The cholesterol/phospholipid ratio was found to be significantly higher in the alcohol-fed animals. Although the phospholipid concentrations per cell (erythrocytes) and per milligram protein (synaptosomal membranes) were not different between control and treated animals, cholesterol levels were increased by 15% and 10%, respectively. Such an increase in cholesterol content is not unexpected in view of earlier studies (GRANDE et al., 1960; LIEBER et al., 1963) that demonstrated elevated plasma cholesterol levels following chronic ethanol administration to dogs and man. An increase in the cholesterol/phospholipid ratio appears to decrease membrane fluidity, both in synthetic membranes and erythrocyte membranes from blood of cirrhotic patients (VANDERKOOI, 1979). The stiffening effect of cholesterol on the membrane is also correlated with decreased oxygen diffusion into the membrane (VANDERKOOI, 1979).

LITTLETON and JOHN (1977) and LITTLETON et al. (1979) have analyzed the fatty acid composition of membrane phospholipids from mice (TO Swiss strain) made tolerant to the effects of ethanol. Chronic ethanol treatment was associated with an increase in the saturation of phospholipid fatty acids, most notably in the synaptosomal membrane. A study of the time course of this effect revealed that the change in fatty acid composition occurred as early as 2 h after acute administration of alcohol and that there was little quantitative difference from the fatty acid pattern observed after 10 days after chronic ethanol treatment (LITTLETON et al., 1979). These lipid alterations are similar to those reported in goldfish and lower organisms in adapting to temperature changes (COSSINS, 1977; COSSINS et al., 1977). Alcohol tolerance and increased temperature adaptation both appear to be associated with decreased membrane fluidity. In general, adaptive decreases in membrane fluidity are correlated with lower content of polyunsaturated fatty acids and a relatively greater proportion of saturated and mono-unsaturated fatty acids.

These several studies of the acute and chronic effects of alcohol on membrane lipid composition lend support to the hypothesis advanced by HILL and BANGHAM (1975) as an explanation for tolerance to central depressants. According to their proposed model, biologic membranes should be able to adapt homeostatically to the acute membrane-fluidizing effects of lipophilic agents through "stiffening" of the membranes. Alcohol-induced changes in membrane lipid composition would be consistent with this concept.

Present evidence is insufficient to postulate a mechanism for the shift toward increased cholesterol content or fatty acid saturation during tolerance development. It would be of great importance to know whether this apparent adaptation of neuronal tissue to the effects of ethanol were due to intrinsic changes within the central nervous system or to passive incorporation of membrane-stiffening lipids from the peripheral circulation. Such lipids might arise because of ethanol effects on fat metabolism in adipose tissue or liver rather than as a result of changes in neuronal metabolism. Indeed, the possibility of a primary peripheral effect appears plausible in view of reports that lipids of erythrocytes (CHIN et al., 1978) and mitochondria from liver (IHRIG et al., 1969) and adrenals (SUN and SUN, 1978), as well as cardiac lipids (REITZ et al., 1973; LITTLETON et al., 1979), exhibit similar changes in cholesterol or fatty acid composition following chronic ethanol treatment of experimental animals. SUN and YAU (1976) have demonstrated that exogenous fatty acid precursors can be incorporated into synaptosomal membrane phospholipids in vivo, while MENDENHALL et al., (1969) have found an increase in lysophosphoglyceride: acyl CoA transferase activity in liver following chronic ethanol administration. It is thus possible that *both* increased membrane phospholipid turnover and changes in circulating lipids might be involved in the changes in neuronal membrane fatty acid composition observed during the acute and chronic adaptation of membranes to the fluidizing effect of ethanol.

The rapid change in membrane phospholipid fatty acids reported by LITTLETON et al. (1979) is reminiscent of so-called acute tolerance, also known as the MELLANBY phenomenon. MELLANBY (1919) first described greater impairment, in humans, associated with a given concentration of blood alcohol during the ascending limb of the blood alcohol curve than with the same alcohol concentration during descending blood alcohol levels. Because MELLANBY had sampled venous blood from the arm, his results were subject to the criticism that the alcohol concentration measured probably did not represent the actual concentrations in arterial blood or brain tissue, which are known to be higher during the early phase of absorption and distribution of alcohol. Other investigators, however, have subsequently corroborated MELLANBY's general conclusions in more definitive experiments in which a variety of dependent variables were measured (MIRSKY et al., 1941; EGGLETON, 1942; MAYNERT and KLINGMAN, 1960). Adequate mechanistic explanations for the phenomenon of "acute" tolerance, particularly with respect to rapid alterations in membrane lipid constituents, have yet to be presented.

3. Sodium- and Potassium-Dependent Adenosine Triphosphatase

JÄRNEFELT (1961a) first reported the presence of a Na^+-stimulated ATPase in a rat brain microsomal preparation and described its inhibition by ethanol at high, but nonlethal concentrations (JÄRNEFELT (1961b, 1961c). Inhibition by methanol, ethanol, and *N*-butanol correlated with their relative intoxicating effects. $(Na^+ + K^+)$-ATPase is now thought to be of primary importance in maintaining the normal resting membrane potential by active transport of monovalent cations (SKOU, 1965).

Subsequent reports have confirmed the acute inhibitory effect of ethanol upon this membrane-bound enzyme system. Active transport of ions in rat brain cortex slices was found to be suppressed by moderate concentrations of ethanol (ISRAEL et al., 1965). In a beef brain microsomal preparation, ISRAEL and SALAZAR (1967) demonstrated ethanol inhibition of $(Na^+ + K^+)$-ATPase and found that K^+, but not Na^+, could competitively antagonize the effects of ethanol. SUN and SAMORAJSKI (1970) reported that ethanol noncompetitively inhibited $(Na^+ + K^+)$-ATPase in guinea pig cortex synaptosomes and was significantly less effective in inhibiting the Mg^{2+}-activated ATPase.

Following long-term administration of ethanol, $(Na^+ + K^+)$-ATPase was reported to be increased in preparations from brains of alcohol-tolerant rats and cats (ISRAEL et al., 1970; KNOX et al., 1972; ROACH et al., 1973; AKERA et al., 1973). This apparent sign of membrane tolerance was not found, however, in mouse brain cerebral cortex homogenates (GOLDSTEIN and ISRAEL, 1972) or microsomal preparations of mouse brain (ISRAEL and KURIYAMA, 1971) and rat brain (AKERA et al., 1973). The variability of reported $(Na^+ + K^+)$-ATPase responses to chronic ethanol administration is probably attributable to differences in the preparations used, to the conditions of the assay, and primarily to the duration of withdrawal prior to measurement of ATPase activity. WALLGREN et al. (1975) have measured microsomal $(Na^+ + K^+)$-ATPase and Mg2$^+$-ATPase activities separately during withdrawal. Increased intensity of withdrawal was correlated with alcohol dose and magnitude of change in the activities of the two ATPases. $(Na^+ + K^+)$-ATPase increased, while Mg^{2+}-ATPase decreased; total ATPase remained unchanged. Subsequent studies by RANGARAJ and KALANT (1978) indicate that there was no increase in the $(Na^+ + K^+)$-ATPase until 12–48 h after cessation of alcohol administration. Enhanced ATPase activity was greatest 24 h into withdrawal and was localized in the lysed synaptosomal membrane fraction. The effect could be observed 16 h after a single dose of ethanol and reversed by another dose given 1 h before sacrifice. Other experiments led the investigators to conclude that the increase in $(Na^+ + K^+)$-ATPase activity was not a direct adaptive homeostatic response to tolerance to ethanol, but rather a more rapid effect of increased catecholaminergic activity associated with withdrawal stress (RANGARAJ and KALANT, 1978). Such an explanation is not inconsistent with the concept of $(Na^+ + K^+)$-ATPase activation and inhibition by conformational changes (membrane fluidity) induced by cations, ethanol, or changes in membrane lipid composition (WARREN et al., 1974; KIMELBERG, 1975; SUN et al., 1977; and KALANT et al., 1978).

4. Calcium

Ethanol and general anesthetics have been found to alter both membrane binding and the transmembrane flux of calcium, not only in neurons but also in other cells (SEEMAN, 1972). Calcium is crucial to the electric stability and physiologic responses of cell membranes. Membrane-bound extracellular calcium appears to act as a barrier to monovalent cation entry into the cell (WHITTAM, 1968). The maintenance of low intracellular calcium concentrations by ATPase-dependent exchange with sodium is believed to be essential for functional integrity of neuronal membranes (DUNCAN, 1976). Calcium is required for coupling electric stimuli to the release of neurotransmitters (DOUGLAS, 1968) and affects cyclic nucleotide systems (BROSTROM et al., 1975) as well as enzymatic activity essential to neurotransmitter synthesis (MORGENROTH et al., 1975).

Following an intoxicating dose of ethanol, membrane-bound calcium was reported to increase significantly (EHRENPREIS, 1965; SEEMAN et al., 1971). SEEMAN's data indicate that this might be due to increased affinity rather than an increase in the number of calcium binding sites. It has been suggested that this might be explained by a conformational change in membrane protein or by an ethanol-induced shift toward more optimal spacing of the negative sites of phospholipids for binding the hydrated calcium ion (SEEMAN, 1972).

ROSS and his colleagues (1974) on the other hand, have reported that acute alcohol (and morphine) administration reduces the regional concentrations and total level of calcium in the rat brain. Chronic alcohol treatment resulted in excess calcium accumulation in synaptosomes, increased membrane-bound calcium, and reduced calcium-binding capacity of synaptic membranes (ROSS, 1977; ROSS et al., 1977). Similar results have also been reported by SUN et al. (1977). Such findings are consistent with the development of increased membrane rigidity during chronic ethanol treatment (see Sect. IV.D.1.), as increases in membrane-bound calcium are known to decrease the fluidity of cell membranes (VIRET and LETERRIER, 1976).

Parallel with the changes in membrane-bound calcium found in the brains of ethanol-tolerant rats, ROSS et al. (1977) demonstrated an increase in the amount of neuraminidase-releasable sialic acid, quite like the study reported earlier by NOBLE et al. (1976) who examined membrane glycoproteins in cultured hamster astroblasts treated chronically with alcohol. These results indicate that alterations in the number of negatively charged glycoprotein residues might explain the effects of ethanol on calcium binding. Further studies by ROSS et al. (1979) revealed that an acute intoxicating dose of ethanol increased rat cortex neuraminidase, while chronic treatment reduced its activity. Such changes are consistent with both the acute and chronic effects of ethanol on membrane-bound calcium.

One of the interesting aspects of the studies reported by ROSS (1976) was that, in addition to ethanol, single doses of salsolinol and morphine also caused regional depletion of brain calcium. Naloxone was found to reverse the calcium effects of all three agents. Tolerance could be demonstrated 24 h after a single dose of either alcohol or morphine, and at this time cross-tolerance between these two drugs could be demonstrated for the calcium-depleting effect. To our knowledge these findings have not yet been confirmed by other laboratories.

5. Cyclic Nucleotides and Membrane Receptors

Cyclic AMP is now well-established as a second messenger regulating and mediating the release and actions of many membrane receptor-bound hormones and neurotransmitters. Numerous investigations have focused on the possibility that ethanol might alter neuronal function because of effects on the adenylate cyclase system. More recently attention has also been directed at the effects of alcohol on cGMP, the function of which is less well-understood. Studies of changes in cyclic neucleotides may also indicate alterations in the effective synaptic concentrations of neurotransmitters or the sensitivity of specific receptors. Although such investigations have yielded few definitive answers regarding the primary mechanisms of ethanol effects on the brain, research in this area has revealed several interesting aspects of the acute and chronic consumption of ethanol.

In several tissues, ethanol had been reported to stimulate the adenylate cyclase system (GORMAN and BITENSKY, 1970; GREENE et al., 1971; VOLICER and HYNIE, 1971; MASHITER et al., 1974). However, KURIYAMA and ISRAEL (1973) could detect no acute effect of ethanol on mouse brain cAMP, adenylate cyclase, or phosphodiesterase. All reports of adenylate cyclase stimulation were at such high ethanol concentrations as to be unlikely in vivo, except perhaps in the gastrointestinal tract where ethanol has been shown to affect both phosphodiesterase and adenylate cyclase, and where increases in mucosal cAMP may mediate the stimulatory effect of ethanol on gastric acid secretion (KARPPANEN et al., 1976).

In contrast to the stimulatory effects of alcohol reported in some tissues, and the negative findings with mouse cerebral cortex, acute administration of a large dose of ethanol to the rat produced a significant decrease of cAMP in brain tissues (VOLICER and GOLD, 1973). Ethanol in large doses was found to inhibit the postdecapitation increase in all areas of the brain examined, while lower doses produced regional effects of different magnitudes. Because anoxia normally causes hydrolysis of ATP to adenosine, which is a major factor in the postdecapitation rise in cAMP, VOLICER and GOLD postulated that inhibition of ATPase activity might explain ethanol suppression of the postdecapitation increase in cAMP.

During chronic ethanol administration, adenylate cyclase activity in the mouse cerebral cortex was reported to increase (ISRAEL et al., 1972), although the effect could not be demonstrated when the assay was done in the presence of sodium fluoride, an activator of adenylate cyclase. Phosphodiesterase activities did not appear to be affected by chronic ethanol treatment, and addition of ethanol in vitro had no effect on either cyclase or diesterase activities. When basal and cAMP-dependent protein kinase were measured after an acute dose of ethanol, or upon ethanol addition in vitro, no alteration in enzymatic activity was detectable (KURIYAMA, 1977). But, when mice were treated chronically, a significant increment was found in the cAMP-dependent protein kinase activity of the synaptosomal preparation.

ISRAEL et al. (1972) found that norepinephrine addition in vitro to cerebral cortex slices from control mice stimulated cAMP formation, whereas no increase above already elevated cAMP levels could be demonstrated in chronically treated animals. More extensive data of similar nature have been provided by other investigators (FRENCH and PALMER, 1973 and FRENCH et al., 1975). These and other results agree with the general model that postulates a decrease in the norepinephrine sensitivity of the receptor-adenylate cyclase system to compensate for increased levels of cAMP during chronic ethanol treatment. The net effect would be to maintain intracellular cAMP levels within the normal range. During withdrawal, however, a quick recovery of this system is proposed to occur (KURIYAMA, 1977), causing a rapid rise in cAMP.

Experiments reported by ASKEW and CHARALAMPOUS (1977), who used mice treated chronically with ethanol vapors, with and without the alcohol dehydrogenase inhibitor pyrazole, revealed no rebound of cerebellar cAMP during withdrawal. Instead, cAMP levels were reduced during the development of the dependent state and remained depressed during the expression of withdrawal symptoms.

COLLIER and his colleagues (1976) have suggested a somewhat similar model for compensatory neuronal subsensitivity during dependence and supersensitivity during withdrawal. According to their comprehensive analysis of factors involved in withdrawal, opposing effects of cAMP and cGMP, and the neurotransmitters affecting their steady-state levels, are proposed to explain the abstinence syndrome.

Cyclic GMP was first reported to be involved in the central effects of ethanol when REDOS et al. (1976) showed that a single dose of ethanol depleted the cerebellar content of cGMP in rats to 5% of control levels within 1 h. In more detailed studies (VOLICER and HURTER, 1977; VOLICER et al., 1977) examined several regions of the rat brain for changes in cAMP, cGMP and GABA. Cyclic GMP was reduced by acute ethanol administration in all brain areas, while cAMP levels were suppressed in cerebral cortex, cerebellum, pons, and medulla oblongata. Chronic ethanol treatment appeared to produce tolerance to the lowering of cAMP, while cGMP was still decreased by a further dose of ethanol. During withdrawal, cAMP and cGMP levels were increased in some brain areas but not in others. GABA levels were decreased in withdrawal only in regions where cGMP levels were increased, indicating that the effect on GMP was mediated through changes in GABA and consistent with a proposed reciprocal relationship between GABA and cGMP.

In a more recent report, VOLICER and his co-workers (1979) present new data indicating that the reciprocal changes in cAMP found in the rat cerebral cortex during acute ethanol treatment and withdrawal may be secondary to other effects. They point out that the magnitude and direction of the alcohol effect on regional cAMP concentrations appear to be dependent on the animal strain or species. Because alcohol can perturb neurotransmitter release at concentrations much lower than those required to affect basal adenylate cyclase, altered cAMP concentrations are more likely to be a reflection of acute and chronic effects on catecholamine release (see Sect. D. III. 1) and/or the sensitivity of the receptor/adenylate cyclase system to catecholamines (FRENCH et al., 1975; SHEN et al., 1977; TABAKOFF et al., 1978).

The reduction in levels of cGMP after acute ethanol administration, on the other hand, appears to be similar in all brain areas and animal strains examined (REDOS et al., 1976; HUNT et al., 1977; VOLICER and HURTER, 1977; VOLICER et al., 1977). That this is not likely to be due to a direct effect on guanylate cyclase has been shown by studies in vitro, which produced no evidence for either acute, chronic, or withdrawal effects of ethanol on basal or sodium azide-stimulated guanylate cyclase in homogenates of mouse brain (MIKI et al., 1977). Guanylate cyclase is dependent, however, on the redox potential, being stimulated by oxidized metabolites (GOLDBERG and HADDOX, 1977). Because of evidence that ethanol might decrease the brain NAD/NADH ratio (RAWAT and KURIYAMA, 1972), rats were pretreated with pyrazole to block ethanol metabolism by alcohol dehydrogenase, thus preventing the redox shift. While ethanol significantly lowered the cGMP levels in cerebral cortex and cerebellum of control rats, the pyrazole-treated rats showed a greatly increased concentration of cGMP in these tissues (VOLICER et al., 1979). It was concluded from these results that the changes in cGMP, observed after acute ethanol administration, are more likely to be secondary to a change in the redox potential of brain tissue produced by ethanol oxidation. Considering the lack of specificity of pyrazole, however, there are other possibilities that should also be considered to explain the acute effect of ethanol on cGMP. One of these is the involvement of acetylcholine, which is known to stimulate cGMP production, while its release is inhibited by ethanol (see Sect. D. III. 3).

Changes in cAMP metabolism associated with chronic ethanol administration might be explained in part by the dependence of adenylate cyclase on the lipid composition of the receptor/membrane system. Increased cholesterol content (i.e., decrease in membrane fluidity) suppresses adenylate cyclase activity in cultured fibroblasts (KLEIN et al., 1978), and coupling of the glucagon receptor to adenylate cyclase in liver cells makes the enzyme sensitive to its lipid environment (HOUSLAY et al., 1976).

Cyclic nucleotide metabolism is also regulated by the relative amounts of free and bound calcium, adenylate cyclase and phosphodiesterase activities being activated by free calcium (BROSTROM et al., 1975; SCHULTZ, 1975). Ethanol-induced changes in synaptosomal calcium concentrations (ROSS, 1977) and the effect of calcium in decreasing membrane fluidity (ROUFOGALIS, 1973) might help to explain regional suppression of intracellular cAMP levels during chronic ethanol administration. The data of VOLICER et al. (1979) show, however, that the decrease in cGMP following ethanol cannot be blocked by intraventricular infusion of calcium.

Adaptive refractory changes in catecholamine receptors coupled to the cyclic nucleotide system might involve decreases in the number of receptors as a compensation for elevated intraneuronal catecholamine concentrations. As has been described previously (Sect. D. III. 1), a number of studies have concurred in finding increased catecholamine activity or increased turnover of catecholamines associated with chronic alcohol treatment. Other reports suggest that a decrease in the number of receptors follows elevation of catecholamine concentrations (KEBABIAN et al., 1975; MUKHERJEE et al., 1975). A rapid change in protein synthesis in response to altered catecholamine levels, as shown in vitro by DEVELLIS and BROOKER (1974), might explain changes in the number of receptors.

V. Aldehyde-Biogenic Amine Cyclization Products

McIsaac (1961) suggested that endogenously produced aldehyde condensation products might be involved in mental illness, and he demonstrated that such a compound could be isolated from the urine of rats treated with alcohol or acetaldehyde as well as monoamine oxidase and aldehyde dehydrogenase inhibitors. The concept that such aberrant agents might be involved in the actions of alcohol was supported by further experimental evidence in 1970. Davis and Walsh (1970) and Cohen and Collins (1970), working with brain stem homogenates and perfused adrenal respectively, showed that salsolinol (the dopamine-acetaldehyde condensation product) and tetrahydropapaveroline (the dopamine-dopaldehyde product) could be produced under certain conditions.

One of the hypotheses suggested by Davis and Walsh (1970) was that these alkaloids might mediate alcohol dependence because of opiatelike properties. This concept was refuted in part by the demonstration that naloxone (an opiate antagonist) did not precipitate withdrawal in ethanol-dependent mice (Goldstein and Judson, 1971). Nevertheless, great interest was stimulated and many reports have since been published describing the isolation, identification, synthesis, and pharmacologic properties of aldehyde-amine condensation products.

To demonstrate that such compounds could be formed in vivo during ethanol treatment, it was necessary to treat animals with enzyme inhibitors to assure high endogenous concentration of the aldehyde and biogenic amine precursors (Davis and Walsh, 1970; Cohen and Collins, 1970; Sandler et al., 1973; Turner et al., 1974; Collins and Bigdeli, 1975). In the absence of other drugs, investigators had been unable to detect significant levels of salsolinol formation in brains of ethanol-dependent mice (O'Neill and Rahwan, 1977). More recently, however, sensitive gas chromatographic techniques have been employed to show that methoxysalsolinol, probably a metabolite of salsolinol, could be formed in mouse striatum after 10 days of ethanol vapor exposure, without the use of other drugs (Hamilton et al., 1978).

To assess the significance of these and other similar findings, one needs to know the local levels of the *active* agent and the concentration required for meaningful pharmacologic effects. The concentration of methoxysalsolinol found in the mouse brain (5–8 ng/g tissue) was probably greater than that of salsolinol. Most effects demonstrated for salsolinol and other cyclized neuroamines appear to require higher concentrations (Rahwan, 1975; Cohen, 1978; Hirst et al., 1977), although the actual local concentration in vivo is difficult to determine. Nevertheless, considerably more information is required before dismissing these compounds as being biologically uninteresting. Only a few of the many naturally occurring isoquinoline alkaloids have been tested for their pharmacologic properties, and other more potent compounds may yet be found in biologic systems. Specific involvement of aldehyde-amine condensation alkaloids in the withdrawal syndrome as false neurotransmitters, or as opiatelike agents, has yet to be established as being biologically significant under normal conditions of ethanol intoxication, dependence, or withdrawal. A recent report is that chronic infusion of tetrahydropapaveroline into the cerebral ventricle of rats caused increased preference for ethanol (Melchior and Myers, 1977). Enhanced ethanol ingestion, dependence, and withdrawal symptoms were produced with local concentrations of tetrahydropapaveroline that were undoubtedly below present detection limits.

E. Conclusion

Steady progress in elucidating the mechanism of action of ethanol on the central nervous system has taken place during the past decade. Most advances have been made possible by the development and application of technologies derived from basic scientific disciplines such as biochemistry and molecular biology. The alcohol molecule has a remarkable ability to perturbate central nervous system function with predictable behavioral concomitants. But until a better understanding of those neural processes which regulate the complex expression of such phenomena as mood, memory, perception, and ideation are understood, it will be difficult to explain the pharmacologic aspects of alcohol intoxication and withdrawal.

What does appear to be clear is that alcohol can achieve its effects upon the central nervous system through diverse yet interrelated systems. Further exploration of alcohol effects on metabolic, neurotransmitter, and membrane function will undoubtedly add new understanding of the biochemical pharmacology of alcohol.

Although there is rapid growth of new information about how alcohol may interact with neurochemical systems and membrane function, many questions remain concerning the significance of this information for our understanding of alcohol abuse. To date we have only obtained the barest shreds of evidence for a neurochemical, neurophysical, or molecular biologic basis for alcohol abuse and alcoholism. Those who pursue knowledge about basic alcohol actions upon the nervous system may rightfully argue that systematic study of the "normal" biochemical pharmacology of alcohol is a prerequisite for understanding the biochemical pharmacology of alcohol abuse. Yet the history of science suggests that the study of pathophysiologic processes has contributed a great deal to fundamental knowledge in biochemistry and molecular biology. Thus, studies of the biochemical and biophysical concomitants of alcohol dependence in experimental animals and humans may enrich the scientific disciplines of pharmacology, biochemistry, and molecular biology.

References

Abramson, E.A., Arky, R.A.: Acute antilipolytic effects of ethyl alcohol and acetate in man. J. Lab. Clin. Med. *72*, 105–117 (1968)

Ahtee, L., Eriksson, K.: 5-Hydroxytryptamine and 5-hydroxyindolylacetic acid content in brain of rat strains selected for their alcohol intake. Physiol. Behav. *8*, 123–126 (1972)

Ahtee, L., Svartström-Fraser, M.: Effect of ethanol dependence and withdrawal on the catecholamines in rat brain and heart. Acta Pharmacol. Toxicol. (Kbh.) *36*, 289–298 (1975)

Akera, T., Rech, R.H., Marquis, W.J., Tobin, T., Brody, T.M.: Lack of relationship between brain $Na^+ + K^+$)-activated adenosine triphosphatase and the development of tolerance to ethanol in rats. J. Pharmacol. Exp. Ther. *185*, 594–601 (1973)

Altura, B.M., Carella, A., Altura, B.T.: Acetaldehyde on vascular smooth muscle: Possible role in vasodilator action of ethanol. Eur. J. Pharmacol. *52*, 73–83 (1978)

Ammon, H.P.T., Estler, C.J., Heim, F.: Inactivation of coenzyme-A by ethanol: 1. Acetaldehyde as mediator of the inactivation of coenzyme-A following the administration of ethanol in vivo. Biochem. Pharmacol. *18*, 29–33 (1969)

Askew, W.E., Charalampous, K.D.: Cyclic AMP and ethanol withdrawal in the mouse cerebellum. In: Currents in alcoholism. Seixas, F.A. (ed.), Vol. 1, pp. 111–121. New York: Grune & Stratton 1977

Azmitia, E.C., jr., McEwen, B.S.: Corticosterone regulation of tryptophan hydroxylase in midbrain of the rat. Science *166*, 1274–1276 (1969)

Baraona, E., Lieber, C.S.: Effects of ethanol on hepatic protein synthesis and secretion. In: Currents in alcoholism. Seixas, F.A. (ed.), Vol. 1, pp. 33–46. New York: Grune & Stratton 1977

Barker, J.L.: Activity of CNS depressants related to hydrophobicity. Nature *252*, 52–54 (1974)

Battey, L.L., Heyman, A., Patterson, J.L., jr.: The effects of ethyl alcohol on cerebral blood flow and metabolism. J. Am. Med. Ass. *152*, 6–10 (1953)

Beer, C.T., Quastel, J.H.: The effects of aliphatic alcohols on the respiration of brain cortex slices and rat brain mitochondria. Can. J. Biochem. *36*, 543–556 (1958)

Blum, K., Wallace, J.E.: Effects of catecholamine synthesis inhibition on ethanol-induced withdrawal symptoms in mice. Br. J. Pharmacol. *51*, 109–111 (1974)

Blum, K., Eubanks, J.D., Wallace, J.E., Hamilton, H.: Enhancement of alcohol withdrawal convulsions in mice by haloperidol. Clin. Toxicol. *9*, 427–434 (1976)

Brostrom, C.O., Huang, Y.C., Breckenridge, B. McL., Wolff, D.J.: Identification of a calcium binding protein as a calcium dependent regulator of brain adenylate cyclase. Proc. Natl. Acad. Sci. USA *72*, 64–68 (1975)

Bustos, G., Roth, R.H.: Effect of acute ethanol treatment on transmitter synthesis and metabolism in central dopaminergic neurons. J. Pharm. Pharmacol. *28*, 580–582 (1976)

Büttner, H., Portwich, F., Engelhardt, K.: Der DPN$^+$ – under DPN-H-Gehalt der Rattenleber während des Abbaues von Äthanol und seine Beeinflussung durch Sulfonylharnstoff und Disulfiram. Arch. Exp. Pathol. Pharmakol. *240*, 573–583 (1961)

Carlsson, A., Lindqvist, M.: Effect of ethanol on the hydroxylation of tyrosine and tryptophan in rat brain in vivo. J. Pharm. Pharmacol. *25*, 437–440 (1973)

Carlsson, A., Magnusson, T., Svenson, T.H., Waldeck, B.: Effect of ethanol on the metabolism of brain catecholamines. Psychopharmacology *30*, 27–36 (1973)

Carmichael, F.J., Israel, Y.: Effects of ethanol on neurotransmitter release by rat brain cortical slices. J. Pharmacol. *193*, 824–834 (1975)

Chan, A.W.K.: Gamma aminobutyric acid in different strains of mice. Effects of ethanol. Life Sci. *19*, 597–604 (1976)

Chapman, D.: Phase transitions and fluidity characteristics of lipids and cell membranes. Q. Rev. Biophys. *8*, 185–235 (1975)

Chin, J.H., Goldstein, D.B.: Effects of low concentrations of ethanol on the fluidity of spin-labeled erythrocyte and brain membranes. Mol. Pharmacol. *13*, 435–441 (1977a)

Chin, J.H., Goldstein, D.B.: Drug tolerance in biomembranes: A spin label study of the effects of ethanol. Science *196*, 684–685 (1977b)

Chin, J.H., Parsons, L.M., Goldstein, D.B.: Increased cholesterol content of erythrocyte and brain membranes in ethanol-tolerant mice. Biochim. Biophys. Acta *513*, 358–363 (1978)

Chopde, C.T., Brahamankar, D.M., Shripad, V.N.: Neurochemical aspects of ethanol dependence and withdrawal reactions in mice. J. Pharmacol. Exp. Ther. *200*, 314–319 (1977)

Cohen, G.: The synaptic properties of some tetrahydroisoquinoline alkaloids. Alcoholism *2*, 121–125 (1978)

Cohen, G., Collins, M.: Alkaloids from catecholamines in adrenal tissue: Possible role in alcoholism. Science *167*, 1749–1751 (1970)

Collier, H.O.J., Hammond, M.D., Schneider, C.: Effects of drugs affecting endogenous amines or cyclic nucleotides on ethanol withdrawal head twitches in mice. Br. J. Pharmacol. *58*, 9–16 (1976)

Collins, M.A., Bigdeli, M.G.: Tetrahydroisoquinolines in vivo. I. Rat brain formation of salsolinol, a condensation product of dopamine and acetaldehyde, under certain conditions during ethanol intoxication. Life Sci. *16*, 585–602 (1975)

Cossins, A.R.: Adaptation of biological membranes to temperature. The effect of temperature acclimation of goldfish upon the viscosity of synaptosomal membranes. Biochim. Biophys. Acta *470*, 395–411 (1977)

Cossins, A.R., Friedlander, M.J., Prosser, C.L.: Correlations between behavioral temperature adaptations of goldfish and the viscosity and fatty acid compositions of their synaptic membranes. J. Comp. Physiol. [A] *120*, 109–121 (1977)

Curran, M., Seeman, P.: Alcohol tolerance in a cholinergic nerve terminal: Relation to the membrane expansion-fluidization theory of ethanol action. Science *197*, 910–911 (1977)

Curzon, G., Friedel, J., Knott, P.J.: The effect of fatty acids on binding of tryptophan to plasma proteins. Nature *242*, 198–200 (1973)

Darden, J.H., Hunt, W.A.: Reduction of striatal dopamine release during an ethanol withdrawal syndrome. J. Neurochem. *29*, 1143–1145 (1977)
Davis, V.E., Walsh, M.J.: Alcohol, amines, and alkaloids: A possible biochemical basis for alcohol addiction. Science *167*, 1005–1007 (1970)
Davis, V.E., Brown, H., Huff, H.A., Cashaw, J.L.: The alteration of serotonin metabolism to 5-hydroxytryptophol by ethanol ingestion in man. J. Lab. Clin. Med. *69*, 132–140 (1967a)
Davis, V.E., Brown, H., Huff, J.A., Cashaw, J.L.: Ethanol-induced alterations of norepinephrine in man. J. Lab. Clin. Med. *69*, 787–799 (1967b)
Deitrich, R.A., Erwin, V.G.: Involvement of biogenic amine metabolism in ethanol addiction. Fed. Proc. *34*, 1962–1968 (1975)
Dembiec, D., MacNamee, D., Cohen, G.: The effects of pargyline and other MAO inhibitors on blood acetaldehyde levels in ethanol-intoxicated mice. J. Pharmacol. Exp. Ther. *197*, 332–339 (1976)
DeVellis, J., Brooker, G.: Reversal of catecholamine refractoriness by inhibitors of RNA and protein synthesis. Science *186*, 1221–1223 (1974)
Douglas, W.W.: Stimulus-secretion coupling: The concept and clues from chromaffin and other cells. Br. J. Pharmacol. *34*, 451–474 (1968)
Duncan, C.J.: Properties of the Ca^{++}-ATPase activity of mammalian synaptic membrane preparations. J. Neurochem. *27*, 1277–1279 (1976)
Eccleston, D., Reading, W., Richie, I.: 5-Hydroxytryptamine metabolism in brain and liver slices and the effects of ethanol. J. Neurochem. *16*, 274–276 (1969)
Eggleton, M.G.: The diuretic action of alcohol in man. J. Physiol. (London), *101*, 172–191 (1942)
Ehrenpreis, S.: An approach to the molecular basis of nerve activity. J. Cell. Comp. Physiol. *66*, 159–164 (1965)
Ellingboe, J., Varanelli, C.C.: Ethanol inhibits testosterone biosynthesis by direct action on Leydig cells. Res. Commun. Chem. Pathol. Pharmacol. *24*, 87–102 (1979)
Ellis, F.W.: Effect of ethanol on plasma corticosterone levels. J. Pharmacol. Exp. Ther. *153*, 121–128 (1966)
Erickson, C.K., Graham, D.T.: Alteration of cortical and reticular acetylcholine release by ethanol in vivo. J. Pharmacol. Exp. Ther. *185*, 583–593 (1973)
Feldstein, A., Hoagland, H., Freeman, H., Williamson, O.: The effect of ethanol on serotonin metabolism in man. Life Sci. *6*, 53–61 (1967)
Fernstrom, J.D., Wurtman, R.J.: Brain serotonin content: Physiological dependence on plasma tryptophan levels. Science *173*, 149–152 (1971)
Ferrari, R.A., Arnold, A.: The effect of central nervous system agents on rat-brain γ-aminobutyric acid level. Biochim. Biophys. Acta *52*, 361–367 (1961)
Fleming, E.W., Tewari, S., Noble, E.P.: Effects of chronic ethanol ingestion on brain aminoacyl-tRNA synthetases and tRNA. J. Neurochem. *24*, 553–560 (1975)
Forsander, O.A.: Influence of the metabolism of ethanol on the lactate/pyruvate ratio of rat-liver slices. Biochem. J. *98* 244–247 (1966)
French, S.W., Palmer, D.S.: Adrenergic supersensitivity during ethanol withdrawal in the rat. Res. Commun. Chem. Pathol. Pharmacol. *6*, 651–662 (1973)
French, S.W., Palmer, D.S., Narod, M.E., Reid, P.E., Ramey, C.W.: Noradrenergic sensitivity of the cerebral cortex after chronic ethanol ingestion and withdrawal. J. Pharmacol. *194*, 319–326 (1975)
French, S.W., Palmer, D.S., Wiggers, K.D.: Changes in receptor sensitivity of the cerebral cortex and liver during chronic ethanol ingestion and withdrawal. Adv. Exp. Med. Biol. *85A*, 515–538 (1977)
Gitlow, S.F., Dziedzic, L.M., Dziedzic, S.W., Wong, B.L.: Influence of ethanol on human catecholamine metabolism. Ann. NY. Acad. Sci. *273*, 263–279 (1976)
Goldberg, N.D., Haddox, M.K.: Cyclic GMP metabolism and involvement in biological regulation. Ann. Rev. Biochem. *46*, 823–896 (1977)
Goldfarb, W., Wortis, J.: The availability of ethyl alcohol for human brain oxidations. Q. J. Stud. Alcohol *1*, 268–271 (1940–41)
Goldfarb, W., Bowman, K.M., Wortis, J.: The effect of alcohol on cerebral metabolism. Am. J. Psychiatry *97*, 384–387 (1940)

Goldstein, D.B.: Alcohol withdrawal reactions in mice: Effects of drugs that modify neurotransmission. J. Pharmacol. Exp. Ther. *186*, 1–9 (1973)

Goldstein, D.B.: Physical dependence on alcohol in mice. Fed. Proc. *34*, 1953–1961 (1975)

Goldstein, D.B., Israel, Y.: Effects of ethanol on mouse brain (Na + K)-activated adenosine triphosphatase. Life Sci. *11*, 957–963 (1972)

Goldstein, A., Judson, B.A.: Alcohol dependence and opiate dependence: Lack of realationship in mice. Science *172*, 290–292 (1971)

Goldstein, D.B., Pal, N.: Alcohol dependence produced in mice by inhalation of ethanol: Grading the withdrawal reaction. Science *172*, 288–290 (1971)

Gordon, E.R.: The effect of ethanol on the concentration of γ-aminobutyric acid in the rat brain. Can. J. Physiol. Pharmacol. *45*, 915–918 (1967)

Gorman, R.E., Bitensky, M.W.: Selective activation by short chain alcohols of glucagon responsive adenyl cyclase in liver. Endocrinology *87*, 1075–1081 (1970)

Grande, F., Hay, L.J., Heupel, H.W., Amatuzio, D.S.: Effect of ethanol on serum cholesterol concentration in dog and man. Circ. Res. *8*, 810–819 (1960)

Greene, H.L., Herman, R.H., Kraemer, S.: Stimulation of jejunal adenyl cyclase by ethanol. J. Lab. Clin. Med. *78*, 336–342 (1971)

Grenell, R.G.: The binding of alcohol to brain membranes. Adv. Exp. Med. Biol. *59*, 11–22 (1975)

Griffiths, P.J., Littleton, J.M.: Concentrations of free amino acids in brains of mice during the induction of physical dependence of ethanol and during the ethanol withdrawal syndrome. Br. J. Exp. Pathol. *58*, 19–27 (1977)

Griffiths, P.J., Littleton, J.M., Ortiz, A.: Changes in monoamine concentrations in mouse brain associated with ethanol dependence and withdrawal. Br. J. Pharmacol. *50*, 489–498 (1974)

Guynn, R.W.: Effect of ethanol on brain CoA and acetyl-CoA. J. Neurochem. *27*, 303–304 (1976)

Gysling, K., Bustos, G., Concha, I., Martinez, G.: Effect of ethanol on dopamine synthesis and release from rat corpus striatum. Biochem. Pharmacol. *25*, 157–162 (1976)

Häkkinen, H.-M., Kulonen, E.: Increase in the γ-aminobutyric acid content of rat brain after ingestion of ethanol. Nature *184*, 726 (1959)

Häkkinen, H.-M., Kulonen, E.: The effect of alcohol on the amino acids of the rat brain with a reference to the administration of glutamine. Biochem. J. *78*, 588–593 (1961)

Hamilton, M.G., Blum, K., Hirst, M.: Identification of an isoquinoline alkaloid after chronic exposure to ethanol. Alcoholism *2*, 133–137 (1978)

Hawkins, R.A., Williamson, D.H., Krebs, H.A.: Ketone-body utilization by adult and suckling rat brain in vivo. Biochem. J. *122*, 13–18 (1971)

Higgins, E.S.: The effect of ethanol on GABA content of rat brain. Biochem. Pharmacol. *11*, 394–395 (1962)

Hill, M.W., Bangham, A.D.: General depressant drug dependence: A biophysical hypothesis. Adv. Exp. Med. Biol. *59*, 1–9 (1975)

Himwich, H.E., Nahum, L.H., Rakieten, N., Fazekas, J.F., DuBois, D., Gildea, E.F.: The metabolism of alcohol. J. Am. Med. Ass. *100*, 651–654 (1933)

Hirst, M., Hamilton, M.G., Marshall, A.M.: Pharmacology of isoquinoline alkaloids and ethanol interactions. In: Alcohol and opiates, neurochemical and behavioral mechanisms. Blum, K. (ed)., pp. 167–187. New York: Academic Press 1977

Hoffman, P.L., Tabakoff, B.: Alterations in dopamine receptor sensitivity by chronic ethanol treatment. Nature *268*, 551–553 (1977)

Houslay, M.D., Hesketh, T.R., Smith, G.A., Warren, G.B., Metcalfe, J.C.: The lipid environment of the glucagon receptor regulates adenylate cyclase activity. Biochim. Biophys. Acta *436*, 495–504 (1976)

Hubbell, W.L., McConnell, H.M.: Spin-label studies of the excitable membranes of nerve and muscle. Proc. Natl. Acad. Sci. USA *61*, 12–16 (1968)

Hunt, W.A., Dalton, T.K.: Regional brain acetylcholine levels in rats acutely treated with ethanol or rendered ethanol-dependent. Brain Res. *109*, 628–631 (1976)

Hunt, W.A., Majchrowicz, E.: Alterations in the turnover of brain norepinephrine and dopamine in alcohol-dependent rats. J. Neurochem. *23*, 549–552 (1974)

Hunt, W.A., Redos, J.D., Dalton, T.K., Catravas, G.N.: Alterations in brain guanosine 3′:5′-monophosphate levels after acute and chronic treatment with ethanol. J. Pharmacol. Exp. Ther. *201*, 103–109 (1977)

Ihrig, T.J., French, S.W., Morin, R.J.: Lipid composition of cellular membranes after ethanol feeding. Fed. Proc. *28*, 626 (1969)

Israel, M.A., Kimura, H., Kuriyama, K.: Changes in activity and hormonal sensitivity of brain adenyl cyclase following chronic ethanol administration Experientia *28*, 1322–1323 (1972)

Israel, Y., Salazar, I.: Inhibition of brain microsomal adenosine triphosphatases by general depressants. Arch. Biochem. Biophys. *122*, 310–317 (1967)

Israel, Y., Kuriyama, K.: Effects of in vivo ethanol administration on adenosine triphosphatase activity of subcellular fractions of mouse brain and liver. Life Sci. *10*, 591–599 (1971)

Israel, Y., Kalant, H., Laufer, I.: Effects of ethanol on Na, K, Mg-stimulated microsomal ATPase activity. Biochem. Pharmacol. *14*, 1803–1814 (1965)

Israel, Y., Kalant, H., LeBlanc, E., Bernstein, J.C., Salazar, I.: Changes in cation transport and (Na+K)-activated adenosine triphosphatase produced by chronic administration of ethanol. J. Pharmacol. Exp. Ther. *174*, 330–336 (1970)

Jarlstedt, J.: Experimental alcoholism in rats: Protein synthesis in subcellular fractions from cerebral cortex and liver after long-term treatment. J. Neurochem. *19*, 603–608 (1972)

Jarlstedt, J.: Alcohol and brain protein synthesis. Adv. Exp. Med. Biol. *85A*, 155–171 (1977)

Jarlstedt, J., Hamberger, A.: Experimental alcoholism in rats: Effect of *acute* alcohol intoxication on the in vitro incorporation of ^{3}H-leucine into neuronal and glial cell protein. J. Neurochem. *19*, 2299–2306 (1972)

Järnefelt, J.: Sodium-stimulated adenosine triphosphatase in microsomes from rat brain. Biochim. Biophys. Acta *48*, 104–110 (1961a)

Järnefelt, J.: Inhibition of the brain microsomal adenosine-triphosphatase by depolarizing agents. Biochim. Biophys. Acta *48*, 111–116 (1961b)

Järnefelt, J.: A possible mechanism of action of ethyl alcohol on central nervous system. Ann. Med. Exp. Biol. Fenniae (Helsinki) *39*, 267–272 (1961c)

Jeejeebhoy, K.N., Phillips, M.J., Bruce-Robertson, A., Ho, J., Sodke, U.: The acute effect of ethanol on albumin, fibrogen and transferrin synthesis in the rat. Biochem. J. *126*, 1111–1126 (1972)

Kalant, H., Grose, W.: Effects of ethanol and pentobarbital on release of acetylcholine from cerebral cortex slices. J. Pharmacol. Exp. Ther. *158*, 386–393 (1967)

Kalant, H., Woo, N., Endrenyi, L.: Effect of ethanol on the kinetics of rat brain ($Na^{+}+K^{+}$) ATPase and K^{+}-dependent phosphatase with different alkali ions. Biochem. Pharmacol. *27*, 1353–1358 (1978)

Karoum, F., Wyatt, R.J., Majchrowicz, E.: Brain concentrations of biogenic amine metabolites in acutely treated and ethanol-dependent rats. Br. J. Pharmacol. *56*, 403–411 (1976)

Karppanen, H., Puurunen, J., Kairaluoma, M., Larmi, T.: Effects of ethyl alcohol on the adenosine 3′,5′-monophosphate system of the human gastric mucosa. Scand. J. Gastroenterol. *11*, 603–607 (1976)

Kebabian, J.W., Zatz, M., Romero, J.A., Axelrod, J.: Rapid changes in rat pineal β-adrenergic receptor: Alterations in *l*-[^{3}H] alprenolol binding and adenylate cyclase. Proc. Natl. Acad. Sci. USA *72*, 3735–3739 (1975)

Kety, SS., Schmidt, C.F.: Nitrous oxide method for the quantitative determination of cerebral blood flow in man; theory, procedure and normal values. J. Clin. Invest. *27*, 276–483 (1948)

Khawaja, J.A., Lindhalm, D.B., Niittyla, J.: Selective inhibition of protein synthetic activity of cerebral membrane-bound ribosomes as a consequence of ethanol ingestion. Res. Commun. Chem. Pathol. Pharmacol. *19*, 185–188 (1978)

Kiianmaa, K.: Alcohol intake in the rat after lowering brain 5-hydroxytryptamine content by electrolytic midbrain raphé lesions, 5,6-dihydroxytryptamine or p-chlorophenylalanine. Med. Biol. *54*, 203–209 (1976)

Kimelberg, H.K.: Alterations in phospholipid-dependent ($Na^{+}+K^{+}$)-ATPase activity due to lipid fluidity. Effects of cholesterol and Mg^{2+}. Biochim. Biophys. Acta *413*, 143–156 (1975)

Kirsch, R.E., Frith, L. O'C., Stead, R.H., Saunders, S.J.: Effect of alcohol on albumin synthesis by the isolated perfused rat liver. Am. J. Clin. Nutr. *26*, 1191–1194 (1973)

Klein, I., Moore, L., Pastan, I.: Effect of liposomes containing cholesterol on adenylate cyclase activity of cultured mammalian fibroblasts. Biochim. Biophys. Acta *506*, 42–53 (1978)

Klemm, W.R.: Dissociation of EEG and behavioural effects of ethanol provide evidence for a noncholinergic basis of intoxication. Nature *251*, 234–236 (1974)
Klingman, L.G., Goodall, M.: Urinary epinephrine and levarterenol excretion during acute sublethal alcohol intoxication in dogs. J. Pharmacol. *121*, 313–318 (1957)
Knott, P.J., Curzon, G.: Free tryptophan in plasma and brain tryptophan metabolism. Nature *239*, 452–453 (1972)
Knox, W.H., Perrin, R.G., Sen, A.K.: Effect of chronic administration of ethanol on (Na+K)-activated ATPase activity in six areas of the cat brain. J. Neurochem. *19*, 2881–2884 (1972)
Krebs, H.A., Freedland, R.A., Hems, R.Stubbs, M.: Inhibition of hepatic gluconeogenesis by ethanol. Biochem. J. *112*, 117–124 (1969)
Krebs, H.A., Hems, R., Lund, P.: Accumulation of amino acids by the perfused rat liver in the presence of ethanol. Biochem. J. *134*, 697–705 (1973)
Kuriyama, K.: Ethanol-induced changes in activities of adenylate cyclase, guanylate cyclase and cyclic adenosine 3′,5′-monophosphate dependent protein kinase in the brain and liver. Drug Alcohol Depend. *2*, 335–348 (1977)
Kuriyama, K., Israel, M.A.: Effect of ethanol administration on cyclic 3′,5′-adenosine monophosphate metabolism in brain. Biochem. Pharmacol. *22*, 2919–2922 (1973)
Kuriyama, K., Sze, P.Y., Rauscher, G.E.: Effects of acute and chronic ethanol administration on ribosomal protein synthesis in mouse brain and liver. Life Sci. *10*, 181–189 (1971a)
Kuriyama, K., Rauscher, G.E., Sze, P.Y.: Effect of acute and chronic administration of ethanol on the 5-hydroxytryptamine turnover and tryptophan hydroxylase activity of the mouse brain. Brain Res. *26*, 450–454 (1971b)
Lahti, R. A., Majchrowicz, E.: The effects of acetaldehyde on serotonin metabolism. Life Sci. *6*, 1300–1406 (1967)
Lahti, R.A., Majchrowicz, E.: Acetaldehyde – an inhibitor of enzymatic oxidation of 5-hydroxyindoleacetaldehyde. Biochem. Pharmacol. *18*, 535–538 (1969)
LaManna, J.R., Younts, B.W., jr., Rosenthal, M.: The cerebral oxidative metabolic response to acute ethanol administration in rats and cats. Neuropharmacology *16*, 283–288 (1977)
LeLoir, L.F., Muñoz, J.M.: Ethyl alcohol metabolism in animal tissues. Biochem. J. *31*, 299–307 (1938)
Lieber, C.S., DeCarli, L.M.: Ethanol oxidation by hepatic microsomes: Adaptive increase after ethanol feeding. Science *162*, 917–918 (1968)
Lieber, C.S., Leevy, C.M., Stein, S.W., George, W.S., Cherrick, G.R., Abelmann, W.H., Davidson, C.W.: Effect of ethanol on plasma free fatty acids in man. J. Lab. Clin. Med. *57*, 826–832 (1962)
Lieber, C.S., Jones, D.P., Mendelson, J.H., DeCarli, L.M.: Fatty liver, hyperlipemia and hyperuricemia produced by prolonged alcohol consumption, despite adequate dietary intake. Trans. Assoc. Am. Physicians *76*, 289–300 (1963)
Lin, S.C., Sutherland, V.C.: The regional effects of ethanol on GABA release from Guinea pig brain in vitro. Proc. West. Pharmacol. Soc. *17*, 188–192 (1974)
Littleton, J.M., John, G.: Synaptosomal membrane lipids of mice during continuous exposure to ethanol. J. Pharm. Pharmacol. *29*, 579–580 (1977)
Littleton, J.M., John, G.R., Grieve, S.J.: Alterations in phospholipid composition in ethanol tolerance and dependence. Alcoholism *3*, 50–56 (1979)
Loman, J., Myerson, A.: Alcohol and cerebral vasodilatation. N. Engl. J. Med. *227*, 439–441 (1942)
Lundquist, F., Tygstrup, N., Winkler, K., Mellemgaard, K., Munck-Petersen, S.: Ethanol metabolism and production of free acetate in the human liver. J. Clin. Invest. *41*, 955–961 (1962)
Lundsgaard, E.: Alcohol oxidation as a function of the liver. C. R. Trav. Lab. Carlsberg Ser. Chim. *22*, 333–337 (1938)
Madras, B.K., Cohen, E.L., Munro, H.N., Wurtman, R.J.: Elevation of serum free tryptophan, but not brain tryptophan, by serum nonesterified fatty acids. Adv. Biochem. Psychopharmacol. *11*, 143–151 (1974)
Majchrowicz, E.: Effects of aliphatic alcohols and aldehydes on the metabolism of potassium-stimulated rat brain cortex slices. Can. J. Biochem. *43*, 1041–1051 (1965)
Majchrowicz, E.: Effect of peripheral ethanol metabolism on the central nervous system. Fed. Proc. *34*, 1948–1952 (1975)

Mashiter, K., Mashiter, G.D., Field, J.B.: Effects of prostaglandin E, ethanol and TSH on the adenylate cyclase activity of beef thyroid plasma membranes and cyclic AMP content of dog thyroid slices. Endocrinology *94*, 370–376 (1974)
Maynert, E.W., Klingman, G.I.: Acute tolerance to intravenous anesthetics in dogs. J. Pharmacol. Exp. Ther. *128*, 192–200 (1960)
McIsaac, W.M.: Formation of 1-methyl-6-methoxy-1,2,3,4-tetrahydro-2-carboline under physiological conditions. Biochim. Biophys. Acta *52*, 607–609 (1961)
Melchior, C.L., Myers, R.D.: Preference for alcohol evoked by tetrahydropapaveroline (THP) chronically infused in the cerebral ventricle of the rat. Pharmacol. Biochem. Behav. *7*, 19–35 (1977)
Mellanby, E.: Alcohol: Its absorption into and disappearance from the blood under different conditions. Special Report Series, No. 31, London: Medical Research Committee (1919)
Mendenhall, C.L., Bradford, R.H., Furman, R.H.: Effect of ethanol on fatty acid composition of hepatic phosphatidylcholine and phosphatidylethanolamine and on microsomal fatty acyl-CoA: lysophosphatide transferase activities in rats fed corn oil or coconut oil. Biochim. Biophys. Acta *187*, 510–519 (1969)
Metzger, H., Erdmann, W., Thews, G.: Effect of short periods of hypoxia, hyperoxia and hypercapnia on brain O_2 supply. J. Appl. Physiol. *31*, 751–759 (1971)
Meyer, H.H.: Zur Theorie der Alkoholnarkose. III. Mitt. Der Einfluß wechselnder Temperatur auf Wirkungsstärke und Teilungskoeffizient der Narkotika. Arch. Exp. Pathol. Pharmakol. *46*, 338–350 (1901)
Michaelis, E.K., Mulvaney, M.J., Freed, W.J.: Effects of acute and chronic ethanol intake on synaptosomal glutamate binding activity. Biochem. Pharmacol. *27*, 1685–1691 (1978)
Miki, N., Nagano, M., Kuriyama, K.: Effect of ethanol administration on guanylate cyclase activities in liver and brain. Jpn. J. Pharmacol. *27*, 322–325 (1977)
Miller, A.L., Hawkins, R.A., Veech, R.L.: Decreased rate of glucose utilization by rat brain in vivo after exposure to atmospheres containing high concentrations of CO_2. J. Neurochem. *25*, 553–558 (1975)
Mirsky, I.A., Piker, P., Rosenbaum, M., Lederer, H.: "Adaptation" of the central nervous system to varying concentrations of alcohol in the blood. Q. J. Stud. Alcohol *2*, 35–45 (1941)
Morgenroth, V.H., Boadle-Biber, M.C., Roth, R.H.: Activation of tyrosine hydroxylase from central noradrenergic neurons by calcium. Mol. Pharmacol. *11*, 427–435 (1975)
Moskow, H.A., Pennington, R.C., Knosely, M.H.: Alcohol, sludge and hypoxic areas of nervous system, liver and heart. Microvasc. Res. *1*, 174–185 (1968)
Mukherjee, C., Caron, M.G., Lefkowitz, R.J.: Catecholamine-induced subsensitivity of adenylate cyclase associated with loss of β-adrenergic receptor binding sites. Proc. Natl. Acad. Sci. USA *72*, 1945–1949 (1975)
Murphy, G.E., Guze, S.G., King, L.J.: Urinary excretion of 5-HIAA in chronic alcoholism. J. Am. Med. Ass. *82*, 565 (1962)
Myers, R.D., Veale, W.L.: Alcohol preference in the rat: Reduction following depletion of brain serotonin. Science *160*, 1469–1471 (1968)
Nielsen, R.H., Harkins, R.W., Veech, R.L.: The effects of acute ethanol intoxication on cerebral energy metabolism. Adv. Exp. Med. Biol. *59*, 93–109 (1975)
Noble, E.P., Tewari, S.: Protein and ribonucleic acid metabolism in brains of mice following chronic alcohol consumption. Ann. N.Y. Acad. Sci. *215*, 333–345 (1973)
Noble, E.D., Syapin, P.J., Vigran, R., Rosenberg, L.B.: Neuraminidase-releasable surface sialic acid of cultured astroblasts exposed to ethanol. J. Neurochem. *27*, 217–221 (1976)
Ogata, M., Mendelson, J.H., Mello, N.K., Majchrowicz, E.: Adrenal function and alcoholism II. Catecholamines. Psychosom. Med. *33*, 159–180 (1971)
O'Neill, P.J., Rahwan, R.G.: Absence of formation of brain salsolinol in ethanol-dependent mice. J. Pharmacol. Exp. Ther. *200*, 306–313 (1977)
Ortiz, A., Griffiths, P.J., Littleton, J.M.: A comparison of the effects of chronic administration of ethanol and acetaldehyde to mice: Evidence for a role of acetaldehyde in ethanol dependence. J. Pharm. Pharmacol. *26*, 249–260 (1974)
Overton, E.: Studien über die Narkose: zugleich ein Beitrag zur allgemeinen Pharmakologie. Jena: Fisher 1901
Patel, G.J., Lal, H.: Reduction in brain γ-aminobutyric acid and in barbital narcosis during ethanol withdrawal. J. Pharmacol. Exp. Ther. *186*, 625–629 (1973)

Paterson, S.J., Butler, K.W., Huang, P., Labelle, J., Smith, I.C.P., Schneider, H.: The effects of alcohols on lipid bilayers: A spin label study. Biochim. biophys. Acta *266*, 597–602 (1972)

Pohorecky, L.A.: Effects of ethanol on central and peripheral noradrenergic neurons. J. Pharmacol. *189*, 380–391 (1974)

Pohorecky, L.A., Newman, B.: Effect of ethanol on dopamine synthesis in rat striatal synaptosomes. Drug Alcohol Depend. *2*, 329–334 (1977)

Pohorecky, L.A., Newman, B.: A correlated study of the effects of acute ethanol on serotonin metabolism in rat. In: Currents in alcoholism. Seixas, F.A. (ed.), Vol. III, pp. 119–139. New York: Grune & Stratton 1978

Quastel, D.M.J., Hacket, J.T., Cooke, J.D.: Calcium: Is it required for transmitter secretion? Science *172*, 1034–1036 (1971)

Rahwan, R.G.: Toxic effects of ethanol: Possible role of acetaldehyde, tetrahydroisoquinolines, and tetrahydro-β-carbolines. Toxicol. Appl. Pharmacol. *34*, 3–27 (1975)

Rangaraj, N., Kalant, H.: Effects of ethanol withdrawal, stress and amphetamine on rat brain ($Na^+ + K^+$)-ATPase. Biochem. Pharmacol. *27*, 1139–1144 (1978)

Raskin, N.H., Sokoloff, L.: Enzymes catalysing ethanol metabolism in neural and somatic tissues of the rat. J. Neurochem. *19*, 273–282 (1972)

Rawat, A.K.: Brain levels and turnover rates of presumptive neurotransmitters as influenced by administration and withdrawal of ethanol. J. Neurochem. *22*, 915–922 (1974)

Rawat, A.K., Kuriyama, K.: Ethanol oxidation: Effect on the redox state of brain in mouse. Science *176*, 1133–1135 (1972)

Rawat, A.K., Kuriyama, K., Mose, J.: Metabolic consequences of ethanol oxidation in brains from mice chronically fed alcohol. J. Neurochem. *20*, 23–33 (1973)

Redos, J.D., Catravas, G.N., Hunt, W.A.: Ethanol-induced depletion of cerebellar guanosine 3′,5′-cyclic monophosphate. Science *193*, 58–59 (1976)

Reitz, R.C., Helsabeck, E., Mason, D.P.: Effects of chronic alcohol ingestion on the fatty acid composition of the heart. Lipids *8*, 80–84 (1973)

Roach, M.K., Khan, M.M., Coffman, R., Pennington, W., Davis, D.L.: Brain ($Na^+ + K^+$)-activated adenosine triphosphatase activity and neurotransmitter uptake in alcohol-dependent rats. Brain Res. *63*, 323–329 (1973)

Rogawski, M.A., Knapp, S., Mandell, A.J.: Effects of ethanol on tryptophan hydroxylase activity from striate synaptosomes. Biochem. Pharmacol. *23*, 1955–1962 (1974)

Rosenfeld, G.: Inhibitory influence of ethanol on serotonin metabolism. Proc. Soc. Exp. Biol. Med. *103*, 144–149 (1960)

Ross, D.H.: Selective action of alcohols on cerebral calcium levels. Ann. N.Y. Acad. Sci. *273*, 280–294 (1976)

Ross, D.H.: Adaptive changes in Ca^{++}-membrane interactions following chronic ethanol exposure. Adv. Exp. Med. Biol. *85*, 459–471 (1977)

Ross, D.H., Medina, M.A., Cardenas, H.L.: Morphine and ethanol: Selective depletion of brain calcium. Science *186*, 63–65 (1974)

Ross, D.H., Kibler, B.C., Cardenas, H.L.: Modifications of glycoprotein residues as Ca^{++} receptor sites after chronic ethanol exposure. Drug Alcohol Depend. *2*, 305–315 (1977)

Ross, D.H., Mutchler, T.L., Grady, M.M.: Calcium and glycoprotein metabolism as correlates for ethanol preference and sensitivity. Alcoholism *3*, 64–69 (1979)

Rothschild, M.A., Oratz, M., Mongelli, J., Schreiber, S.S.: Alcohol-induced depression of albumin synthesis: Reversal by tryptophan. J. Clin. Invest. *50*, 1812–1818 (1971)

Roufogalis, B.D.: Properties of a ($Mg^{+2} + Ca^{+2}$) dependent ATPase of bovine brain cortex: Effects of detergents, freezing, cations and local anesthetics. Biochim. Biophys. Acta *318*, 360–370 (1973)

Rubin, E., Lieber, C.S., Altman, K., Gordon, G.G., Southren, A.L.: Prolonged ethanol consumption increases testosterone metabolism in the liver. Science *191*, 563–564 (1976)

Sandler, M., Carter, S.B., Hunter, K.R., Stern, G.M.: Tetrahydroisoquinoline alkaloids: In vivo metabolites of L-Dopa in man. Nature *241*, 439–443 (1973)

Schlapfer, W.S., Woodson, P.B.J., Smith, G.A., Tremblay, J.P., Barondes, S.H.: Marked prolongation of posttetanic potentiation at a transition temperture and its adaptation. Nature *258*, 623–625 (1975)

Schultz, J.: Cyclic adenosine 3′,5′-monophosphate in Guinea pig cerebral cortical slices: Possible regulation of phosphodiesterase activity by cyclic adenosine 3′,5′-monophosphate and calcium ions. J. Neurochem. *24*, 495–501 (1975)
Seeber, U., Kuschinsky, K.: Dopamine-sensitive adenylate cyclase in homogenates of rat striata during ethanol and barbiturate withdrawal. Arch. Toxicol. (Berl.) *35*, 247–253 (1976)
Seeman, P.: The membrane actions of anesthetics and tranquilizers. Pharmacol. Rev. *24*, 583–655 (1972)
Seeman, P., Lee, T.: The dopamine-releasing actions of neuroleptics and ethanol. J. Pharmacol. Exp. Ther. *190*, 131–140 (1974)
Seeman, P., Chau, M., Goldberg, M., Sauks, T., Sax, L.: The binding of Ca^{2+} to the cell membrane increased by volatile anesthetics (alcohols, acetone, ether) which induce sensitization of nerve or muscle. Biochim. Biophys. Acta *225*, 185–193 (1971)
Shen, A., Jacobyansky, A., Smith, T., Pathman, D., Thurman, R.G.: Cyclic adenosine 3′,5′-monophosphate, adenylate cyclase and physical dependence on ethanol: Studies with dranylcypromine. Drug Alcohol Depend. *2*, 431–440 (1977)
Sinensky, M.: Temperature control of phospholipid biosynthesis in *Escherichia coli*. J. Bacteriol. *106*, 449–455 (1971)
Sippel, H.W.: The acetaldehyde content in rat brain during ethanol metabolism. J. Neurochem. *23*, 451–452 (1974)
Sippel, H.W., Eriksson, C.J.P.: The acetaldehyde content in rat brain during ethanol oxidation. The Finnish Foundation for Alcohol Studies *23*, 149–157 (1975)
Skou, J.C.: Enzymatic basis for active transport of Na^+ and K^+ across cell membrane. Physiol. Rev. *45*, 596–617 (1965)
Smith, C.M.: The pharmacology of sedative/hypnotics, alcohol, and anesthetics: Sites and mechanisms of action. In: Drug addiction I. Morphine, sedative/hypnotic and alcohol dependence. Martin, W.R., (ed.), pp. 413–587. Berlin, Heidelberg, New-York: Springer 1977
Sun, A.Y., Samorajski, T.: Effect of ethanol on adenosine triphosphatase and acetylcholinesterase activity in isolated synaptosomes of guinea pig brain. J. Neurochem. *17*, 1365–1372 (1970)
Sun, A.Y., Seaman, R.N., Middleton, C.C.: Effects of acute and chronic alcohol administration on brain membrane transport systems. Adv. Exp. Med. Biol. *85A*, 123–138 (1977)
Sun, G.Y., Sun, A.Y.: The effects of chronic ethanol administration on acyl group composition of mitochondrial phospholipids from guinea pig adrenal. Res. Commun. Chem. Pathol. Pharmacol. *21*, 355–358 (1978)
Sun, G.Y., Yau, T.M.: Incorporation of 1-^{14}C oleic acid and 1-^{14}-arachidonic acid into lipids of the subcellular fractions of mouse brain. J. Neurochem. *27*, 87–92 (1976)
Sze, P.Y., Neckers, L.: Requirement for adrenal glucocorticoid in the ethanol-induced increase of tryptophan hydroxylase activity in mouse brain. Brain Res. *72*, 375–378 (1974)
Tabakoff, B., Boggan, W.O.: Effects of ethanol on serotonin metabolism in brain. J. Neurochem. *22*, 759–764 (1974)
Tabakoff, B., Ritzmann, R.F., Boggan, W.O.: Inhibition of the transport of 5-hydroxyindoleacetic acid from brain by ethanol. J. Neurochem. *24*, 1043–1051 (1975)
Tabakoff, B., Anderson, R.A., Ritzmann, R.F.: Brain acetaldehyde after ethanol administration. Biochem. Pharmacol. *25*, 1305–1309 (1976)
Tabakoff, B., Hoffman, P.L., Ritzmann, R.F.: Dopamine receptor function after chronic ingestion of ethanol. Life Sci. *23*, 643–648 (1978)
Tewari, S., Noble, E.P.: Ethanol and brain protein synthesis. Brain Res. *26*, 469–474 (1971)
Tewari, S., Noble, E.P.: Alteration in cerebral polynucleotide metabolism following chronic ethanol ingestion. Adv. Exp. Med. Biol. *59*, 37–53 (1975)
Tewari, S., Noble, E.P.: Brain polynucleotide metabolism following longterm ethanol ingestion. Adv. Exp. Med. Biol. *85A*, 139–154 (1977)
Thomas, C.B.: The cerebral circulation. XXXI. Effect of alcohol on cerebral vessels. Arch. Neurol. Psychiatr. *38*, 321–339 (1937)
Traynor, M.E., Woodson, P.B.J., Schlapfer, W.T., Barondes, S.H.: Sustained tolerance to a specific effect of ethanol on posttetanic potentiation in *Aplysia*. Science *193*, 510–511 (1976)
Traynor, M.E., Schlapfer, W.T., Woodson, P.B.J., Barondes, S.H.: Crosstolerance to effect of ethanol and temperature in *Aplysia*: Preliminary observations. Alcoholism *3*, 57–59 (1979)

Trudell, J.R.: A unitary theory of anesthesia based on lateral phase separations in nerve membranes. Anesthesiology *46*, 5–10 (1977)

Turner, A.J., Baker, K.M., Algeri, S., Grigerio, A., Garattini, S.: Tetrahydropapaveroline: Formation in vivo and in vitro in rat brain. Life Sci. *14*, 2247–2257 (1974)

Tytell, M., Myers, R.D.: Metabolism of [^{14}C]-serotonin in the caudate nucleus, hypothalamus and reticular formation of the rat after ethanol administration. Biochem. Pharmacol. *22*, 361–371 (1973)

Vanderkooi, J.M.: Effect of ethanol on membranes: A fluorescent probe study. Alcoholism *3*, 60–63 (1979)

Vanderkooi, J.M., Landesburg, R., Selick, H., McDonald, G.G.: Interaction of general anesthetics with phospholipid vesicles and biological membranes. Biochim. Biophys. Acta *464*, 1–16 (1977)

Veloso, D., Passonneau, J.V., Veech, R.L.: The effects of intoxicating doses of ethanol upon intermediary metabolism in rat brain. J. Neurochem. *19*, 2679–2686 (1972)

Viret, J., Leterrier, F.: A spin label study of rat brain membranes-effects of temperature and divalent cations. Biochim. Biophys. Acta *436*, 811–824 (1976)

Volicer, L., Gold, B.I.: Effect of ethanol on cyclic AMP levels in rat brain. Life Sci. *13*, 269–280 (1973)

Volicer, L., Hurter, B.P.: Effects of acute and chronic ethanol administration and withdrawal on adenosine 3′:5′-monophosphate and guanosine 3′:5′-monophosphate levels in the rat brain. J. Pharmacol. Exp. Ther. *200*, 298–305 (1977)

Volicer, L., Hynie, S.: Effects of catecholamines and angiotensin on cyclic AMP in rat aorta and tail artery. Eur. J. Pharmacol. *15*, 214–220 (1971)

Volicer, L., Hurter, B.P., Williams, R., Puri, S.K., Volicer, B.J.: Relationship between brain levels of cyclic nucleotides and γ-aminobutyric acid during ethanol withdrawal in rats. Drug Alcohol Depend. *2*, 317–327 (1977)

Volicer, L., Schmidt, W.K., Hartz, T.P., jr., Klosowicz,B.A., Meichner, R.: Cyclic nucleotides and ethanol tolerance and dependence. Druc Alcohol Depend. *3*, 295–305 (1979)

Wallgren, H., Kulonen, E.: Effect of ethanol on respiration of rat brain cortex slices. Biochem. J. *75*, 150–158 (1960)

Wallgren, H., Nikander, P., Virtanen, P.: Ethanol-induced changes in cation-stimulated ATPase activity and lipid-proteolipid labeling of brain microsomes. Adv. Exp. Med. Biol. *59*, 23–36 (1975)

Walsh, M.J., Truitt, E.B., jr.: Acetaldehyde mediation in the mechanisms of ethanol-induced changes in norepinephrine metabolism. Mol. Pharmacol. *6*, 416–424 (1970)

Warren, G.B., Toon, P.A., Birdsall, N.J.M., Lee, A.G., Metcalfe, J.C.: Reversible lipid titrations of the activity of pure adenosine triphosphatase-lipid complexes. Biochemistry *13*, 5501–5507 (1974)

Whittam, R.: Control of membrane permeability to potassium in rat blood cells. Nature *219*, 610 (1968)

Wilson, D.F., Stubbs, M., Veech, R.L., Ericinska, M., Krebs, H.A.: Equilibrium relations between the oxidation reduction reactions and the ATP synthesis in suspensions of isolated liver cells. Biochem. J. *140*, 57–64 (1974)

Woodson, P.B.J., Traynor, M.E., Schlapfer, W.T., Barondes, S.H.: Increased membrane fluidity implicated in acceleration of decay of post-tetanic potentiation by alcohols. Nature *260*, 797–799 (1976)

CHAPTER 12

Dependence-Producing Effects and Alcohol Dependence Syndrome

T. L. Chruściel

A. Introduction

Ethyl alcohol (ethanol, C_2H_5OH) is one of the most widely disputed dependence-producing drugs. Knowledge of its biologic properties is essential for research workers in all fields of medicine, because it belongs to the endogenous substances as well as to the exogenous biologically active compounds used in various medical procedures. The knowledge of ethanol pharmacology is important for all physicians and health workers, from the professors in various fields of medicine down to the "bare-foot doctors" working in the bush. The widespread, worldwide use of ethanol causes it to be the substance which most frequently may enter into interaction with medicaments. Thus its clinically important interactions should be well known to health workers at all levels. Its influence upon human psychological activity and behavior has been the subject of study by psychologists and sociologists. The consequences of its use, including particularly long-term use leading to dependence, are enormous and must be taken into consideration by all research disciplines and political sciences dealing with the problems of modern society. Morbidity and mortality associated with alcohol use make it a major public health problem.

The concept of alcohol dependence is relatively new, particularly since already in the time in which homo faber appeared alcohol was used and, indeed, overused. It has been known for centuries, however, that repetitive use of alcohol produces habitual use, and the consequences of chronic use of alcohol were described even in medieval textbooks of medicine. The first use of the term "dependence" in connection with chronic use of alcohol is credited to Eddy and his co-workers (Eddy et al., 1965), who drafted a general paper on drug dependence for an early meeting of the World Health Organization Committee on Drug Dependence, called at that time the WHO Committee on Addiction-Producing Drugs. In their paper the following definition of drug dependence was given:

"Drug dependence is a state, psychic and sometimes also physical, resulting from the interaction between a living organism and a drug, characterized by behavioural and other responses that always include a compulsion to take the drug on a continuous or periodic basis in order to experience its psychological effects, and sometimes also to avoid the discomfort of its absence. Tolerance may or may not be present. A person may be dependent on more than one drug" (World Health Organization, 1969).

By the term "drug" there is understood "any substance, that when taken into the living organism, may modify one or more of its functions" (World Health Organization, 1969). Drug abuse can be considered as "persistent or sporadic excessive drug use inconsistent with or unrelated to acceptable medical practice" (World Health Organization, 1969).

In such a general scheme alcohol, considered as a drug under this definition, joined other dependence producing substances. Alcohol dependence was originally described under the general heading alcohol-barbiturate like dependence. EDDY and co-workers (ELLIS and PICK, 1971; World Health Organization, 1964; World Health Organization, 1969) were apparently of the opinion that many similarities in the type of dependence produced by both alcohol and barbiturates (including barbiturate like medicaments) justify this "umbrella" term; moreover it was much easier in a general paper dealing with numerous types of drugs with different properties to group several drugs together. It is true that many similarities exist in the type of dependence to alcohol and that to barbiturates.

Alcohol dependence syndrome is now recognized as a disease in its own right, and as a major health hazard of worldwide distribution and significance. Even in the countries in which religion prohibits use of alcohol, in reality, a number of people use locally produced alcoholic beverages at the risk of both punishment and social disregard or condemnation and development of dependence. Excessive medical use of alcohol and dependence have both social and medical overtones and the comprehensive care of the alcoholic is an important health care problem in all highly developed as well as in many developing, including the least developed, countries. Large proportions of the population are continuously exposed to dangers resulting from both acute and chronic use of alcohol, and yet in many societies the social use of alcohol is deeply rooted into the habits and mores and the state of light drunkenness is almost everywhere not disregarded, while social drinking is approved. The network of services needed for users of alcohol is widened and increased by the governments and from private funds and donations almost everywhere in the world. New laws are being drafted and the responsibility for drunken offenders is being recognized by social and medical services. However, the complexity of the problems related to alcohol use and resulting from alcohol dependence call for in-depth study of alcohol, its biological properties, and effects.

B. The Concept of Alcoholism

DAVIES (1974) emphasized that the approach to alcoholism is mostly through pharmacology and pathology, bypassing the psychological and social aspects of what is essentially a medicosocial problem. The study of alcoholism as well as the treatment of alcoholics is frequently left entirely in the hands of highly specialized physicians, and general practitioners and other specialists are relieved from concerning themselves with it. The concept of disease is based on several variables: (1) the physical variable; (2) the personal variable; and (3) the social variable (MELLOR, 1974). Thus, when we say that a person is sick, ill, or diseased, he has something physically wrong with him, he feels bad and he is socially designated as sick. However, it is possible for somebody to have a physical disease (e.g., myopia) without personal discomfort (because eye glasses can correct the condition), and without being socially defined as ill.

DAVIES (1974) proposes a working definition of alcoholism as the intermittent or continual ingestion of alcohol leading to dependence or harm to the individual or to others. Under this definition acute intoxication resulting from overdose cannot be considered.

There is enormous variety in the drinking patterns of alcoholics (JELLINEK, 1960).

The United States National Council on Alcoholism Criteria Committee in 1972 defined alcoholism as a pathological dependence on alcohol (National Council on Alcoholism, Criteria Committee, 1972). SEEVERS (1968) points out that in the development of dependence, quantity and frequency of administration are all-important. DELINT and SCHMIDT (1971) suggest that the daily consumption of alcohol beverages equal to the alcohol content in half a bottle of whiskey over an extended period, months and years, may be enough to establish dependence or harm. With heroin, of course, much shorter time intervals are involved (ELLIS and PICK, 1971).

C. Etiology of Alcoholism

There are considerable problems in defining the condition of alcoholism, and hence there are difficulties in establishing the time of onset of its effects. The etiological hypotheses are considered under the heading of genetic, psychological, and social factors (ROEBUCK and KESSLER, 1972).

I. Genetic Hypotheses

Alcoholism has always been recognized as a familial disorder. The family environment has usually been cited as a cause of alcoholism. Such an environmental causation of the condition has in general appeared more "reasonable" and even more attractive than genetic hypotheses (MELLOR, 1974).

Enzyme deficiency, related to vitamins of the B group, has been postulated by several authors (BRADY and WESTERFIELD, 1947; MARDONES, 1951; WILLIAMS, 1959).

JELLINEK (1945) was of the opinion that it is not the disposition to alcoholism which is inherited but a weak constitution unable to resist the social risk of inebriety.

More recent studies using twins have concentrated on the investigation of progeny who are separated from their biological parents shortly after birth and are raised by adoptive parents. KAIJ (1960) found that 10 of 14 pairs of monozygotic twins (over 71%) were concordant for chronic alcoholism and there were 31 pairs of dizygotic twins with a concordance of 32% for chronic alcoholism. PARTANEN et al. (1966) and JONSSON and NILSSON (1968) suggest that there is a genetic contribution to heavy alcohol consumption. The subjects of SCHUCKIT et al. (1972) were more likely to have a drinking problem if their parent was an alcoholic. They found that 62% of their alcoholics had an alcoholic parent compared with 20% of their nonalcoholics. GOODWIN et al. (1973) studied a group of 55 men, separated from their biological parents 6 weeks after birth and who had one parent with a diagnosis of alcoholism. Significantly more (18%) of the group with alcoholic parents were alcoholics, compared with 5% for the matched control group of the adoptees. This study suggests that physical dependence on alcohol may reflect a genetic predisposition. Obviously some people were especially prone to the development of alcohol dependence, and there is now increasing evidence that predisposition to dependence may be, at least in part, genetically determined (LIEBER and DECARLI, 1974).

OMENN and MOTULSKY (1972) have formulated the possible ways in which genes might contribute to the development of alcoholism as follows: (1) personalities with a predisposition to alcoholism; (2) taste preference for alcoholic beverages; (3) effects of alcohol intoxication; (4) development of physical dependence; and (5) physical consequences of alcoholism, e.g., liver cirrhosis.

II. Psychological Hypotheses

The psychological reasons for excessive drinking can be listed as follows: (1) to counter disappointment and hurt; (2) to bolster courage; (3) to alleviate feelings of isolation and loneliness; (4) to reduce ethical restraints; and (5) to blot out the sense of an existence without meaning.

Psychological etiological hypotheses are not mutually exclusive: they are interdependent. MELLOR (1974) subdivides these hypotheses into four groups.

1. Alcohol Effect Hypotheses

The effect of alcohol is such that it leads to excessive use and eventually to dependence. COLEMAN described the psychological effects of alcohol in the following way: The intoxicated person typically experiences a sense of warmth, expansiveness and well-being. In such a mood unpleasant realities are wiped out and the drinker's feelings of self-esteem and adequacy rise. The user enters a generally pleasant new world in which his worries are temporarily left behind (ROEBUCK and KESSLER, 1972). Alcohol was shown to reduce the level of anxiety in man (MELLOR, 1974; National Council on Alcoholism, Criteria Committee, 1972; TAMERIN and MENDELSON, 1969). BENNETT et al. (1969) were unable to demonstrate that alcohol potentiates aggression.

2. Learning Theory Hypotheses

Perpetuation of drinking behavior results from reinforcement by the effects of alcohol. The effect of alcohol is considered to reward, to reinforce the learning of an association between the stimulus and response. When a certain response leads to a reduction in strength of the drive, the individual would be more likely to repeat the response when confronted with a similar situation. Only a few supporters of this hypothesis provided some experimental evidence (BANDURA, 1969; CONGER, 1956; KINGHAM, 1958; SMART, 1965).

3. Personality Hypotheses

Certain personality traits predispose some people to excessive alcohol use. One can postulate that there exist one or more types of personalities who find excessive drinking rewarding. Such personalities are likely to develop alcoholism. These hypotheses are, however, unlikely to be accepted (BOWMAN and JELLINEK, 1941; NATHAN et al., 1970; SYME, 1957), although the belief in an "alcoholic personality" was held by clinicians for a considerable time. MELLOR (1974) underlines that until a prospective follow-up study can be undertaken it is unlikely that the personality hypothesis can be empirically supported or refuted.

4. Other Hypotheses

Some schools using psychotherapeutic techniques have developed particular hypotheses focusing upon personality dynamics. A review of psychoanalytic theories of alcoholism etiology is given by Blum (1966).

III. Sociological Hypotheses

If one assumes a relationship between the structure of society, drinking behavior, and alcoholism rate one can construct sociological theories of the etiology of alcoholism. Such theories may be universal, cultural, subcultural, or alienation hypotheses (Mellor, 1974).

1. Universal Hypotheses

No society, regardless of its state of development, remained indifferent to their members' use of alcohol. Each society worked out its acceptable drinking practices and in a number of countries at certain stages a loose set of observed habits or an explicit set of rules, given in the form of orders and instructions or laws, govern the time, place, type of alcoholic beverage, rate of consumption, and even the behavior appropriate to drinking. Anthropologists search for evidence clarifying the links between the high level of alcohol consumption and the high (or adversely low) rate of alcoholism. An interesting example is provided by the Gambas of Central America who apparently consume large amounts of strong alcoholic beverages at their gatherings and yet are said to have little alcoholism (Mellor, 1974).

2. Cultural Hypotheses

Classical studies pointing to cultural differences associated with different rates of alcoholism are those of Horton (1943) and Bales (1946). Horton (1943) in his survey of 77 societies proposed that the strength of the drinking response varies directly with the level of anxiety in a given society. Bales (1946) studied Irish and Jewish populations, known to have very high (the former) and very low (the latter) rates of alcoholism, and concluded that alcoholism rates vary positively with the degree to which a culture induces feelings of tension and anxiety. He also emphasised the importance of drinking attitudes by postulating that where utilitarian use of alcohol is more frequent alcoholism rates will be higher.

There are also several hypotheses based on preference to drink by some subgroups or subcultures. A number of epidemiological studies have demonstrated an association between high rates of alcoholism and being an unmarried male, member of a particular ethnic group, an urban dweller, having a certain occupation, etc.

3. Alienation Hypotheses

These hypotheses derive from some of the ideas outlined above and complete the list. It may be assumed that there exist a number of people who do not feel themselves to be members of their respective societies and have no sense of affinity to it. They consequently do not feel bound by the society's rules and habits which govern drinking behavior.

MELLOR (1974) emphasizes that the strength of sociological hypotheses derives in part from the inability of both genetic and psychological hypotheses to provide a completely self-sufficient cause for alcoholism. An all-inclusive causal hypothesis would state that an individual who consumes too much alcohol and hence runs the risk of becoming an alcoholic, might belong to a society which is permissive or unable to enforce the sanctions regulating alcohol use. He may belong to a subculture which prescribes alcohol, and this overrides the prescriptions of the larger society. Finally, he may be uninfluenced by society and therefore experience no external constraints upon his use of alcohol (MELLOR, 1974). As in all cases of drug dependence, in alcohol dependence there is always a multiple causation and in etiology one cannot search for one unique factor: it is rather a factor on top of the others, multiple causal agents, that decides the issue. The combination of causal elements to produce alcoholism has been little studied. The etiology of alcoholism presents considerable methodological problems, because the cause and effect relationships are difficult to identify with reasonable certainty, particularly for population groups. The means by which the genetic, psychological, and sociological factors play a part in the development of alcoholism in a given individual or a population group and act together to produce alcoholism is an area undergoing continuous changes as time passes in our continuously changing world, and requires further, perhaps continuous investigation. Two studies (PLANT, 1967; ROGERS et al., 1979) have achieved classical status in pointing to cultural differences associated with different rates of alcoholism. HORTON (1943) directly linked the degree of insobriety with the level of anxiety in a particular societal group. He claimed that the strength of the drinking response was higher in societies with a subsistence economy. On the contrary, FIELD (1962) was of the opinion that the level of social organization less structured in subsistence economies was a better explanation of the higher frequency of drunkenness. BALES (1946), in comparing the drinking patterns of the Irish and the Jews, observed that the former always had a very high rate and the latter very low rates of alcoholism. He suggested that alcoholism rates vary positively with the degree to which a culture induces feelings of tension and anxiety. He considered the drinking attitudes important and postulated that where utilitarian use of alcohol is more frequent alcoholism rates will be higher. MELLOR (1974) concluded that it is difficult to advance a higher-level hypothesis which might explain differences in drinking levels among different cultures without invoking sociological hypotheses. The necessity of postulating constitutional differences between the members of different cultures in their response to alcohol and alcohol tolerance was not supported by evidence. Only WOLFF (1972) has found differences between Caucasian and Mongolian children in the reactivity of their autonomic nervous system to ethanol.

4. Subcultural Hypotheses

The rules governing the drinking habits of discrete social groups vary considerably. Men almost always drink more than women. In ancient times the warriors and shamans were expected to drink heavily. In modern times the physicians, clergymen, and judges are indeed subclasses of the population who strongly discourage heavy drinking, although many members of these societal groups do not abstain. It has already been indicated that people alienated from a particular society do not feel themselves bound by the society's rules governing drinking behavior. It is likely that such individuals would develop alcoholism (KINSEY and PHILLIPS, 1968). Sociopathic individuals have a high rate of alcoholism.

It is clear from the considerations in this section that a single etiological factor as a cause of alcoholism is highly improbable. Genetic, psychological, and sociological causes are all operating in conjunction with alcohol to produce alcoholism. An all-inclusive multicausal hypothesis refers to an individual who consumes too much alcohol and hence runs the risk of becoming an alcoholic. He might be genetically predetermined, psychologically easy to influence, and in an appropriate permissive environment ready to fall into the trap of alcoholism. It is highly probable that in the etiology of alcoholism, genetic, psychological, and sociological factors all play a part, but the relative contribution of each may be considerably different in individual cases and among different societal groups.

D. Alcohol Dependence Syndrome

The definition of dependence on alcohol has been a source of considerable confusion in the literature (CICERO, 1978). It has been used to describe numerous features related to alcohol use and frequently understood in different ways by various researchers.

Alcohol tolerance develops when it is necessary to drink increasing amounts in order to experience equivalent changes in feeling state and behavioral effects. The degree of tolerance to alcohol-induced effects and toxicity, however, does not develop parallelly, and, for example, the LD_{50} for ethanol changed very little, even with very long periods of ethanol exposure, while a formidable degree of tolerance to behavioral effects develops rapidly. In addition to developing tolerance, the chronic alcohol user may become psychologically and physically dependent on alcohol.

The biochemical bases for craving for alcohol are not yet known, but it is interesting that a recent study showed that a craving for ethanol in ethanol-dependent rats could be significantly reduced by a selective lesion of the ventral ascending noradrenaline bundle by 6-OH-dopamine, while a corresponding lesion of the ascending dopamine bundle caused only a small decrease in craving (BROWN and AMIT, 1977).

Physical dependence on alcohol is understood as those adaptive biological changes induced by chronic alcohol exposure that are reflected in the various behavioral and physiological responses expressed upon withdrawal of alcohol. Hippocrates was the first to point out that tremor of the hands was associated with chronic use of wine (MENDELSON and MELLO, 1974); he did not recognize yet that these symptoms were due not to drinking but to abrupt cessation of alcohol use. In the nineteenth century delirium tremens was described. At the present, the alcohol withdrawal syndrome is recognized as the complex of symptoms, ranging from hangover to delirium tremens, which often emerge in a severe form when alcohol intake is stopped or considerably reduced after a prolonged drinking bout. The withdrawal symptoms may include tremulousness, psychomotor and autonomic overactivity, gastric distress, seizures, delirium tremens, and alcoholic hallucinations, sometimes associated with headache, fever, sweating, vomiting, diarrhea, hypertension, hyperreflexia and nystagmus.

ISBELL et al. (1955) demonstrated that the full-blown alcohol withdrawal reaction could be observed in a man by keeping him continuously intoxicated for several weeks. This experiment established the principle that maintenance of continuous intoxication is the key to the development of physical dependence (GOLDSTEIN 1976). GROSS correlated the severity of the human abstinence syndrome with the cumulative blood alcohol level maintained over 5–7 days (GOLDSTEIN, 1976). The abstinence syndrome may be prevented or relieved by alcohol or other depressants of the central nervous system, such as barbiturates, chloral hydrate, paraldehyde, and benzodiazepines.

The study of physical dependence on alcohol has been complicated by the fact that dependence generally evolves over a long period of time, commonly over years of continuous drinking.

Alcohol dependence syndrome belongs to the disabilities related to alcohol consumption. The word "alcoholism", introduced in 1849 by MAGNUS HUS (1849), is synonymous with alcohol dependence (EDWARDS et al., 1979). Alcoholism is conceived of as an uncontrollable behavior consisting of the repetitive ingestion of alcohol-containing beverages to the degree that harms the user. Alcohol dependence syndrome appears to be advantageous as a diagnostic term.

Alcohol dependence syndrome is manifested by alterations at the behavioral, subjective, and psychobiological levels with, as a leading symptom, an impaired control over intake of ethanol (EDWARDS et al., 1979). The alcohol dependence syndrome exists in degrees. It is an alcohol-related disability which predicates the likelihood of drinking behavior resulting over time in a clustering of other disabilities (EDWARDS et al., 1979). The degree of disability in an individual that ensues from his alcohol dependence is determined by the general context of his health and ill-health. The fact that an individual is alcohol dependent implies a probably impaired responsiveness of his behavior to social control. Not all people with alcohol-related disabilities are alcohol dependent, but they may be at an increased risk of developing dependence (EDWARDS et al., 1979).

Alcohol dependence syndrome should be seen as conceptually distinct from the alcohol-related disability. The individual with social, physical, or mental alcohol-related disabilities need not necessarily be alcohol dependent. Alcohol disabilities can exist without alcohol dependence; however, severe dependence is always connected with drinking at such a level as to result in a cluster of alcohol disabilities. Not all alcohol-related disability is alcohol-dependence related. The alcohol dependence syndrome is a diagnosable condition. The syndrome is multifactorial and exists in degrees. Interacting personal and environmental factors are important in the development of the syndrome.

I. Animal Models for Physical Dependence on Ethanol

An acute physical dependence on ethanol can be demonstrated after a single injection of the drug. For example, motor activity depression by ethanol is followed shortly thereafter by a rebound response above control level (WALLGREN and BARRY, 1970). MCQUARRIE and FINGL (1958) found that, 8–12 h after an injection of alcohol, the dose of metrazol required to induce seizures in rats was reduced by 25%–30% in alcohol treated rats. GOLDSTEIN (1974) found that handling-induced seizures could be produced in mice treated with a single injection of alcohol 10–14 h earlier. These data

Table 1. Methods used for the induction of physical dependence in animals (After FENNESY, 1979)

Species	Technique	Duration of exposure (days)	Dose
Mouse	Gavage	14	$5.4\ g\ kg^{-1}\ day^{-1}$
	Ethanol liquid diet	4	0.5 ml absolute ethanol
	Ethanol liquid diet	4	$15–18\ mg\ g^{-1}$
	Inhalation ethanol vapour	1–3	$11\ mg\ l^{-1}$ of air
Rat	Intubation of ethanol		
	Fluid	37	$3–7\ g\ kg^{-1}\ day^{-1}$
	Ethanol liquid diet	4–21	4 ml absolute ethanol
	Ethanol – sole fluid	35–49	–
	Polidipsia	90	$13\ g\ kg^{-1}\ day^{-1}$
Dog	Intragastric infusion	40–54	$4.5\ ml\ kg^{-1}\ day^{-1}$
	Nasogastric intubation	14–56	$3.7\ g\ kg^{-1}\ day^{-1}$
Rhesus	Intravenous self-administration	>120	$8.6\ g\ kg^{-1}\ day^{-1}$
Monkey	Intravenous self-administration	90–360	$6–8\ g\ kg^{-1}\ day^{-1}$
	Shock avoidance	20–200	$2.5\ g\ kg^{-1}\ day^{-1}$
	Ethanol liquid diet	40	$5–7\ g\ kg^{-1}\ day^{-1}$

seem to indicate that even after a single dose of ethanol a measurable degree of physical dependence can be observed.

Chronic physical dependence and tolerance develop simultaneously (CICERO, 1978). The degree of tolerance (depending on the response measured) and physical dependence are dependent both on the length of the alcohol exposure period and on the total dose of ethanol to which the organism was exposed (CICERO, 1978; GOLDSTEIN, 1976; KALANT et al., 1971). The degree of tolerance and dependence which can be developed is limited, and at some point, no further enhancement of tolerance and dependence can be achieved, despite increased exposure to ethanol. Tolerance to and dependence on ethanol develop quickly and dissipate very shortly. Residual physical dependence and tolerance may be present for months and years. The mechanisms underlying the development and persistance of tolerance and physical dependence have been excellently reviewed by CICERO (1978).

An animal model of physical dependence on ethanol can be designed as in the case of other physical dependence-producing drugs. A considerable obstacle in developing methods based on repeated administration of ethanol is to circumvent the animals' inherent aversion to the irritating taste of ethanol. The chronicity of experiments differs considerably from one method to another; in some cases a 1-day administration period is considered sufficient to study acute dependence phenomena while in other methods using small animals, up to 90 days' treatment is recommended. In the monkey, longer experiments are usual.

A number of methods using oral, intragastric, intravenous, and inhalational routes of administration for the induction of physical dependence on ethanol in experimental animals have been developed within the past decade. FENNESY's (1979) review provides details of the methods applied. The behavioral (self-administration) techniques allow one to examine those factors which contribute to the development

Table 2. Ethanol withdrawal signs in mice (from GOLDSTEIN, 1973)

Sign	Minimum degree	Maximum degree
Tremor	Twitching, occasional trembling	Continuous tremor
Tail lift	One per hour	Four or more per hour
Lethargy	Slow movement, dragging limbs	Coma
Startle to tap on cage	Twitch	Convulsion
Spontaneous convulsion	Mild, tonic; jumping	Three or more generalized tonic-clonic convulsions per hour
Convulsion on handling	Mild, tonic	Severe, tonic-clonic

of the dependence process as a function of time. More classical pharmacological methods applying forced administration permit the more rapid inducement of physical dependence and provide an important tool for assessing physical dependence.

The first successful animal model for physical dependence on ethanol was reported in 1968 by ESSIG and LAM (1968). Later on, several models for alcohol physical dependence have been developed in at least five animal species: dogs (ELLIS and PICK, 1973; ELLIS and PICK, 1971, ESSIG and LAM, 1968), monkeys (DENEAU et al., 1969; ELLIS and PICK, 1973; ELLIS and PICK, 1970), rats (FALK et al., 1972; GIBBINS et al., 1971), mice (FREUND, 1969; GOLDSTEIN, 1973; GOLDSTEIN, 1974; GOLDSTEIN and NAKAJIMA, 1967), and chimpanzee (PIEPER et al., 1972). None of these, however, can be considered a model for alcoholism as a whole, because they do not reflect all its complex behavioral and social aspects. Nevertheless a straightforward model to elicit and examine physical dependence with pharmacological techniques is very useful, particularly in screening for treatment techniques. One such model (HAUBEK and LEE, 1979) is described below.

GOLDSTEIN (1973, 1974) conducted her experiment in two phases: an intoxication phase of a few days' duration and a withdrawal period during which the intensity of abstinence signs was measured. GOLDSTEIN (1973) emphasized that intermittent intoxication with alcohol does not produce physically dependent animals. On the contrary, it was shown by ISBELL et al. (1955) that physical dependence results from periods of continuous intoxication both in man and in the laboratory animals. Ethanol, therefore, is administered by inhalation to maintain stable blood alcohol levels. The mice were housed in a vapor chamber where there was a constant low concentration of ethanol in the circulating air. The mice were treated with a small daily dose of pyrazole (68 $mg.kg^{-1}$ i.p. every 24 h) to partially inhibit liver alcohol dehydrogenase. At the start of the experiment the mice were injected with ethanol to establish the blood level that was later to be maintained by inhalation. The withdrawal phase was initiated by simply removing the animals from the vapor chamber. Table 2 indicates the signs of a characteristic withdrawal syndrome.

The sign called "convulsions on handling" elicited by picking the mouse up by the tail, was considered sufficiently reliable to serve as the sole basis for grading the withdrawal reaction. The fits were scored on a standard rating system with a range of 0–4 points. A plot of the mean scores at each time point showed the time course and intensity of the withdrawal reaction for each experimental group. The whole syndrome of withdrawal signs, including the elicited convulsions, developed over the first 10 h

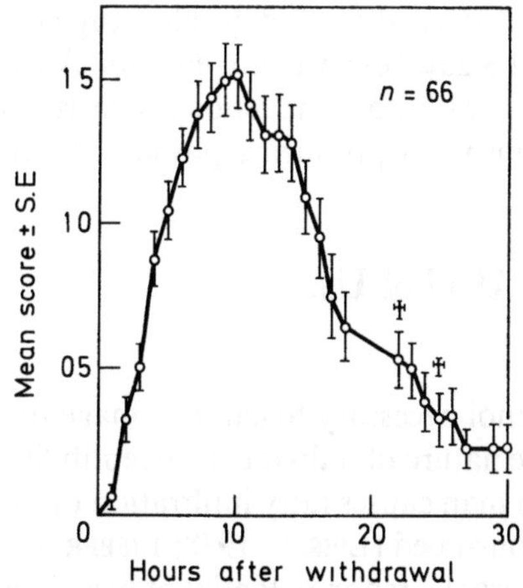

Fig. 1. Graded withdrawal reaction. Mice were exposed to ethanol by inhalation, removed from the vapor chamber, and scored repeatedly for elicited convulsions. The line is drawn through the mean scores (±S.E.) at each observation time. Data from 66 animals in seven different experiments are included. Two deaths are indicated (†); there was one more death at 49 h after withdrawal (After GOLDSTEIN, 1973)

after withdrawal and then regressed during the subsequent 24 h (Fig. 1). Computed area under the curve (AUC) indicating the overall intensity and duration of the withdrawal reaction and the peak height, indicating the maximum severity, can be used as parameter for ordinary statistical procedures.

In mice, the intensity of the withdrawal reaction was determined by the total dose of ethanol, regardless of the duration of the intoxication. The same amount of ethanol delivered during 13 days, resulting in a high blood level, produced the same intensity of elicited convulsions after withdrawal (GOLDSTEIN, 1973).

GOLDSTEIN (1973) has found in mice that both ethanol and any of the sedative or anxiolytic drugs applied in her experiments (meprobamate, paraldehyde, pentobarbital) suppressed the withdrawal seizures. Diazepam suppressed the convulsions for several hours (at a dose of 20 $mg.kg^{-1}$) or abolished them completely (at a dose of 50 $mg.kg^{-1}$). On the other hand phenothiazines (chlorpromazine and promazine) increased the intensity of the withdrawal seizures (GOLDSTEIN, 1973; KAIM et al., 1969).

Substances influencing GABA receptors or GABA metabolism modify the withdrawal seizures. Aminooxyacetic acid, which raises brain GABA levels, suppressed the seizures effectively, while picrotoxin, a GABA antagonist, caused a brief increase in seizures (GOLDSTEIN, 1974).

Drugs that act on catecholamine pathways increase the severity of withdrawal reactions. Both phentolamine and propranolol transiently increase the scores. Reserpine, which depletes catecholamines, greatly increases both the intensity and the duration of the withdrawal (GOLDSTEIN, 1974). α-Methyltyrosine, another catecholamine depletor, causes, however, only a slight increase in seizures scores (GOLDSTEIN, 1973).

More recently, MCCOMB and GOLDSTEIN (1979) described an experimental model that may be used for cross-dependence studies. They found that t-butanol substituted for ethanol at equipotent concentrations in 3 or 6 days inhalation of either t-butanol or ethanol vapor. t-Butanol inhaled for 3 days also augmented the abstinence syndrome produced by the first 3 days' exposure to ethanol. An additive effect of ethanol and t-butanol in producing a withdrawal reaction is consistent with the hypothesis of a single underlying mechanism for producing physical dependence on alcohols.

E. Chronic Effects of Alcohol Use

I. Hepatotoxic Effects

The average intake of ethanol necessary to cause damage to any of the organs is becoming established, but the nature of individual susceptibility remains to be clarified. A high intake of ethanol in man causes fatty infiltration of the liver. Its degree is proportional to the amount consumed (LIEBER, 1978; LIEBER and RUBIN, 1968). The deposition of fat occurs because the redox potential of liver is deranged by the constant drain on the coenzyme NAD required in the oxidation of ethanol through acetaldehyde to acetic acid. Thus, the ratio NAD/NADH is decreased and the consequent reduction in fatty acid oxidation results in hepatic fat deposition (LIEBER and DAVIDSON, 1962). Structurally, electron microscopic studies have shown that at early stages of fatty infiltration, swelling and cavitation as well as other changes of the mitochondria occur (SVOBODA and MANNING, 1964). Such abnormal mitochondria have a reduced capacity to oxidize fatty acids and to metabolize intermediary products. This impaired oxidation is probably why fat is deposited in the liver cells. Numerous observations in animals confirm liver toxicity of ethanol. LIEBER et al. (1975) fed baboons for several months with alcohol. The animals developed fatty liver and progressed to alcohol hepatitis and cirrhosis. Considerable epidemiological evidence links diseases of the liver, as well as the pancreas and the heart to excessive ethanol consumption (LELBACH, 1975; TURNER et al., 1977).

The relation between the severity of liver pathology and amounts of ethanol consumed is difficult to establish. Gathering data concerning the amount consumed is difficult, and patient self-reporting is unreliable, particularly in women, because of the reluctance of the patients to accuse themselves in view of the social stigma attached to alcoholism. There is a tendency to minimize the amount consumed. Furthermore, individual consumption varies considerably according to the life habits of the patient. Such factors as availability and cost of the preferred alcohol beverages related to frequently changeable income of the user may influence the drinking pattern and hence the amount of ethanol consumed. Consequently the duration of time during which the user is exposed to the liver-damaging levels of ethanol is extremely difficult to calculate. This level seems to be more stable in wine-producing countries, where the availability of wine is universal, its cost low, and social acceptance complete. Not surprisingly, most research which has attempted to measure alcohol intake and relate it to human disease has come from wine-producing countries. Attempts to measure the toxic dose of ethanol have mainly referred to its effects on the liver. LELBACH (1974) in 1960–1963 studied 319 liver biopsies in men in whom the history of ethanol intake was collected. The mean daily ethanol intake of those with normal livers was 139,5 g (equivalent to eight pints of beer, a bottle of sherry, or two-thirds of a bottle of high-percentage alcoholic beverage). The patients with fatty liver, chronic hepatitis, and cirrhosis had mean intakes of 172 g, 203,5 g, and 245,5 g, respectively. No patient with cirrhosis had an average daily intake of less than 190 g. This report provided an excellent confirmation of the direct dose-effect relation of ethanol in man, measured by clinically important and objective evidence. It also indicated a thin margin of safety between the relatively well-tolerated high level intake (eight pints of beer) and the toxic level. It reconfirms that all attempts to reduce the individual intake of alcohol remains the main preventive factor, while prophylactic attempts to reduce the level of other factors contributing to alcohol toxicity have a secondary importance.

The positive association between amount of ethanol consumed and degree of liver damage is strong evidence in support of a direct hepatotoxic effect of ethanol. The establishment of the hepatotoxic level is, however, not completed and several more recent papers report lower hepatotoxic levels. Some patients, especially women, may develop advanced liver disease after consuming much less than the amounts calculated by LELBACH (1974). Apparently nutritional, genetic, or immunological factors, concomitant diseases, and intrinsic or extrinsic environmental chemical substances may lower the threshold dose required to initiate damage of liver and/or favor its progression. Thus, PEQUIGNOT (1974) concluded that there is an increased prevalence of cirrhosis when daily alcohol consumption exceeds 60 g for men and 20 g for women. These levels will be underestimates, however, since some of his patients were cirrhotic with nonalcoholic disease. KRASNER et al. (1977) confirmed that women are more susceptible to alcoholic liver disease. They have found an increase in the incidence of smooth muscle and antinuclear antibodies and higher mean IgG and IgM concentrations. BAILEY et al. (1976) have shown a higher prevalence of the histocompatibility antigen HLA-B8 in alcoholics with cirrhosis than in those with fatty changes only. Regular drinking increased the liver damage, while intermittent patterns of heavy drinking produced less severe histological abnormalities (BRUNT et al., 1974). In most countries cirrhosis now ranks among the five leading causes of death for persons between the ages of 25 and 64 years. In Sri Lanka, for example, the contribution of alcohol cirrhosis to total cirrhosis rates rose from 24% in 1948 to 55% in 1968. The cirrhosis death rate in Anchorage, Alaska, increased by 142% between 1953 and 1975 (World Health Organization, 1978).

II. Pancreatotoxic Effects

Heavy ethanol consumption produces both acute and chronic pancreatitis (BENJAMIN et al., 1977; JAMES et al., 1974). The relation between the amount of intake and pancreatic damage has been scarcely documented. SARLES et al. (1965) noted that the mean daily alcohol intake in 55 patients with chronic pancreatitis was 175 g. Another survey (SCHNALL and WIENER, 1958) indicated the mean daily intake of about 150 g.

Acute alcoholic pancreatitis, by contrast, tends to be a disease related to acute overdose, and the patients are usually young men rather than chronic alcoholics (BENJAMIN et al., 1977)

III. Brain Damage

Intellectual impairment is a devastating complication of alcohol abuse. The extreme form of alcoholic dementia was described by WERNICKE (1881) a century ago. The correlation between intellectual damage and organic brain damage in chronic alcoholism is suspected but not definitively proven. Some evidence concerning alcohol-induced brain damage (BREWER and PARRETT, 1971; CALA et al., 1978; FOX et al., 1976; VON GALL et al., 1978; HAUBEK and LEE, 1979; HANG, 1968; LEE et al., 1979; TUMARKIN et al., 1955) is being accumulated due to modern diagnostic techniques (CALA et al., 1978; FOX et al., 1976; VON GALL et al., 1978; HAUBEK and LEE, 1979; LEE et al., 1979). LEE et al. (1979) examined 37 alcoholic males by psychometric tests, by liver biopsy, and by computerized tomography (CT scans). Factors other than alcoholism that might have caused brain damage were excluded. The prevalence of brain damage in this group was far greater than that of severe liver damage: 59% were intellectually impaired and 49% had cerebral atrophy on CT scan whereas only 19% had cirrhosis. LEE et al. (1979) did not find a significant correlation between the degree of intellectual impairment and the presence of cerebral atrophy. The CT scan seems to be an inadequate measure of functional brain damage, and psychometric tests are preferable (LEE et al., 1979).

IV. Cardiotoxic Effects

Relatively low level of ethanol cardiac toxicity was described in older textbooks. Alcoholic cardiomyopathy is a well-established, but infrequent and rather uncommon sequel to chronic alcoholism. It is seen most often in patients who have drunk heavily for a long period of time (DEMAKIS et al., 1974). The incidence of ischemic heart disease seems to be less in people who drink than in total abstainers (Editorial, 1978). In both the Framingham (STASON et al., 1976) and Kaiser-Permanente (KLATSKY et al., 1977) long-term prospective studies, the incidence of ischemic heart disease was lower in people with a moderate intake of alcohol. The same, even stronger, negative correlation was shown by YANO et al. (1977) more recently. However, more evidence is needed to reconfirm these observations. There is some evidence that alcohol may directly damage muscle tissue, including the heart muscle, particularly in the state of malnutrition.

The Kaiser-Permanente epidemiological studies (KLATSKY et al., 1974; KLATSKY et al., 1977) have also found that a raised blood pressure (both systolic and diastolic) was more common among those consuming 40 g of alcohol per day than in abstainers. However, other research data did not indicate a correlation between ethanol intake and blood pressure level (BARBORIAK et al., 1977).

F. Epidemiology of Alcohol Use and Overuse

In a number of countries detailed epidemiological studies concerning both alcohol use and overuse have been done in the past, and considerable relevant literature can be easily consulted in any medical library. In some countries efforts were made to collect and discuss available epidemiological data at some points in time, thus creating a foundation for studies of trends and enabling evaluation of results of antialcoholism activities and programs implemented. In some countries, mostly developing ones, however, in-depth alcohol epidemiological studies have never been undertaken and consequently the global picture is not available. The magnitude of the problem of alcohol consumption and overuse of alcohol and particularly the magnitude of the medical, social, economic, etc., problems related to alcohol use, can therefore be evaluated and presented on the basis of incomplete data only. The incompleteness of vocabulary in the whole area of nonmedical use of drugs, frequent use of terms with slight differences in meaning and understanding and particularly the lack of general international agreements concerning definitions of terms used in statistical studies almost totally prevent, at the present time, the presentation of the worldwide scale of problems of alcohol dependence with the necessary scientific exactitude.

On the other hand it can be assumed that tendencies and trends of human behavior tend to repeat themselves when environmental conditions of human settings and lifestyle are getting closer. The analysis of trends and studies of the history of alcohol use in a country may, therefore, be extremely useful for decision-making personnel and developers of health and social services programs in other countries. The interested reader may wish to conduct an in-depth study of the relevant literature using services of the largest alcohol research abstracting service, organized by Rutgers University.

As an example of the kind of data that are commonly collected within developed, highly industrialized countries and used for evaluation of trends in use of alcohol, a few lines are quoted from the report of the Canadian Commission of Inquiry into the Non-medical Use of Drugs (Le Dain's Commission) in 1972 (Government of Canada, 1972):

"It is estimated that in Canada in 1969 5,45% of the drinking population (that is, about 617,000 persons) consumed a "hazardous" amount of alcohol, defined as 100 ml (about 3,5 ounces), equivalent to about five social drinks of absolute alcohol daily."

"Between the years 1959–1968, deaths in Canada due to alcoholism increased by 74,8% for males and 107,4% for females. In 1969 there were 905 deaths in Canada due to alcoholism, including those caused by poisoning and cirrhosis of the liver."

Another important factor may be helpful in epidemiological studies: a good indication of the extent of alcohol use is given by road accidents data. Excessive drinking contributes to traffic accidents. Over the years 1965–1975, road accidents rates in Kuwait, for example, have tripled. A study of autopsies in Zambia revealed that 27% of road accident victims had ethanol levels above 0,8 g per liter blood, and in two-thirds of these cases the blood level was above 2 g-%. Alcohol was implicated in 36%–60% and 80% of cases of letal traffic accidents in Venezuela and Alaska, respectively.

G. Alcohol-Related Criminality

There is an acknowledged association between alcohol and crime, particularly crimes of violence. Criminality due to and related to use of alcohol differs from that related to the use of other dependence-producing drugs. First of all, the use of alcoholic beverages although not forbidden, compared with nonmedical use of narcotics, does not enjoy the same social recognition, acceptance, and approval, and, in a large majority of social strata it is considered to violate the ethical and/or moral code. The social and financial cost of use of alcohol has been known and discussed by legislators for centuries, while the socioeconomic consequences of other dependence-producing drugs are a relatively new phenomenon. Alcohol is universally available; its purchase, sale, and possession are legal in most countries (except in some

Islamic states); other dependence-producing substances, particularly those narcotic and psychotropic drugs thus are under international control, cannot move in commerce outside some specifically devised channels and their private possession, except for legitimate personal use, is illegal almost everywhere in the world. Criminal acts to procure money for the purchase of alcoholic beverages are rare in the courts and if occurring at all, are usually of negligible importance. On the contrary, the majority of criminal offences related to narcotic and psychotropic drugs under international control concern illicit trade and activities aiming at the quick appropriation of salable goods or liquid money for the purchase of drugs.

Some countries reported in 1979 to the World Health Organisation that 50% of their crime is alcohol related (World Health Organisation, 1978). Studies of the relationship between alcohol and crimes of violence implicate alcohol in 13%–50% of rapes, 24%–72% of assaults, and 28%–86% of homicides (World Health Organisation, 1978).

H. The Treatment of Alcoholism

The World Health Organization has estimated that in many countries the prevalence of dependence on alcohol is much greater than that of narcotics. For example in both Canada and the United States the prevalence of dependence on alcohol is 100 times greater than dependence on all controlled narcotic and psychotropic drugs. The life expectancy of an alcoholic is 10–12 years less than the average (Jaffe, 1975). These indications point to the seriousness which should be attached to the treatment of alcoholism – the most widespread drug-dependence problem in the world. In many countries alcoholism is among the four or five leading causes of mortality and in some of these countries it is moving up the scale. Alcoholism constitutes a global problem, spreading rapidly over previously relatively immune developing countries, and should be seen as a worldwide threat. Alcoholism is not restricted to any one social class; it affects the poor and those who were not poor (Edwards, 1979).

The main pathological disabilities resulting from or connected with the overuse of alcohol and requiring medical and/or social therapy include (Glasscote et al., 1972; Jaffe, 1975):

1) Intoxication, including poisoning;

2) Alcohol dependence, including the problems of abstinence syndrome during withdrawal;

3) Malnutrition, often resulting in neurological disorders;

4) Cirrhosis and other liver diseases;

5) Psychiatric problems, both those underlying the disease and those arising from the use of alcohol; and

6) Social maladjustement, including both microenvironment and family problems.

A comprehensive community alcoholism treatment and rehabilitation program must provide multiple methods of treatment and rehabilitation (Blum and Blum, 1967). The rehabilitation of an alcoholic must be considered as a problem of the social system itself (Holder and Stratas, 1972; Nathan et al., 1968; Pattison, 1974a; Pattison, 1974b).

Historically, the development of alcoholism rehabilitation programs was based on the assumption that there was *one* population of alcoholics, to be treated by *one* best method, resulting in *one* therapeutic outcome – complete abstinence for ever (PEQUIGNOT et al., 1974). This model is too simplistic and is no longer acceptable. There are major differences among individual users, groups of users, treatment facilities, and treatment outcomes, and the evaluation of results of treatment requires acceptance of a set of criteria.

The treatment of persons dependent on alcohol has produced encouraging results. However, it has often been viewed with pessimism. Evaluation of the results of treatment provided data differing considerably. BOWMAN and JELLINEK (1941) and PATTISON (1966) reported a success rate of 20%–30% only. Lack of consideration of criteria for evaluation of the results of treatment and acceptance of abstinence as a sole criterion of successful treatment produced unjustified nihilistic interpretations of treatment results (EINSTEIN and GARITANO, 1972; PATTISON, 1974b). The WHO Expert Committee on Mental Health in its fourteenth report (1967) stated that a marked improvement of social recovery has been reported in up to 50%–70% of cases, depending mainly on the underlying personality of the person treated. A skid-row population has a low rehabilitation potential and we can expect only a 5% success rate. On the contrary, an industrial population of employed alcoholics has an 80%–90% rehabilitation potential (PATTISON, 1974b). Therapeutic failures are commonly more frequent among abusers of other drugs, and the social and cultural factors as well as the extent of alcoholism within the population affect the treatment results.

Detoxification of the dependent person constitutes only one aspect of the total treatment and rehabilitation process. This procedure is less time consuming and difficult in alcoholism than in other drug dependencies, and it is more succesful than the other essential therapeutic steps. Intensive treatment of psychological dependence and of drug-induced and other physical accompanying disorders and social and vocational rehabilitation and long follow-up are all needed in the majority of cases if the alcoholic is to have an optimal chance of complete recovery to a productive healthy life (World Health Organization, 1967). The treatment should be easily accessible, should exist in the vicinity and easily reach the people. The best treatment, therefore, was the treatment that reached the alcohol-using people (EDWARDS, 1979). The treatment must seek to reach the early cases and must be multimodal (EDWARDS, 1979).

In all stages of treatment and rehabilitation of alcoholics there is a need for team work. The professions involved in a treatment program include general practitioners, psychiatrists, internal medicine specialists, psychologists, sociologists, occupational therapists, social workers, including probation officers, clergy men and, above all, the members of the family. These various categories represent a great strength in any treatment unit if they are well coordinated and if leadership of the team is provided by those with organizational abilities and humanity. For all team professions flexibility of operation and an excellent knowledge of local legal, cultural, and socioeconomic factors are important stepping stones for success. Organizations such as Alcoholics Anonymous have their role to play. The leadership of the treatment and rehabilitation team must not necessarily be by physicians. However, the treatment of individuals dependent on alcohol and/or other drugs is, or should be, to a large extent a medical problem, and a physician must assume the ultimate responsibility for the medical treatment of the alcoholic. During other phases of the treatment and particularly during rehabilitation, other professionals have important contributions to make and members of the team other than physicians may appropriately carry the major role (World Health Organization, 1967). Nonmedical personnel are heavily involved in the rehabilitation phase.

The therapists representing various disciplines and even philosophies should accept the patient, emotionally as well as intellectually as a sick person and avoid a moralistic and condemnatory attitude (World Health Organization, 1967).

Treatment must start with withdrawal of alcohol. This should be abrupt and complete. After withdrawal and detoxification, the patient should be treated with a combination of the available psychological, physical, and social methods best suited and adapted to his individual needs. The duration of treatment may be long and is measured in months or even years. It overlaps early with the rehabilitation phase. It is followed and also overlaps with follow-up services during which the patient is helped to return to normal and socially appropriate, productive life without relying on alcohol. A great variety of treatment methods and types of services are available. They differ among countries, and even among cities within a country, and are subject to prevailing attitudes and societal approaches to the problem of alcoholism, social mores, and local medical schools. Pharmacological treatment may be used both in detoxification and rehabilitation phases. Individual and group psychotherapy and psychodrama have been employed in the treatment. Numerous organizations, consisting mainly of former alcoholics, exist in many countries. Many persons dependent on alcohol have been helped by these organizations with little, if any, medical collaboration. Such organizations can also be instrumental in the case-finding and in the rehabilitation phases.

I. Current Methods of Treatment

Treatment of alcohol users, including dependent users, requires treatment facilities. Treatment encompasses procedures in intoxication, including acute medical emergencies as well as procedures necessary for long-term therapy and social rehabilitation and readaptation. Treatment facilities must be multipurpose and must range from very simple facilities to diagnostic and treatment centers with highly sophisticated equipment in the laboratory and in the clinical ward. The number of needed treatment facilities for various stages of the treatment and rehabilitation program depends very much on the dimension of the problem and can be based on the results of epidemiological studies. It depends also heavily on the economic resources of the country and to a certain extent on policy decisions. Medical care for cases requiring emergency treatment can be provided and assured by intensive care wards, if they are sufficient in number. In a number of countries, however, special outpatient stations have been developed to provide specialized services in acute intoxication. They remain in close contact with the hospitals and provide short-term bed facilities and sufficient expertise to cope with the most acute cases. Medical problems resulting from and related to both acute overuse and long-term, chronic use can be treated in the hospital wards dealing with particular internal disorders. What cannot be treated in any ward is the main problem resulting from alcohol overuse over a long period of time, namely alcohol dependence. Alcohol dependence treatment, although dissappointingly commonly evaluated as insatisfactory, is normally provided in special alcoholism treatment wards (or institutions). Such treatment is closely linked and interwoven with both medical and social readaptation and aims at the social reintegration of the user. The concepts of treatment and social readaptation are closely linked, and in fact, alcoholism treatment means both medical treatment and social readaptation.

The legal framework within a country is instrumental in developing facilities and giving them wide or narrow accessibility. Human beliefs, traditions, and cultural habits considerably influence the creation of facilities by decision makers and the use of existing facilities. The effectiveness of treatment of alcohol dependence relies heavily upon motivation of the dependent individual, hence a great value of microenvironment and the particular treatment difficulty; the need is for the creation of surroundings oriented toward social reintegration not only in the treatment facility but also in the future microenvironment of the treated person.

Virtually anyone who becomes alcoholically intoxicated in a public place may find himself, in any country, under police custody and may then "sleep it off" in primitive police premises, usually without the benefit of medical care. Whether a dependent user, or an "at risk of developing dependence" chronic user, is than referred to any treatment facility depends largely on the country (or territory of the country) in which his arrest occurred and under what circumstances. In most countries there are no organized means of reaching problem drinkers who are unwilling to seek help. The socioeconomic status of drinkers also influences their projected chances for recovery in a number of countries. CHAFETZ et al. (1962) have demonstrated that the failure of treatment programs is not the alcoholic's lack of motivation; more often it is the failure to provide an appropriate program to which the alcoholic can respond.

II. Referral for Treatment

The problem drinker, including the dependent alcohol user, can be referred for assistance by legal, industrial, medical, or other channels. The alcohol law in a number of countries specifies the conditions under which treatment becomes obligatory. A small but constantly growing number of industrial companies now include clinical alcoholism treatment referral services for their employees. The family physician or the general practitioner still play the vital role in the referral of alcohol-related disabilities because the general practitioners usually have much greater and easier contact with the user and his family and have greater persuasive powers on the basis of detailed knowledge of the microenvironment. The decision as to what kind of services may be helpful and indeed are needed must be timely. A variety of other formal or informal routes may be created that may serve as a system for detecting problem drinkers: clergymen, family counselors, social welfare workers, youth organization leaders, and interested relatives and friends. The effectiveness of such networks is unknown, due in part to their informality.

III. Treatment Facilities

1. General Hospitals

The treatment typically provided in general hospitals is very limited; in most cases it deals only with the patient's intoxication and other urgent medical problems or medical complications related to alcohol use and connected behavior. Only rarely are at-

Table 3. Existing facilities for prevention and treatment of dependence on alcohol and/or other drugs. Each of the facilities carries out one or more of the following functions: Case-finding, diagnosis, assessment, detoxification, withdrawal, active treatment, rehabilitation, after-care, follow-up, long-term care (World Health Organization, 1967)

Facilities as part of other services

General health services: general hospitals, outpatient departments, health centers, day-care centers, family physicians.

Mental health services: mental hospitals, institutions for long-term care, outpatient departments, community mental health centers, day hospitals, night hospitals, halfway houses, private psychiatrists.

Industrial health services: social and wefare services (including sheltered workshops).

Educational institutions

Religious agencies

Law-enforcement agencies

Special facilities

Information centers (United Kingdom, United States, other countries)

Sobriety boards (Scandinavia)

Hang-over clinics (Finland)

Sobering-up stations (Poland)

Medical consultation bureaux (Netherlands)

Special withdrawal facilities

- Ex-patients organizations (e.g., Alcoholics Anonymous)
- Halfway houses for ex-patients
- Clubs for ex-patients
- Rehabilitation farms and work colonies

tempts made to deal with the drinking problem or to develop a plan for the patient's continued treatment. Referral to psychiatric or social service departments or to a specialized treatment agency depends on local administrative arrangements and the general policy. General hospitals, while suffering a continuous burden of services rendered to patients treated because of ailments related to alcohol use, make a limited contribution toward solving the problems of alcohol-related disabilities and alcohol dependence.

2. Mental Hospitals

Only a limited number of mental hospitals have specialized wards or programs for treatment of alcohol-dependent drinkers. Milieu therapy and intensive individual psychotherapy are usually employed. Most specialized wards deal with selected patients. The selection ensures that there is no serious psychiatric or physical condition present that would make admission to an alcoholic ward inadvisable.

3. Detoxification Centers

Detoxification centers serve a limited but increasingly important function as the first stage in a system of alcoholism treatment facilities. Such centers, usually established in major urban areas, frequently provide the most needed first contact. Their structure and staffing are vital for further referral and considerably influence users' attitudes.

Usually upon arrival at a detoxification center clients are simply cleaned up, treated with necessary psychoactive and cardiovascular drugs, put to bed, and kept under observation. After this "drying up" procedure, which usually takes about 1 day, counseling should be given by appropriate staff. In practice many such centers have no formal system of referral for further services and serve as primary help centers. In some countries the names of clients are forwarded to employers, in the hope of creating a negatively reinforcing environment arount the client.

4. Transitional Facilities

Halfway houses have qualities useful in the treatment of alcoholics. Their managers frequently set up detailed conditions of admissions, and the internal rules are followed with an iron hand. Residents are expected to find employment and be involved in the resocialization and reintegration efforts. The treatment milieu and goal of all halfway houses is total abstinence. However, the methods applied and the internal arrangements, financing, and incorporation into general medical services by referral systems differ considerably among countries. Many halfway houses make extensive use of Alcoholics Anonymous. The inmates are expected to modify their behavior patterns.

5. Alcoholics Anonymous

Alcoholics Anonymous (AA) and similar groups have been helpful in the rehabilitation of certain types of drinkers. The organization is usually operated by former alcohol users. The new members are confronted by persons who at once convey understanding and concern and provide models for correct behavior. Each member participates in meetings and other activities. It helps to avoid contact with the previous environment in which drinking occurred, to keep the new member away from the former microsociety and in the company of people who share his concern about excessive drinking. However, only a small percentage of compulsive users seem motivated enough to seek admission to such groups; fewer still enter after learning what is expected of members, and many leave within some weeks after joining. Those who remain in residential programs do well while they are members and many continue to do well after they leave. The evaluation of effectiveness of AA activities is rarely undertaken, and opinions concerning their value and impact upon the results of curative and reintegrative services provided differ in the literature. One should underline that even the mere existence of such groups provides opportunities for those in need of discussing their problems, and such psychological support frequently becomes an invaluable incentive for further treatment.

6. Pharmacological Methods in the Treatment of Alcohol Dependence Syndrome

In general, drugs play a limited role in the overall management of alcohol dependence syndrome, but are necessary adjuncts in the control of alcohol withdrawal reactions. Hollister (1976) singles out two major principles of treatment of alcohol withdrawal reactions: (1) a replacement of alcohol with a pharmacologically equivalent drug, and (2) a gradual withdrawal of the equivalent drug. Dosage of the maintenance (substitutive) drug must be flexible and adapted to individual and varying needs of the patient. Benzodiazepines (chlordiazepoxide, diazepam) and clomethiazole edisylate (chlormethiazole) are frequently used. Very high doses may be required to counteract the withdrawal symptoms. Since these drugs are themselves dependence producing, their use should be short time; weaning from the sedative drug should be gradual and guided by the clinical symptoms. The low-dosage continuation of such medication is recommended by HOLLISTER (1976), among others, for a limited period in the early recovery phase to relieve tension and to prevent the return of drinking. Higher doses may be necessary to manage psychiatric complications.

Good supportive treatment prevents more serious withdrawal complications, such as convulsions and delirium tremens. Very detailed and careful medical supervision is essential.

a) Disulfiram

Disulfiram (Antabuse) was developed in Denmark in the late 1940 s. It alters the metabolism of ethyl alcohol. With its introduction the destruction of acetaldehyde is retarded, and the accumulation of this highly toxic compound provokes intensely unpleasant effects, which may include nausea and vomiting and sometimes also dangerous cardiovascular effects. The patient who understands what disulfiram is doing realizes that, "if he takes a drink it is no longer whiskey, rum, wine or beer that he is drinking but acetaldehyde." Disulfiram thus has a deterrent effect on the alcoholic.

Disulfiram inhibits the activity of the enzymes alcohol dehydrogenase and aldehyde dehydrogenase, resulting in the accumulation of ethanol and its major metabolite, acetaldehyde (MUSACCHIO et al., 1966). In the organism, ethanol and acetaldehyde, in concentrations comparable to those seen in man after ingestion of ethanol, have sympathomimetic effects that are dependent on release of catecholamines (EADE, 1959). After disulfiram treatment, depletion of noradrenaline and accumulation of its precursor, dopamine, has been demonstrated in the heart and in the central nervous system (GOLDSTEIN et al., 1964; GOLDSTEIN and NAKAJIMA, 1966). Disulfiram inhibits also dopamine β-hydroxylase activity. Disulfiram is slowly and incompletely absorbed from the gastrointestinal tract, or from tablets (Esperal) implanted under the skin. Its maximum effect is achieved in 12–24 h after oral ingestion; the effect lasts for 3–4 days.

A major metabolite of disulfiram, diethyldithiocarbamate, chelates copper, which is essential for the activity of the enzyme dopamine β-hydroxylase (GOLDSTEIN and PAL, 1971). In animals dopamine β-hydroxylation constitutes a rate-limiting step in noradrenaline synthesis. It has been suggested that altered synthesis disturbs adrenergic function and plays a role in the hypotensive aspect of the ethanol – disulfiram reaction in man. ROGERS et al. (ROGERS et al., 1979) evaluated adrenergic function in seven normal subjects before and during disulfiram administration (500 mg/day orally for 2 weeks). The decrease of excretion in urine of vanilmandelic acid (VMA) and noradrenaline and the increase of excretion of homovanillic acid (HVA) were consistent with reduced noradrenaline synthesis during disulfiram administration. ROGERS et al. (1979) stated that the cardiovascular responses to usual activities were unchanged by disulfiram and only with extreme hypotensive stress was there evidence of impaired response.

The main drawback of disulfiram use is that the patient has to take the deterring medicament continuously and regularly. If he fails to do so, he can easily relapse into his drinking habit. Attempts were made to introduce long-term effect pharmaceutical forms. Tablets (Esperal) to be inserted under the skin enjoy a certain popularity. They provide a monthly supply through slow release of the tablet and can be quite helpful in less well-motivated users.

Several drugs (e.g., Dipsan, Temposil) producing sensitization to alcohol effects have been recommended and are in a use on a small scale in a number of countries; none, however, was shown to be better than disulfiram.

b) Psychoactive Medicaments

Tranquilizers (ataractics, anxiolytics) combined not infrequently with antidepressants are prescribed to alleviate anxiety and depression. This mode of treatment might serve as a kind of maintenance therapy. The tranquilizers would be substituted for alcohol much as methadone is being used in the substitution maintenance treatment of heroin dependence. Such long-term cure may make it easier to eventually achieve a complete cure with the help of long-continued psychotherapy.

c) Aversive Conditioning

Many methods of conditioning alcoholics against the consumption of liquor have been tried. Most frequently, drugs which induce nausea and vomiting are given just before the patient is encouraged to drink alcohol. Painful electric shocks have been also used as conditioning stimuli. Apomorphine and emetine were administered. Short-term muscle nerve endings paralyzing drugs (e.g., suxamethonium) were also applied by some teams. However, FRANKS (1966) has shown that this form of conditioning did not bring about any long-term improvements.

References

Bailey, R.J., Krasner, N., Eddleston, A., Williams, R., Tee, D., Doniach, D., Kennedy, L., Batchelor, J.: Histocompatibility antigens, autoantibodies and immunoglobulins in alcoholic liver disease. Brit. Med. J. *1976 II*, 727–729

Bales, R.F.: Cultural differences in rates of alcoholism. Q. J. Stud. Alcohol *6*, 480–489 (1946)

Bandura, A.: Principles of behaviour modification. New York: 1969

Barboriak, J., Rimm, A., Anderson, A., Schmidhoffer, M., Tristani, F.: Coronary occlusion and alcohol intake. Brit. Heart J. *39*, 289–293 (1977)

Benjamin, I.S., et al. In: Alcoholism – new knowledge and new responses. Edwards, G., Grand, M. (eds.), p. 198. London: Cromm Helm 1977

Bennett, R.M., Bussard, A.H., Carpenter, J.A.: Alcohol and human physical aggression. Q. J. Stud. Alcohol. *30*, 870–876 (1969)

Blum, E.M.: Psychoanalytic views on alcoholism. Q. J. Stud. Alcohol. *27*, 259–299 (1966)

Blum, R.H., Blum, E.M.: Alcoholism: modern psychological approaches to treatment. San Francisco: Jossey-Bass 1967

Bowman, K.M., Jellinek, E.M.: Alcohol addiction and its treatment. Q. J. Stud. Alcohol. *2*, 98–176 (1941)

Brady, R.A., Westerfield, W.W.: The effect of B complex vitamins on voluntary consumption of alcohol by rats. Q. J. Stud. Alcohol. *7*, 499–505 (1947)

Brewer, C., Parrett, L.: Brain damage due to alcohol consumption: an air-encephalographic, psychometric and electroencephalographic study. Brit. J. Addict. *66*, 170–182 (1971)

Brown, Z.W., Amit, Z.: The effect of selective catecholamine depletion by 6-hydroxydopamine on ethanol preference in rats. Neurosci. Letters *5*, 333 (1977)

Brunt, P.W., Kew, M.C., Scheuer, P.I., Sherlock, S.: Studies in alcoholic liver disease in Britain. 1. Clinical and pathological patterns related to natural history. Gut *15*, 52–58 (1974)
Cahn, S.: The treatment of alcoholics: an evaluation study. New York: Oxford Univ. Press 1970
Cala, L.A., et al.: Aust. N. Z. J. Med. *8*, 147 (1978)
Chafetz, M.E., Blane, H.T., Abraham, H.S., Golner, J., Lacy, E., McCourt, W.F., Clark, E., Meyers, W.: Establishing treatment relations with alcoholics. J. Nerv. Ment. Dis. *134*, 395–409 (1962)
Cicero, T.J.: Tolerance to and psychical dependence on alcohol: behavioral and neurobiological mechanisms. In: Psychopharmacology. A generation of progress. Lipton, M.A., Di Mascio, A., Killam, K.F. (eds.), p. 1603. New York: Raven Press 1978
Conger, J.J.: Reinforcement theory and the dynamics of alcoholism. Q. J. Stud. Alcohol. *17*, 296 (1956)
Davies, D.L.: Implications for medical practice of an acceptable concept of alcoholism. In: Alcoholism: a medical profile. Kessel, N., Hawker, A., Chalke, H. (eds.), pp. 13–19. London: B. Edsall and Co. Ltd. 1974
Demakis, J.G., Proskey, A., Rahimtoola, S., Jamil, M., Sutton, G., Rosen, K., Gunnar, R., Tobin, J.: The natural course of alcoholic cardiomyopathy. Ann. Int. Med. *80*, 293–297 (1974)
Deneau, G., Yanagita, T., Seevers, M.H.: Self-administration of psychoactive substances by the monkey. Psychopharmacology *16*, 30–48 (1969)
Eade, N.R.: Mechanism of sympathomimetic action of aldehydes. J. Pharm. Exp. Ther. *127*, 29–34 (1959)
Eddy, N.B., Halbach, H., Isbell, H., Seevers, M.H.: Drug dependence: its significance and characteristics. Bull. Wld. Hlth Org. *32*, 721–733 (1965)
Editorial: Brit. Med. J. *1978 II*, 381–382
Edwards, G., Gross, M.M., Keller, M., Moser, J., Room, R.: Alcohol-related disabilities. WHO Offset Publ. No. 32, Geneva, World Health Organization, 1977
Edwards, G.: Discussion. WHO Document EB.63/SR/24, p. 7, 24 Jan. 1979
Einstein, S., Garitano, W.W.: Treating the drug abuser: problems, factors and alternatives. Int. J. Addict. *7*, 321–331 (1972)
Ellis, F.W., Pick, J.R.: Animal models of ethanol dependency. Ann. N. Y. Acad. Sci. *215*, 215–217 (1973)
Ellis, F.W., Pick, J.R.: Dose and time-dependent relationship in ethanol-induced withdrawal reactions. Fed. Proc. *30*, 568 (1971)
Ellis, F.W., Pick, J.R.: Experimentally induced ethanol dependence in Rhesus monkeys. J. Pharmacol. Exp. Ther. *175*, 88–93 (1970)
Essig, C.F., Lam, R.C.: Convulsions and hallucinatory behaviour following alcohol withdrawal in the dog. Arch. Neurol. *18*, 626–633 (1968)
Falk, L.L., Samson, H.H., Winger, G.: Behavioural maintenance of high concentrations of blood ethanol and physical dependence in the rat. Science *177*, 811–813 (1972)
Fennesy, M.R.: Induction of physical dependence on ethanol using animal models. Trends Pharmacol. Sci. *1*, 52–54 (1979)
Field, P.B.: A new cross-cultural study of drunkenness. In: Society, culture and drinking patterns. Pittman, D., Snyder, C. (eds.). New York: 1962
Fox, J.H., Ramsey, R., Huckmann, M., Proske, A.: Cerebral ventricular enlargement. J. Am. Med. Assoc. *236*, 365–367 (1976)
Franks, C.M.: Conditioning and conditioned aversion therapy in the treatment of the alcoholic. Int. J. Addict. *1*, 62–98 (1966)
Freund, G.: Alcohol withdrawal syndrome in mice. Arch. Neurol. *21*, 315–320 (1969)
Gall, M. von, Becker, H., Artmann, H., Lerch, G., Nemeth, N.: Results of computer tomography on chronic alcoholics. Neuroradiology *16*, 329–331 (1978)
Gibbins, R.J., Kalant, H., LeBlanc, A.E., Clark, J.W.: The effect of chronic administration of ethanol on startle thresholds in rats. Psychopharmacology *19*, 95–104 (1971)
Glasscote, R., Sussex, J.N., Jaffe, J.H., Brill, L.: The treatment of drug abuse: Programs, problems, prospects. Washington: Joint Information Service 1972
Goldstein, D.B.: Quantitative study of alcohol withdrawal signs in mice. Ann. N. Y. Acad. Sci. *215*, 218–223 (1973)
Goldstein, D.B.: Experimental studies on physical dependence on alcohol. Intra-Sci. Chem. Rep. *8*, No. 1–3, 165–174 (1974)

Goldstein, D.B.: An animal model for testing effects of drugs on alcohol withdrawal reactions. J. Pharmacol. Exp. Ther. *190*, 377–383 (1974)
Goldstein, D.B.: Pharmacological aspects of physical dependence on ethanol. Life Sci. *18*, 553–562 (1976)
Goldstein, D.B., Pal, N.: Alcohol dependence produced in mice by inhalation of ethanol: grading the withdrawal reaction. Science *172*, 288–290 (1971)
Goldstein, M., Anagnoste, B., Lauber, E., McKereghan, M.R.: Inhibition of dopamine β-hydroxylase by disulfiram. Life Sci. *3*, 763–767 (1964)
Goldstein, M., Nakajima, K.: The effects of disulfiram on the repletion of brain catecholamine stores. Life Sci. *5*, 1133–1138 (1966)
Goldstein, M., Nakajima, K.: The effects of disulfiram on catecholamine levels in the brain. J. Pharmacol. Exp. Ther. *157*, 96–102 (1967)
Goodwin, D.W., Schulsinger, F., Hermansen, L., Guze, S.B., Winokur, G.: Alcohol problems in adoptees raised apart from alcohol biological parents. Arch. Gen. Psychiat. *28*, 238–243 (1973)
Government of Canada. Treatment. A report of the Commission of Inquiry into the Non-medical Use of Drugs. LeDain, G. et al. (eds.). Ottawa: Information Canada 1972
Haubek, A., Lee, K.: Computed tomography in alcoholic cerebellar atrophy. Neuroradiology *18*, 77–79 (1979)
Hang, J.O.: Pneumoencephalographic evidence of brain damage in chronic alcoholics. A preliminary report. Acta Psychiat. Scand. *203*, Suppl., 135–143 (1968)
Holder, H.D., Stratas, N.E.: A systems approach to alcoholism programming. Am. J. Psychiat. *129*, 32–37 (1972)
Hollister, L.E.: Psychiatric disorders. In: Drug treatment. Avery, G.S. (ed.), p. 796. Sydney: Adis Press 1976
Horton, D.: The functions of alcohol in primitive societies. A cross cultural study. Q. J. Stud. Alcohol. *4*, 199–320 (1943)
Huus, M.: Alcoholismus chronicus eller chronisk alkoholsjukdom. Stockholm 1849
Isbell, H., Fraser, H.F., Wikler, A., Belleville, R.E., Eisenman, A.J.: An experimental study of the etiology of "rum fits" and delirium tremens. Q. J. Stud. Alcohol. *16*, 1–33 (1955)
Jaffe, J.H.: Drug addiction and drug abuse. In: The pharmacological basis of therapeutics. Goodman, L.S., Gilman, A. (eds.), pp. 284–324. New York: MacMillan 1975
James, O., Agnew, J.E., Bouchier, I.A.D.: Chronic pancreatitis in England. A changing picture? Brit. Med. J. *1974 II*, 34–38
Jellinek, E.M.: Heredity of the alcoholic. In: Alcohol, science and society. New Haven: 1945
Jellinek, E.M.: The disease concept of alcoholism. New Brunswick, Highland Park, NY: Hillhouse Press 1960
Jonsson, E., Nilsson, T.: Alkoholkonsumtion hos monozygota dizygota zvillingpor. Nord. Hyg. Tideskr. *49*, 21–25 (1968)
Kaij, L.: Alcoholism in twins: studies on the etiology and sequel of abuse of alcohol. Stockholm: Almquist and Wiksell 1960
Kaim, S., Klett, C.J., Rothfield, B.: Treatment of the acute alcohol withdrawal state: A comparison of few drugs. Am. J. Psychiat. *125*, 1640–1646 (1969)
Kalant, H., LeBlanc, A.E., Gibbins, R.J.: Tolerance to, and dependence on, some non-opiate psychotropic drugs. Pharm. Rev. *23*, 135–191 (1971)
Kingham, R.J.: Alcoholism and reinforcement theory of learning. Q. J. Stud. Alcohol. *19*, 320–330 (1958)
Kinsey, B., Phillips, L.: Evaluation of anomy as a predisposing or developmental factor in alcohol addiction. Q. J. Stud. Alcohol. *29*, 892–898 (1968)
Klatsky, A., Friedman, G., Siegelbaum, A., Gérard, M.: Alcohol consumption and blood pressure (Kaiser-Permanente multiphasic health examination data). New Engl. J. Med. *296*, 1194–1200 (1977)
Klatsky, A.L., Friedman, G., Siegelaur, A.: Alcohol consumption before myocardial infarction. Ann. Intern. Med. *81*, 294–301 (1974)
Krasner, N., Davis, M., Portmann, B., Williams, R.: Changing pattern of alcoholic liver disease in Great Britain: relation to sex and signs of autoimmunity. Brit. Med. J. *1977 I*, 1497–1500
Lee, K., Müller, L., Hardt, F., Haubek, A., Jensen, E.: Alcohol-induced brain damage and liver damage in young males. Lancet *1979 II*, 759–761

Lelbach, W.K.: Organic pathology related to volume and pattern of alcohol use. In: Research advances in alcohol and drug problems. Gibbins, R.J., Israel, Y., Kalant, H. (eds.), vol. I, pp. 93–198. New York: J. Wiley 1974
Lelbach, W.K.: Quantitative aspects of drinking in alcoholic liver cirrhosis. In: Alcoholic liver pathology. Khanna, J.M., Israel, Y., Kalant, H. (eds.). Ontario: Addiction Research Foundation of Ontario 1975
Lieber, C.S.: Alcoholism and liver injury (correspondence). New Engl. J. Med. *229*, 260 (1978)
Lieber, C.S., DeCarli, L.M.: An experimental model of alcohol feeding and liver injury in the baboon. J. Med. Primatol. *3*, 153–163 (1974)
Lieber, C.S., Davidson, C.S.: Some metabolic effects of ethyl alcohol. Am. J. Med. *33*, 319 (1962)
Lieber, C.S. et al.: Effect of chronic alcoholic consumption on ethanol and acetaldehyde metabolism. In: Alcohol intoxication and withdrawal. Experimental studies. II. Gross, M.M. (ed.). New York: Plenum Press 1975
Lieber, C.S., Rubin, E.: Alcoholic fatty liver in man on a high protein and low fat diet. Am. J. Med. *44*, 200–206 (1968)
De Lint, J., Schmidt, W.: Consumption averages and alcoholism prevalence: a brief review of epidemiological investigation. Brit. J. Addict. *66*, 97–107 (1971)
Mardones, J.: On the relationship between the deficiency of B vitamins and alcohol intake in rats. Q. J. Stud. Alcohol. *12*, 563–575 (1951)
McComb, J.A., Goldstein, D.B.: Additive physical dependence: Evidence for a common mechanism in alcohol dependence. J. Pharmacol. Exp. Ther. *210*, 87–90 (1979)
McQuarrie, D.G., Fingl, E.: Effects of single doses and chronic administration of ethanol on experimental seizures in mice. J. Pharmacol. Exp. Ther. *124*, 264–271 (1958)
Mellor, C.S.: Aetiology in alcoholism. In: Alcoholism: a medical profile. Kessel, N. et al. (eds.), pp. 30–38. London: Edsall B. and Co. Ltd. 1974
Mendelson, J.H., Mello, N.: Alcohol, aggression and androgens. Nerv. Ment. Dis. *52*, 225–236 (1974)
Musacchio, J.M., Goldstein, D.B., Anagnoste, B., Poch, G., Kopin, I.J.: Inhibition of dopamine β-hydroxylase by disulfiram in vivo. J. Pharmacol. Exp. Ther. *152*, 56–61 (1966)
Nathan, P.E., et al.: Int. J. Addict. *3*, 55 (1968)
Nathan, P.E., O'Brien, J.S., Norten, D.: Comparative study of the interpersonal and affective behaviour of alcoholics and non alcoholics during prolonged experimental drinking. In: Rec. Adv. in Studies of alcoholism. Mello, N.K., Mendelson, J.H. (eds.). Washington: 1970
National Council on Alcoholism, Criteria Committee: Criteria for the diagnosis of alcoholism. Am. J. Psychiatry *129*, 127–135 (1972)
Omenn, G.S., Motulsky, A.G.: A biochemical and genetic approach to alcoholism. Ann. N. Y. Ac. Sci. *197*, 16–23 (1972)
Partanen, J., Bruun, K., Markkanen, T.: Inheritance of drinking behaviour. Helsinki, Finnish Foundation for Alcohol Studies, Publ. No. 14, 1966
Pattison, M.E.: A critique of alcoholism treatment concepts with special reference to abstinence. Q. J. Stud. Alcohol *27*, 49–71 (1966)
Pattison, M.: Discussion. In: Alcoholism: a medical profile. Kessel, N., et al. (eds.), p. 20. London: Edsall and Co. Ltd., 1974a
Pattison, M.: Drinking outcome of alcoholism treatment. Abstinence, social, modified, controlled, and normal drinking. In: Alcoholism: a medical profile. Kessel, N., Hawker, A., Chalke, H. (eds.), p. 57. London: B. Edsall and Co. Ltd., 1974b
Pequignot, G., et al.: Rev. Alcoolisme *20*, 191 (1974)
Pieper, W.A., Sheen, M.J., McClure, H.M., Bourne, P.G.: The chimpanzee as an animal model for investigating alcoholism. Science *176*, 71–73 (1972)
Plant, T.F.: Alcohol problems: a report to the nation. New York, Oxford: Oxford Univ. Press 1967
Roebuck, J.B., Kessler, R.G.: The etiology of alcoholism. Springfield, Ill.: Ch. C. Thomas, Publ. 1972
Rogers, W.K., Benowitz, N.L., Wilson, M., Abbott, J.A.: Effects of disulfiram on adrenergic function. Clin. Pharmacol. Ther. *25*, 469–477 (1979)

Sarles, H., Sarles, I.C., Camatte, R., Muratore, R., Gaini, M., Guien, C., Pastor, J., Le Roy, F.: Observation on 205 confirmed cases of acute pancreatitis, recurring pancreatitis and chronic pancreatitis. Gut *6*, 545–559 (1965)
Sarles, H.: An international survey on nutrition and pancreatitis. Digestion *9*, 389–403 (1973)
Schnall, C., Wiener, J.S.: Clinical evaluation of blood pressure in alcoholics. Q. J. Stud. Alcohol. *19*, 432–446 (1958)
Schuckit, M.A., Goodwin, D.W., Winokur, G.: A study of alcoholism in half siblings. Am. J. Psychiat. *128*, 122–126 (1972)
Seevers, M.H.: Psychopharmacological elements of drug dependence. J. Am. Med. Assoc. *206*, 1263–1266 (1968)
Smart, R.J.: Effects of alcohol on conflict and avoidance behaviour. Q. J. Stud. Alcohol. *26*, 187–205 (1965)
Stason, W.B., Neff, R., Miettinen, O., Jick, H.: Alcohol consumption and non fatal myocardial infarction. Am. J. Epidemiol. *104*, 603–608 (1976)
Svoboda, D.J., Manning, R.T.: Am. J. Pathol. *44*, 645 (1964)
Syme, L.: Personality characteristics of the alcoholic. Q. J. Stud. Alcohol *18*, 288–302 (1957)
Tamerin, J.S., Mendelson, J.H.: The psychodynamics of chronic inebriation: observations of alcoholics during the process of drinking in an experimental group setting. Am. J. Psychiat. *125*, 886–889 (1969)
Tumarkin, B., Wilson, J.D., Snyder, G.: Cerebral atrophy due to alcoholism in young adults. U. S. Armed Forces Med. J. *6*, 67–74 (1955)
Turner, T.B., Mezey, E., Kimball, A.: Measurements of alcohol-related effects in man: chronic effects in relation to levels of alcohol consumption. John Hopkins Hosp. Med. J. *141*, 235–243 (1977)
Wallgren, H., Barry, H.: Actions of alcohol. Amsterdam: Elsevier 1970
Wernicke, C.: Die akute hämorrhagische Polioencephalitis superior. Lehrbuch der Gehirnkrankheiten 1881, p. 229.
Williams, R.J.: Biochemical individuality and cellular nutrition. Q. J. Stud. Alcohol. *20*, 452–463 (1959)
Wolff, P.H.: Ethnic differences in alcohol sensitivity. Science *175*, 449–450 (1972)
World Health Organization. Wld Hlth Org. techn. Rep. Ser. No. 273, Annex 1 (1964)
World Health Organization. WHO Expert Committee on Drug Dependence. Sixteenth Report. Wld Hlth Org. techn. Rep. Ser. No. 407, p. 6 (1969)
World Health Organization. Services for the prevention and treatment of dependence on alcohol and other drugs. Wld. Hlth. Org. techn. Rep. Ser. No. 363 (1967)
World Health Organization. Alcohol-related problems: the need to develop further the WHO initiative. Report by the Director General. WHO Document EB 63/23, 27 Nov. 1978
Yano, K., Rhoads, G., Kagan, A.: Coffee, alcohol and risk of coronary heart disease among Japanese men living in Hawaii. New Engl. J. Med. *297*, 405–409 (1977)

Psychotropic Effects of Central Acting Drugs

CHAPTER 13

Psychotropic Effects of Opioids and Opioid Antagonists

S.R. GOLDBERG, R.D. SPEALMAN, and H.E. SHANNON

A. Introduction

The discovery that morphine and related drugs combine with specific receptors in nervous tissue and the subsequent indentification of endogenous peptides with high affinity for these receptors (GOLDSTEIN, 1976; HUGHES and KOSTERLITZ, 1977; SNYDER and SIMANTOV, 1977; TERENIUS, 1978; BEAUMONT and HUGHES, 1979) have served to enhance interest in the psychotropic effects of opioids and opioid antagonists.[1] In recent years there has been a rapid increase in the development of new opioids and antagonists which have proved to be effective therapeutic agents as well as useful experimental tools. In the present chapter we will review the psychotropic effects of these drugs. The chapter is divided into two major sections: 1) signs, symptoms, and subjective effects in humans; and 2) experimental analysis of behavioral effects in laboratory animals.

B. Evaluation of Signs, Symptoms, and Subjective Effects in Humans

I. Introduction

The importance of characteristic patterns of drug-induced changes in signs, symptoms, and subjective effects for assessing morphine-like drugs was recognized very early. ISBELL and co-workers first attempted to define and assess the subjective changes produced specifically by morphine and related drugs (ISBELL, 1948). These changes included increased talkativeness, reports of satisfaction with the effects of the drug, requests for increased doses of the drug, and, with larger doses, slurring of speech, motor ataxia, and evidence of marked sedation. Prior to 1960, however, drug-induced changes in subjective effects were evaluated primarily by clinical judgment. FRASER and ISBELL (1960) introduced the first questionnaires into studies of drugs for morphine-like abuse liability. FRASER et al. (1961) developed, among other questionnaires, the "single-dose opiate questionnaires" for subjects and trained observers in

---

The views expressed by the authors do not necessarily reflect the opinions, official policy, or position of the Addiction Research Center, the National Institute on Drug Abuse, the Alcohol, Drug Abuse and Mental Health Administration, or the U.S. Department of Health, Education and Welfare.

1 There is no fully accepted way to classify drugs as opioids or opioid antagonists. After JAFFE and MARTIN (1980), the term "opioid" is used here in the generic sense to designate drugs that to varying degrees have morphine-like actions. The term "opioid antagonist" designates drugs that to varying degrees block the actions of opioids. Many of the drugs discussed here have both types of effects

order to assess systematically the signs, symptoms, and reports of subjective effects resulting from administration of various opiates. These questionnaires are still among the basic instruments utilized to measure the subjective effects of opioids and opioid antagonists.

It was also recognized that standardized questionnaire scales were needed to distinguish changes in reports of subjective effects produced by drugs from different classes. To this end, the Addiction Research Center Inventory (ARCI) was developed and validated statistically in postaddict subjects (HAERTZEN et al., 1963; HAERTZEN, 1974a). From the ARCI, which contains 550 true-false items, short scales were empirically developed which discriminated placebo from particular drug conditions. The original scales distinguished subjective effects induced by morphine, pentobarbital, chlorpromazine, LSD, pyrahexyl, amphetamine, and alcohol from placebo and no-drug conditions (HILL et al., 1963a, b). Subsequently, pattern, or drug group, scales were developed because of the commonality of a large number of items among the empirical scales (HAERTZEN, 1966). The three most commonly used group scales are: the morphine-benzedrine group (MBG) scale, which measures reports of morphine-like subjective effects; the pentobarbital-chlorpromazine-alcohol group (PCAG) scale, which measures effects produced by sedative-hypnotics; and the LSD scale, which measures psychotomimetic effects. The profile of scores on these three scales has been used to evaluate an extensive series of opioids, opioid antagonists, and other psychoactive drugs (HAERTZEN, 1974b).

Operationally, then, drug-induced subjective effects have been defined as statistically reliable, dose-related changes in responses to items on specifically designed questionnaires. The procedures have been described in detail elsewhere (e.g., JASINSKI et al., 1971a). Drugs are administered to nondependent subjects with a history of opiate abuse under double-blind conditions and according to a crossover design. Each subject receives placebo, two or three doses of a standard drug such as morphine, and two or three doses of the test drug. The drugs are administered in random order with a minimum 7-day interval between each drug administration. At timed intervals after drug or placebo administration, subjects and trained observers complete the single-dose opiate questionnaire and subjects also complete a "subjective drug-effects questionnaire" containing items from the MBG, PCAG, and LSD scales. Concurrently, pupil diameter is measured photographically as a physiologic measure of drug action. The responses on the questionnaires are quantified using a standard scoring system. Dose-response curves are constructed using the group mean scores for the standard and test drugs for each of the measurements, and relative potencies are calculated from these dose-response curves with statistical methods for parallel-line bioassays.

II. Opioid Analgesics

1. Effects of Single Doses in Nondependent Subjects

Single-dose opiate questionnaires have been used extensively to assess the signs, symptoms, and reports of subjective effects following the administration of opioid analgesics. One question asked of the subjects (and observers) is to identify the drugs administered to the subject from among a list of drugs [including the possible answers of opiate ("dope"), barbiturate ("goofballs"), LSD ("acid"), "blank", and "other"]. Subjects rarely identify placebo as active drug. In a direct comparison of graded doses of morphine and heroin, MARTIN and FRASER (1961) demonstrated that the percentage of subjects who recognized and correctly identified either morphine or heroin as an opiate was linearly related to dose. In general, about 50% of subjects identify 6 mg/70 kg morphine administered subcutaneously or intramuscularly as an opiate with the other half reporting a "blank"; about 90% of the subjects correctly identify 20 mg/70 kg morphine as an opiate (see also MARTIN, 1966). Subjects also are able to discriminate morphine from other psychoactive drugs. Morphine has been directly compared in double-blind crossover experiments with pentobarbital (MARTIN et al., 1974), D-amphetamine (JASINSKI and NUTT, 1972), nalorphine, and cyclazocine (MARTIN et al., 1965). Subjects often confused lower doses of these drugs, but with larger doses, subjects correctly discriminated morphine from the other drugs.

With the single-dose opiate questionnaires, subjects and observers also are asked to report which signs and symptoms occur after drug administration from among a list of items. The frequency with which subjects report the symptoms "itchy skin," "relaxed," "coasting," and "drive" and with which observers report the signs "scratching," "coasting," and "nodding" have been shown to increase with dose of an opioid (MARTIN and FRASER, 1961). Additionally, subjects are asked to rate their degree of "liking" for the drug on a five-point ordinal scale. Morphine produces both dose- and time-related changes in the "liking" scores, with higher doses producing higher average scores.

The subjective drug-effect questionnaire containing 40 items from the MBG, PCAG, and LSD scales of the ARCI was first introduced into assessment studies of opiate derivatives by JASINSKI et al. (1971 a). Morphine produces dose-related increases in scores on the MBG scale but not on the PCAG or LSD scales. Items on the MBG scale primarily relate to reports of well-being, self-esteem, satisfaction, and competence. Although morphine may on some occasions produce increases in the PCAG scale related to sedative-like subjective effects, this is not typical and tends to occur several hours after drug administration. For example, in a direct comparison of morphine and buprenorphine (JASINSKI et al., 1978), 30 mg/70 kg morphine produced significant increases in MBG scale scores but not in PCAG scale scores during the first 6 h following acute administration. From 12 to 30 h after drug administration, the subjects continued to identify the drug as opiate-like, but scores on the PCAG scale were significantly elevated while MBG scale scores were not.

2. Effects in Tolerant Subjects

In subjects tolerant to morphine, single acute doses of morphine produce much smaller changes in scores on the MBG scale than are produced in nontolerant subjects. The effects of an acute dose of morphine in tolerant subjects also differ qualitatively in that symptoms primarily related to apathy and sedation are reported and scores are elevated on the PCAG scale (HAERTZEN and HOOKS, 1969). Subjects report feeling tired and are observed to be hypochondriacal and withdrawn. "Liking" scores also may decrease during chronic administration of morphine (FRASER et al., 1961). Similar findings have been obtained for chronically administered heroin (HAERTZEN and HOOKS, 1969) and methadone (MARTIN et al., 1973a). During abrupt withdrawal of morphine, heroin, or methadone, subjects report tiredness, lack of motivation, tenseness, irritability, and inefficient physical, social, and intellectual functioning, and scores are elevated on the PCAG and opiate withdrawal scales of the ARCI (HAERTZEN et al., 1970). During withdrawal from morphine and related opioids, subjects repeatedly request drugs for relief of their symptoms. Scores on the PCAG and opiate withdrawal scales generally return to control values within 6 to 8 weeks, but a protracted abstinence syndrome, defined primarily in terms of physiologic changes, has been reported to persist for as long as 24 weeks (MARTIN and JASINSKI, 1969; MARTIN et al., 1973 a). During protracted abstinence from methadone, scores on the narcotic antagonist scale of the ARCI are significantly elevated (but scores on the opiate withdrawal scales are not). Scores also tend to be elevated on scales related to apathy and sedation (e.g., PCAG) and decreased on scales related to feelings of well-being (e.g., the MBG).

3. Opioid Analgesics of Low Abuse Liability

Codeine, meperidine, and D-propoxyphene have a low incidence of illicit use relative to the extent of licit use (JASINSKI, 1977). Pharmacologically these three drugs are quite similar. All produce morphine-like subjective effects in that they are identified as an opiate and produce dose-related increases in opiate signs and symptoms and increases in "liking" scores. Scores are elevated on the MBG scale but not the LSD scale; meperidine, but not codeine or D-propoxyphene, increases PCAG scale scores. All three drugs suppress abstinence in morphine-dependent subjects, although meperidine and propoxyphene appear to only partially suppress morphine abstinence. During withdrawal from each of these three drugs, subjects identify the abstinence symptoms as opiate-like and request drugs for relief. The lower abuse liability of these drugs appears to be related to factors such as their low potency, tissue irritant properties, low solubility, and toxic side effects which limit their effectiveness in producing strong morphine-like effects.

4. Dextrorphan and Dextromethorphan

Dextrorphan (D-3-hydroxy-*N*-methylmorphinan) and dextromethorphan (D-3-methoxy-*N*-methylmorphinan) are dextrorotatory isomers of opiates but are generally devoid of opiate-like properties. ISBELL and FRASER (1953) reported that single doses of dextrorphan and dextromethorphan administered both orally and subcutaneously up to 100 mg per dose produced neither opiate-like subjective effects nor pupillary constriction in nondependent subjects. JASINSKI et al. (1971 b) compared dextromethorphan directly with morphine and nalorphine in a double-blind crossover study. In doses up to 240 mg/70 kg, dextromethorphan did not produce significant opiate signs and symptoms scores, significant increases in "liking" scores, nor significant increases in MBG scale scores. Subjects frequently identified dextromethorphan as a barbiturate. Oral dextromethorphan produced significant increases in LSD and PCAG scale scores, although subcutaneously administered dextromethorphan significantly elevated only LSD scale scores. These effects of dextromethorphan were similar to those observed with high doses of nalorphine (30 mg/70 kg) in the same subjects. Dextromethorphan could be distinguished from nalorphine, however, in that the former drug produced mydriasis whereas the latter produced miosis.

5. Subject Population

The quantitative assessment of subjective effects of opioids and related drugs has been conducted almost exclusively with subjects sophisticated in the use of opioids and other psychoactive drugs (see MARTIN, 1966, for a detailed description of this subject population). On the other hand, subjects with either no experience or only limited experience with opioids usually describe their effects as unpleasant when these drugs have been given in structured experimental settings. Students, for example, frequently reported drowsiness, tiredness, and sleepiness, as well as nausea and itching after morphine or heroin, while symptoms such as friendliness, geniality, peacefulness, satisfaction, and detachment were reported less frequently (SMITH and BEECHER, 1959, 1962; SMITH et al., 1962). Symptoms such as nausea, dizziness, headache, inability to concentrate, loss of interest, and sleepiness, which are reported as unpleasant by nonaddict subjects (e.g., LASAGNA et al., 1955), may be reported as desirable by addict subjects.

III. Partial Agonists of the Morphine Type

A partial agonist acts on the same receptors as an agonist, but due to its lower degree of efficacy or intrinsic activity cannot produce the same magnitude of effect (TALLARIDA and JACOB, 1979). Under appropriate conditions, therefore, a partial agonist may antagonize the actions of an agonist. Subjects dependent on 240 mg/70 kg per day of morphine have been considered to have near-maximal dependence (ANDREWS and HIMMELSBACH, 1944) and therefore near-maximal receptor occupation. Consequently, a partial agonist would displace morphine and reduce the degree of agonist activity, thereby precipitating abstinence signs and symptoms (e.g., JASINKSI et al., 1971a). In subjects dependent on only 60 mg/70 kg per day of morphine, however, a much smaller proportion of the receptors would be occupied and the displacement of morphine by a partial agonist could be offset by the partial agonist occupying more receptor sites and thus substituting for morphine.

1. Profadol and Propiram

In a series of studies by JASINSKI et al. (1971 a), the effects of profadol and propiram were evaluated in nondependent and in morphine-dependent subjects. In subjects dependent on 240 mg/70 kg per day of morphine, profadol and propiram precipitated abstinence signs and symptoms; in contrast, these drugs suppressed signs and symptoms of abstinence in subjects dependent on 60 mg/70 kg per day of morphine. Subjects identified single doses of profadol or propiram as an opiate, and both drugs produced dose-related increases in opiate symptom and sign scores, "liking" scores, and MBG scale scores. Neither drug produced PCAG and LSD scale scores greater than those observed with morphine. When profadol and propiram were administered chronically, subjects identified both drugs as opiate-like. Nalorphine precipitated abstinence in subjects dependent on either profadol or propiram. The subjects identified abstinence symptoms from these agents as opiate-like and requested opiate administration for relief.

2. Buprenorphine

On the basis of clinical and experimental studies in animals, buprenorphine appears to be a partial agonist of the morphine type. In the chronic spinal dog (MARTIN et al., 1976), buprenorphine produced typical morphine-like effects in single doses and physical dependence with chronic administration. Lower doses of buprenorphine suppressed morphine abstinence whereas higher doses precipitated a mild abstinence syndrome in morphine-dependent dogs. In addition, ceiling effects occurred with single doses of buprenorphine, and the slopes of the dose-response curves for suppression and precipitation of abstinence were relatively flat.

In man, single doses of buprenorphine also produced typical morphine-like effects (JASINSKI et al., 1978; MELLO and MENDELSON, 1980). Subjects identified buprenorphine as an opiate, and it produced dose-related increases in opiate symptom and sign scores. During the first 5 h after administration, this drug produced dose-related increases in "liking" scores and MBG scale scores, while scores on the PCAG and LSD scales were comparable to those obtained with morphine. From approximately 6 to 36 h after an acute dose of buprenorphine, however, PCAG scale scores were significantly elevated, but buprenorphine was still identified as an opiate by the subjects. During chronic administration, subjects identified buprenorphine as an opiate, and "liking" scores were comparable to those obtained with the chronic administration of morphine. Acute administration of morphine up to 120 mg/70 kg was without effect during chronic buprenorphine administration. Naloxone failed to precipitate abstinence at a dose (4 mg/70 kg) well above that required to precipitate abstinence in morphine-dependent subjects. Interestingly, upon abrupt discontinuation of chronically administered buprenorphine, abstinence signs and symptoms were not reported in some subjects until day 15 of withdrawal. During the time that each of the subjects reported abstinence symptoms, they requested opioids for relief.

IV. Pentazocine-Like Opioids

Pentazocine, nalbuphine, and butorphanol produce many effects in common with morphine although they are opioid antagonists in laboratory animals (e.g., BLUMBERG and DAYTON, 1974; PACHTER, 1974). These three compounds differ from profadol and propiram, however, in that they fail to suppress abstinence in human subjects dependent on 60 mg/70 kg per day of morphine as well as in the qualitative nature of the subjective effects they produce. The profile of subjective effects which these compounds produce distinguishes them from morphine-like agents as well as from cyclazocine- or nalorphine-like agents.

1. Effects of Acute Doses

Pentazocine in doses up to approximately 40 mg/70 kg produced typical morphine-like effects which were similar to those produced by 10 mg/70 kg morphine (JASINSKI et al., 1970). In this dose range, pentazocine was identified by subjects predominantly as opiate-like and produced dose-related increases in opiate symptom and sign scores as well as increases in "liking" scores. The 40-mg dose of pentazocine increased MBG scale scores comparable to those obtained with 10 mg morphine. No increases in

PCAG and LSD scale scores were observed up to 40 mg pentazocine. When the dose of pentazocine was increased to 60 mg/70 kg, the overall pattern of subjective effects changed. Although opiate symptom and sign scores remained elevated, the source of the points differed between 60 mg pentazocine and 10 or 20 mg morphine. Morphine primarily increased the frequency of reports of the symptoms "itchy skin," "relaxed," and "coasting" whereas reports of the symptoms "nervous," "drunken," and "other" were frequently reported with the high dose of pentazocine. While "liking" scores remained elevated with the 60-mg dose of pentazocine, MBG scale scores were not. Moreover, scores on the PCAG and LSD scale were elevated. This pattern of effects obtained with the larger dose of pentazocine resembles that obtained with nalorphine and cyclazocine (see Sect. V).

The subjective effects produced by nalbuphine are similar in most respects to those produced by pentazocine (JASINSKI and MANSKY, 1972). Low doses (up to 24 mg/70 kg) were identified by subjects as opiate-like and produced increases in opiate symptom and sign scores as well as "liking" scores. Only small increases were seen in MBG scale scores, however, along with slight increases in PCAG scale scores. LSD scale scores were not elevated by low doses of nalbuphine. Increasing the dose of nalbuphine to 72 mg/70 kg produced a qualitative change in the subjective effects similar to that observed with the 60 mg/70 kg dose of pentazocine. The symptoms and signs "sleepy," "drunken," and "other" were more frequently reported with the highest dose of nalbuphine than with morphine. In contrast to pentazocine, the item "nervous" was reported infrequently, although more often for nalbuphine than for morphine. The highest dose of nalbuphine did not further increase the MBG scale scores, but did produce a significant increase in PCAG scale scores and a small increase in LSD scale scores. JASINSKI and MANSKY (1972) concluded that, because of the small increases in MBG scale scores, significant increases in PCAG scale scores and slight increases in LSD scale scores, the subjective effects of nalbuphine more closely resemble those of pentazocine than those of morphine, but include less psychotomimetic effects than those of pentazocine.

Acute doses of butorphanol produced some effects in common with morphine, including significant dose-related "liking" scores and opiate symptom and sign scores (JASINSKI et al., 1975). As for pentazocine and nalbuphine, reports of the symptoms "nervousness" and "drunkenness" were more frequent for butorphanol than morphine. Subjects identified butorphanol as an opiate or as a barbiturate or alcohol with approximately equal frequency. Moreover, butorphanol did not increase MBG scale scores, but did produce significant increases in PCAG and LSD scale scores.

2. Chronic Administration

During chronic administration, subjects predominantly identified pentazocine, nalbuphine, and butorphanol as nonopiates whereas observers typically identified these drugs as opiate-like (JASINSKI et al., 1970; JASINSKI and MANSKY, 1972; JASINSKI et al., 1976). Subjects typically were unable or refused to identify pentazocine, identified nalbuphine as an opiate or nonopiate with approximately equal frequency (when identifications were given), and identified butorphanol predominantly as a barbiturate. Observers also frequently identified chronically administered butorphanol as a barbiturate. During chronic administration, particulary with higher doses, subjects reported irritability, nervousness, and inability to sleep, as well as strange and vivid dreams. Subjects also complained of racing and uncontrollable thoughts. Typically, subjects were indifferent toward these drugs as supported by the predominance of "don't care" reponses to the question, "Would you like to take the drug every day?", and a lack of increases in "liking" scores. Subjects tended to identify abstinence symptoms from these agents as opiate-like although clear differences existed between the characteristics of the morphine abstinence syndrome and the abstinence syndromes of pentazocine, nalbuphine, and butorphanol. However, subjects reported withdrawal from these drugs as uncomfortable and requested drugs for relief of symptoms.

V. Nalorphine- and Cyclazocine-Like Antagonists

1. Effects of Acute Doses

The profile of the subjective effects of the narcotic antagonists nalorphine and cyclazocine is readily distinguishable from that of morphine. Early studies utilizing the singe-dose opiate questionnaire (MARTIN et al., 1965) determined that lower doses of these two drugs are frequently identified as an opiate, although they may also be identified as a barbiturate. Higher doses of both nalorphine and cyclazocine were predominantly identified as a barbiturate. Both drugs significantly increased "liking" scores as well as opiate symptom and sign scores, but with the items "sleepy" and "drunkenness" contributing relatively more to the scores for nalorphine and cyclazocine than for morphine. In more recent studies using the ARCI questionnaire, cyclazocine and nalorphine produced no significant increases in responses on items generally taken as related to a sense of well-being, but significantly increased responses on items related to the sedative, drunkenness, and disorienting effects of barbiturates as well as to psychotomimetic phenomena (HAERTZEN, 1970). Subsequently, nalorphine and cyclazocine were evaluated using the MBG, PCAG, and LSD scales (JASINSKI et al., 1968a; JASINSKI et al., 1971a; JASINSKI et al., 1975). Both drugs failed to increase MBG scale scores, but significantly increasd PCAG and LSD scale scores.

2. Chronic Administration

During chronic administration of nalorphine or cyclazocine, observers predominantly identified the effects as opiate-like, whereas subjects less readily identified the effects of these drugs (MARTIN et al., 1965; MARTIN and GORODETZKY, 1965). When subjects reported identifications, nalorphine was identified most frequently as an opiate whereas cyclazocine was identified predominantly as a barbiturate. Subjects were indifferent to these drugs during chronic administration, as evidenced by the answer "don't care" to the question "Would you like to take the drug every day?". Tolerance as well as cross-tolerance developed to the subjective effects of both nalorphine and cyclazocine as evaluated by scores on the opiate symptoms and signs scales. Upon abrupt withdrawal of either antagonist, subjects reported abstinence symptoms, but made no requests for drugs for relief of these symptoms. While the qualitative natures of the abstinence syndromes for nalorphine and cyclazocine were similar, they could be differentiated from the morphine abstinence syndrome on the basis of signs and symptoms which contributed points to the abstinence scores.

VI. Naloxone and Naltrexone

Neither naloxone (JASINSKI et al., 1967) nor naltrexone (MARTIN et al., 1973 b) in doses up to 24 and 30 mg/70 kg, respectively, produced measurable changes in responses on the single-dose opiate questionnaire, or on the MBG, PCAG, and LSD scales. Few if any behavioral or physiologic changes were observed during chronic administration and withdrawal of naloxone or naltrexone in doses of 90 and 50 mg/70 kg per day, respectively. These findings led to the conclusion that naloxone and naltrexone are opioid antagonists with little agonist activity.

VII. Discussion

1. Quantitative Evaluation of Subjective Effects

Drug-induced changes in reports of subjective effects are central elements in predicting the therapeutic usefulness as well as the abuse liability of pharmacologic agents. Quantitative methods using questionnaires for assessing reports of subjective effects have been developed and validated both statistically and pharmacologically. The pattern of dose-related changes in scores on these questionnaires distinguishes among classes of psychoactive drugs, including opioid agonists and antagonists. Table 1 summarizes these patterns for representative opioid agonists, partial agonists, and antagonists. Results have been reproducible across studies, even when conducted several years apart, and across different routes of drug administration. In addition, there has been good concordance among potency estimates for subjective effects, changes in pupil diameter, suppression of abstinence, and analgesia (JASINSKI, 1977). These operational methods for assessing subjective effects have been of major importance in assessing opioids and synthetic analgesics.

2. Evaluation of Morphine-Like Abuse Liability

The underlying principle in evaluating the abuse liability of opioid agonists and antagonists has been that drugs which are pharmacologically equivalent will have a similar liability for abuse. The actual frequency of abuse of a drug depends on many factors, including legal controls, the overall availability of the drug, and its physicochemical properties (e.g., water solubility), as well as the prevailing attitudes and customs of society. Other factors of importance include side effects or toxicity, which may be unique to a particular congener. In subjects with a high degree of physical dependence on an opiate, partial agonists and antagonists can precipitate an abstinence syndrome which renders these drugs unacceptable to them. The relative degree of opioid, and other drug, abuse also may be a function of the subject or patient population. As discussed earlier, persons without a history of opioid abuse often report that the subjective effects of morphine are unpleasant.

Drugs which (1) produce morphine-like effects on the single-dose opiate questionnaire, (2) elevate scores on the MBG but not PCAG or LSD scales, (3) suppress morphine abstinence, and (4) produce a morphine-like physical dependence have generally been assessed as having a high abuse liability similar to that of morphine. Methadone and heroin are examples of such drugs. On the other hand, the morphine-like

Table 1. Comparison of representative opioid agonists, partial agonists, and antagonists[a]

	Subjective effects				Substitution in morphine-dependent subjects		Direct addiction			
	MBG	PCAG	LSD	ID[b]	60 mg/day	240 mg/day	Abstinence syndrome	Drug-seeking	Nalorphine P	Naloxone P
Narcotic agonists										
Morphine [1]	+	0	0	M	S	S	+(M)	+	+	+
Methadone [2]	+	0	0	M		S	+(M)	+		+
Codeine [3]	+	0	0	M		S	+(M)	+	+	
Meperidine [4]	+	+	0	M		S (Partial)	+(M)		+	
Propoxyphene [5]	+	0	0	M	S	S (Partial)	+(M)	+	+	
Partial agonists										
Profadol [6]	+	0	0	M	S	P	+(M)	+	+	
Buprenorphine [7]	+	(+)	0	MB			+	(+)		(0)
Pentazocine-like agents										
Pentazocine [8]	+	+	+	MB	0	P	+(M, N)	+	0	+
Nalbuphine [9]	+	+	+	MB	P	P? (Probable)	+(M, N)	+	0	+
Butorphanol [10]	0	+	+	MB	0		+(N)	+	+	+
Narcotic antagonists										
Nalorphine [11]	0	+	+	MB	P	P	+(N)	0	S	?
Cyclazocine [12]	0	+	+	MB	P? (Probable)	P	+(N)	0	S	?
Naloxone [13]	0	0	0	0	P	P	0	0		

[a] Modified and expanded from Jasinski, 1973
[b] Drug identification by subjects
+, Significantly increased or occurrence; 0, not significantly increased or nonoccurrence; M, morphine-like; B, barbiturate-like; N, nalorphine-like; S, suppression; P, precipitation
[1] JASINSKI, 1977. [2] MARTIN et al., 1973a. [3] JASINSKI et al., 1971a; HIMMELSBACH et al., 1940; KAY et al., 1967; FRASER et al., 1961. [4] HIMMELSBACH, 1942; JASINSKI and NUTT, 1973. [5] FRASER and ISBELL, 1960; JASINSKI et al., 1971; JASINSKI et al., 1975. [6] JASINSKI et al., 1971a. [7] JASINSKI et al., 1978. [8] JASINSKI et al., 1970. [9] JASINSKI and MANSKY, 1972. [10] JASINSKI et al., 1975; JASINSKI et al., 1976. [11] MARTIN et al., 1965; HAERTZEN, 1970. [12] MARTIN and GORODETZKY, 1965. [13] JASINSKI et al., 1967

properties of codeine and D-propoxyphene are well recognized, but both drugs would be expected to have an abuse liability lower than that of morphine on the basis of lesser solubility, tissue-irritant properties, availability predominantly as oral preparations in low dosage units, and side effects which limit the ability to attain strong morphine-like effects (see JASINSKI, 1977, for discussion). Epidemiologic measures have supported the conclusion that codeine and D-propoxyphene have lower abuse liabilities compared with morphine (JASINSKI, 1977).

3. Psychotomimetic Effects

The psychotomimetic effects of nalorphine and cyclazocine as well as pentazocine-like agents have been widely recognized. The capacity of these agents to produce psychotomimetic effects differs, however, particularly when compared at doses which are approximately equimiotic. Equimiotic doses often are used for comparisons because changes in pupil diameter have been measured concurrently with subjective effects and because equimiotic doses are approximately equianalgesic and thus are predictive of therapeutic doses. At approximately equimiotic doses, cyclazocine (1.0 mg/70 kg) clearly has the most psychotomimetic effects and produces large increases in LSD scale scores, whereas nalorphine (10 mg/70 kg) produces only slight, but significant, increases in LSD scale scores, as does butorphanol (2 mg/70 kg). Pentazocine (40 mg/70 kg) does not increase LSD scale scores within this dose range; rather, psychotomimetic effects occur only at doses which are above the usual therapeutic range (BROGDEN et al., 1973). Nalbuphine does not produce dose-related changes in pupil diameter, but clearly produces the smallest increases in LSD scale scores; psychotomimetic effects have been encountered only rarely in therapeutic use (MILLER, 1980). Thus, these drugs differ both with respect to their effectiveness in producing psychotomimetic effects and in the dose range over which such effects occur.

MARTIN et al. (1976) have suggested that there are three types of specific receptors in nervous tissue which mediate the agonistic effects of opioids and opioid antagonists. These receptors have been termed "mu," "kappa," and "sigma" on the basis of distinct patterns of physiologic effects. The mode of action of pentazocine- and nalorphine-like compounds in producing psychotomimetic effects has been attributed to actions at the putative sigma receptor (MARTIN et al., 1976). That these are agonistic and not antagonistic actions is supported by the findings that tolerance develops to these effects upon chronic administration and there is cross-tolerance between nalorphine and cyclazocine (MARTIN et al., 1965; JASINSKI et al., 1970). Evidence is not currently available on cross-tolerance between pentazocine and nalorphine or cyclazocine with respect to their psychotomimetic components of action. The question of whether naloxone is an antagonist at the sigma receptor is controversial. In a study of the interactions between cyclazocine and naloxone (JASINSKI et al., 1968a), cyclazocine alone produced significant elevations in mean scores on the PCAG and MBG scales but not on the LSD scale. Naloxone antagonized the effects of cyclazocine on the MBG and PCAG scales. Although the mean scores on the LSD scale were not elevated, JASINSKI et al. (1968a) reported that naloxone antagonized the effects of cyclazocine for those subjects in which cyclazocine produced an elevated LSD scale score and also that naloxone was effective in terminating psychotomimetic episodes which occurred outside the structured experimental setting.

4. Barbiturate-Like Effects

The barbiturate-like effects of opioid derivatives have been less widely recognized, perhaps because effects such as tiredness and drunkenness are not totally unexpected effects of drugs which depress central nervous system function. Yet, morphine, particularly at higher doses, rarely is identified as a barbiturate or produces significant PCAG scores. Moreover, subjects were able to distinguish between morphine and pentobarbital in a double-blind crossover study (MARTIN et al., 1974). As with psychotomimetic effects, opioid derivatives differ in their effectiveness in producing barbiturate-like effects, as well as the dose ranges over which such effects occur. At equimiotic doses, cyclazocine and nalorphine are approximately equieffective in elevating PCAG scale scores. Pentazocine and butorphanol produce relatively small increases in PCAG scores in the therapeutic dose range, although significant PCAG scores are obtained at higher doses. Nalbuphine increases PCAG scores only at doses well above the therapeutic range. Buprenorphine also increases PCAG scores, but these effects are not greater than those observed with morphine in the same subjects. During chronic administration, cyclazocine and butorphanol are most frequently identified as barbiturates, whereas subjects typically have difficulty in identifying chronically administered nalorphine, pentazocine, and nalbuphine.

The mode of action of opioid derivatives in producing sedative or barbiturate-like effects has been attributed to actions at the kappa receptor (MARTIN et al., 1976). The prototypic kappa receptor agonist ketocyclazocine has not been evaluated in humans. Morphine has been postulated to be an agonist at both the mu and kappa receptors, whereas cyclazocine has been postulated to be an agonist at both the kappa and sigma receptors (MARTIN et al., 1976). Naloxone has been postulated to be an antagonist at both the mu and kappa receptors, since naloxone clearly antagonizes the effects of morphine (JASINSKI et al., 1967) as well as the increase in PCAG scale scores produced by cyclazocine (JASINSKI et al., 1968a).

5. Summary

Acute doses of morphine and related opioids produce subjective effects which are readily discriminated by nondependent addict subjects. Operationally, morphine-like subjective effects are measured by the single-dose opiate questionnaire and the subjective drug-effects questionnaire containing items from the MBG, PCAG, and LSD scales of the Addiction Research Center Inventory. Morphine-like drugs increase "liking" scores as well as opiate signs and symptoms scores on the single-dose opiate questionnaires, increase scores on the MBG scale, but not on the PCAG and LSD scales, and suppress abstinence in morphine-dependent subjects. Acute doses of pentazocine-like drugs increase "liking" scores and usually increase MBG scores. In contrast to morphine, pentazocine-like drugs increase PCAG and LSD scale scores and fail to suppress abstinence in morphine-dependent subjects. During withdrawal from morphine- or pentazocine-like drugs, subjects request drugs for relief. Nalorphine-like drugs may increase "liking" scores but do not increase MBG scores. These latter drugs do increase PCAG and LSD scale scores and precipitate abstinence in morphine-dependent subjects. In marked contrast to the observations with morphine- and pentazocine-like drugs, subjects do not request drugs for relief during withdrawal from nalorphine or cyclazocine, although subjects report abstinence symptoms.

C. Experimental Analysis of Behavioral Effects in Laboratory Animals

Opioids and opioid antagonists exhibit a wide spectrum of behavioral actions in laboratory animals, ranging from marked changes in locomotor activity to subtle alterations in the frequency of occurrence and temporal patterns of learned behavior. Because the effects of opioids and opioid antagonists can change dramatically with repeated administration, there has been a continuing need for objective and quantitative techniques that provide reproducible patterns of behavior, which can be studied over long periods of time and are sensitive to the effects of pharmacologic interventions. Methods developed by B. F. Skinner and used successfully in the experimental analysis of operant behavior meet such criteria. Over the last 30 years, these methods have been used increasingly in studies of the behavioral pharmacology of psychoactive drugs, including opioids and opioid antagonists.

Operant behavior can be defined simply as behavior controlled by its consequences (SKINNER, 1937, 1938). When an environmental event occurs as a consequence of a specified response by an experimental subject, the frequency of occurrence of that response may increase, and this increased frequency may be maintained on subsequent occasions. For example, delivery of food to a food-deprived rat immediately after it presses a lever may result in an increased frequency of lever pressing. In this case, the lever-pressing response is defined as an operant, the increased frequency of the response is defined as the process of operant conditioning or reinforcement, and the delivery of food is defined as a reinforcer. Events as diverse as the presentation of food or water, the electrical stimulation of the brain, the termination of a stimulus associated with electric shock, the delivery of electric shock, or the intravenous injection of various drugs can function as reinforcers to maintain operant behavior.

I. Opioids and Opioid Antagonists as Discriminative Stimuli

As discussed in an earlier section, human volunteers sophisticated in the use of opioids and other drugs are able to reliably discriminate the subjective effects produced by morphine-like drugs from the subjective effects produced by pentazocine and nalorphine as well as nonopioid psychoactive drugs when single doses are administered to them on a double-blind basis. Laboratory animals can be trained to discriminate between a drug and its vehicle by requiring them to emit one operant response following the administration of that drug and another operant response following the administration of drug vehicle, presumably on the basis of drug-induced interoceptive stimuli. Stimuli which set the occasion for differential responding are termed "discriminative stimuli" (e.g., TERRACE, 1966). Reinforcement of responses in the presence of one stimulus increases the tendency to respond not only in the presence of that stimulus but also in the presence of similar stimuli. When this occurs, the behavior is said to generalize among stimuli. Stimulus generalization is defined functionally: behavior is said to generalize to all those stimuli in whose presence the probability of responding increases after the response has been reinforced in the presence of another stimulus. Thus, the probability of occurrence of a response may covary with different values of a stimulus presented along a continuum. The function thus generated, which relates responding to stimulus value, is termed a "stimulus generalization gradient." The discriminative stimulus properties of opioids and opioid antagonists have been studied extensively in several species of animals.

1. Opioid Agonists

The discriminative stimulus effects of opioid agonists have been extensively investigated in animals trained to discriminate between vehicle and either morphine or fentanyl. The stimulus control of behavior by morphine and fentanyl meets four generally accepted criteria for a specific opioid effect (RETHY et al., 1971; DOMINO and WILSON, 1973). Firstly, morphine- or fentanyl-like stimulus control is dose related and produced by other opioid analgesics from diverse chemical families in several species, including rats (HIRSCHHORN and ROSECRANS, 1974; 1976; GIANUTSOS and LAL, 1975; COLPAERT et al., 1975a, b; WINTER, 1975; SHANNON and HOLTZMAN, 1976a; 1977), gerbils (JARBE and ROLLENHAGEN, 1978), pigeons (JARBE, 1978; HERLING et al., 1980), squirrel monkeys (SCHAEFER and HOLTZMAN, 1977), and rhesus monkeys (WOODS et al., 1980). The relative potencies of these opioids for producing morphine- or fentanyl-like discriminative stimuli agree well with their relative potencies for producing analgesia (LAL et al., 1977; COLPAERT, 1978).

Secondly, stimulus control by morphine or fentanyl exhibits stereospecificity in that levorphanol but not its nonopioid enantiomer dextrorphan produces morphine-like stimulus control (WINTER, 1975; SHANNON and HOLTZMAN, 1976a; SCHAEFER and HOLTZMAN, 1977; HERLING et al., 1980), and dextromoramide but not its nonopioid enantiomer laevormoramide produces fentanyl-like stimulus control (COLPAERT, 1978). Structural analogs and metabolites of opioid analgesics that lack opioid activity in other procedures, i.e., thebaine, normetazocine, and morphine-3-glucuronide, also fail to produce morphine-like stimulus control (SHANNON and HOLTZMAN, 1976a; 1977).

Thirdly, the discriminative stimulus effects of morphine and fentanyl are blocked by the specific narcotic antagonists naloxone and naltrexone administered parenterally or orally (ROSECRANS et al., 1973; HIRSCHHORN and ROSECRANS, 1974; WINTER, 1975; SHANNON and HOLTZMAN, 1976a, b; COLPAERT et al., 1976; GIANUTSOS and LAL, 1976; SCHAEFER and HOLTZMANN, 1977; JARBE and ROLLENHAGEN, 1978; JARBE, 1978; OVERTON and BATTA, 1979; TEAL and HOLTZMAN, 1980a). The development of tolerance to the discriminative stimulus effects of opioids upon repeated administration of an opioid, the fourth criterion, has not as yet been studied in sufficient detail to warrant general conclusions. Tolerance has been reported not to develop in rats to the discriminative stimulus effects of morphine (HIRSCHHORN and ROSECRANS, 1974) or fentanyl (COLPAERT et al., 1976; 1978) when discrimination training was continued during chronic opioid administration. In contrast, shifts to the right in the dose-response curves for both morphine and methadone were observed following chronic morphine administration when rats were maintained in their home cages and discrimination training was discontinued during chronic administration (SHANNON and HOLTZMAN, 1976a).

The specificity of the stimulus control by morphine and fentanyl has been well documented. Nonopioid psychoactive drugs which do not produce morphine- or fentanyl-like stimulus control include pentobarbital, amphetamine, mescaline, LSD, chlorpromazine, haloperidol, clonidine, scopolamine, and physostigmine (HIRSCHHORN and ROSECRANS, 1974; COLPAERT et al., 1975a, b; GIANUTSOS and LAL, 1975; SHANNON and HOLTZMAN, 1976a; 1977; SCHAEFER and HOLTZMAN, 1977; HERLING et al., 1980). Similarly, the centrally active antagonists atropine, cyproheptadine, and methysergide neither produce morphine-like stimulus control nor antagonize the discriminative stimulus effects of morphine (HIRSCHHORN and ROSECRANS, 1974).

2. Pentazocine

In humans, the subjective effects produced by pentazocine are complex in that lower doses are predominantly morphine-like whereas higher doses are predominantly cyclazocine-like (see Sect. B.IV). The discriminative stimulus effects of pentazocine in laboratory animals are also complex as evidenced by the sometimes seemingly inconsistent results in various studies. In rats trained to discriminate between vehicle and pentazocine, morphine has been reported both to produce (KUHN et al., 1976) and not to produce (HIRSCHHORN, 1977; OVERTON and BATTA, 1979) pentazocine-like stimulus control; nalorphine and cyclazocine also failed to produce pentazocine-like stimulus control (HIRSCHHORN, 1977; OVERTON and BATTA, 1979). Similarly, in rats, pigeons, and squirrel and rhesus monkeys trained to discriminate between morphine and saline, pentazocine has been reported both to produce (SHANNON and HOLTZMAN, 1976a; 1979; COLPAERT et al., 1976) and not to produce (HIRSCHHORN and ROSECRANS, 1976; HOLTZMAN et al., 1977; OVERTON and BATTA, 1979; HERLING et al., 1980; WOODS et al., 1980) morphine-like stimulus control. Further, in rats trained to dicriminate between saline and a relatively low training dose of cyclazocine (TEAL and HOLTZMAN, 1980b), pentazocine produced cyclazocine-like stimulus control; however, pentazocine failed to produce cyclazocine-like stimulus control in rats and squirrel monkeys trained to discriminate between saline and a relatively higher training dose of cyclazocine (HIRSCHHORN, 1977; SCHAEFER and HOLTZMAN, 1978; TEAL and HOLTZMAN, 1980b). Regardless of whether or not pentazocine produced morphine- or cyclazocine-like stimulus control in these studies, the average percentage of morphine- or cyclazocine-appropriate responses emitted following the administration of pentazocine generally was quite high and usually increased in a dose-related fashion. These findings suggest that, concordant with the results in man, the discriminative stimulus effects of pentazocine have commonalities with both morphine and cyclazocine.

3. Cyclazocine-Like Antagonists

The pharmacologic characteristics of the discriminative stimulus effects of cyclazocine differ from those of morphine in a manner consistent with the difference in the profiles of subjective effects of these two drugs in humans. In monkeys trained to discriminate between cyclazocine and saline, the opioid antagonists with agonist activity levallorphan, oxilorphan, and ketocyclazocine produced cyclazocine-like stimulus control whereas nalorphine, pentazocine, and morphine produced only intermediate percentages of cyclazocine-appropriate responding (SCHAEFER and HOLTZMAN, 1978). In rats, the pharmacologic characteristics of the discriminative stimulus effects of cyclazocine vary with the magnitude of the training dose of cyclazocine (HIRSCHHORN and ROSECRANS, 1977; ROSECRANS et al., 1978; OVERTON and BATTA, 1979; TEAL and HOLTZMAN, 1980b) in a manner consistent with the observations that in man low doses of cyclazocine produce somewhat different subjective effects than higher doses. In the study by TEAL and HOLTZMAN (1980b), which compared a low and a high training dose of cyclazocine directly, the opioid antagonists ketocyclazocine and SKF 10,047 as well as the nonopioids phencyclidine and ketamine produced cyclazocine-like stimulus control at both training doses. The antagonists ethylketocyclazocine, pentazocine, and levallorphan produced cyclazocine-like stimulus control at the lower but not the higher training dose of cyclazocine. In addition, morphine and nalorphine produced intermediate percentages of responding in rats trained with the lower dose of cyclazocine but only saline-appropriate responding in rats trained with the higher dose of cyclazocine. Nonopioid psychoactive drugs such as mescaline, LSD, and amphetamine did not produce cyclazocine-like stimulus control at either training dose of cyclazocine.

In squirrel monkeys, naloxone effectively antagonized the discriminative stimulus effects of cyclazocine (SCHAEFER and HOLTZMAN, 1978), but the dose of naloxone was approximately 30-fold higher than the dose required to antagonize the effects of morphine (SCHAEFER and HOLTZMAN, 1977). In the rat, naltrexone did not completely antagonize the effects of cyclazocine (TEAL and HOLTZMAN, 1980b).

On the basis of these findings in cyclazocine-trained animals, as well as other considerations, TEAL and HOLTZMAN (1980b) postulated that cyclazocine has both an opioid and a nonopioid component of action. The opioid component is antagonized by naloxone or naltrexone and is thus apparently mediated through opioid receptors. The nonopioid component is not blocked by naloxone or naltrexone and is mimicked by phencyclidine but not LSD or mescaline. In this regard, dexoxadrol, a piperidinol dissociative anesthetic similar to phencyclidine, has been demonstrated to produce subjective effects similar to those of nalorphine in humans (JASINSKI et al., 1968b).

II. Effects of Opioids and Opioid Antagonists on Schedule-Controlled Behavior

Since the classification of opioids and opioid antagonists into subgroups on the basis of their effects as discriminative stimuli in laboratory animals has been generally consistent with classifications obtained using subjective rating scales in humans, these techniques provide a meaningful way to analyze their effects on behavior. Another meaningful way to analyze the behavioral actions of opioids and opioid antagonists in laboratory animals is to study their effects on operant behavior maintained under various schedules of reinforcement. Schedules of reinforcement can be defined as those rules that govern the temporal and sequential relations between responses and reinforcers (FERSTER and SKINNER, 1957). Schedules often are classified on the basis of whether the reinforcer follows a specified number of responses (ratio schedules) or follows a response only after a specified interval of time has elapsed (interval schedules). The response requirement or interval time may remain constant (fixed-ratio or fixed-interval schedules) or may vary around a predetermined mean value (variable-ratio or variable-interval schedules). Although there are many possible schedules of reinforcement, these four types have been studied most extensively. Each type of schedule engenders its own characteristic rate and temporal pattern of responding that can be reproduced across different species, different response topographies, and different events as reinforcers (see reviews by FERSTER and SKINNER, 1957; MORSE, 1966; MORSE and KELLEHER, 1970, 1977; NEVIN, 1973; ZEILER, 1977). These characteristic schedule-controlled performances can be maintained throughout nearly the entire lifetime of an experimental subject and yet are extremely sensitive to treatment with psychotropic drugs.

1. Effects of Morphine on Schedule-Controlled Behavior

a) Behavior Maintained by Schedule Presentation of Food

Over a wide range of conditions, acute administration of morphine decreases schedule-controlled behavior maintained by food presentation. In early studies by HILL et al. (1957) and WEISSMAN (1959), for example, morphine produced dose-related decrements in the rate of responding by rats when each response produced a pellet of food. In subsequent studies, morphine also decreased responding when food was presented more intermittently under fixed- or variable-ratio schedules in rats (TSOU, 1963; THOMPSON et al., 1970), pigeons (MCMILLAN and MORSE, 1967; MCMILLAN et al., 1970; DYKSTRA et al., 1974; DOWNS and WOODS, 1976; GOLDBERG et al., 1976b), rhesus monkeys (HOLTZMAN and VILLARREAL, 1973; DOWNS and WOODS, 1976), squirrel monkeys (GOLDBERG et al., 1976b), and baboons (BYRD, 1975). Although minor exceptions to the usual rate-decreasing effects of morphine under ratio schedules occasionally have been observed (for example, 1 mg/kg often slightly increased responding in the THOMPSON et al. study), an important exception was reported by BYRD (1975). In his study, a tenfold range of doses (0.1–1 mg/kg) increased fixed-ratio responding by chimpanzees to as much as 160% of the control rate, but only decreased fixed-ratio responding by baboons.

Under fixed-interval schedules, morphine can either increase or decrease rates of responding maintained by food presentation. In rhesus monkeys (DOWNS and WOODS, 1976), squirrel monkeys (MCKEARNEY, 1974; GOLDBERG et al., 1976b), baboons (BYRD, 1975), and in several studies with pigeons (MCMILLAN et al., 1970; DYKSTRA et al., 1974; DOWNS and WOODS, 1976; GOLDBERG et al., 1976b), for example, morphine decreased fixed-interval responding in a dose-related manner. In rats (TSOU, 1963; THOMPSON et al., 1970), cats (DJAHANGUIRI et al., 1966), and in one study with pigeons (MCMILLAN and MORSE, 1967), on the other hand, low and intermediate doses of morphine increased responding, whereas higher doses decreased responding. The increases in responding produced by morphine in these studies were generally small compared to the large increases produced by psychomotor stimulants such as amphetamine or cocaine under similar schedules (GOLDBERG et al., 1976b; GONZALEZ and GOLDBERG, 1977; SPEALMAN et al., 1979a). However, much more striking increases in responding have been reported in chimpanzees (BYRD, 1975). In this species, a wide range of doses (0.3–5.6 mg/kg) increased fixed-interval responding to as much as 534% of the control rate; these same doses only decreased fixed-interval responding by baboons. Under variable-interval schedules of food presentation, morphine has been found to only decrease responding in both rats (HILL et al., 1957; TSOU, 1963; THOMPSON et al., 1970) and rhesus monkeys (HOLTZMAN and VILLARREAL, 1973).

In summary, the predominant effect of morphine on schedule-controlled behavior maintained by food presentation is to produce dose-related decrements in rates of responding. Although it has been tempting to attribute these decrements to morphine's anorectic actions (cf. WEISSMAN, 1959), this interpretation is not readily compatible with the increased rates of responding produced by morphine under suitable schedule conditions and in some species.

b) Behavior Maintained by Scheduled Delivery of Electric Shock

Because a prominent action of morphine is the relief of clinical pain, there has been a continuing interest in examining its effects on behavior controlled by noxious stimuli such as electric shock. Several early studies used a signaled avoidance-escape schedule. Under this schedule, an exteroceptive stimulus (e.g., a tone or light) is presented for a specified period of time, during which a response (e.g., climbing a pole or pressing a lever) prevents delivery of an impending electric shock (avoidance); if an avoidance response is not made, electric shock then is delivered continuously until a response terminates the shock (escape). Although high doses of morphine have been found to decrease both avoidance and escape responding by rats under these schedules, morphine characteristically decreases avoidance responding at doses lower than those required to decrease escape responding (VERHAVE et al., 1959; CHITTAL and SHETH, 1963; COOK and CATANIA, 1964). Interestingly, morphine shares this action with many drugs used clinically as antipsychotic agents (COOK and CATANIA, 1964; COOK and DAVIDSON, 1978), though morphine has no recognized antipsychotic efficacy.

Other studies involving electric shock delivery have used a continuous avoidance schedule. Under this schedule, brief electric shocks are delivered at regular intervals in the absence of responding, and each response postpones delivery of electric shock for a specified period of time; no exteroceptive preshock stimulus is presented (SIDMAN, 1953). Morphine often has been found to decrease continuous avoidance responding by rats in a dose-related manner (WEISSMAN, 1959; HEISE and BOFF, 1962; TSOU, 1963; HOLTZMAN and JEWETT, 1972), and these decreases typically occur at doses that decrease signaled avoidance responding. Under some conditions, however, morphine can increase responding under continuous avoidance schedules. In rats, for example, HOLTZMAN and JEWETT (1971, 1972) found that 1–4 mg/kg morphine produced dose-related increases in responding when a high shock intensity was used, but only decreased responding when a lower shock intensity was used.

The effects of morphine on responding in squirrel monkeys have been investigated under several different schedules of electric shock delivery. Under a continuous avoidance schedule, HOLTZMAN (1976) found that low and intermediate doses of morphine (0.3–1 mg/kg) increased responding, whereas higher doses decreased responding. MCKEARNEY (1975) found that 0.3 mg/kg morphine increased responding by squirrel monkeys under a fixed-interval schedule in which responding terminated a visual stimulus associated with periodic electric shocks (stimulus-shock termination; MORSE and KELLEHER, 1966). MCKEARNEY (1974) also reported that this same dose of morphine increased responding by squirrel monkeys under a fixed-interval schedule when responding was maintained by the presentation, rather than termination, of electric shock. These findings are important because they show that, in the same species, suitable doses of morphine can alter schedule-controlled behavior in similar ways regardless of whether responding results in a decreased frequency of shock delivery (as under the continuous avoidance and stimulus-shock termination schedules) or does not change the frequency of shock delivery (as under the shock presentation schedule). Such findings indicate that the effects of morphine on behavior controlled by postponement, termination, or presentation of electric shock are determined largely by factors other than analgesia.

c) Behavior Suppressed by Scheduled Delivery of Electric Shock

Two types of procedures have been used to study the effects of morphine on behavior suppressed by electric shock delivery. In the first type (conditioned suppression; ESTES and SKINNER, 1941), responding typically is maintained under a schedule of food presentation. An exteroceptive stimulus (e.g., a tone or light) which regularly precedes an unavoidable electric shock then is superimposed periodically on this baseline. The result is a characteristic decline in response rate during the preshock stimulus, even though responding has no specified effect on shock delivery. Early studies with rats indicated that morphine (e.g., 1–11 mg/kg) could increase responding that had been suppressed during the preshock stimulus (HILL et al., 1954, 1957; YAMAHIRO et al., 1961). Later studies with both rats (LAUENER, 1963) and rhesus monkeys (HOLTZMAN and VILLARREAL, 1969), however, found that morphine did not increase suppressed responding at any dose tested. The factors responsible for these different effects of morphine are presently unclear, but may involve differences in the adventitious temporal relations that can exist between responding and shock delivery under conditioned suppression procedures (KELLEHER and MORSE, 1968).

In contrast to conditioned suppression procedures, punishment procedures explicitly specify the extant temporal relations between responding and shock delivery (AZRIN, 1956, 1960; AZRIN and HOLZ, 1966). In these procedures, responding typically is maintained under a schedule of food presentation. Delivery of electric shock then is scheduled as an additional consequence of responding; no preshock stimulus is presented. The result is an overall suppression of responding. In several species and under various schedule conditions, drugs used clinically as antianxiety agents, such as barbiturates, benzodiazepines, and meprobamate, characteristically produce marked increases in punished responding (MCMILLAN, 1975; MORSE et al., 1977; HOUSER, 1978). In contrast, morphine generally does not increase punished responding at any dose tested in rats (GELLER et al., 1963), pigeons (KELLEHER and MORSE, 1964; MCMILLAN, 1973b, but see MCMILLAN, 1973a), or rhesus monkeys (HOLTZMAN and VILLARREAL, 1973) and often further decreases punished responding.

The failure of morphine to consistently increase suppressed responding under either the conditioned suppression or punishment procedures is not incompatible with its known analgesic actions. Morphine often decreases schedule-controlled responding maintained by food presentation (Sect. C.II.1.a), and these decreases can occur at doses lower than those required to produce analgesia. Moreover, several studies (e.g., AZRIN, 1960; KELLEHER and MORSE, 1964; COOK and DAVIDSON, 1973) have shown that removal of electric shock typically does not result in an immediate increase in previously suppressed responding. Thus, even if morphine completely eliminated responsiveness to electric shock, it would not, through this action, be expected to abruptly increase suppressed responding.

d) Behavior Maintained by Titration of Electric Shock Intensity

The role of the analgesic actions of morphine in altering schedule-controlled behavior has been studied explicitly under schedules in which experimental subjects regulate the intensity of a continuously presented electric shock (titration schedules). Under one type of titration schedule (escape titration), responding reduces the intensity of an electric shock which otherwise increases at a specified rate (WEISS and LATIES, 1959, 1961). Several studies with rhesus and squirrel monkeys have shown that morphine and related drugs can increase the intensity at which electric shock is maintained (WEISS and LATIES, 1964; MALIS, 1973; MALIS and GLUCKMAN, 1974; MALIS et al., 1975; DYKSTRA and MCMILLAN, 1977; SMITH and MCKEARNEY, 1977). In these studies, doses of morphine that markedly increased shock intensity also decreased rates of responding. Thus, increases in the intensity of electric shock may have been the result of morphine's direct rate-decreasing effects on escape responding (Sect. C.II.1.b) rather than its effects on responsiveness to painful stimulation. Recently, DYKSTRA (1979) used a modified escape titration schedule which minimizes the role of altered response rates in determining shock intensity. Under this schedule, the intensity of electric shock increases at a specified rate, and a response terminates the shock for a fixed period of time; at the end of this period, shock resumes at a lower intensity (cf. MARKOWITZ et al., 1976). DYKSTRA found that suitable doses of morphine as well as pentazocine and cyclazocine increased the intensity at which shock was maintained, but had little or no effect on the rate of responding in the presence of shock. These findings suggest that morphine-induced changes in the maintained intensity of electric shock are not exclusively due to changes in the rate of responding.

Another type of titration schedule (punishment titration) has been used to study the effects of morphine on behavior controlled by electric shock. In this case, responding is maintained under a schedule of food presentation; additionally, responding *increases* the intensity of an electric shock which otherwise *decreases* at a specified rate (RACHLIN and LOVELAND, 1971; RACHLIN, 1972). SMITH and MCKEARNEY (1977) found that morphine, as well as methadone, nalorphine, and naloxone, only decreased the rate of responding by squirrel monkeys under this schedule and, hence, only decreased the intensity at which shock was maintained. While these findings might be interpreted as showing a "hyperalgesic" action of morphine, it is much more likely that they reflect the direct rate-decreasing effects of morphine on punished behavior (Sect. C.II.1.c).

The results of studies using both punishment and escape titration schedules clearly indicate that morphine can have pronounced effects on the regulation of electric shock that do not depend simply on its actions as an analgesic. Although altered responsiveness to noxious stimulation may contribute to the behavioral effects of morphine under some titration schedules (e.g., DYKSTRA, 1979), it may not under others (e.g., SMITH and MCKEARNEY, 1977). In general, titration schedules do not appear to routinely screen for the analgesic effects of morphine.

2. Tolerance to the Behavioral Effects of Morphine

Tolerance to the effects of morphine can develop rapidly in standardized tests of analgesia in laboratory animals. KAYAN et al. (1973), for example, found that acute administration of 5 or 10 mg/kg morphine increased reaction time of rats placed on a heated surface, but that complete tolerance to this effect developed after only two to six treatments. A similarly rapid development of tolerance has been reported for the effects of morphine on schedule-controlled behavior maintained by food presentation. In rats (BABBINI et al., 1972, 1976), cats (DJAHANGUIRI et al., 1966), and pigeons (MCMILLAN and MORSE, 1967; HEIFETZ and MCMILLAN, 1971; SMITH, 1979), tolerance to the rate-decreasing effects of morphine under fixed-ratio and fixed-interval schedules can occur within 4 to 10 days when morphine is administered once or twice daily. Moreover, after several months of chronic administration, the morphine dose-effect curves can be shifted six to tenfold to the right in pigeons and rhesus monkeys responding under these schedules (WOODS and CARNEY, 1978).

Differences in rate of development and magnitude of tolerance have been reported with different species and different schedules of reinforcement. In rats, for example, tolerance appears to develop more slowly under fixed-ratio schedules (BABBINI et al., 1972) or under schedules that differentially reinforce low rates of responding (ADAM-CARRIERÉ et al., 1978) than under fixed-interval schedules (BABBINI et al., 1976). Even under fixed-interval schedules, clear development of tolerance is not always observed in rats (RHODUS et al., 1974). In rhesus monkeys, marked tolerance to the rate-decreasing effects of morphine has been reported under variable-interval schedules of food presentation, but it requires from 1 to 8 weeks to develop (HOLTZMAN and VILLARREAL, 1973).

Following long-term exposure to morphine, abruptly discontinuing morphine treatment or administering a morphine antagonist such as naloxone or nalorphine can produce marked disruptions in schedule-controlled behavior that parallel other signs of the morphine abstinence syndrome. In rats, responding maintained by food presentation may be either decreased (BABBINI et al., 1972; GELLERT and SPARBER, 1977) or increased (BABBINI et al., 1976; FORD and BALSTER, 1976), depending on the schedule of reinforcement and the duration of morphine abstinence. In rhesus monkeys, either discontinuing morphine treatment or administering naloxone or nalorphine markedly decreases rates of schedule-controlled responding maintained by food presentation or avoidance of electric shock (THOMPSON and SCHUSTER, 1964; GOLDBERG and SCHUSTER, 1967, 1970; HOLTZMAN and VILLARREAL, 1973). In contrast to the effects observed in rats and monkeys, discontinuing morphine treatment produces little or no disruption of schedule-controlled behavior in pigeons (HEIFETZ and MCMILLAN, 1971; Woods and CARNEY, 1978).

3. Self-Administration of Morphine

Early studies of morphine self-administration by laboratory animals used subjects that were made physically dependent by repeated injections of the drug prior to testing (SPRAGG, 1940; HEADLEE et al., 1955; NICHOLS et al., 1956; BEACH, 1957; WEEKS, 1962; THOMPSON and SCHUSTER, 1964; WEEKS and COLLINS, 1964). This emphasis on physical dependence strengthened the belief that morphine was self-administered chiefly because it terminated or postponed the characteristic abstinence syndrome induced by morphine withdrawal. Although physical dependence may profoundly affect morphine self-administration, it is not necessary for either the acquisition or maintenance of that behavior. In rhesus monkeys with no drug or experimental history, DENEAU et al. (1969) found that responding could be initiated and subsequently maintained when each response produced an intravenous injection of morphine. Although the monkeys in the DENEAU et al. study eventually self-administered sufficient doses of morphine to develop a high level of physical dependence, other studies have shown that morphine self-administration can be maintained in the absence of physical dependence (SCHUSTER, 1968; WOODS and SCHUSTER, 1968, 1971; HOFFMEISTER and

Schlichting, 1972; Hoffmeister and Goldberg, 1973). In these latter studies, persistent responding by rhesus monkeys was maintained under either interval or ratio schedules of intravenous morphine injection even though the doses were so low that demonstrable physical dependence did not develop.

Although schedule-controlled responding can be reliably maintained by intravenous injections of morphine, rates of responding often have been low compared to those maintained by other consequent events such as food presentation or electric shock delivery. These low rates of responding most likely reflect the cumulative effects of repeated injections of morphine in decreasing schedule-controlled behavior (previous sections). Yet, such low rates are not inevitable. Several recent studies have shown that intravenous or intramuscular injections of morphine can maintain high rates of responding under schedules in which injections occur infrequently (Goldberg, 1975; Goldberg et al., 1976a, 1979; Goldberg and Tang, 1977a, b; Sanchez-Ramos and Schuster, 1977). In the Goldberg (1975) and Goldberg and Tang (1977a, b) studies, for example, rhesus monkeys and squirrel monkeys responded under a second-order schedule in which every 30th response during a 60-min interval produced a brief light; the first 30-response unit completed after 60 min elapsed produced several consecutive pairings of the light and intravenous injection of morphine and ended the session. Under this schedule, several thousand responses occurred during each 60-min interval and overall rates of responding usually exceeded one response per second.

Brief visual stimuli that are occasionally paired with morphine injections have been found to be important in maintaining high rates of responding under second-order schedules. Either omitting the brief stimuli (Goldberg and Tang, 1977a; Goldberg et al., 1979) or replacing them with brief stimuli that were never paired directly with morphine injections (Goldberg et al., 1979) resulted in markedly reduced rates of responding; reinstating the paired brief stimuli restored responding at high rates. These findings suggest that second-order schedules can be particularly useful in assessing the role of environmental stimuli associated with morphine injections in maintaining persistent self-administration behavior.

4. Opioid Antagonists

a) Antagonism of the Effects of Morphine on Schedule-Controlled Behavior

Antagonism of the behavioral effects of morphine has been studied most extensively under fixed-ratio and fixed-interval schedules of food presentation. As described previously, high doses of morphine can markedly decrease responding under these schedules in most species of laboratory animals. In pigeons, the rate-decreasing effects of morphine can be blocked by several opioid antagonists, including naloxone, naltrexone, nalorphine, cyclazocine, and diprenorphine (McMillan et al., 1970; McMillan and Harris, 1972; Dykstra et al., 1974; Downs and Woods, 1976; Goldberg et al., 1976b). The relative potencies for these drugs as opioid antagonists have been found to differ somewhat depending on the schedule and dose of morphine in question, but are in general: naltrexone ≈ diprenorphine > D-cyclazocine > D,L-cyclazocine > naloxone > D-cyclazocine > nalorphine. Similar results also have been reported for naloxone and nalorphine in rhesus and squirrel monkeys responding under fixed-interval and fixed-ratio schedules of food presentation (Downs and Woods, 1976; Goldberg et al., 1976b). In contrast, pentazocine appears to produce little or no antagonism of the behavioral effects of morphine in either pigeons (McMillan et al., 1970; McMillan and Harris, 1972) or rhesus monkeys (Downs and Woods, 1976).

Antagonism of the behavioral effects of morphine is not restricted to responding under schedules of food presentation. Naloxone, naltrexone, and nalorphine have been found to block the rate-decreasing effects of morphine in squirrel monkeys responding under a continuous avoidance schedule (Holtzman, 1976) or under a fixed-interval schedule of electric shock presentation (Byrd, 1976). Naloxone and naltrexone also can block the effects of morphine in rats responding under various schedules in which morphine serves as a discriminative stimulus (Rosecrans et al., 1973; Winter, 1975; Shannon and Holtzman, 1976b). Again, the approximate relative order of potencies in antagonizing these various behavioral effects of morphine has been found to be: naltrexone > naloxone > nalorphine. With the possible exception of pentazocine, the potency relations observed for antagonizing the effects of morphine on schedule-controlled behavior are similar to those observed for antagonizing various physiologic effects of morphine in rodents (Blumberg and Dayton, 1973, 1974) and for antagonizing the inhibitory effects of morphine on electrically induced contractions of the guinea pig ileum (Kosterlitz et al., 1973).

b) Direct Effects of Opioid Antagonists on Schedule-Controlled Behavior

Opioid antagonists usually have been found to produce few direct effects on schedule-controlled behavior at low doses that can effectively block the behavioral effects of morphine. Nonetheless, high doses of many opioid antagonists can markedly alter schedule-controlled behavior when given to drug-free animals. In a series of studies with pigeons, McMillan and his co-workers (McMillan and Morse, 1967; McMillan et al., 1970; McMillan and Harris, 1972; Dykstra et al., 1974) compared the effects of morphine, methadone, and several opioid antagonists on responding under fixed-ratio and fixed-interval schedules of food presentation. In these studies, low and intermediate doses of morphine, methadone, naloxone, or its 6-hydroxy analog (EN-2265), naltrexone, nalorphine, cyclazocine, and pentazocine had little or no effect on fixed-ratio responding and sometimes slightly increased fixed-interval responding. Higher doses of each drug, on the other hand, decreased both fixed-ratio and fixed interval responding in a dose-related manner. The approximate order of potency in producing these direct rate-decreasing effects was: L-cyclazocine > D,L-cyclazocine > methadone > morphine > D-cyclazocine > L-pentazocine > D,L-pentazocine > D-pentazocine > naloxone > naltrexone ≈ EN 2265 > nalorphine. Similar effects have been reported for naloxone, nalorphine, and pentazocine in rhesus and squirrel monkeys responding under fixed-ratio and fixed-interval schedules of food presentation (Downs and Woods, 1976; Goldberg et al., 1976b). In monkeys, however, nalorphine was at least ten times more potent than naloxone in decreasing responding (Goldberg et al., 1976b). With the exception of nalorphine, which is relatively inactive in pigeons, the potency relations observed for the behavioral effects of opioid antagonists compare favorably with those observed for their physiologic effects in rodents (Blumberg and Dayton, 1973), their inhibitory effects in the guinea pig ileum preparation (Kosterlitz et al., 1973), and their subjective and analgesic effects in man (Sect. B III–VI).

Although most opioid antagonists have qualitatively similar effects on schedule-controlled behavior maintained by food presentation, differences in the behavioral effects of opioid antagonists have been observed under schedules involving electric shock delivery. In an extensive study with squirrel monkeys, HOLTZMAN (1976) compared the effect of morphine and several opioid antagonists on responding under a continuous avoidance schedule. Morphine, nalorphine, and cyclazocine had qualitatively similar effects on avoidance responding; low and intermediate doses of each drug increased responding, whereas higher doses decreased responding and occasionally produced salivation or vomiting. In contrast, naloxone and naltrexone did not alter the rate of responding at any dose tested, even though the highest doses often produced tremors and vomiting.

c) Self-Administration of Opioid Antagonists

Perhaps the most striking differences in the behavioral effects of opioid antagonists have been observed in studies of self-administration. In a series of experiments by HOFFMEISTER and his co-workers (GOLDBERG et al., 1972; HOFFMEISTER and SCHLICHTING, 1972; HOFFMEISTER and WUTTKE, 1974), rhesus monkeys responded under a fixed-ratio schedule in which every tenth response resulted in an intravenous injection of 50 μg/kg codeine. Experimental sessions were limited to 3 h per day to prevent the development of physical dependence. Injections of codeine then were replaced by injections of either saline, morphine (0.1–500 μg/kg), heroin (0.1–50 μg/kg), codeine (0.1–500 μg/kg), pentazocine (1–500 μg/kg), nalorphine (1–10 μg/kg), or cyclazocine (5–500 μg/kg). With this substitution procedure, suitable doses of morphine, heroin, codeine, and pentazocine maintained responding well above the level maintained by saline. Furthermore, each drug maintained similar maximum rates of responding, though pentazocine was less potent than the three other opioids. In contrast, nalorphine and cyclazocine failed to maintain responding at any dose tested, and higher doses often suppressed responding below the level maintained by saline.

Differences in the behavioral effects of opioid antagonists also have been observed under a signaled avoidance-escape schedule in which responding terminated a visual stimulus associated with intravenous drug injection. In two studies (HOFFMEISTER and WUTTKE, 1973, 1974), rhesus monkeys initially were trained to terminate a stimulus associated with electric shock. Electric shocks then were replaced by injections of either saline, nalorphine (1–500 μg/kg), cyclazocine (0.1–10 μg/kg) or naloxone (5–100 μg/kg). Suitable doses of nalorphine and cyclazocine maintained responding above the level maintained by saline. Naloxone, on the other hand, failed to maintain responding at any dose tested, as did 50-μg/kg injections of morphine and pentazocine.

Although naloxone and pentazocine did not maintain responding under the signaled avoidance-escape schedule in nondependent subjects, these drugs, as well as nalorphine, have been found to maintain persistent responding under similar schedules in monkeys that were physically dependent on morphine (GOLDBERG et al., 1971, 1972; DOWNS and WOODS, 1975a, b; TANG and MORSE, 1976). In the GOLDBERG et al. (1972) and HOFFMEISTER and WUTTKE (1974) studies, for example, rhesus monkeys were made dependent on morphine by administering periodic infusions totaling about 18 mg/kg morphine per day. In these subjects, naloxone (1–10 μg/kg per injection), nalorphine (5–10 μg/kg per injection), and pentazocine (50–1,000 μg/kg per injection) reliably maintained responding under the signaled avoidance-escape schedule. The different findings observed in morphine-dependent and nondependent monkeys demonstrate that the behavioral effects of morphine antagonists can depend critically on the extant physiologic state of the subject.

In addition to the presence or absence of physical dependence, the schedule under which opioid antagonists are administered can be important in determining their behavioral effects. In the GOLDBERG et al. (1971) study described previously, responding by morphine-dependent monkeys was maintained by termination of a stimulus associated with injections of nalorphine. Nonetheless, when conditions were arranged so that each response *produced* an injection of nalorphine, responding was reliably maintained even though injections resulted in signs of severe abstinence. Similar effects also have been reported for naloxone (DOWNS and WOODS, 1975b). In that study, morphine-dependent rhesus monkeys responded under a schedule in which every 30th response terminated a stimulus associated with the injection of naloxone (0.2–20 μg/kg per injection). The schedule was then changed so that every 30th response produced a brief visual stimulus, and the completion of 10 or 15 30-response units produced both the brief stimulus and a 2 μg/kg injection of naloxone. Under this second-order schedule, high rates of responding were maintained by injections of naloxone for as many as 15 days. Although responding eventually declined, these results suggest that under suitable conditions naloxone can maintain responding that leads to its injection. These findings emphasize the importance of factors other than the intrinsic pharmacologic properties of opioid antagonists in determining their effects on behavior.

d) Supersensitivity to the Behavioral Effects of Opioid Antagonists

Although higher doses of morphine antagonists are usually required to produce noticeable changes in schedule-controlled behavior of morphine-free animals, very low doses can markedly alter responding in animals that have been made physically dependent on morphine (GOLDBERG and SCHUSTER, 1967, 1970; WOODS et al., 1973; VILLARREAL and KARBOWSKI, 1974; GELLERT and SPARBER, 1977). In morphine-dependent rhesus monkeys, for example, WOODS et al. (1973) and VILLARREAL and KARBOWSKI (1974) found that doses of naloxone as low as 0.1 mg/kg produced behavioral changes similar to those produced by abrupt withdrawal of morphine. Other studies have shown that low doses of naloxone also can have marked behavioral effects in animals that have received only brief exposures to morphine (JACOB et al., 1974; MEYER and SPARBER, 1977; SPARBER et al., 1978; KELLEHER and GOLDBERG, 1979). In rats responding under a fixed-ratio schedule of food presentation, for example, SPARBER et al. (1978) found that a previously ineffective dose of naloxone (2.5 mg/kg) markedly decreased responding when given 3 h after the animals had received an injection of morphine (15 or 30 mg/kg) which itself had little effect on responding. While these findings demonstrate that low doses of naloxone can have clear behavioral effects in animals that have received only a single injection of morphine, it is not yet clear whether such findings are best interpreted in terms of naloxone producing a morphine-abstinence syndrome by revealing a rapidly developing state of dependence or in terms of morphine enhancing the behavioral effects of naloxone. At an empirical level, the results are most simply described as a shift to the left of the naloxone dose-effect curve after pretreatment with morphine.

Similar shifts in dose-effect curves also have been reported for naloxone and nalorphine in animals that have previously received morphine but remained morphine free for several days to several months prior to testing (GOLDBERG and SCHUSTER, 1969; KELLEHER and GOLDBERG, 1979). In the GOLDBERG and SCHUSTER (1969) study, for example, morphine-dependent rhesus monkeys were withdrawn from morphine for 3 months and then trained to respond under a fixed-ratio schedule of food presentation. With these previously dependent monkeys, the nalorphine dose-effect curves were displaced to the left of the curves obtained with other monkeys that had never received morphine, indicating that chronic administration of morphine can produce long-term supersensitivity to the behavioral effects of nalorphine.

Supersensitivity to the behavioral effects of morphine antagonists also can be produced by chronic administration of naloxone or naltrexone (KELLEHER and GOLDBERG, 1979; SPEALMAN et al., 1979b, 1981; Goldberg et al., 1981). In these studies, rhesus monkeys, squirrel monkeys, and rats responded under a fixed-ratio schedule of food presentation, and dose-effect curves were determined for naloxone (rhesus monkeys) or naltrexone (squirrel monkeys and rats) both before and after a 3-week period during which the drugs were administered daily. In most cases, chronic administration of naloxone (10 mg/kg per day in rhesus or squirrel monkeys) or naltrexone (3–17 mg/kg per day in squirrel monkeys; 30–100 mg/kg per day in rats) shifted the dose-effect curves by about 1 log unit or more to the left. In squirrel monkeys, supersensitivity to the effects of naltrexone on food-maintained behavior persisted for as long as 6 months after chronic administration had ended (KELLEHER and GOLDBERG, 1979; GOLDBERG et al., 1981). Other studies have shown that chronic administration of naloxone or nalorphine can produce supersensitivity to the analgesic effects of morphine in rats (ORAHOVATS et al., 1953; TANG and COLLINS, 1978) and to the inhibitory effect of opioids in the guinea pig ileum preparation (SCHULZ et al., 1979), concomitant with an increase in opiate receptor binding (LAHTI and COLLINS, 1978; SCHULZ et al., 1979). Taken together, these findings suggest that supersensitivity to the effects of opioid antagonists on food-maintained behavior may develop as a result of chronic receptor blockade.

5. Discussion

Early studies of the behavioral pharmacology of morphine emphasized that the analgesic and dependence-inducing actions of the drug were pertinent to evaluating its effects on behavior. As techniques improved and data accumulated, it became clear that other factors were equally important. It is now known that the temporal and sequential relations between behavior and its consequences (i.e., the schedule) can be fundamental in determining whether opioids and opioid antagonists increase or decrease rates of responding. Similarly, the schedule under which these drugs are administered can be critical in determining whether they maintain responding that leads to their injection or maintain responding that terminates their injection. Such findings represent an important initial step in understanding how environmental conditions alter the behavioral effects of opioids and opioid antagonists. Since opioid antagonists can block opiate receptors, which mediate the actions of endorphins, the behavioral effects of these drugs might reveal functional characteristics of the endorphin system. Although opioid antagonists typically have few effects on schedule-controlled behavior at low doses that block opiate receptors, higher doses can markedly alter responding. Moreover, under suitable conditions, the behavioral effects of these drugs can become more pronounced or can occur at relatively low doses in animals that have previously received morphine or opioid antagonists. Clearly, further research is required to elucidate the role of drug-environment interactions in modulating the functions of the endorphin system.

D. Summary and Conclusions

Drug-induced changes in reports of subjective effects are central elements in predicting the therapeutic usefulness as well as the abuse liability of psychotropic drugs. Quantitative methods using standardized questionnaires for assessing reports of subjective effects have been developed and validated; they provide reproducible results across studies and across different routes of drug administration. The pattern of dose-related changes in scores on these questionnaires reliably distinguishes among the patterns of signs, symptoms, and subjective effects produced in human volunteers by different subgroups of opioid agonists, partial agonists, and antagonists.

Laboratory animals can be trained to discriminate between administration of a drug and its vehicle using methods developed for the study of operant behavior. Reinforcement of responses in the presence of the effects of one drug increases the tendency of the animal to respond not only in the presence of that drug but also in the presence of similar drugs. The classification of opioid agonists, partial agonists, and antagonists into subgroups on the basis of their effects as discriminative stimuli in laboratory animals has been generally consistent with classifications obtained using questionnaires for assessing subjective effects in humans.

Another approach to the analysis of the psychotropic effects of opioids and opioid antagonists is to study their effects on operant behavior maintained under various schedules of reinforcement. Studies of this type have emphasized the importance of the temporal and sequential relations between behavior and its consequences in determining the behavioral effects of opioids and opioid antagonists. They provide a meaningful way to evaluate how environmental conditions can modify the psychotropic effects of opioids and opioid antagonists.

Acknowledgements. Preparation of this paper was supported in part by U. S. Public Health Service grants DA00499, MH02094, MH02658, MH07658, and RR00168.

References

Adam-Carrière, D., Merali, Z., Stretch, R.: Effects of morphine, naloxone, D,L-cyclazocine, and D-amphetamine on behavior controlled by a schedule of inter-response time reinforcement. Can. J. Physiol. Pharmacol. *56*, 707–720 (1978)

Andrews, H.L., Himmelsbach, C.K.: Relation of the intensity of the morphine abstinence syndrome to dosage. J. Pharmacol. Exp. Ther. *81*, 288–293 (1944)

Azrin, N.H.: Some effects of two intermittent schedules of immediate and non-immediate punishment. J. Psychol. *42*, 3–21 (1956)

Azrin, N.H.: Effects of punishment intensity during variable-interval reinforcement. J. Exp. Anal. Behav. *2*, 123–142 (1960)

Azrin, N.H., Holz, W.C.: Punishment. In: Operant behavior: Areas of research and application. Honig, W.K. (ed.), pp. 380–447. New York: Appleton-Century-Crofts 1966
Babbini, M., Gaiardi, M., Bartoletti, M.: Changes in operant behavior as an index of a withdrawal state from morphine in rats. Psychon. Sci. *29*, 142–144 (1972)
Babbini, M., Gaiardi, M., Bartoletti, M.: Changes in fixed-interval behavior during chronic morphine treatment and morphine abstinence in rats. Psychopharmacology *45*, 255–259 (1976)
Beach, H.D.: Morphine addiction in rats. Can. J. Psychol. *11*, 104–112 (1957)
Beaumont, A., Hughes, J.: Biology of opioid peptides. Ann. Rev. Pharmacol. Toxicol. *19*, 245–267 (1979)
Blumberg, H., Dayton, H.B.: Naloxone and related compounds. In: Agonist and antagonist actions of narcotic analgesic drugs. Kosterlitz, H.W., Collier, H.O.J., Villarreal, J.E. (eds.), pp. 110–119. Baltimore, London, Tokyo: University Park Press 1973
Blumberg, H., Dayton, H.B.: Naloxone, naltrexone and related noroxymorphones. In: Narcotic antagonists. Adv. Biochem. Psychopharmacol. *8*, 33–43 (1974)
Brogden, R.N., Speight, T.M., Avery, G.S. Pentazocine, a review of its pharmacological properties, therapeutic efficacy and dependence liability. Drugs. *5*, 6–91 (1973)
Byrd, L.D.: Contrasting effects of morphine on schedule-controlled behavior in the chimpanzee and baboon. J. Pharmacol. Exp. Ther. *193*, 861–869 (1975)
Byrd, L.D.: Effects of morphine alone and in combination with naloxone or D-amphetamine on shock-maintained behavior in the squirrel monkey. Psychopharmacology *49*, 225–234 (1976)
Chittal, S.M., Sheth, U.K.: Effects of drugs on conditioned avoidance response in rats. Arch. Int. Pharmacodyn. *144*, 471–480 (1963)
Colpaert, F.C., Lal, H., Niemegeers, C.J.E., Janssen, P.A.J.: Investigations on drug produced and subjectively experienced discriminative stimuli. 1. The fentanyl cue, a tool to investigate subjectively experienced narcotic drug actions. Life Sci. *16*, 705–716 (1975a)
Colpaert, F.C., Niemegeers, C.J.E., Lal, H., Janssen, P.A.J.: Investigations on drug produced and subjectively experienced discriminative stimuli. 2. Loperamide, an antidiarrheal devoid of narcotic cue producing action. Life Sci. *16*, 717–728 (1975b)
Colpaert, F.C., Niemegeers, C.J.E., Janssen, P.A.J.: On the ability of narcotic antagonists to produce the narcotic cue. J. Pharmacol. Exp. Ther. *197*, 180–187 (1976)
Colpaert, F.C.: Discriminative stimulus properties of narcotic analgesic drugs. Pharmacol. Biochem. Behav. *9*, 863–887 (1978)
Cook, L., Weidley, E.: Behavioral effects of some psychopharmacological agents. Ann. N. Y. Acad. Sci. *66*, 740–752 (1957)
Cook, L., Catania, A.C.: Effects of drugs on avoidance and escape behavior. Fed. Proc. *23*, 818–835 (1964)
Cook, L., Davidson, A.B.: Effects of behaviorally active drugs in a conflict-punishment procedure in rats. In: The benzodiazepines. Garattini, S., Mussini, E., Randall, L.O. (eds.), pp. 327–345. New York: Raven Press 1973
Cook, L., Davidson, A.B.: Behavioral pharmacology: Animal models involving aversive control of behavior. In: Psychopharmacology: A generation of progress. Lipton, M.A., DiMascio, A.D., Killam, K.S. (eds.), pp. 563–567. New York: Raven Press 1978
Deneau, G.A., Yanagita, T., Seevers, M.H.: Self-administration of psychoactive substances by the monkey: A measure of psychological dependence. Psychopharmacologia *16*, 30–48 (1969)
Djahanguiri, B.M., Richelle, M., Fontaine, O.: Behavioral effects of prolonged treatment with small doses of morphine in cats. Psychopharmacology *9*, 363–372 (1966)
Domino, E.F., Wilson, A.: Effects of narcotic analgesic agonists and antagonists on rat brain acetylcholine. J. Pharmacol. Exp. Ther. *184*, 18–32 (1973)
Downs, D.A., Woods, J.H.: Fixed-ratio escape and avoidance-escape from naloxone in morphine-dependent monkeys: Effects of naloxone dose and morphine pretreatment. J. Exp. Anal. Behav. *23*, 415–427 (1975a).
Downs, D.A., Woods, J.H.: Naloxone as a negative reinforcer in rhesus monkeys: Effects of dose, schedule, and narcotic regimen. Pharmacol. Rev. *27*, 397–406 (1975b)

Downs, D.A., Woods, J.H.: Morphine, pentazocine and naloxone effects on responding under a multiple schedule of reinforcement in rhesus monkeys and pigeons. J. Pharmacol. Exp. Ther. *196*, 298–306 (1976)
Dykstra, L.A., McMillan, D.E., Harris, L.S.: Antagonism of morphine by long acting narcotic antagonists. Psychopharmacology *39*, 151–162 (1974)
Dykstra, L.A., McMillan, D.E.: Electric shock titration: Effects of morphine, methadone, pentazocine, nalorphine, naloxone, diazepam and amphetamine. J. Pharmacol. Exp. Ther. *202*, 660–669 (1977)
Dykstra, L.A.: Effects of morphine, pentazocine and cyclazocine alone and in combination with naloxone on electric shock titration in the squirrel monkey. J. Pharmacol. Exp. Ther. *211*, 722–732 (1979)
Estes, W.R., Skinner, B.F.: Some quantitative properties of anxiety. J. Exp. Psychol. *29*, 390–400 (1941)
Ferster, C.B., Skinner, B.F.: Schedules of reinforcement. New York: Appleton-Century-Crofts 1957
Ford, R.D., Balster, R.L.: Schedule-controlled behavior in the morphine-dependent rat. Pharmacol. Biochem. Behav. *4*, 569–573 (1976)
Fraser, H.F., Isbell, H.: Pharmacology and addiction liability of D,L- and D-propoxyphene. Bull. Narc. *12*, 9–14 (1960)
Fraser, H.F., Van Horn, G.D., Martin, W.R., Wolbach, A.B., Isbell, H.: Methods for evaluating addiction liability. (A) "Attitude" of opiate addicts toward opiate-like drugs, (B) A short-term "direct" addiction test. J. Pharmacol. Exp. Ther. *133*, 371–387 (1961)
Geller, I., Bachman, E., Seifter, J.: Effects of reserpine and morphine on behavior suppressed by punishment. Life Sci. *4*, 226–231 (1963)
Gellert, V.F., Sparber, S.B.: A comparison of the effects of naloxone upon body weight loss and suppression of fixed-ratio operant behavior in morphine-dependent rats. J. Pharmacol. Exp. Ther. *201*, 44–54 (1977)
Gianutsos, G., Lal, H.: Effect of loperamide, haloperidol and methadone in rats trained to discriminate morphine from saline. Psychopharmacology *41*, 267–270 (1975)
Gianutsos, G., Lal, H.: Selective interaction of drugs with a discriminable stimulus associated with narcotic action. Life Sci. *19*, 91–98 (1976)
Goldberg, S.R., Schuster, C.R.: Conditioned suppression by a stimulus associated with nalorphine in morphine-dependent monkeys. J. Exp. Anal. Behav. *10*, 235–242 (1967)
Goldberg, S.R., Schuster, C.R.: Nalorphine: Increased sensitivity of monkeys formerly dependent on morphine. Science *166*, 1548–1549 (1969)
Goldberg, S.R., Woods, J.H., Schuster, C.R.: Morphine: Conditioned increases in self-administration in rhesus monkeys. Science *166*, 1306–1307 (1969)
Goldberg, S.R., Schuster, C.R.: Conditioned nalorphine-induced abstinence changes: Persistence in post morphine-dependent monkeys. J. Exp. Anal. Behav. *14*, 33–46 (1970)
Goldberg, S.R., Hoffmeister, F., Schlichting, U.U., Wuttke, W.: Aversive properties of nalorphine and naloxone in morphine-dependent rhesus monkeys. J. Pharmacol. Exp. Ther. *179*, 268–276 (1971)
Goldberg, S.R., Hoffmeister, F., Schlichting, U.U.: Morphine antagonists: Modification of behavioral effects by morphine dependence. In: Drug addiction. I. Experimental pharmacology. Singh, J.M., Miller, L., Lal, H. (eds.), pp. 31–48. Mount Kisco, N.Y.: Futura Publishing Co. 1972
Goldberg, S.R.: Stimuli associated with drug injections as events that control behavior. Pharmacol. Rev. *27*, 325–340 (1975)
Goldberg, S.R., Morse, W.H., Goldberg, D.M.: Behavior maintained under a second order schedule by intramuscular injection of morphine or cocaine in rhesus monkeys. J. Pharmacol. Exp. Ther. *199*, 278–286 (1976a)
Goldberg, S.R., Morse, W.H., Goldberg, D.M.: Some behavioral effects of morphine, naloxone and nalorphine in the squirrel monkey and the pigeon. J. Pharmacol. Exp. Ther. *196*, 625–636 (1976b)
Goldberg, S.R., Tang, A.H.: Behavior maintained under second-order schedules of intravenous morphine injection in squirrel and rhesus monkeys. Psychopharmacology *51*, 235–242 (1977a)

Goldberg, S.R., Tang, A.H.: Reinforcement of behavior by morphine injections. In: Alcohol and opiates. Blum, K., Ross, D.H. (eds.), pp. 341–357. New York: Academic Press 1977b

Goldberg, S.R., Spealman, R.D., Kelleher, R.T.: Enhancement of drug-seeking behavior by environmental stimuli associated with cocaine or morphine injections. Neuropharmacology *18*, 1015–1017 (1979)

Goldberg, S.R., Morse, W.H., Goldberg, D.M.: Acute and chronic effects of naltrexone and naloxone on schedule-controlled behavior of squirrel monkeys and pigeons. J. Pharmacol. Exp. Ther. *216*, 500–509 (1981)

Goldstein, A.: Opioid peptides (endorphins) in pituitary and brain. Science *193*, 1081–1086 (1976)

Gonzalez, F.A., Goldberg, S.R.: Effects of cocaine and *d*-amphetamine on behavior maintained under various schedules of food presentation in squirrel monkeys. J. Pharmacol. Exp. Ther. *201*, 33–43 (1977)

Haertzen, C.A., Hill, H.E., Belleville, R.E.: Development of the Addiction Research Center Inventory (ARCI): Selection of items that are sensitive to the effects of various drugs. Psychopharmacology *4*, 155–166 (1963)

Haertzen, C.A.: Development of scales based on patterns of drug effects, using the Addiction Research Center Inventory (ARCI). Psychopharmacology *18*, 163–194 (1966)

Haertzen, C.A., Hooks, N.T., Jr.: Changes in personality and subjective experience associated with the chronic administration and withdrawal of opiates. J. Nerv. Ment. Dis. *148*, 606–614 (1969)

Haertzen, C.A.: Subjective effects of narcotic antagonists cyclazocine and nalorphine on the Addiction Research Center Inventory (ARCI). Psychopharmacology *18*, 366–377 (1970)

Haertzen, C.A., Meketon, M.J., Hooks, N.T., Jr.: Subjective experiences produed by withdrawal of opiates. Br. J. Addict. *65*, 245–255 (1970)

Haertzen, C.A.: Subjective effects of narcotic antagonists. In: Narcotic antagonists. Adv. Biochem. Psychopharmacol. *8*, 383–398 (1974a)

Haertzen, C.A.: An overview of Addiction Research Center Inventory scales (ARCI): an appendix and manual of scales. DHEW Publication No. (ADM) 74–92. Rockville, Maryland: National Institute on Drug Abuse 1974b

Headlee, C.P., Coppock, H.W., Nichols, J.R.: Apparatus and technique involved in a laboratory method of detecting the aversiveness of drugs. J. Am. Pharm. Ass. (Sci. Ed.) *44*, 229–231 (1955)

Heifetz, S.A., McMillan, D.E.: Development of behavioral tolerance to morphine and methadone using the schedule-controlled behavior of the pigeon. Psychopharmacology *19*, 40–52 (1971)

Heise, G.A., Boff, E.: Continuous avoidance as a base-line for measuring behavioral effects of drugs. Psychopharmacology *3*, 264–282 (1962)

Herling, S., Coale, E.H., Valentino, R.J., Hein, D.W., Woods, J.H.: Narcotic discrimination in pigeons. J. Pharmacol. Exp. Ther. *214*, 139–146 (1980)

Hill, H.E., Belleville, R.E., Wikler, A.: Reduction of pain conditioned anxiety by analgesic doses of morphine in rats. Proc. Soc. Exp. Biol. Med. *86*, 881–884 (1954)

Hill, H.E., Pescor, F.T., Belleville, R.E., Wikler, A.: Use of differential bar-pressing rates of rats for screening analgesic drugs. I. Techniques and effects of morphine. J. Pharmacol. Exp. Ther. *120*, 388–397 (1957)

Hill, H.E., Haertzen, C.A., Wolbach, A.B., Miner, E.J.: The Addiction Research Center Inventory: Standardization of scales which evaluate subjective effects of morphine, amphetamine, pentobarbital, alcohol, LSD-25, pyrahexyl and chlorpromazine. Psychopharmacology *4*, 167–183 (1963a)

Hill, H.E., Haertzen, C.A., Wolbach, A.B., Jr., Miner, E.J.: The Addiction Research Center Inventory: Appendix. I. Items comprising empirical scales for seven drugs. II. Items which do not differentiate placebo from any drug condition. Psychopharmacology *4*, 184–205 (1963b)

Himmelsbach, C.K.: Studies of the addiction liability of "Demerol" (D-140). J. Pharmacol. Exp. Ther. *75*, 64–68 (1942)

Himmelsbach, C.K., Andrews, H.L., Felix, R.H., Oberst, F.W., Davenport, L.F.: Studies on codeine addiction. Publ. Health Rep. (Wash.) Suppl. *158* (1940)

Hirschhorn, I.D.: Pentazocine, cyclazocine and nalorphine as discriminative stimuli. Psychopharmacology *54*, 289–294 (1977)

Hirschhorn, I.D., Rosecrans, J.A.: A comparison of the stimulus effects of morphine and lysergic acid diethylamide (LSD). Pharmacol. Biochem. Behav. *2*, 361–366 (1974)

Hirschhorn, I.D., Rosecrans, J.A.: Generalization of morphine and lysergic acid diethylamide (LSD) stimulus properties to narcotic analgesics. Psychopharmacology *47*, 65–69 (1976)

Hoffmeister, F., Schlichting, U.U.: Reinforcing properties of some opiates and opioids in rhesus monkeys with histories of cocaine and codeine self-administration. Psychopharmacology *23*, 55–74 (1972)

Hoffmeister, F., Goldberg, S.R.: A comparison of chlorpromazine, imipramine, morphine and *d*-amphetamine self-administration in cocaine-dependent rhesus monkeys. J. Pharmacol. Exp. Ther. *187*, 8–14 (1973)

Hoffmeister, F., Wuttke, W.: Negative reinforcing properties of morphine antagonists in naive rhesus monkeys. Psychopharmacology *33*, 247–258 (1973)

Hoffmeister, F., Wuttke, W.: Self-administration: Positive and negative reinforcing properties of morphine antagonists in rhesus monkeys. In: Narcotic antagonists. Adv. Biochem. Psychopharmacol. *8*, 361–369 (1974)

Holtzman, S.G., Villarreal, J.E.: The effects of morphine on conditioned suppression in rhesus monkeys. Psychon. Sci. *17*, 161–162 (1969)

Holtzman, S.G., Jewett, R.E.: Interactions of morphine and nalorphine with physostigmine on operant behavior in the rat. Psychopharmacology *22*, 384–395 (1971)

Holtzman, S.G., Jewett, R.E.: Shock intensity as a determinant of the behavioral effects of morphine in the rat. Life Sci. *11*, 1085–1091 (1972)

Holtzman, S.G., Villarreal, J.E.: Operant behavior in the morphine-dependent rhesus monkey. J. Pharmacol. Exp. Ther. *184*, 528–541 (1973)

Holtzman, S.G.: Tolerance to the stimulant effects of morphine and pentazocine on avoidance responding in the rat. Psychopharmacology *39*, 23–37 (1974)

Holtzman, S.G.: Effects of morphine and narcotic antagonists on avoidance behavior of the squirrel monkey. J. Pharmacol. Exp. Ther. *196*, 145–155 (1976)

Holtzman, S.G., Shannon, H.E., Schaefer, G.J.: Discriminative properties of narcotic antagonists. In: Discriminative stimulus properties of drugs. Lal, H. (ed.), pp. 47–72. New York: Plenum Publishing Corp. 1977

Houser, V.P.: The effects of drugs on behavior controlled by aversive stimuli. In: Contemporary research in behavioral pharmacology. Blackman, D.E., Sanger, D.J. (eds.), pp. 69–157. New York: Plenum Press 1978

Hughes, J., Kosterlitz, H.W.: Opioid peptides. Br. Med. Bull. *33*, 157–161 (1977)

Isbell, H.: Methods and results of studying experimental human addiction to the newer synthetic analgesics. Ann. N.Y. Acad. Sci. *51*, 108–122 (1948)

Isbell, H., Fraser, H.F.: Actions and addiction liabilities of dromoran derivatives in man. J. Pharmacol. Exp. Ther. *107*, 524–530 (1953)

Jacob, J.J.C., Barthelemy, C.D., Tremblay, E.C., Colombel, M.-C.L.: Potential usefulness of single-dose acute physical dependence on and tolerance to morphine for the evaluation of narcotic antagonists. In: Narcotic antagonists. Adv. Biochem. Psychopharmacol. *8*, 299–318 (1974)

Jaffe, J.H., Martin, W.R.: Narcotic analgesics and antagonists. In: The pharmacological basis of therapeutics. Goodman, L.S., Gilman, A. (eds.), pp. 245–283. New York: MacMillan Co. 1975

Jarbe, T.U.C.: Discriminative effects of morphine in the pigeon. Pharmacol. Biochem. Behav. *9*, 411–416 (1978)

Jarbe, T.U.C., Rollenhagen, C.: Morphine as a discriminative cue in gerbils: Drug generalization and antagonism. Psychopharmacology *58*, 271–275 (1978)

Jasinski, D.R., Martin, W.R., Haertzen, C.A.: The human pharmacology and abuse potential of N-allylnoroxymorphone (naloxone). J. Pharmacol. Exp. Ther. *157*, 420–426 (1967)

Jasinski, D.R., Martin, W.R., Sapira, J.D.: Antagonism of the subjective, behavioral, pupillary, and respiratory depressant effects of cyclazocine by naloxone. Clin. Pharmacol. Ther. *9*, 215–222 (1968a)

Jasinski, D.R., Martin, W.R., Sapira, J.D.: Progress report on the dependence-producing properties of GPA-1657, profadol hydrochloride (CI-572), propiram fumarate (BAY-4503) and dexoxadrol. Reported to the 30th Meeting, Committee on Problems of Drug Dependence – National Research Council, Indianapolis, Ind. (1968b)

Jasinski, D.R., Martin, W.R., Hoeldtke, R.D.: Effects of short- and long-term administration of pentazocine in man. Clin. Pharmacol. Ther. *11*, 385–403 (1970)
Jasinski, D.R., Martin, W.R., Hoeldtke, R.D.: Studies of the dependence-producing properties of GPA-1657, profadol, and propiram in man. Clin. Pharmacol. Ther. *12*, 613–649 (1971 a)
Jasinski, D.R., Martin, W.R., Mansky, P.: Progress report on the assessment of the antagonists nalbuphine and GPA-2087 for abuse potential and studies of the effects of dextromethorphan in man. Reported to the 33rd Meeting of the Committee on Problems of Drug Dependence – National Research Council, Toronto, Canada (1971 b)
Jasinski, D.R., Mansky, P.A.: Evaluation of nalbuphine for abuse potential. Clin. Pharmacol. Ther. *13*, 78–90 (1972)
Jasinski, D.R., Nutt, J.G.: Progress report on the assessment program of the NIMH Addiction Research Center. Reported to the 34th Meeting of the Committee on Problems of Drug Dependence – National Research Council, Washington, D.C., 1972
Jasinski, D.R., Nutt, J.G.: Progress report on the clinical assessment program of the Addiction Research Center. Reported to the 35th Meeting, Committee on Problems of Drug Dependence – National Research Council, Chapel Hill, N.C., 1973
Jasinski, D.R.: Effects in man of partial morphine agonists. In: Agonist and antagonist actions of narcotic analgesic drugs. Kosterlitz, H.W., Collier, H.O.J., Villarreal, J.E. (eds.), pp. 94–103. Baltimore: University Park Press and London-Tokyo: MacMillan Press 1973
Jasinski, D.R., Griffith, J.D., Pevnick, J.S., Clark, S.C.: Progress report on studies from the clinical pharmacology section of the Addiction Research Center. Reported to the 37th Meeting of the Committee on Problems of Drug Dependence, National Academy of Sciences – National Research Council, Washington, D.C., 1975
Jasinski, D.R., Pevnick, J.S., Griffith, J.D., Gorodetzky, C.W., Cone, E.J.: Progress report on studies from the clinical pharmacology section of the Addiction Research Center. Reported to the 38th Meeting of the Committee on Problems of Drug Dependence, 1976
Jasinski, D.R.: Assessment of the abuse potentiality of morphine-like drugs. In: Drug addiction. I. Morphine, sedative-hypnotic and alcohol dependence. Handbook of Experimental Pharmacology. Martin, W.R. (ed.), vol. 45, pp. 197–258. Berlin-Heidelberg-New York: Springer 1977
Jasinski, D.R., Pevnick, J.S., Griffith, J.D.: Human pharmacology and abuse potential of the analgesic buprenorphine. Arch. Gen. Psychiat. *35*, 501–516 (1978)
Jasinski, D.R.: Human pharmacology of narcotic antagonists. Br. J. Pharmacol. *7*, (Suppl. 3) 287 s–290 s (1979)
Kay, D.C., Gorodetzky, C.W., Martin, W.R.: Comparative effects of codeine and morphine in man. J. Pharmacol. Exp. Ther. *156*, 101–106 (1967)
Kayan, S., Ferguson, R.K., Mitchell, C.L.: An investigation of pharmacologic and behavioral tolerance to morphine in rats. J. Pharmacol. Exp. Ther. *185*, 300–306 (1973)
Kelleher, R.T., Morse, W.H.: Escape behavior and punished behavior. Fed. Proc. *23*, 808–817 (1964)
Kelleher, R.T., Morse, W.H.: Determinants of the specificity of behavioral effects of drugs. Ergebn. Physiol. Biol. Chem. Exp. Pharmacol. *60*, 1–56 (1968)
Kelleher, R.T., Goldberg, S.R.: Effects of naloxone on schedule-controlled behavior in monkeys. In: Endorphins in mental health research. Usdin, E., Bunney, W.E., Jr., Kline, N.S. (eds.), pp. 461–472. London-Basingstoke: MacMillan Press 1979
Kosterlitz, H.W., Lord, J.A.H., Watt, A.J.: Morphine receptor in the myenteric plexus of the guinea-pig ileum. In: Agonist and antagonist actions of narcotic analgesic drugs. Kosterlitz, H.W., Collier, H.O.J., Villarreal, J.E. (eds.), pp. 45–61. Baltimore: University Park Press and London-Tokyo: MacMillan Press 1973
Kuhn, D.M., Greenberg, I., Appel, J.B.: Stimulus properties of the narcotic antagonist pentazocine: similarity to morphine and antagonism by naloxone. J. Pharmacol. Exp. Ther. *196*, 121–127 (1976)
Lahti, R.A., Collins, R.J.: Chronic naloxone results in prolonged increases in opiate binding sites in brain. Eur. J. Pharmacol. *51*, 185–186 (1978)
Lal, H., Gianutsos, G., Miksic, S.: Discriminable stimuli produced by analgesics. In: Discriminative stimulus properties of drugs. Lal, H. (ed.), pp. 23–45. New York: Plenum Press 1977
Lasagna, L., Von Felsinger, J.M., Beecher, H.K.: Drug-induced mood changes in man. 1. Observation on healthy subjects, chronically ill patients, and "postaddicts". J. Am. Med. Ass. *157*, 1006–1020 (1955)

Lauener, H.: Conditioned suppression in rats and the effect of pharmacological agents thereon. Psychopharmacology *4*, 311–325 (1963)

Malis, J.L.: Analgesic testing in primates. In: Agonist and antagonist actions of narcotic analgesic drugs. Kosterlitz, H.W., Collier, H.O.J., Villarreal, J.E. (eds.), pp. 106–109. Baltimore: University Park Press and London-Tokyo: MacMillan Press 1973

Malis, J.L., Gluckman, M.I.: Assaying narcotic-antagonist drugs for analgesic activity in rhesus monkeys. In: Narcotic antagonists. Adv. Biochem. Psychopharmacol. *8*, 225–233 (1974)

Malis, J.L., Rosenthale, M.E., Gluckman, M.I.: Animal pharmacology of Wy-16,225, a new analgesic agent. J. Pharmacol. Exp. Ther. *194*, 488–498 (1975)

Markowitz, R., Jacobson, J., Bain, G., Kornetsky, C.: Naloxone blockade of morphine analgesia: A dose-effect study of duration and magnitude. J. Pharmacol. Exp. Ther. *199*, 385–388 (1976)

Martin, W.R., Fraser, H.F.: A comparative study of physiological and subjective effects of heroin and morphine administered intravenously in postaddicts. J. Pharmacol. Exp. Ther. *133*, 388–399 (1961)

Martin, W.R., Fraser, H.F., Gorodetzky, C.W., Rosenberg, D.E.: Studies of the dependence-producing potential of the narcotic antagonist 2-cyclopropylmethyl-2′-hydroxy-5,9-dimethyl-6,7-benzomorphan (cyclazocine, WIN-20,740, ARC II-C-3). J. Pharmacol. Exp. Ther. *150*, 426–436 (1965)

Martin, W.R., Gorodetzky, C.W.: Demonstration of tolerance to and physical dependence on N-allylnormorphine (nalorphine). J. Pharmacol. Exp. Ther. *150*, 437–442 (1965)

Martin, W.R.: Assessment of the dependence-producing potentiality of narcotic analgesics. In: International Encyclopedia of Pharmacology and Therapeutics. Radouco-Thomas, C., Lasagna, L. (eds.), Vol. 1, pp. 155–180. Glasgow: Pergamon Press 1966

Martin, W.R., Jasinski, D.R.: Physiological parameters of morphine dependence in man – tolerance, early abstinence, protracted abstinence. J. Psychiat. Res. *7*, 9–17 (1969)

Martin, W.R., Jasinski, D.R., Haertzen, C.A., Kay, D.C., Jones, B.E., Mansky, P.A., Carpenter, R.W.: Methadone – A reevaluation. Arch. Gen. Psychiat. *28*, 286–295 (1973 a)

Martin, W.R., Jasinski, D.R., Mansky, P.A.: Naltrexone, an antagonist for the treatment of heroin dependence. Arch. Gen. Psychiat. *28*, 784–791 (1973 b)

Martin, W.R., Thompson, W.O., Fraser, H.F.: Comparison of graded single intramuscular doses of morphine and pentobarbital in man. Clin. Pharmacol. Ther. *15*, 623–630 (1974)

Martin, W.R., Eades, C.G., Thompson, J.A., Huppler, R.E., Gilbert, P.E.: The effects of morphine- and nalorphine-like drugs in the nondependent and morphine-dependent chronic spinal dog. J. Pharmacol. Exp. Ther. *197*, 517–532 (1976)

McKearney, J.W.: Effects of *d*-amphetamine, morphine, and chlorpromazine on responding under fixed-interval schedules of food presentation or electric shock presentation. J. Pharmacol. Exp. Ther. *190*, 141–153 (1974)

McKearney, J.W.: Effects of morphine, methadone, nalorphine and naloxone on responding under fixed-interval (FI) schedules in the squirrel monkey. Fed. Proc. *34*, 766 (1975)

McMillan, D.E., Morse, W.H.: Some effects of morphine and morphine antagonists on schedule-controlled behavior. J. Pharmacol. Exp. Ther. *157*, 175–184 (1967)

McMillan, D.E., Wolf, P.S., Carchman, R.A.: Antagonism of the behavioral effects of morphine and methadone by narcotic antagonists in the pigeon. J. Pharmacol. Exp. Ther. *175*, 443–458 (1970)

McMillan, D.E., Harris, L.S.: Behavioral and morphine-antagonist effects of the optical isomers of pentazocine and cyclazocine. J. Pharmacol. Exp. Ther. *180*, 569–579 (1972)

McMillan, D.E.: Drugs and punished responding. I: Rate-dependent effects under multiple schedules. J. Exp. Anal. Behav. *19*, 133–145 (1973 a)

McMillan, D.E.: Drugs and punished responding. III. Punishment intensity as a determinant of drug effect. Psychopharmacology *30*, 61–74 (1973 b)

McMillan, D.E.: Determinants of drug effects on punished responding. Fed. Proc. *34*, 1870–1879 (1975)

Mello, N.K., Mendelson, J.H.: Buprenorphine suppresses heroin use by heroin addicts. Science *207*, 657–659 (1980)

Meyer, D.R., Sparber, S.B.: Evidence of possible opiate dependence during the behavioral depressant action of a single dose of morphine. Life Sci. *21*, 1087–1094 (1977)

Miller, R.R.: Evaluation of nalbuphine hydrochloride. Am. J. Hosp. Pharm. *37*, 942–949 (1980)
Morse, W.H.: Intermittent reinforcement. In: Operant behavior: Areas of research and application. Honig, W.K. (ed.), pp. 52–108. New York: Appleton-Century-Crofts 1966
Morse, W.H., Kelleher, R.T.: Schedules using noxious stimuli. I. Multiple fixed-ratio and fixed-interval termination of schedule complexes. J. Exp. Anal. Behav. *9*, 267–290 (1966)
Morse, W.H., Kelleher, R.T.: Schedules as fundamental determinants of behavior. In: The theory of reinforcement schedules. Schoenfeld, W.N. (ed.), pp. 139–185. New York: Appleton-Century-Crofts 1970
Morse, W.H., Kelleher, R.T.: Determinants of reinforcement and punishment. In: Operant behavior. Honig, W.K., Staddon, J.E.R. (eds.), pp. 174–200. New York: Prentice Hall 1977
Morse, W.H., McKearney, J.W., Kelleher, R.T.: Control of behavior by noxious stimuli. In: Handbook of psychopharmacology, principles of behavioral pharmacology. Iversen, L.L., Iversen, S.D., Snyder, S.H. (eds.), pp. 151–180. New York: Plenum Press 1977
Nevin, J.A.: The maintenance of behavior. In: The study of behavior: Learning, motivation, emotion and instinct. Nevin, J.A., Reynolds, G.S. (eds.), pp. 201–236. Glenville, Ill.: Scott, Foresman 1973
Nichols, J.R., Headlee, C.P., Coppock, H.W.: Drug addiction. I. Addiction by escape training. J.Am. Pharm. Ass. (Sci. Ed.) *45*, 788–791 (1956)
Orahovats, P.D., Winter, L.A., Lehman, E.G.: The effect of N-allylnormorphine upon the development of tolerance to morphine in the albino rat. J. Pharmacol. Exp. Ther. *109*, 413–416 (1953)
Overton, D.A., Batta, S.K.: Investigation of narcotics and antitussives using drug discrimination techniques. J. Pharmacol. Exp. Ther. *211*, 401–408 (1979)
Pachter, I.J.: Synthetic 14-hydroxymorphinan narcotic antagonists. In: Narcotic antagonists. Adv. Biochem. Psychopharmacol. *8*, 57–62 (1974)
Rachlin, H., Loveland, D.: Titration of punishment. Psychon. Sci. Sect. Anim. *22*, 39–40 (1971)
Rachlin, H.: Response control with titration of punishment. J. Exp. Anal. Behav. *17*, 147–157 (1972)
Rethy, C.R., Smith, C.B., Villarreal, J.E.: Effects of narcotic analgesics upon the locomotor activity and brain catecholamine content of the mouse. J. Pharmacol. Exp. Ther. *176*, 472–479 (1971)
Rhodus, D.M., Elsmore, T.F., Manning, F.J.: Morphine and heroin effects on multiple fixed-interval schedule performance in rats. Psychopharmacology *40*, 147–155 (1974)
Rosecrans, J.A., Goodloe, M.H., Bennett, G.J., Hirschhorn, I.: Morphine as a discriminative cue: Effects of amine depletors and naloxone. Eur. J. Pharmacol. *21*, 252–256 (1973)
Rosecrans, J.A., Chance, W.T., Spencer, R.M.: The discriminative stimulus properties of cyclazocine: Generalization studies involving nalorphine, morphine and LSD. Res. Commun. Chem. Path. Pharmacol. *20*, 221–237 (1978)
Sanchez-Ramos, J.R., Schuster, C.R.: Second-order schedules of intravenous drug self-administration in rhesus monkeys. Pharmacol. Biochem. Behav. *7*, 443–450 (1977)
Schaefer, G.J., Holtzman, S.G.: Discriminative effects of morphine in the squirrel monkey. J. Pharmacol. Exp. Ther. *201*, 67–75 (1977)
Schaefer, G.J., Holtzman, S.G.: Discriminative effects of cyclazocine in the squirrel monkey. J. Pharmacol. Exp. Ther. *205*, 291–301 (1978)
Schulz, R., Wurster, M., Herz, A.: Supersensitivity to opioids following the chronic blockade of endorphin action by naloxone. Naunyn-Schmiedebergs Arch. Pharmacol. *306*, 93–96 (1979)
Schuster, C.R.: Variables affecting the self-administration of drugs by rhesus monkeys. In: Use of nonhuman primates in drug evaluation. Vagtborg, H. (ed.), pp. 283–299. Austin-London: University of Texas Press 1968
Shannon, H.E., Holtzman, S.G.: Evaluation of the discriminative effects of morphine in the rat. J. Pharmacol. Exp. Ther. *198*, 54–65 (1976a)
Shannon, H.E., Holtzmann, S.G.: Blockade of the discriminative effects of morphine in the rat by naltrexone and naloxone. Psychopharmacology *50*, 119–124 (1976b)
Shannon, H.E., Holtzman, S.G.: Further evaluation of the discriminative effects of morphine in the rat. J. Pharmacol. Exp. Ther. *201*, 55–66 (1977)
Shannon, H.E., Holtzman, S.G.: Morphine training dose: A determinant of stimulus generalization to narcotic antagonists in the rat. Psychopharmacology *61*, 239–244 (1979)

Sidman, M.: Avoidance conditioning with brief shock and no exteroceptive warning stimulus. Science *118*, 157–158 (1953)
Skinner, B.F.: Two types of conditioned reflex: a reply to Konorski and Miller. J. Gen. Psychol. *16*, 272–279 (1937)
Skinner, B.F.: The behavior of organisms. New York: Appleton-Century-Crofts 1938
Smith, G.M., Beecher, H.K.: Measurement of "mental clouding" and other subjective effects of morphine. J. Pharmacol. Exp. Ther. *126*, 50–62 (1959)
Smith, G.M., Beecher, H.K.: Subjective effects of heroin and morphine in normal subjects. J. Pharmacol. Exp. Ther. *136*, 47–52 (1962)
Smith, G.M., Semke, C.W., Beecher, H.K.: Objective evidence of mental effects of heroin, morphine and placebo in normal subjects. J. Pharmacol. Exp. Ther. *136*, 53–58 (1962)
Smith, J.B., McKearney, J.W.: Effects of morphine, methadone, nalorphine and naloxone on responding under schedules of electric shock titration. J. Pharmacol. Exp. Ther. *200*, 508–515 (1977)
Smith, J.B.: Prevention by naltrexone of tolerance to the rate-decreasing effects of morphine on schedule-controlled responding in the pigeon. Psychopharmacologia *63*, 49–54 (1979)
Snyder, S.H., Simantov, R.: The opiate receptor and opioid peptides. J. Neurochem. *28*, 13–20 (1977)
Sparber, S.B., Gellert, G.F., Lichtblau, L., Eisenberg, R.: The use of operant behavioral methods to study aggression and effects of acute and chronic morphine administration in rats. In: Factors affecting the action of narcotics. Adler, M.W., Mahara, L., Samanin, R. (eds.), pp. 63–91. New York: Raven Press 1978
Spealman, R.D., Goldberg, S.R., Kelleher, R.T., Morse, N.H., Goldberg, D.M., Hakansson, C.G., Nieferth, K.A., Lazer, E.S.: Effects of norcocaine and some norcocaine derivatives on schedule-controlled behavior of pigeons and squirrel monkeys. J. Pharmacol. Exp. Ther. *210*, 196–205 (1979 a)
Spealman, R.D., Kelleher, R.T., Goldberg, D.M., Goldberg, S.R., Hakansson, C.G.: Supersensitivity to the behavioral effects of naloxone and naltrexone after chronic administration in rhesus monkeys, squirrel monkeys and rats. Fed. Proc. *38*, 741 (1979 b)
Spealman, R.D., Kelleher, R.T., Morse, W.H., Goldberg, S.R.: Supersensitivity to the behavioral effects of opiate antagonists. Psychopharmacol. Bull. *17*, 54–56 (1981)
Spragg, S.D.S.: Morphine addiction in chimpanzees. Comparative psychology monographs, Vol. 15, No. 7, Ser. 79. Baltimore: Johns Hopkins Press 1940
Tallarida, R.J., Jacob, L.S.: Dose-response relation in pharmacology. New York: Springer 1979
Tang, A.H., Morse, W.H.: Termination of a schedule complex associated with intravenous injections of nalorphine in morphine-dependent rhesus monkeys. Pharmacol. Rev. *27*, 407–417 (1975)
Tang, A.H., Collins, R.J.: Enhanced analgesic effects of morphine after chronic administration of naloxone in the rat. Eur. J. Pharmacol. *47*, 473–474 (1978)
Teal, J.J., Holtzman, S.G.: Stimulus effects of morphine in the monkey: Quantitative analysis of antagonism. Pharmacol. Biochem. Behav. *12*, 587–593 (1980 a)
Teal, J.J., Holtzman, S.G.: Discriminative stimulus effects of cyclazocine in the rat. J. Pharmacol. Exp. Ther. *212*, 368–376 (1980 b)
Terenius, L.: Endogenous peptides and analgesia. Ann. Rev. Pharmacol. Toxicol. *18*, 189–204 (1978)
Terrace, H.S.: Stimulus control. In: Operant behavior: Areas of research and application. Honig, W.K. (ed.), pp. 271–344. Englewood Cliffs, N.J.: Prentice-Hall, Inc. 1966
Thompson, T., Schuster, C.R.: Morphine self-administration, food-reinforced and avoidance behaviors in rhesus monkeys. Psychopharmacology *5*, 87–94 (1964)
Thompson, T., Trombley, J., Luke, D., Lott, D.: Effects of morphine on behavior maintained by four simple food-reinforcement schedules. Psychopharmacology *17*, 182–192 (1970)
Tsou, K.: Effects of morphine upon several types of operant conditionings in the rat. Acta Physiol. Sinica *26*, 143–150 (1963)
Verhave, T., Owen, J.E., Jr., Robbins, E.B.: The effect of morphine sulfate on avoidance and escape behavior. J. Pharmacol. Exp. Ther. *125*, 248–251 (1959)
Villarreal, J.E., Karbowski, M.G.: The actions of narcotic antagonists in morphine-dependent rhesus monkeys. In: Narcotic antagonists. Adv. Biochem. Psychopharmacol. *8*, 273–289 (1974)

Weeks, J.R.: Experimental morphine addiction: Method for autonomic intravenous injections in unrestrained rats. Science *138*, 143–144 (1962)

Weeks, J.R., Collins, R.J.: Factors affecting voluntary morphine intake in self-maintained addicted rats. Psychopharmacology *6*, 267–279 (1964)

Weiss, B., Laties, V.G.: Titration behavior on various fractional escape programs. J. Exp. Anal. Behav. *2*, 227–248 (1959)

Weiss, B., Laties, V.G.: Changes in pain tolerance and other behavior produced by salicylates. J. Pharmacol. Exp. Ther. *131*, 120–129 (1961)

Weiss, B., Laties, V.G.: Analgesic effects in monkeys of morphine, nalorphine and a benzomorphan narcotic antagonist. J. Pharmacol. Exp. Ther. *143*, 169–173 (1964)

Weissman, A.: Differential drug effects upon a three-ply multiple schedule of reinforcement. J. Exp. Anal. Behav. *2*, 271–287 (1959)

Winter, J.C.: The stimulus properties of morphine and ethanol. Psychopharmacology *44*, 209–214 (1975)

Woods, J.H., Schuster, C.R.: Reinforcement properties of morphine, cocaine, and SPA as a function of unit dose. Int. J. Addict. *3*, 231–237 (1968)

Woods, J.H., Schuster, C.R.: Opiates as reinforcing stimuli. In: Stimulus properties of drugs. Thompson, T., Pickens, R. (eds.), pp. 163–175. New York: Appleton-Century-Crofts 1971

Woods, J.H., Downs, D.A., Villarreal, J.E.: Changes in operant behavior during deprivation- and antagonist-induced withdrawal states. In: Psychic dependence, Bayer-Symposium IV. Goldberg, L., Hoffmeister, F. (eds.), pp. 114–121. Berlin, Heidelberg, New York: Springer 1973

Woods, J.H., Carney, J.: Narcotic tolerance and operant behavior. In: Behavioral tolerance: Research and treatment implications. NIDA Res. Monog. No. 18. Krasnegor, N.A. (ed.), pp. 54–66. Washington, D.C.: U.S. Government Printing Office 1978

Woods, J.H., Herling, S., Valentino, R.J., Hein, D.W., Coale, E.H.: Narcotic drug discriminations by rhesus monkeys and pigeons. In: Proceedings of the 41st Annual Scientific Meeting, The Committee on Problems of Drug Dependence, Inc. Ed. by Harris, L.S., NIDA Res. Monog. No. 27, pp. 128–134, U.S. Government Printing Office, Washington, D.C., 1980

Yamahiro, R.S., Bell, E.C., Hill, H.E.: The effect of reserpine on a strongly conditioned emotional response. Psychopharmacology *2*, 197–202 (1961)

Zeiler, M.: Schedules of reinforcement: The controlling variables. In: Handbook of operant behavior. Honig, W.K., Staddon, J.E.R. (eds.), pp. 201–232. Englewood Cliffs, N.J.: Prentice-Hall 1977

CHAPTER 14

Hypnotics

W. R. MARTIN

A. Hypnotics and Sleep Disorders

The general concept of hypnotic drugs is a vague one. Hypnotics alter the function of many parts of the brain which results not only in the more rapid onset and persistence of sleep, but changes in levels of consciousness, arousability, and mood, as well as in cognitive and motor function. Furthermore, most hypnotics have been subject to abuse, induce tolerance, and produce or satisfy dependencies. In general, hypnotics are used to treat patients who complain of sleep disorders which are commonly associated with discomforting anxieties or emotional and psychic trauma. Thus, the treatment of sleep disorders cannot be dissociated from the treatment of anxiety and affective disorders. Approximately one-fifth to one-third of the general population has sleep disorders (BIXLER et al., 1976). At one time or another, 85% of patients complaining of sleep disorders have psychopathology as indicated by abnormal Minnesota Multiphasic Personality Inventory (MMPI) profiles (KALES and KALES, 1974).

The characterization of sleep disorders has been recently reviewed by SOLDATOS et al. (1979). The most common sleep disorder is staying asleep followed in frequency by difficulties in falling asleep and early wakening (KALES et al., 1974). This characterization of sleep disorders should provide guidance in the use of hypnotics, particularly as it relates to their duration of action. Insomnia is associated with a variety of other pathologies including depression, anxieties, suffering, fear, pain and discomfort associated with other illnesses, sociopathy, obsessive-compulsive characteristics, and schizophrenia. Sleep problems become more prevalent in the elderly, who are especially subject to loss of self-image, depression, and feelings of anxiety.

A variety of drugs can cause insomnia, including caffeine in coffee, tea and colas, as well as amphetamine-type bronchodilators and anorexigenics (amphetamine, methamphetamine, ephedrine, phenmetrazine, methylphenidate). Despite enormous increases in knowledge about the neurophysiology and neurochemistry of sleep, the treatment of insomnia remains empiric as does therapeutic research. Although, some causes of sleep disorders can be dealt with definitively, such as excessive ingestion of caffeine and amphetamines by limiting ingestion, the treatment of depression with antidepressants or the treatment of schizophrenia with tranquilizers, most patients

---

This effort was partially supported by a grant from the National Institute of Drug Abuse DA 02195-01.

List of Abbreviations

ACh Acetylcholine, DA Dopamine, DLH dl Homocysteic acid, EPSP Excitatory postsynaptic potential, GABA γ Aminobutyric acid, IPSP Inhibitory postsynaptic potential, MDR Maximum depression rating, NE Norepinephrine

must be treated with a variety of hypnotics that have been introduced into clinical medicine. Although knowledge about sleep is developing at a rapid rate, its physiologic significance is not well understood and is a complex phenomenon.

Electroencephalographic and physiologic studies have revealed that sleep has several stages. Stage 1 is characterized by loss of alpha activity; stage 2 by spindles and K-complexes; stage 3 by spindles and delta rhythms; stage 4 by 50% delta rhythms in the absence of spindles; and rapid eye movement sleep (REMS). The effects of hypnotics on these stages of sleep can be measured in a variety of ways (see KAY et al., 1976), including time spent in waking state, delta sleep, and REM sleep as well as time of total sleep and sleep latency. The physiologic and pathologic significance of these measurements as well as the therapeutic implications of altering these measures is not known. This is in part a consequence of the lack of understanding of the physiologic significance of sleep. There are several excellent collections of articles dealing with various facets of sleep (WEITZMAN, 1974; KETY et al., 1967; LEVIN and KOELLA, 1975; WILLIAMS and KARACAN, 1976). It is known that severe sleep deprivation can alter affect and produce emotional lability, deterioration of intellectual processes, and possibly psychotic states. Selective deprivation of REMS also causes irritability, anxiety, difficulties in concentrating, and REMS rebound (DEMENT, 1960). One of the theories of sleep is that it is a resting state which allows the recuperation of neurons. Several lines of evidence indicate that this is at best an oversimplification. Not only is sleep a complex phenomena, but active processes are also involved. Further, there is little difference in oxygen consumption between the wakening and sleeping brain (MANGOLD et al., 1955).

Many advances have been made in the neurophysiology and neurochemistry of sleep. Detailed accounts and summaries of some of these important areas of research can be found in the previously mentioned volumes. JOUVET (1966) has proposed that a serotoninergic process involving raphe nuclei mediates slow wave sleep while catecholaminergic processes of the locus ceruleus mediate the atonia of paradoxical sleep (REMS). Other transmitters or processes may also be involved in REMS (RAMM, 1979). Rapid eye movements and pontogeniculate occipital (PGO) spikes may be modulated by both catecholaminergic and serotoninergic influences. Consciousness is also viewed as an active process, and the concept of MAGOUN and MORRUZZI (1949) (see D. III) of a rostrally projecting midbrain activating system which in turn is acted upon by both collateral ascending sensory pathways and corticofugal activity is still heuristic.

Currently the sleep-wakeful cycle is regarded as an instinctual adaptive mechanism and as a need in its own right and that both sleep and wakefulness are active processes. The alternation from one state to another results also in reciprocal sparing of their brain substrates. A variety of neurohumoral processes may be involved in waking (dopaminergic, noradrenergic, cholinergic) and in sleep (serotoninergic, noradrenergic, GABAergic). Recent observations suggest that there may be endogenous brain sleep-producing substances, possibly polypeptides (MONNIER and HOSLI, 1964; MONNIER et al., 1974; NAGASAKI et al., 1974; PAPPENHEIMER et al., 1974; PAPPENHEIMER et al., 1975; KRUEGER et al., 1978). These observations, taken with the recent observations that there are benzodiazepine receptors which may have central nervous system activity in their own right or which modulate GABAergic activity, suggest that the brain may have special synaptic systems involved in sleep processes.

Despite these elegant advances, they have not thus far been helpful in delineating pathologic processes responsible for insomnia nor in the development of therapeutic measures for treating insomnia. In part, this may be a consequence of the fact that much of sleep research has been aimed at characterizing sleep and establishing norms. Many of the adverse consequences of insomnia are related to unpleasant feelings and socially maladjusted behavior which in turn also has affective consequences.

B. Commonly Used Hypnotics

Some of the drugs commonly employed as hypnotics are summarized in Table 1; this table presents only a small portion of the drugs that have been used as hypnotics. Omitted are the atropine-like anticholinergics, antihistaminics, all benzodiazepines except flurazepam, which has earned a unique reputation as a hypnotic, and the monoureides.

I. Barbiturates

Pentobarbital, butabarbital, secobarbital, and amobarbital are most commonly classified as short to intermediate in duration of action. Their plasma half-lives range from 12 to over 40 h. The half-time of the pharmacologic actions of pentobarbital and secobarbital, administered intramuscularly, as measured by their ability to produce subjective changes and enhance the frequency and prolong the duration of post-rational nystagmus, is in excess of 5 h and probably about 12 h (JASINSKI, 1973; MARTIN et al., 1974; FRASER and JASINSKI, 1977). Phenobarbital, a long-acting barbiturate, has a plasma half-life of 24–96 h, while the half-time for its effects on subjective effects and post-rational nystagmus when administerd intramuscularly is also about 12 h. However, effects were seen several days after its administration (FRASER and JASINSKI, 1977).

The effects of barbiturates on sleep have been most intensively studied of all types of hypnotics (KAY et al., 1976). The consensus of findings indicate that, when barbi-

Table 1. Commonly used hypnotics[a]

Barbiturates	Benzodiazepines
Secobarbital, Na (100 mg)	Flurazepam (15–30 mg)
Pentobarbital, Na (100 mg)	Piperidinediones
Butabarbital, Na (50–100 mg)	Glutethimide (250–500 mg)
Amobarbital, Na (65–200 mg)	Methyprylon (200–400 mg)
Phenobarbital (100–300 mg)	Carbamates
Chloral derivatives	Ethinamate (500–1 000 mg)
Chloral Hydrate (500–1 000 mg)	Meprobamate
Chloral Betaine (870–1 700 mg)	Others
Triclofos, Na (1 500 mg)	Methaqualone (150–400 mg)
	Ethchlorvynol (500–1 000mg)
	Paraldehyde (5–10 ml)

[a] Figures in parentheses indicate commonly employed therapeutic doses

turates are administered occasionally for sleep, they decrease the latency of sleep onset and the number of body movements during sleep while increasing total sleep time, spindle sleep, and drowsiness (see KAY et al., 1976, for primary references). Barbiturates also decrease REMS by increasing the latency to onset and decreasing the number and duration of REM episodes. These changes are more profound during the early part of the night than later. Most of the literature suggests that these changes are dose related (KAY et al., 1972); however, many studies of the effects of barbiturates on sleep were aimed at determining the effects of therapeutic dose and not for determining dose-response relationship. When barbiturates are administered chronically, tolerance develops to their ability to facilitate sleep. Thus, OGUNREMI et al., (1973) found that chronic administration of various dose levels of amobarbital (137.5–550 mg/day) resulted in tolerance to its ability to decrease restlessness, and when the administration of amobarbital was terminated, REMS and delta sleep were increased as were plasma levels of growth hormone. KALES et al. (1975) administered pentobarbital (100 mg nightly) for 4 weeks and found that total wakefulness and delta sleep returned to the baseline level, although total awakening remained decreased. No change in REMS occurred.

It has been established that therapeutic doses of pentobarbital, secobarbital, and amobarbital (see KAY et al., 1976, and Table 1) produce significant effects on sleep. Further, the effects of pentobarbital on sleep are dose related (KAY et al., 1972), and it may be presumed that a dose-dependent effect exists for other barbiturate. There is a large variability in the effects of barbiturates on sleep between patients. Thus, examination of data (KAY et al. 1972) on the suppression of REMS shows that there was a two- to threefold difference in effect between subjects. This degree of variability between patients has also been seen in the effect of pentobarbital on subjective state and postrotational nystagmus (MARTIN, unpublished observations, 1962). This large variability in response to barbiturates should be taken into consideration in selecting the dose. The dose should be adjusted to achieve the desired therapeutic effect. Flexibility of dose probably can be best achieved using elixirs.

II. Chloral Hydrate

Chloral hydrate is the oldest of the hypnotics whose popularity has waxed and waned since its introduction. Both it and its metabolite, trichlorethanol, readily enter the brain and are active in altering the EEG (GRUNER et al., 1973). Chloral hydrate is irritating to the mucosa and may cause indigestion, nausea, and vomiting if taken on an empty stomach. Trichlorethanol is also irritating and suffers from the further disadvantage that it is a liquid. Chloral, in addition to being hydrated to yield chloral hydrate, has also been prepared as the phosphate (triclofos) and the betaine (chloral betaine) ester. These forms also are degraded in vivo to yield trichlorethanol and are thought to be therapeutically equivalent to chloral hydrate.

Chloral hydrate in doses of 500–1500 mg, according to several investigators, failed to alter any sleep parameter when recovery nights were interspersed between doses (KALES et al., 1970a; LEHMANN and BAY 1968; JOVANOVIC, 1974). On the other hand, when chloral hydrate was administered nightly in doses of 500–1000 mg, sleep latency was decreased and total sleep increased (KALES et al., 1970b; HARTMANN and CRA-

VENS, 1975). By and large, most investigators have found that REMS is not markedly altered by chloral hydrate even in the presence of decreased sleep latency and an increase in total sleep, drowsiness, and spindle sleep.

III. Benzodiazepines

Perhaps no other group of hypnotics role in the treatment of sleep disorders is as arbitrary as that of the benzodiazepines. Flurazepam is employed as a hypnotic while most of the other benzodiazepines are employed as sedatives and antianxiety drugs. Certainly, when anxiety is a major cause of insomnia, its treatment will facilitate sleep.

A fairly extensive literature indicates that flurazepam increases total sleep time and spindle sleep, decreases sleep latency and delta sleep, and may produce some depression of REMS which is not usually associated with REMS rebound when it is stopped (see review by KAY et al., 1976). Flurazepam does not seem to differ to a significant degree from other benzodiazepines with regard to its effects on various stages of sleep except that it may have a greater effect on REMS than diazepam or chlordiazepoxide.

IV. Piperidinediones

1. Glutethimide

Glutethimide is a highly lypophilic drug which is erratically absorbed from the gastrointestinal tract. Therapeutic and twice therapeutic dose levels have been shown to decrease REMS, but have little effect on other sleep parameters.

2. Methyprylon

The effects of methyprylon on sleep are similar to those of glutethimide.

V. Carbamates

1. Ethinamate

Although ethinamate is employed as a hypnotic, its effect on sleep stages does not appear to have been studied. It is a carbamic acid ester that has a rapid onset and a short duration of action. Because of this property, it is thought to be especially useful in the treatment of insomniacs who have difficulty in falling asleep.

2. Meprobamate

Meprobamate is a carbamic acid ester of propanediol not used primarily as a hypnotic, but most commonly for treatment of anxieties and related states. Dose levels of 800–1200 mg produce modest decreases in REMS and increase spindle sleep, but do not appear to alter other sleep parameters. In a comparison of meprobamate and pentobarbital in addict subjects, meprobamate was found to be $^{1}/_{10}$–$^{1}/_{17}$ as potent as pentobarbital in increasing the frequency of postrotational nystagmus and producing signs of sleepiness and relaxation (MCCLANE and MARTIN, 1976).

VI. Methaqualone

Methaqualone has a very complicated pharmacology. In addition to its hypnotic effects,it has antitussive, anticonvulsant, local anesthetic, and antispasmodic activity. It produces delirium, hyperactive reflexes, and convulsions in large doses. Methaqualone in a dose of 150 mg has liminal effects on sleep, while 300 mg decreases REMS and delta sleep.

VII. Ethchlorvynol

Ethchlorvynol is reported to have a rapid onset and short duration of action. Its effect on sleep does not seem to have been studied.

VIII. Paraldehyde

Paraldehyde, a cyclic polymer of acetaldehyde, is an unstable liquid with a strong characteristic odor and unpleasant taste. Its effects on sleep have not been studied.

C. Mode of Action of Hypnotics

The mode of action of barbiturates has been more thoroughly studied than that of any other group of hypnotics. The literature on their mode of action has been recently reviewed (SMITH, 1977; NICOLL, 1978) to which the interested reader is referred for many primary references. The issue of the mode of action of barbiturates is a complex one which cannot be divorced from their site of action in producing sleep. In anesthetic doses, pentobarbital depresses transmission at the myoneural junction (see below), the sympathetic ganglion (LARRABEE and POSTERNAK, 1952), spinal cord mono- and polysynaptic reflexes (ECCLES, 1946; BROOKS and ECCLES, 1947; LÖYNING et al., 1964; SHAPOVALOV, 1963; WEAKLY, 1969), cuneate nucleus (GALINDO, 1969; POLC and HAEFELY, 1976), and olfactory bulb and cortex (RICHARDS, 1972; SCHOLFIELD and HARVEY, 1975). Whether the effects of very large doses of hypnotics that produce anesthesia are related to hypnotic effects cannot be answered. Certainly, hypnosis should not be considered a liminal anesthetic state.

Even the concept of hypnosis is difficult to operationally define in animals (see GOGERTY, 1976). The cat, which is most commonly used for electrophysiologic and neuropharmacologic studies, normally spends over two-thirds of the time sleeping. In the succinylcholine immobilized cat, which shows predominantly an activated EEG, 4 mg/kg of pentobarbital produces a significant increase in δ and α EEG activity (MARTIN and EADES, 1960). The definition of a hypnotic dose in man is equally difficult. Thus, KAY et al. (1972), who studied the effects of 75, 150, and 300 mg (ca. 1, 2 and 4 mg/kg) of pentobarbital in man found a dose-related decrease in REMS and increase in stage 2 sleep. No dose-related changes in time awake or in drowsy or δ sleep during a standard sleep night were observed. Accepting an ill-defined hypnotic dose of pentobarbital as 1–4 mg/kg in cat and man may place some of the following observations in perspective.

I. Excitatory Processes

1. Acetylcholine

Pentobarbital decreases the depolarizing effect of acetylcholine (ACh) at the myoneural junction as well as the inward and outward flow of membrane currents (SEYAMA and NARAHASHI, 1975). ADAMS (1976) argues that barbiturates block the active ACh channel converter. NICOLL and IWAMOTO (1978) in an extensive analysis of the actions of pentobarbital on the frog lumbar sympathetic ganglion found (1) that the fast excitatory postsynaptic potential (EPSP) was the most sensitive to the depressant action of pentobarbital; (2) that EPSPs evoked by the iontophoretic application of carbachol were depressed to the same extent as those evoked by nerve stimulation; (3) that the number of quanta of ACh released was not changed by pentobarbital; and (4) that pentobarbital depolarized presynaptic nerve terminal and that the depolarization was antagonized by picrotoxin.

Pentobarbital decreases spontaneous firing of as well as firing evoked by the iontophoretic application of ACh to neurons in the pericruciate (CATCHLOVE et al., 1972; CRAWFORT and CURTIS, 1966) and prepiriform (SMAJE, 1976) cortices as well as the thalamus (PHILLIS and TEBECIS, 1967). There is no concurrence as to whether the action of pentobarbital and other barbiturates on ACh depolarizing and stimulating action is selective. Although some investigators have found selective depression of ACh stimulation by barbiturates (PHILLIS and TEBECIS, 1967), others have not (CRAWFORD and CURTIS, 1966). CRAWFORT and CURTIS (1966) and CRAWFORD (1970) found that whereas intravenously administered pentobarbital was equieffective in depressing both ACh and dl-homocysteic acid (DLH) stimulation of cortical neurons, pentobarbital administered iontophoretically was more effective in antagonizing DLH than ACh stimulation. This observation, taken with the observation of JOHNSON et al. (1969) that the percentage of sigmoid cortex neurons excited by the iontophoretic application of ACh was the same in pentobarbital-anesthetized cats and unanesthetized *encephale isolé* cats, raises the question as to whether the depressant action of barbiturates on the responsivity of cortical neurons to ACh is a consequence of an indirect action.

2. NE

Pentobarbital tends to antagonize the excitatory effects of NE and other α agonists. Doses of less than 5 mg/kg prevent methoxamine from evoking the stepping reflex in the chronic spinal dog (MARTIN, unpublished observation, 1967). JOHNSON et al. (1969) found that pentobarbital anesthesia (25 mg/kg) decreased the number of sigmoid cortex neurons that were exited by NE. The percentage of neurons inhibited by NE was increased in pentobarbital-anesthetized cats.

3. Serotonin

In the pentobarbital anesthetized cat, fewer sigmoid cortex neurones were stimulated by serotonin (5HT) and more were depressed by 5HT than in the *encéphale isolé* cat.

4. Glutamate

Pentobarbital depressed the depolarizing effect of glutamate on tissue cultured mouse spinal cord neurons (RANSOM and BARKER, 1975).

II. Inhibitory Processes

The actions of hypnotic and barbiturate on neuronal inhibitory processes have not been studied as thoroughly as their actions on excitatory processes nor are they as easily studied. It is known that barbiturates and benzodiazepines do alter inhibitory process and the identification of brain benzodiazepine binding sites (see Chap. HAEFELY et al.) has opened new ways of thinking about the mode of action of hypnotics.

1. Postsynaptic Inhibition

LARSON and MAJOR (1970) found that hexobarbital prolonged the duration of inhibitory postsynaptic potentials (IPSPs) evoked in unanesthetized decerebrate cat motoneurons by recurrent stimulation. Similarly, IPSPs evoked in hippocampal neurons of pentobarbital and halothane- and NO_2-anesthetized cats were similarly prolonged by pentobarbital (ca. 15–33 mg/kg) (NICOLL et al., 1975). NICOLL (1972) also found that pentobarbital prolonged the IPSPs of mitral cells of the olfactory bulb. SCHOLFIELD (1978) studied the effects of pentobarbital on the guinea pig olfactory cortex and found that IPSPs were prolonged and enhanced (0.02–1.0 m*M*). Lower concentrations did not change resting membrane conductance. POLC and HAEFELY (1976) found that phenobarbital, diazepam, and flunitrazepam increase GABA-mediated postsynaptic inhibition in cuneate nucleus of the decerebrate cat.

2. Presynaptic Inhibition

ECCLES et al. (1963), in their important study which implicated GABA in presynaptic inhibitions and picrotoxin as its antagonist, found that pentobarbital in anesthetic doses, as well as chloralosane and thiamylal, increased, enhanced, and prolonged indirect inhibition as well as the dorsal root potential in the cat (also ECCLES and MALCOLM, 1946). This later finding was confirmed by SCHMIDT (1963) in toads. Pentobarbital, like GABA, depolarizes primary afferents of the frog, and this effect was blocked by picrotoxin and bicuculline (NICOLL, 1975). NICOLL (1975) concludes that this action of pentobarbital decreases the amount of excitatory transmitter released. Other barbiturate and anesthetics as well as chloral hydrate enhance presynaptic inhibition (MIYAHARA et al., 1966). Pentobarbital and phenobarbital increase presynaptic inhibition in the caudate (BANNA and JABBUR, 1969; POLC and HAEFELY, 1976).

3. γ-Aminobutyric Acid (GABA)

The profound influences of hypnotics and related drugs on inhibitory processes suggested that one of their modes of action was to increase endogenous inhibitory processes. Study of interactions of hypnotics, anesthetics, and minor tranquilizers with GABAergic processes has been a particularly active area of investigation. Barbiturates enhance and prolong both GABA-mediated pre- and postsynaptic inhibitory potentials (see C.II.1. and 2.). In addition, several investigators have shown that pentobarbital enhances recurrent inhibition in the hippocampus (WOLF and HAAS, 1977; TSUCHIYA and FUKUSHIMA, 1978). Studying isolated cultured neurons, RANSOM and BARKER (1975) found that pentobarbital prolonged the effect of GABA without altering GABA's ability to decrease membrane resistance.

Although pentobarbital markedly enhances GABA-mediated inhibition, it does not appear to prevent the binding of GABA to Na^{+}-independent saturable GABA binding sites in the brain and/or spinal cord of frogs (ENNA and SNYDER, 1977) or the rat brain (OLSEN et al., 1977). However, pentobarbital as well as other anticonvulsant and convulsant barbiturates do competitively antagonize the saturable binding of radiolabeled dihydropicrotoxinin to rat brain homogenates (TICKU and OLSEN, 1978).

III. Release of Neurotransmitters

Pentobarbital inhibits the uptake of Ca^{++} by rat brain synaptosome in the presence of K^{+}, veratridine, or gramacidin D (BLAUSTEIN and ECTOR, 1975). HAYCOCK et al. (1977) have shown that pentobarbital depressed synaptosomal release of NE and GABA in the presence of CA^{++}, K^{+}, and veratridine.

IV. Stereoisomers of Barbiturates

The stereoisomers of pentobarbital as well as other barbiturates differ in potency as well as in pharmacologic activity. WADDEL and BAGGETT (1973) found that the S(−)-isomer of pentobarbital was more potent than the R(+)-isomer in producing anesthesia. Furthermore, the S(−) isomer produced a smooth anesthesia while the R(+)-isomer produced a syndrome of excitement and jumping before the induction of anesthesia. The R(+)-isomer of methylphenobarbital also produces excitation (BUCH et al., 1969). CHRISTENSEN and LEE (1973) compared the lethality of the R(+)- and S(−)-isomers and the racemic mixtures of pentobarbital, secobarbital, thiopental, and thioamylal in the rat by both the intraperitoneal and intravenous route and found the S(−)-isomer about twice as potent as the R(+)-isomer while the racemic mixture had an intermediate potency. HALEY and GIDLEY (1970) found that the S(−)-isomer of secobarbital was twice as potent as the R(+)-isomer in producing sleep in mice, although both isomers were equieffective in antagonizing strychnine and pentylenetetrazole seizures. Although the R(+)-isomers are metabolized more rapidly than the S(−)-isomers (BUCH et al., 1970), brain levels of the R(+)- and S(−)-isomers are the same (FREUDENTHAL and MARTIN, 1975). The R(+)-isomer of hexobarbital has a more rapid onset and is more potent, but has a shorter duration of action than the S(−)-isomer (WAHLSTROM, 1966; FURNER et al., 1969).

D. Site of Action

I. Spinal Cord

Pentobarbital and other hypnotics are known to depress spinal cord reflexes. WIKLER (1945), and ESPLIN (1963) observed that pentobarbital depressed the mono- and polysynaptic segmental reflex of the cat. HOUDE and WIKLER (1951) and HOUDE et al. (1951) demonstrated that pentobarbital (21–30 mg/kg) and thiopental (21–60 mg/kg) depressed the patellar, extensor thrust, flexor, crossed extensor, skin twitch, and Phillipson's reflex of the chronic spinal dog. In these studies, the barbiturates were compared with morphine and an interneuron depressant. Pentobarbital and thiopental exhibited less specificity than the other two drugs. ABDULLIAN et al. (1960) compared pentobarbital with several interneuron depressants and meprobamate on the modulation of the patellar reflex of the acute spinal cat. Both pentobarbital (5 and 15 mg/kg) and meprobamate (25, 50, and 100 mg/kg) depressed the patellar reflex as well as its inhibition and facilitation by stimulation of the ipsi- and contralateral sciatic nerves. Pentobarbital (24 mg/kg) has also been compared with interneuron depressants, benzodiazepines and anesthetics on the ipsi- and contralateral polysynaptic extensor reflexes evoked by stimulating the sciatic nerve of the acute decerebrate and spinal cat (NGAI et al., 1966). The site of pentobarbital's depressant action was at a spinal level while that of the benzodiazepines was supraspinal. In this regard, MULLER et al. (1978) have shown the presence of benzodiazepine binding sites in rat spinal cord synaptosomes.

Pentobarbital does not selectively depress posttetanic potentiation of the segmental monosynaptic reflex but does prolong its recovery cycle (ESPLIN, 1963). Anesthetic doses of pentobarbital slow the rate of rise of the motor neuron synaptic potential in the cat (SOMJEN and GILL, 1963). Thiopental seems to act on the segmental monosynaptic reflex by stabilizing the postsynaptic membrane (SOMJEN, 1963).

Barbiturates, like opioid analgesics, depress polysynaptic and nociceptive reflexes. In this regard, thiopental produced a dose-dependent decrease of spontaneous and evoked interneuron activity in spinal cord Rexed laminae I and V and spontaneous activity in lamina VI, indicating a selective analgesic activity (KITAHATA et al., 1975).

II. Brain Stem and Cerebellum

Pentobarbital and other barbiturates depress respiration in most species. Thus, pentobarbital (60 and 180 mg) and secobarbital (70 and 210 mg) administered orally produce a dose-related decrease in the respiratory response to CO_2 in man. In this regard, secobarbital is 1.38 times more potent than pentobarbital (BROWN et al., 1973).

In the succinylcholine-immobilized cat, pentobarbital in doses of 4 and 8 mg/kg increased blood pressure and did not alter reflex bradycardia associated with vasopressor responses. Doses of 4, 8, and 12 mg/kg did not alter heart rate and produced a dose-related increase in the threshold of mesencephalic electrical stimulation necessary to produce vasomotor responses and a dose-related depression of the slope of the stimulus-vasopressor response relationship (MARTIN and EADES, 1960).

The effects of pentobarbital and other barbiturates on the spontaneous firing of cerebellar Purkinje cells have been variously describe. The firing rate is decreased (BLOEDEL and ROBERTS, 1969; MURPHY and SABAH, 1970) and fewer cells are active (LATHAM and PAUL, 1972). Barbiturates, paraldehyde, chloral hydrate, glutethimide, ethinamate, methaqualone, clonazepam, and meprobamate produce a dose-related slowing of cerebellar rhythm (GOGALÁK et al., 1972).

Pentobarbital also produces rhythmic activity in the red nucleus which is slowed in a dose-related manner (GOGALÁK, 1970; GOGALÁK et al., 1970) and which is synchronous with burst of unit activity and cerebellar rhythmic activity (GOGALÁK et al., 1970; GOGALÁK and STUMPF, 1972).

Pentobarbital (150, 200, and 250 mg) produced a modest degree of miosis and prolonged the duration and increased the frequency of postrotational nystagmus in a dose-related manner in man (JASINSKI, 1973; MARTIN et al., 1974; MCCLANE and MARTIN, 1976). RASHBASS and RUSSELL (1961) observed that amylobarbital enhanced calorically induced nystagmus when the eyes were open, but not when they were closed. The observations are in keeping with the hypothesis that barbiturates diminishe the ability of subjects to inhibit nystagmus by fixation. MARTIN, JASINSKI, and MCCLANE (unpublished observations, 1966) were unable to clearly demonstrate that fixation inhibited or shortened postrotational nystagmus. Meprobamate, secobarbital, and phenobarbital also produce a dose-related increase in frequency and prolongation of duration of postrotational nystagmus (FRASER and JASINSKI, 1977; JASINSKI, 1973; MCCLANE and MARTIN, 1976).

III. Reticular-Activating System and EEG

The demonstration by MORUZZI and MAGOUN (1949) that there was a midbrain behavioral activating system which when stimulated desynchronized the EEG and inhibited EEG slow-wawe activity aroused great interest in the possibility that this center was necessary for consciousness and was a critical site of action of anesthetics. It was probably a tacit assumption that this activating system was also an important site of action of hypnotics. The effects of barbiturates and other hypnotics on the activating system have been reviewed by KILLAM (1962) and DOMINO (1962). There is general agreement that barbiturates in anesthetic doses virtually abolish EEG activation produced by stimulating the reticular activating system. In hypnotic doses, pentobarbital (less than 5 mg/kg) does increase the threshold for EEG activation as defined by suppression of delta activity (ARDUINI and ARDUINI, 1954; MARTIN and EADES, 1960). Higher doses of pentobarbital and thiopental produce more profound effects on the threshold for EEG activation (DOMINO, 1955; KING, 1956). The effects of barbiturates on the recruiting response, which is thought to be related to EEG spindle activity, are more complex. Small doses of thiopental (3–5 mg/kg) and pentobarbital (10 mg/kg) enhance the recruitment response. Pentobarbital is also known to enhance evoked potentials in the dorsal column (HAGBARTH and KERR, 1954), cochlear nucleus (KILLAM and KILLAM, 1958), and the trigeminal nerve nucleus (HERNANDEZ-PEON and SCHERRER, 1955). These data have been interpreted as a reflection of the reticular activating system's inhibitory effect on these neuronal circuits and a barbiturate-induced release from this inhibition.

Pentobarbital prolongs the refractory period of potentials evoked in the reticular formation and the internal capsule by peripheral nerve and lemniscal stimulation. The recovery cycle of the reticular formation was prolonged by a hypnotic dose (5 mg/kg), while anesthetic doses were required to suppress the thalamic recovery cycle (KING et al., 1957).

Although barbiturates exert a selective action in depressing the inhibitory action of the reticular activating system on certain evoked potentials and slow wave activity, they facilitate or release certain cortical rhythmic activity. The ability of barbiturates to enhance spindle activity and to produce relatively high voltage, fast EEG activity is well known and thought to be related (see BRAZIER, 1963). In a study of the effects of graded doses of pentobarbital and stimulation of the midbrain reticular activating

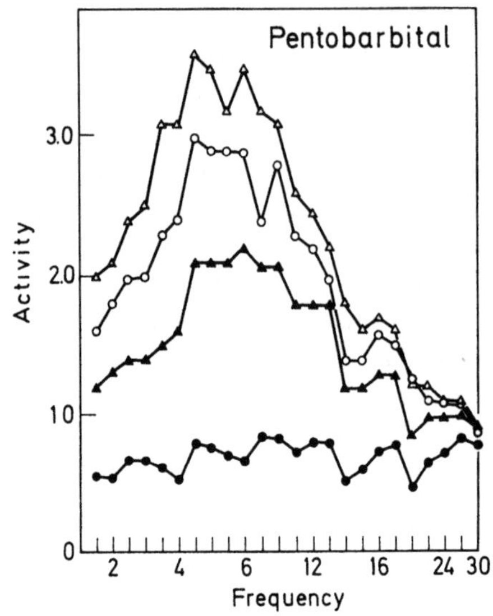

Fig. 1. The EEG frequency spectra of the succinylcholine-immobilized cat before and after graded cumulative doses of pentobarbital. ●, control; ▲, 4 mg/kg; ○, 8 mg/kg; and △, 12 mg/kg. (From MARTIN and EADES, 1960)

system on frequency analysis of the EEG of the succinylcholine-immobilized cat, MARTIN and EADES (1960) made several relevant observations. As can be seen in Fig. 1, increasing doses of pentobarbital produced increasing amounts of spindle and slow wave activity and slowed spindle frequency. Stimulation of the midbrain reticular activating system, on the other hand, produced a voltage-related increase in the frequency of rhythmic cortical activity (see Fig. 2). These data suggest that the reticular formation has a facilitatory influence on the rhythmicity of certain cortical and perhaps thalamic circuits and that this influence is especially apparent in the presence of hypnotic to moderate doses of barbiturates.

E. Tolerance and Dependence

Tolerance to and dependence on sedative hypnotics have many dimensions. There are a number of excellent reviews of the nature of tolerance to and dependence on depressant drugs. Several stand out with regard to their comprehensiveness and their relevance to hypnotics (KALANT et al., 1971; HUG, 1972; LEBLANC and CAPPELL, 1975; SMITH, 1977).

I. Tolerance

From the standpoint of decreased responsiveness to the actions of hypnotics at least three general phenomena are of importance, the first of which is a degree of responsiveness to hypnotics on the part of the individual that is markedly less than that of the general population and which is not obviously related to a history of hypnotic ingestion. This type of tolerance, which is of great clinical importance, has not been

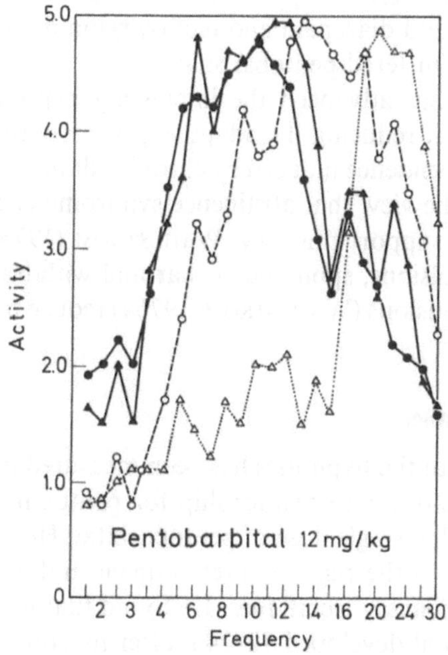

Fig. 2. EEG frequency spectral changes during stimulation of the mesencephalic reticular formation in the pentobarbital treated (12 mg/kg) succinylcholine-immobilized cat. ●, control; ▲, 4.0 V; 0, 4.5 V; and △, 5.0 V. (From MARTIN and EADES, 1960)

studied in any great depth. Speculations about the causes of this type of tolerance include genetic, congenital, developmental, environmental, drug metabolism, and pharmacologic influences.

The second factor is the ability of individuals to rapidly adapt to the effects of hypnotics. This type of tolerance undoubtedly calls into play a large variety of adaptive mechanisms that are related to detoxification, metabolic, redistribution, and excretory processes as well as brain compensatory mechanisms that probably involve phenomena such as homeostatis and motivation. This type of tolerance also has received limited attention particularly in relation to hypnotics. The role of redistribution of pentothal as a mechanism for its relatively short duration of action and the Mellanby phenomena of alcohol intoxication are examples of these types of tolerance.

Third, many authorities restrict the definition of tolerance to the decrease in responsivitity that is a consequence of previous exposure to the same or similar drugs. This type of tolerance can be appropriately called pharmacologic and may be metabolic, which is due to increased rate of metabolism, or functional, which is presumed to be a consequence of altered brain function (see STEVENSON and TURNBULL, 1970). STEVENSON and TURNBULL (1974) have shown that rats administered barbital chronically showed tolerance to intracerebrally administered pentobarbital. Alteration of the liver's ability to metabolize pentobarbital had little effect on intracerebrally administered pentobarbital depression. The chronic administration of chlordiazepoxide, nitrazepam, ethanol, a mixture of methaqualone and diphenhydramine, or chlorpromazine also induced tolerance to intracerebrally administered pentobarbital, whereas chronically administerd morphine and amphetamine did not. Withdrawal from chronically administerd diazepam and methyprylon did not result in tolerance to intraventricularly administered pentobarbital.

WAHLSTROM (1976a) has advanced the interesting hypothesis that withdrawal convulsions are a means of reducing the adaptive processes that are responsible for tolerance and physical dependence induced by chronic administration of barbiturates. This is at variance with the view that abstinence syndrome is a sign of a pathologic adaptive mechanism. To support this view WAHLSTROM (1976a, b) has shown that electrically induced convulsions, spontaneous barbital withdrawal convulsions, and pilocarpine-induced convulsions (WAHLSTROM, 1976a) reduce barbital cross tolerance to hexabarbital.

1. Measurement of Tolerance

Pharmacologic tolerance to the hypnotics has been measured in several ways. ASTON (1965) determined a dose-response relationship for pentobarbital in untreated rats and in rats pretreated with a single dose of pentobarbital. He noted that the dose-response curve was shifted to the right by pretreatment and calculated their relative potency using standard bioassay techniques. He found that maximum tolerance to a single dose of pentobarbital developed 12–24 h after its administration.

ROSENBERG and OKAMOTO (1974) performed a systematic neurologic examination measuring the level of consciousness, arousability, nictitating membrane tone, several reflexes (corneal, nociceptive, and righting), respiratory pattern, and motor performance. Some signs were either present or absent, and others were graded on an ordinal scale (0–3). Using these data, 15 syndromes of depression were defined which were rated on a scale of 0–14 with a score of 14 being maximum depression. The highest score obtained following a dose of a depressant was defined as the maximum depression rating (MDR). OKAMOTO et al.(1975), using this technique, showed that the maximal degree of tolerance developed to pentobarbital in the cat is 2.28; i.e., 2.28 times as much pentobarbital is required to produce a maximal degree of intoxication in the maximally tolerant cat as in the nontolerant cat. It took approximately 2–3 weeks for maximal tolerance to develop. Maximal metabolic tolerance occurred during the 1st week and accounted for approximately half of the tolerance that developed; the remaining tolerance was functional.

4. Acute Tolerance

TURNBULL and WATKINS (1976) have shown that an 8-h intraperitoneal infusion of pentobarbital or repeated intracerebral injections of pentobarbital over a 10-h period in the rat resulted in an increase (approximately 30%) in brain levels of pentobarbital on awakening following a test dose of 50 mg/kg.

II. Physical Dependence

Physical dependence on hypnotics and other depressants has been studied in a variety of species. Regulatory agencies, pharmacologists, and psychiatrists have become enamored of this phenomena to the extent that the concept and its relevance to psychopathology and drug development are frequently lost sight of. The concept of physical dependence emerged during the late 1920s and the 1930s, principally due to the work of SEEVERS and TATUM (1931), LIGHT and TORRANCE (1929), and HIMMELSBACH (1937). These investigators showed that the chronic administration of barbital or narcotic analgesics produced a state which was manifested by an explosive syndrome when the drug was withdrawn. The abstinence syndrome is overtly discomforting in man and is associated with drug-seeking behavior. Thus, the dependence responsible for the drug-seeking behavior was termed physical because (1) it was induced by a chemical agent, and (2) it was associated with a primary syndrome of physiologic abnormalities. Although an abstinence syndrome is generally believed to be the sine qua non of physical dependence, it now is known that an abstinence syndrome need not be associated with drug-seeking behavior (MARTIN et al., 1965; MARTIN and GORODETZKY, 1965). Furthermore, the need for a hypnotic in patients suffering from insomnia or anxiety may be just as "physical" as that demonstrated by patients experiencing an abstinence syndrome. Regardless, abstinence syndromes have been characterized in several species, and extensive studies have been conducted into the basic pathophysiology underlying the abstinence syndrome.

1. Man

The problem of an abstinence syndrome following the withdrawal of barbiturates in individuals who had used them chronically was well recognized by the 1930s by German investigators (see POHLISCH and PANSE, 1934; and review by ISBELL and FRASER, 1950). However, this view did not become generally accepted until the important controlled experiments of ISBELL (ISBELL et al., 1950; FRASER et al., 1954). In these studies, it was found that with chronic administration of barbiturates (secobarbital, pentobarbital, and amorbarbital), cumulation occurred and patients showed signs of intoxication including ataxia, dysarthria, nystagmus, past-pointing and impaired superficial reflexes and psychomotor performance, as well as wide changes in mood ranging from euphoria and pleasantness to hostility, aggressiveness, irritability, and depression. They became disheveled, paying little attention to their personal habits. Their living quarters were neglected and they withdrew from other patients.

When barbiturates were withdrawn, they improved for the first 12 or so hours following which both minor and major signs and symptoms of abstinence emerged. Minor signs and symptoms included weakness, tremor and involuntary twitches, nausea and vomiting, loss of appetite, weight loss, insomnia, orthostatic hypotension, and dizziness. Major signs included grand mal seizures and delirium tremens. Grand mal seizures when they occur usually precede delirium tremens. Delirium tremens may be associated with a fever. In an important study that provides guidance to physicians who are prescribing barbiturates for a protracted period or are treating patients who take barbiturates chronically, FRASER et al. (1958) found that doses of pentobarbital and secobarbital below 0.4 g/day did not produce a clinically significant level of physical dependence.

2. Cat

JAFFE and SHARPLESS (1965) showed that cats that were continuously intoxicated with pentobarbital for 26 h showed a reduction in pentylenetetrazol seizure threshold upon withdrawal. After 5 days of intoxication a near maximum reduction of pentylenetetrazol seizure threshold was seen as well as tremors, increased startle response, and myoclonic jerks following withdrawal of pentobarbital. The time course of reduction of pentylenetetrazol seizure threshold correlated well with the time course of denervation supersensitivity produced surgically or pharmacologically.

ROSENBERG and OKAMOTO (1974), OKAMOTO et al. (1976), and BOISSE and OKAMOTO (1978), using the MDR technique to establish a reproducible and maximal level of tolerance, established and validated a rating system for quantitatively assessing the intensity of the barbiturate abstinence syndrome. The signs observed were twitches, tremor, weakness, muscle function, motor activity, seizures, body shakes, piloerections, body temperature, pupillary diameter and light reflex, eating behavior, and body weight. These were rated using either ordinal scales or quantal measures. These observations and scorings allow both the characterization of the syndrome and the quantitation of the abstinence syndrome. Thus, BOISSE and OKAMOTO (1978) have shown that the pentobarbital abstinence syndrome was twice as intense as the barbital abstinence syndrome.

ROSENBERG and OKAMOTO (1976) studied changes in spinal cord reflex activity in abstinent, pentobarbital-dependent, acute spinal cats. In brief, they found that the amplitude of the monosynaptic reflex was not changed but its recovery cycle was shortened and recovery rate increased. Further, post tetanic potentiation of the monosynaptic reflex was enhanced. The polysynaptic reflex was enhanced and ventral root after-discharge was prolonged. These changes were maximal 1.5–2 days following withdrawal, a time at which many other abstinence signs, including grand mal convulsions, are maximal (OKAMOTO et al., 1976).

ESSIG and FLANARY (1961) studied seizures and EEG changes in cats with permanently implanted epidural electrodes during a cycle of addiction to barbital. The EEG of sleeping barbital-intoxicated cats showed 5–7 Hz activity while active but ataxic cats showed 18–32 Hz spindle activity. This high frequency pattern activity can be evoked by stimulating the midbrain reticular formation in cats who have received graded doses of pentobarbital (see Sect. D.III). During withdrawal of barbital, myoclonic jerks were seen which were associated with short generalized bursts of high voltage spikes and waves. Twitches and jerks were not, always associated with EEG changes. Grand mal convulsions were always associated with high voltage rhythmic spikes. The clonic phase was characterized by rhythmic high voltage slow waves.

3. Dog

Barbital dependence was first demonstrated in experimental animals by SEEVERS and TATUM (1931) in the dog. Grand mal seizures and weight loss were signs of abstinence. FRASER and ISBELL (1954) identified behavior that they interpreted as canine delirium. Other signs of barbiturate abstinence include decreased food and water intake, tremors, nervousness, exaggerated startle response, twitches, and jerks (DENEAU and WEISS, 1968, JONES et al. 1976). These signs can be graded, and the ability of drugs to suppress either barbital or pentobarbital dependence have been assessed. Barbital dependence can be produced in decorticate dogs, although this requires higher stabilization doses (ESSIG, 1962a). Abstinence signs include grand mal seizures and sham rage. Barbital-dependent dogs with $Al(OH)_3$ cortical lesions may have focal cortical seizures during withdrawal (Essig, 1962b).

4. Monkey

YANAGITA and TAKAHASHI (1970) studied tolerance to and physical dependence on barbital and pentobarbital in rhesus monkeys. The ability of barbiturates to impair motor function and depress arousability was assessed on an ordinal scale (0–8). Abstinence signs were observed and classified as mild (apprehension, irritability, mild tremor, anorexia and piloerection), intermediate (marked tremoring, rigidity, impaired motor activity, retching, vomiting, and weight loss) or severe (convulsions, delirium, and hyperthermia). Barbiturates, administered intramuscularly or intravenously by self-administration techniques, produced physical dependence. YANAGITA and TAKAHASHI (1973) used these methods for studying the ability of a variety of drugs to suppress the barbiturate abstinence syndrome.

5. Rat

CROSSLAND and LEONARD (1963) first produced dependence on barbital which was placed in the drinking solution of water-restricted rats. When barbital was abruptly withdrawn, spontaneous and auditory-evoked convulsions were observed. ESSIG (1966) extended these observations and those of SCHMIDT and KLEINMAN (1964) by showing that food and water intake was decreased and weight was lost following withdrawing of barbital from dependent rats. SCHMIDT and KLEINMAN (1964) employed phenobarbital instead of pentobarbital. Of interest is the fact that chronic phenobarbital administration (SCHMIDT and KLEINMAN, 1964) increased water intake, a finding that may be related to the increased food intake seen in the pentobarbital-dependent dog (JONES et al. 1976).

F. Abuse of Sedative Hypnotics

The patterns of abuse of hypnotics based on epidemiologic studies can only be roughly approximated for there is no acceptable consensus as to which agents should be classified as hypnotic. The concepts of hypnosis and sedation are not clearly delineated in either the minds of the physician, user, patient, or epidemiologist. Since most sedative hypnotics are used both for the production of sleep and the relief of anxieties and other discomforting states, the distinction may not be of great importance in this discussion.

I. Prescription

In general, the following statements and generalizations can be made about prescriptions of sedative hypnotics. The use and prescription of psychoactive and psychotherapeutic drugs have been increasing. The prescription of hypnotics (predominantly barbiturates) represents approximately 18% of all psychotherapeutic drugs prescribed. This percentage has been relatively stable and may be decreasing. In contrast minor tranquilizers (mostly benzodiazepines) have been increasingly prescribed and now represent nearly 40% of all prescriptions for psychoactive drugs (MELLINGER et al. 1973). Approximately 10% of all adults use hypnotics, and the incidence of their use increases with age, being highest in patients over 50. They are more commonly used by women than men (PARRY et al. 1973). Most prescriptions for hypnotics are written by general practioners (39%), followed by internists (20%), psychiatrists and neurologists (16%), and surgeons (11%) (MELLINGER et al. 1973).

II. Abuse

Approximately 4% of adults are involved in the nonmedical use of hypnotics. The incidence of nonmedical use is highest in the 18–25 age group and is higher in men than women. A recent survey (JOHNSTON et al. 1979) on prevalence of elicit drug use by high school seniors for the years 1975 through 1978 revealed that 16% of the class of 1978 had used sedatives at least once, although only 0.2% were using them on a regular basis. This prevalence of use has remained nearly constant for the last 4 years. Barbiturates are the most commonly used hypnotic (ca. 66%). The prevalence of daily use of sedative-hypnotics of 0.2% compares with a prevalence of 27.5% for cigarettes, 10.7% for marihuana, 5.7% for alcohol, and 0.5% for stimulants. The prevalence of all other types of drugs of abuse was less than 0.1%.

The perniciousness of the abuse of hypnotics is not readily estimated. There are at least four areas of concern: (1) the impact of motor incoordination on accidents and complex social interactions; (2) the use of hypnotics in suicide attempts; (3) toxic interactions between hypnotics and alcohol and other depressants and, (4) the induction of tolerance and physical dependence. To provide information on the adverse consequences of misuse of drugs, the National Institute of Drug Abuse and the Drug Enforcement Agency of the United States Departments of Health, Education, and Welfare and Justice have jointly supported a survey of drug-associated admissions to emergency rooms and deaths coming to the attention of medical examiners. The reports come from approximately 600 examining rooms and 100 medical examiners from standard metropolitan statistical areas. During the period of April through June of 1978, there were approximately 30,000 visits to emergency rooms in which a drug was involved (see Dawn Quarterly Report, 1978). Approximately 15% of these admissions involved sedative-hypnotics, and 6% involved barbiturates. From January through March of 1978, there were 885 deaths in which drug were identified. Sedative hypnotics were identified in 25% of these deaths and barbiturates in 19%.

G. Conclusions

The role of hypnotic drugs in the management of sleep disorders and the processes and methods by which new hypnotics are identified are both in a stage of active evolution. Insomnia must be viewed from several perspectives: (1) When it is the consequence of a pathologic process, two ingredients are necessary for successful management: an accurate diagnosis and the availability of an efficacious therapeutic modality. (2) When no definable pathologic process can be identified, the judgement of whether the insomnia itself is pathologic must be made. In this regard two questions are important: (a) does the insomnia itself give rise to physiologic pathologies such as a decrement in performance or changes in mood, and (b) does the impact of the insomnia on interpersonal relationships and social interactions secondarily create significant problems for the patient?

Methods for assessing hypnotics in animals have been recently reviewed by GOGERTY (1976). Methods currently employed basically are directed toward identifying drugs that produce or enhance behavioral depression or that increase one or more of the stages of sleep in young or mature animals. It is not unrealistic to assume that patients with sleep disorders may have diverse yet selective neurologic, neurophysiologic, and neurochemical abnormalities. If this be so, then the search for new hypnotics should include methods that identify agents that selectively rectify pathologic processes rather than identifying drugs with general depressant actions in the hope that they will be nontoxic and devoid of physical dependence-producing properties. *With regard to dependence it is important to emphasize that many patients who are chronic insomniacs do have a need of one sort or another for sleep and that even a truly effective and selective hypnotic would be of necessity reinforcing to such patients and would appropriately give rise to drug-seeking behavior or compliance.*

Ageing is one common global pathologic process that frequently gives rise to sleep disorders and hypnotic use. The experimental use of ageing as a variable in the study of hypnotics would be both relevant and expedient. Other animal models of pathologic processes which disturb sleep can be investigated and identified.

The very large number of patients with sleep problems and the fact that most hypnotics currently used are liminally effective in safe clinical dose levels make disordered sleep one of the more important mental health problems and one that is likely to increase in magnitude as the population becomes older and as social compliance becomes more necessary.

References

Abdulian, D.H., Martin, W.R., Unna, K.R.: Effects of central nervous system depressants on inhibition and facilitation of the patellar reflex. Arch. Int. Pharmacodyn. *128*, 169–186 (1960)

Adams, P.R.: Drug blockade of open end-plate channels. J. Physiol. (Lond.) *260*, 531–552 (1976)

Arduini, A., Arduini, M.G.: Effects of drugs and metabolic alterations on brain stem arousal mechanism. J. Pharmacol. Exp. Ther. *110*, 76–85 (1954)

Aston, R.: Quantitative aspects of tolerance and posttolerance hypersensitivity to pentobarbital in the rat. J. Pharmacol. Exp. Ther. *150*, 253–258 (1965)

Banna, J.R., Jabbur, S.J.: Pharmacological studies on inhibition in the cuneate nucleus of the cat. Int. J. Neuropharmacol. *8*, 299–307 (1969)

Bixler, E.O., Kales, J.D., Scharf, M.B., Kales A., Leo, L.: Incidence of sleep disorders in medical practice. A physicians survey. Sleep Res. *5*, 160 (1976)

Blaustein, M.P., Ector, A.C.: Barbiturate inhibition of calcium uptake by depolarized nerve terminals in vitro. Molec. Pharmacol. *1975 II*, 369–378

Bloedel, J.R., Roberts, W.J.: Functional relationship among neurons of the cerebellar cortex in the absence of anesthesia. J. Neurophysiol. *32*, 75–84 (1969)

Boisse, N.R., Okamoto, M.: Physical dependence to barbital compared to pentobarbital, III Withdrawal characteristics. J. Pharmacol. Exp. Ther. *204*, 514–525 (1978)

Brazier, M.A.B.: The Electrophysiological Effects of Barbiturates on the Brain, In: Physiological pharmacology. Root, W.S., Hoffman, W.G. (eds.), pp. 219–238. Academic Press: New York 1963

Brooks, C. MCC., Eccles, J.C.: Electrical investigations of the monosynaptic pathway through the spinal cord. J. Neurophysiol. *10*, 251–273 (1947)

Brown, C.R., Forrest, W.H. and Hayden, J.: The respiratory effects of pentobarbital and secobarbital in clinical doses. J. Clin. Pharmacol. *13*, 28–35 (1973)

Buch, H., Grund, J., Buzello, W. and Rummel, W.: Narkotische Wirksamkeit und Gewebsverteilung der optischen Antipoden des Pentobarbital bei der Ratte. Biochem. Pharmacol. *18*, 1005–1009 (1969)
Buch, H., Knabe, J., Bruzello, W., Rummel, W.: Stereospecificity of anesthetic activity, distribution, inactivation and protein binding of the optical antipodes of two N-methylated barbiturates. J. Pharmacol. Exp. Ther. *175*, 709–716 (1970)
Catchlove, R.F.H., Krnjević, K., Maretic, H.: Similarity between effects of general anestethics and dinitrophenol on cortical neurones. Can. Physiol. Pharmacol. *50*, 111–114 (1972)
Christensen, H.D., Lee, I.S.: Anesthetic potency and acute toxicity of optically active disubstituted barbituric acids. Toxicol. App. Pharmacol. *26*, 495–503 (1973)
Crawford, J.M.: Anesthetic agents and the chemical sensitivity of cortical neurones. Neuropharmacology *9*, 31–46 (1970)
Crawford, J.M., and Curtis, D. R.: Pharmacologic studies of feline Betz cells. J. Physiol. (Lond.) *186*, 121–138 (1966)
Crossland, J., Leonard, B.E.: Barbiturate withdrawal convulsions in the rat. Biochem. Pharmacol. Suppl. *12*, 103 (1963)
Dawn Quarterly Report: A report from the drug abuse warning network; April–June, 1978; U.S. Dept. of Justice, D.E.A. and U.S. Dept. of H.E.W., NIDA
Dement, W.C.: The effect of dream deprivation. Science, *131*, 1705–1707 (1960)
Deneau, G.A., Weiss, S.: A substitution technique for determining barbiturate-like physiological dependence capacity in the dog. Pharmakopsychiatr. Neuropsychopharmakol. *1*, 270–275 (1968)
Domino, E.F.: A pharmacological analysis of the functional relationship between the brainstem arousal and diffuse thalamic projection systems. J. Pharmacol. Exp. Ther. *115*, 449–463 (1955)
Domino, E.F.: Sites of action of some central nervous system depressants. Annu. Rev. Pharmacol. *2*, 215–250 (1962)
Eccles, J.C.: Synaptic potentials of motoneurones. J. Neurophysiol. *9*, 87–120 (1946)
Eccles, J.C., Malcolm, J.L.: Dorsal root potentials of the spinal cord. J. Neurophysiol. *9*, 139–160 (1946)
Eccles, J.C., Schmidt, R., Willis, W.D.: Pharmacological studies on presynaptic inhibition. J. Physiol. (Lond.), *168*, 500–530 (1963)
Enna, S.J., Snyder, S.H.: GABA receptor binding in frog spinal cord and brain. J. Neurochem. *28*, 857–860 (1977)
Esplin, D.W.: Criteria for assessing effects of depressant drugs on spinal cord synaptic transmission with examples of drug selectivity. Arch. Int. Pharmacodyn. Ther. *143*, 479–497 (1963)
Essig, C.F.: Convulsive and sham rage behaviors in decorticate dogs during barbiturate withdrawal. Arch. Neurol. *7*, 471–475 (1962a)
Essig, C.F.: Focal convulsions during barbiturate abstinence in dogs with cerebrocortical lesions. Psychopharmacology *3*, 432–437 (1962b)
Essig, C.F.: Barbiturate withdrawal in white rats. Int. J. Neuropharmacol. *5*, 103–107 (1966)
Essig, C.F., Flanary, H.G.: Convulsive aspects of barbital sodium withdrawal in the cat. Exp. Neurol. *3*, 149–159 (1961)
Fraser, H.F., Isbell, H.: Abstinence syndrome in dogs after chronic barbiturate medication. J. Pharmacol. Exp. Ther. *112*, 261–267 (1954)
Fraser, H.F., Jasinski, D.R.: The assessment of the abuse potentiality of sedative hypnotics (depressants). (Methods used in animals and man). In: Drug addiction I. Martin, W.R. (ed.), pp. 589–612. Berlin, Heidelberg, New York: Springer 1977
Fraser, H.F., Isbell, H., Eisenman, A.J., Wikler, A., Pescor, F.T.: Chronic barbiturate intoxication; further study. Arch. Int. Med. *94*, 34–41 (1954)
Fraser, H.F., Wikler, A., Essig, C.F.: Degree of physical dependence induced by secobarbital or pentobarbital. J. Am. Med. Assoc. *166*, 126–229 (1958)
Freudenthal, R.I., Martin, J.: Correlation of brain levels of barbiturate enantiomers with reported differences in duration of sleep. J. Pharmacol. Exp. Ther. *193*, 664–668 (1975)
Furner, R.L., McCarthy, J.S., Stitzel, R.E., Anders, M.W.: Stereoselective metabolism of the enantiomers of hexobarbital. J. Pharmacol. Exp. Ther. *169*, 153–158 (1969)

Galindo, A.: Effects of procaine, pentobarbital and halothane on synaptic transmission in the central nervous system. J. Pharmacol. Exp. Ther. *169*, 185–195 (1969)

Gogalák, G.: Die Wirkung von Pentobarbital auf die Zelltätigkeit des Nucleus Ruber. Naunyn-Schmiedebergs Arch. Pharmak. *267*, 249–264 (1970)

Gogalák, G., Stumpf, C.: Action of anesthetics on the firing pattern of nucleus ruber neurons. Naunyn-Schmiedebergs Arch. Pharmacol. *272*, 387–394 (1972)

Gogalák, G., Liebeswar, G., Stumpf, C., Williams, H.L.: The relationship between barbiturate-induced activities in the cerebellum and red nucleus of the rabbit. Electroencephalogr. Clin. Neurophysicol. *29*, 67–73 (1970)

Gogalák, G., Krijzer, F., Stumpf, C.: Action of central depressant drugs on the electrocerebellogram of the rabbit. Naunyn-Schmiedebergs Arch. Pharmacol. *272*, 378–386 (1972)

Gogerty, J.H.: Preclinical methodologies related to the development of hypnotic substances. In: Pharmacology of sleep. Williams, R.L., Karacan, I. (eds.), pp. 33–52. New York: John Wiley & Sons 1976

Gruner, J., Krieglstein, J., Rieger, H.: Comparison of the effects of chloral hydrate and trichlorethanol on the EEG of the isolated perfused rat brain. Naunyn-Schmiedebergs Arch. Pharmacol. *277*, 333–348 (1973)

Hagbarth, K.E., Kerr, D.F.B.: Central influences on spinal afferent conduction. J. Neurophysiol. *17*, 295–307 (1954)

Haley, T.J., Gidley, J.T.: Pharmacological comparison of R(+), S(−) and racemic secrobarbital in mice. Eur. J. Pharmacol. *9*, 358–361 (1970)

Hartmann, E., Cravens, J.: The effects of long term administration of psychotropic drugs on human sleep: The effects of chloral hydrate. Psychopharmacology *33*, 233–245 (1975)

Haycock, J.W., Levy, W.B., Cotman, Carl W.: Pentobarbital depression of stimulus-secretion coupling in brain. Selective inhibition of depolarization-induced calcium-dependent release. Chem. Pharmacol. *26*, 159–161 (1977)

Herńańdez-Peón, R., Scherrer, H.: Inhibitory influence of brain stem reticular formation upon synaptic transmission in trigeminal nucleus. Fed. Proc. *14*, 71 (1955)

Himmelsbach, C.K.: Clinical studies of drug addiction II "Rossium" treatment of drug addiction. Publ. Hlth. Rp. (Wash.), Suppl. 125 (1937)

Houde, R.W., Wikler, A.: Delineation of the skin twitch response in dogs and the effects thereon of morphine, thiopental and mephenesin. J. Pharmacol. Exp. Ther. *103*, 236–242 (1951)

Houde, R.W., Wikler, A., Irwin, S.: Comparative actions of analgesic, hypnotic and paralytic agents on hindlimb reflexes in chronic spinal dogs. J. Pharmacol. Exp. Ther. *103*, 243–248 (1951)

Hug, C.E.: Characteristics and theories related to acute and chronic tolerance development. In: Chemical and biological aspects of drug dependence. Mule, S.J., Brill, H. (eds.), pp. 307–358. Cleveland, Ohio: CRC Press 1972

Isbell, H., Fraser, H.F.: Addiction to analgesics and barbiturates. Pharmacol. Rev. *2*, 355–397 (1950)

Isbell, H., Altschul, S., Kornetsky, C.H., Eisenman, E.J., Flanary, H.G., Fraser, H.F.: Chronic barbiturate intoxication; An experimental study. Arch. Neurol. Psychiatry *64*, 1–28 (1950)

Jaffe, J.H., Sharpless, S.K.: The rapid development of physical dependence on barbiturates. J. Pharmacol. Exp. Ther. *150*, 140–145 (1965)

Jasinski, D.R.: Assessment of the dependence liability of opiates and sedative-hypnotics. In: Psychic dependence: Definition, assessment in animals and man, theoretical and clinical implications. Goldberg, L., Hoffmeister, F. (eds.). Berlin, Heidelberg, New York: Springer 1973

Johnson, E.S., Roberts, M.H.T., Straughan, D.W.: The responses of cortical neurones to monoamines under differing anesthetic conditions. J. Physiol. (Lond.) *203*, 261–280 (1969)

Johnston, L.D., Bachman, J.G., O'Malley, P.M.: Drugs and the Class of '78: Behaviors, attitudes and recent national trends. DHEW Publication No. (ADM) 79–877 (1979)

Jones, B.E., Prada, J.A., Martin, W.R.: A method for bioassay of physical dependence on sedative drugs in dog. Psychopharmacology *47*, 7–15 (1976)

Jouvet, M.: Biogenic amines and the states of sleep. Science *163*, 32–41 (1969)

Jovanović, U.J.: Zum Problem der Effekte zentral-wirkender Pharmaka auf den REM-Anteil des Schlafs. Fortschr. Med. *92*, 1090–1094 (1974)
Kalant, H., Leblanc, A.E., Gibbins, R.J.: Tolerance to and dependence on some non-opiate psychotropic drugs. Pharmacol. Rev. *23*, 135–191 (1971)
Kales, A., Kales, J.D.: Sleep disorders. Recent findings in the diagnosis and treatment of disturbed sleep. New Engl. J. Med. *290*, 487–499 (1974)
Kales, A., Allen, C., Scharf, M.B., Kales, J.D.: Hypnotic drugs and their effectiveness. III. All-night EEG studies of insomniac subjects. Arch. Gen. Psychiatry *23*, 226–232 (1970a)
Kales, A., Kales, J.D., Scharf, M.B., Tan, T.L.: Hypnotics and altered sleep-dream patterns. II. All night EEG studies of chloral hydrate, flurazepam and methaqualone. Arch. Gen. Psychiatry *23*, 219–225 (1970b)
Kales, A., Bixler, E.O., Leo, L.A., Healy, S., Slye, T.: Incidence of insomnia in the Los Angeles metropolitan area. Sleep Res. *3*, 139 (1974)
Kales, A., Kales, J.D., Bixler, E.O., Scharf, M.B.: Effectiveness of hypnotic drugs with prolonged use: Flurazepam and pentobarbital. Clin. Pharmacol. Ther. *18*, 356–363 (1975)
Kay, D.C., Jasinski, D.R., Eisenstein, R.B., Kelly, O.A.: Quantified human sleep after pentobarbital. Clin. Pharmacol. Ther. *13*, 221–231 (1972)
Kay, D.C., Blackgurn, A.B., Buckingham, J.A., Karacan, I.: Human pharmacology of sleep. In: Pharmacology of sleep, Williams, R.L., Karacan, I. (eds.). New York: John L. Wiley 1976
Kety, S.S., Evarts, E.V., Williams, H.L.: Sleep and altered states of consciousness, Proceedings of the Association December 3 and 4, 1965, New York. In: Res. Publ. Ass. Nerv. Ment. Dis., vol. XLV, Baltimore: Williams and Wilkins Co. 1967
Killam, E.K.: Drug action on the brain stem reticular formation. Pharmacol. Rev. *14*, 175–223 (1962)
Killam, K.F., Killam, E.K.: Drug action on pathways involving the reticular formation. In: Reticular formation of the brain. Jasper, H.H., Proctor, L.D., Knighton, R.S., Noshay, W.C., Costello, R.T. (eds.), pp. 111–122. Boston: Little Brown and Co. 1958
King, E.E.: Differential action of anesthetics and interneuron depressants upon EEG arousal and recruitment responses. J. Pharmacol. Exp. Ther. *116*, 404–417 (1956)
King, E.E., Naquet, R., Magoun, H.W.: Alterations in somatic afferent transmission through the thalamus by central mechanisms and barbiturates. J. Pharmacol. Exp. Ther. *119*, 48–63 (1957)
Kitahata, L.M., Ghazi-Saidi, K., Yamashita, M., Kosaka, Y., Bonikos, C., Taub, A.: The depressant effect of halothane and sodium thiopental on the spontaneous and evoked activity of dorsal horn cells: lamina specificity time course and dose dependence. J. Pharmacol. Exp. Ther. *195*, 515–521 (1975)
Krueger, J.M., Pappenheimer, J.R., Karnovsky, M.L.: Sleep-promoting factors: Purification and properties. Proc. Natl. Acad. Sci. USA *75*, 5235–5238 (1978)
Larrabee, M.G., Posternak, J.M.: Selective action of anesthetics on synapses and axons in mammalian sympathetic ganglia. J. Neurophysiol. *15*, 91–114 (1952)
Larson, M.D., Major, M.A.: The effect of hexobarbital on the duration of the recurrent IPSP in cat motoneurons. Brain Res. *21*, 309–311 (1970)
Latham, A., Paul, D.H.: Effects of sodium thiopentone on cerebellar neurone activity. Brain Res. *25*, 212–215 (1972)
Leblanc, A.E., Cappell, H.D.: Historical antecedents as determinants of tolerance to and dependence upon psychoactive drugs. In: Biologic and behavioral approaches to drug dependence. Cappell, H.D., LeBlanc, A.E. (eds.), pp. 43–51. Toronto Ontario: Addiction Research Foundation, House of Lind 1975
Lehmann, H.E., Ban, T.A.: The effects of hypnotics on rapid eye movement (REM). Int. Zeit. Klin. Pharmakol. Ther. Toxik. *1*, 424–427 (1968)
Levin, P., Koella, W.P.: Sleep 1974. Instinct, neurophysiology, endocrinology, episodes, dreams, epilepsy and intracranial pathology. Proceedings of the Second European Congress on Sleep Research, Rome, April 8–11, 1974. Basel: S. Karger AG 1975
Light, D.B., Torrance, E.G.: Opium addiction VI. The effects of abrupt withdrawal followed by administration of morphine in human addicts with special reference to the composition of the blood, the circulation and metabolism. Arch. Intern. Med. *44*, 1–16 (1929)

Löyning, Y., Oshima, T., Yokota, T.: Site of action of thiamylal sodium on the monosynaptic spinal reflex pathway in cats. J. Neurophysiol. *27*, 408–427 (1964)
Mangold, R., Sokoloff, L., Conner, E., Kleinerman, J., Therman, P.G., Kety, S.S.: The effect of sleep and lack of sleep on the cerebral circulation and metabolism of normal young men. J. Clin. Invest. *34*, 1092–1100 (1955).
Martin, W.R., Eades, C.G.: A comparative study of the effect of drugs on activating and vasomotor responses evoked by midbrain stimulation: atropine, pentobarbital, chlorpromazine and chlorpromazine sulfoxide. Psychopharmacology *1*, 303–335 (1960)
Martin, W.R., Gorodetzky, C.W.: Demonstration of tolerance to and physical dependence on N-allylnormorphine (nalorphine). J. Pharmacol. Exp. Ther. *150*, 437–442 (1965)
Martin, W.R., Fraser, H.F., Gorodetzky, C.W., Rosenberg, D.E.: Studies of the dependence-producing potential of the narcotic antagonist 2-cyclopropylmethyl-2-hydroxy-5,9-dimethyl-6, 7-benzomorphan (cyclazocine, Win 20, 740, ARC II-C-3). J. Pharmacol. Exp. Ther. *150*, 426–436 (1965)
Martin, W.R., Thompson, W.O., Fraser, H.F.: Comparison of graded single intramuscular doses of morphine and pentobarbital in man. Clin. Pharmacol. Ther. *15*, 623–630 (1974)
McClane, T.K., Martin, W.R.: Subjective and physiologic effects of morphine, pentobarbital and meprobamate. Clin. Pharmacol. Ther. *20*, 192–198 (1976)
Mellinger, G.D., Balter, M.B., Parry, H.J., Manheimer, D.J., Cisin, I.H.: An overview of psychotherapeutic drug use in the United States: Presented at Epidemiology of Drug Abuse Conference, San Juan, Puerto Rico, 1973
Miyahara, J.T., Esplin, D.W., Zablocka, B.: Differential effects of depressant drugs on presynaptic inhibition. J. Pharmacol. Exp. Ther. *154*, 119–127 (1966)
Monnier, M., Hosli, L.: Dialysis of sleep and waking factors in blood of the rabbit. Science *146*, 796–798 (1964)
Monnier, M., Schoenenberger, G.A., Dudler, L., Herkert, B.: Production isolation and further characterization of the "sleep peptide delta." Biological aspects. In: Sleep, 1974. Instinct, neurophysiology, endocrinology, episodes, dreams, epilepsy and intracranial pathology. Levin, P., Koella, W.P. (eds.), Proceedings of the Second European Congress on Sleep Research, Rome, April 8–11, 1974. Basel: S. Karger AG 1975
Moruzzi, G., Magoun, H.W.: Brain stem reticular formation and activation of the EEG. Electroencephalogr. Clin. Neurophysiol. *1*, 455–473 (1949)
Muller, W.E., Schlafer, V., Wollert, V.: Benzodiazepine receptor binding in rat spinal cord membranes. Neurosci. Lett. *9*, 239–243 (1978)
Murphy, J.T., Sabah, N.H.: Spontaneous firing of cerebellar perkinje cells in decerebrated and barbiturate anesthetized cats. Brain Res. *17*, 515–519 (1970)
Nagasaki, H., Iriki, M., Inoue, S., Uchizono, K.: The presence of sleep promoting material in the brain of sleep deprived rats. Proc. Jpn. Acad. *50*, 241–246 (1974)
Ngai, S.A., Tseng, D.T.C., Wang, S.C.: Effect of diazepam and other central nervous system depressants on spinal reflexes in cats. A study of the site of action. J. Pharmacol. Exp. Ther. *153*, 344–351 (1966)
Nicoll, R.A.: The effects of anesthetics on synaptic excitation and inhibition in the olfactory bulb. J. Physiol. (Lond.) *223*, 803–814 (1972)
Nicoll, R.A.: Presynaptic actions of barbiturates in the frog spinal cord. Proc. Natl. Acad. Sci. USA *72*, 1460–1463 (1975)
Nicoll, R.A.: Selective actions of barbiturates on synaptic transmission. In: Psychopharmacology: a generation of progress. Lipton, M.A., DiMascio, A., Killam, K.F. (eds.). New York: Raven Press 1978
Nicoll, R.A., Iwamoto, E.T.: Action of pentobarbital on sympathetic ganglion cells, J. Neurophysiol. *41*, 977–986 (1978)
Nicoll, R.A., Eccles, J.C., Oshima, T., Rubia, F.: Prolongation of hippocampal in inhibitory potsynaptic potentials by barbiturates. Nature *258*, 625–627 (1975)
Ogunremi, O.O., Adamson, L., Brezinova, V., Hunter, W.M., Maclean, A.W., Oswald, I., Percy-Robb, I.W.: Two anti-anxiety drugs: A psychoneuroendocrine study. Br. Med. J. *1973 II*, 202–205
Okamoto, M., Rosenberg, H.C., Boisse, N.R.: Tolerance characteristics produced during the maximally tolerable chronic pentobarbital dosing in the cat. J. Pharmacol. Exp. Ther. *192*, 555–564 (1975)

Okamoto, M., Rosenberg, H.C., Boisse, N.R.: Withdrawal characteristics following chronic pentobarbital dosing in cat. Eur. J. Pharmacol. *40*, 107–119 (1976)
Olsen, R.W., Greenlee, D., Vanness, P., Ticku, M.K.: Studies on the Gamma-aminobutyric acid receptor ionophore protein in mammalian brain. In: Amino acids as chemical transmitter. Fonnum, F. (ed.). New York, London: Plenum Press 1977
Pappenheimer, J.R., Fencl, V., Karnovsky, M.L., Koski, G.: Peptides in cerebrospinal fluid and their relation to sleep and activity. Brain dysfunction in metabolic disorders. F. Plum (ed.). Res. Publ. Assoc. Res. Nerv. Ment. Dis. *53*, 201–210 (1974)
Pappenheimer, J.R., Koski, G., Fencl, V., Karnovsky, M.L., Krueger, J.: Extraction of sleep-promoting factors from cerebrospinal fluid and from brains of sleep-deprived animals. J. Neurophysiol. *38*, 1299–1311 (1975)
Parry, H.J., Balter, M.B., Mellinger, G.D., Cisin, I.H., Manhiemer, M.A.: National patterns of psychotherapeutic drug use. Arch. Gen. Psychiatry *28*, 769–783 (1973)
Phillis, J.W., Tebecis, A.K.: The effects of pentobarbitone sodium on acetylcholine excitation and noradrenaline inhibition of thalamic neurons. Life Sci. *6*, 1621–1625 (1967)
Pohlisch, K., Panse, F.: Schlafmittelmißbrauch. Leipzig: Georg Thieme 1934
Polc, P., Haefely, W.: Effects of two benzodiazepines, phenobarbitone and baclofen on synaptic transmission in the cat cuneate nucleus. Naunyn Schmiedebergs Arch. Pharmacol. *294*, 121–131 (1976)
Ramm, P.: The locus coeruleus, catecholamines, and REM sleep: A critical review. Behav. Neur. Biol. *25*, 415–448 (1979)
Ransom, B.R., Barker, J.L.: Pentobarbital modulates transmitter effects on mouse spinal neurones grown in tissue culture. Nature (Lond.) *254*, 703–705 (1975)
Rashbass, C., Russell, C.F.M.: Action of a barbiturate drug (amylobarbitone sodium) on the vestibulo-ocular reflex. Brain *84*, 329–335 (1961)
Richards, C.D.: On mechanism of barbiturate anesthesia. J. Physiol. (Lond.) *227*, 749–767 (1972)
Rosenberg, H.C., Okamoto, M.: A method for producing maximal pentobarbital dependence in cats: dependency characteristics. In: Drug addiction: Neurobiology and influences on behavior. Singh, J.M., Lal, H. (eds.), vol. 3. Miami: Miami's Symposium Specialists 1974
Rosenberg, H.C., Okamoto, M.: Electrophysiology of barbiturate withdrawal in the spinal cord. J. Pharmacol. Exp. Ther. *199*, 189–197 (1976)
Schmidt, R.F.: Pharmacological studies on the primary afferent depolarization of the toad spinal cord. Pfluegers Arch. *277*, 325–346 (1963)
Schmidt, H., Kleinman, K.M.: Effect of chronic administration and withdrawal of barbiturates upon drinking in the rat. Arch. Int. Pharmacodyn. Ther. *151*, 142–149 (1964)
Schofield, C.N.: A barbiturate induced intensification of the inhibitory potential of guinea pig olfactory cortex. J. Physiol. (Lond.) *275*, 559–566 (1978)
Scholfield, C.N., Harvey, J.A.: Local anesthetics and barbiturates: Effects in evoked potentials in isolated mammalian cortex. J. Pharmacol. Exp. Ther. *195*, 522–531 (1975)
Seevers, M.H., Tatum, A.L.: Chronic experimental barbital poisoning. J. Pharmacol. Exp. Ther. *42*, 217–231 (1931)
Seyama, I., Narahashi, T.: Mechanism of blockade of neuromuscular transmission by pentobarbital. J. Pharmacol. Exp. Ther. *192*, 95–104 (1975)
Shapovalov, A.I.: Intracellular microelectrode investigation of effects of anesthetics on transmission of excitation in the spinal cord. Fed. Proc. *23*, T 113–T 116 (1963)
Smaje, J.C.: General anesthetics and the acetylcholine-sensitivity cortical neurons. Br. J. Pharmacol. *58*, 359–366 (1976)
Smith, C.M.: The pharmacology of sedative/hypnotics, alcohol and anesthetics: Sites and mechanisms of action. In: Drug addiction I. Martin, W.R. (ed.). Berlin, Heidelberg, New York: Springer 1977
Soldatos, C.R., Kales, A., Kales, J.D.: Management of insomnia. Annu. Rev. Med. *30*, 301–312 (1979)
Somjen, G.G.: Effects of ether and thiopental on spinal presynaptic terminals. J. Pharmacol. Exp. Ther. *140*, 396–402 (1963)
Somjen, G.G., Gill, M.: The mechanism of blockade of synaptic transmission in the mammalian spinal cord by diethylether and by thiopental. J. Pharmacol. Exp. Ther. *140*, 19–30 (1963)

Stevenson, I.H., Turnbull, M.J.: The sensitivity of the brain to barbiturate during chronic administration and withdrawal of barbitone sodium in the rat. Brit. J. Pharmacol. *39*, 325–333 (1970)

Stevenson, I.H., Turnbull, M.J.: A study of the factors affecting the sleeping time following intracerebroventricular administration of pentobarbitone sodium: effect of prior administration of centrally acting drugs. Brit. J. Pharmacol. *50*, 499–511 (1974)

Ticku, M.K., Olsen, R.W.: Interaction of barbiturates with dihydropicrotoxinin binding sites related to the GABA receptor-ionophore system. Life Sci. *22*, 1643–1651 (1978)

Tsuchiya, T., Fukushima, H.: Effects of benzodiazepines and pentobarbitone on the GABA-ergic recurrent inhibition of hippocampal neurones. Eur. J. Pharmacol. *48*, 421–424 (1978)

Turnbull, M.J., Watkins, J.W.: Acute tolerance to barbiturates in the rat. Eur. J. Pharmacol. *36*, 15–20 (1976)

Waddell, W.J., Baggett, B.: Anesthetic and lethal activity in mice of the stereoisomers of 5-ethyl-5-(1-methylbutyl) barbituric acid (pentobarbital). Arch. Int. Pharmacodyn. Ther. *205*, 40–44 (1973)

Wahlstrom, G.: Differences in anesthetic properties between the optical antipodes of hexobarbital in the rat. Life Sci. *5*, 1781–1790 (1966)

Wahlstrom, G.: The interaction between spontaneous convulsions and tolerance to hexobarbital in the abstinence after chronic barbital treatments in the rat. Life Sci. *19*, 1817–1826 (1976a)

Wahlstrom, G.: The interaction between electrically induced convulsions and tolerance in the abstinence period after chronic barbital treatment in the cat. Psychopharmacology *48*, 239–245 (1976b)

Weakly, J.N.: Effect of barbiturates on "quantal" synaptic transmission in spinal montoneurones. J. Physiol. (Lond.) *204*, 63–77 (1969)

Weitzman, E.D. (ed.): Advances in sleep research, Vol. 1. Flushing: Spectrum Publications, Inc. 1974

Wikler, A.: Effects of morphine, nembutal, ether and eserine in two-neuron and multineuron reflexes in the cat. Proc. Soc. Exp. Biol. Med. *58*, 193–196 (1945)

Williams, R.L., Karacan, I.: Pharmacology of sleep. New York: John Wiley & Sons 1976

Wolf, P., Haas, H.L.: Effects of diazepines and barbiturates on hippocampal recurrent inhibition. Naunyn-Schmiedebergs Arch. Pharmacol. *299*, 211–218 (1977)

Yanagita, T., Takahashi, S.: Development of tolerance to and physical dependence on barbiturates in rhesus monkeys. J. Pharmacol. Exp. Ther. *172*, 163–169 (1970)

Yanagita, T., Takahashi, S.: Dependence liability of several sedative-hypnotic agents evaluated in monkeys. J. Pharmacol. Exp. Ther. *185*, 307–316 (1973)

CHAPTER 15

Anticholinergics

L. G. ABOOD

A. Introduction

The use of the term anticholinergics by definition implies that this class of drugs acts primarily on cholinergic synapses, which, on the basis of our understanding of the parasympathetic nervous system, can be either muscarinic or nicotinic. Since most of the so-called anticholinergic drugs employed by neuropharmacologists and other investigators are primarily antimuscarinic, the term has generally referred to antagonists of muscarinic sites, particularly those in the parasympathetic nervous system. Although the term theoretically includes antinicotinic drugs, such as hexamethonium and other bis-quaternary amines, the discussion in this chapter will be restricted to antimuscarinic agents. Bis-quaternary agents evidently do not permeate the blood-brain barrier; however, when they are injected intraventricularly into specific brain regions, they produce severe prolonged seizures and other neurologic symptoms (FELDBERG, 1963).

There are a number of naturally occurring anticholinergics whose psychotomimetic effects have been known for centuries. Included among these are the solanaceous alkaloids, such as (−)-hyoscyamine, atropine (racemic hyoscyamine), and scopolamine (hyoscine). Among the better known plants containing the alkaloids are henna *(Hyocyamus niger)*, deadly nightshade *(Atropa belladonna)*, and jimson weed *(Datura stramonium)*. Extracts from such plants have been employed by primitive cultures both for their medicinal purposes and to produce delirium and other psychotomimetic effects, often as a punitive measure.

B. Structure–Activity Relationships

The structure–activity relationships of an extensive number and variety of anticholinergics have been described in a number of reviews (BIEL et al., 1961; ABOOD and BIEL, 1962; ABOOD, 1968); only the general features will be described here. The main difficulty in comparing chemical structure with the psychopharmacologic potency of the drugs is the deficiency of unequivocal behavioral measurements for assessing potency. Although a number of the anticholinergics have been evaluated for their psychotomimetic potency in man (ABOOD and BIEL, 1962; GERSHON, 1966), the comparisons are based largely on a battery of quantifiable psychopharmacologic measurements in animals including such parameters as hyperactivity (LIPMAN et al., 1963), swim maze (KOSMAN, 1964), characteristic exploratory head movements (ABOOD and BIEL, 1962), and operant conditioning paradigms (POLIDORA, 1963; WEISS and HELLER, 1969; LOWY et al., 1974). The limitations and reliability of these comparisons

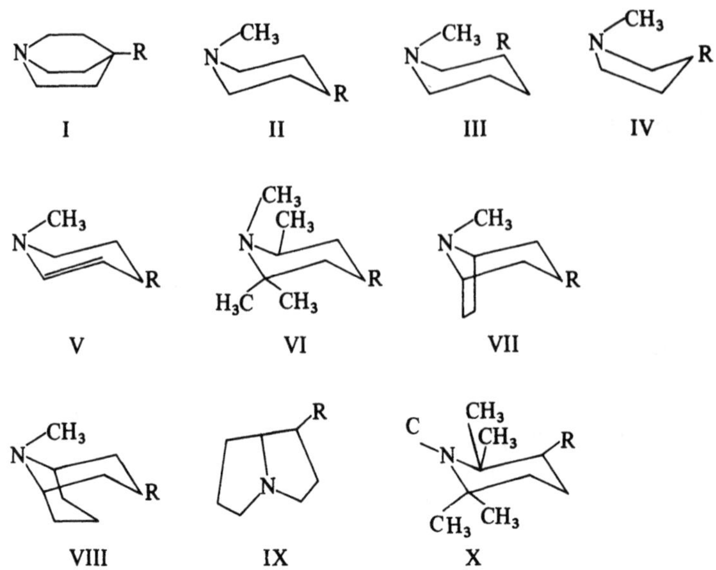

Fig. 1. Chemical structure of various heterocyclic amino esters of benzilic acid. I = 3-quinuclidinyl, II = *N*-methyl-4-piperidyl, III = *N*-methyl-3-piperidyl, IV = *N*-methyl-3-pyrrolidyl, V = *N*-methyl-*N*-methyl-2,3-piperidienyl, VI = 1,2,2,6-tetramethylpiperidyl, VII = *N*-methyl-3-tropanyl, VIII = *N*-methyl-3-granatonyl, IX = 1-pyrrolizidinyl, X = 1,2,2,6,6-pentamethyl-3-piperidyl. R = benzilate. Psychotomimetic potency decreases from I to X

have been discussed elsewhere (ABOOD, 1968), and they do permit certain generalizations concerning the relative ability of the anticholinergics to produce behavioral disturbances in animals that may reflect their psychotogenic potency in man. Structural variations in the heterocyclic amino alcohol result in marked changes in potency with the most potent being 3-quinuclidinyl with its rigid conformation (Fig. 1).

With respect to the acid moiety of the anticholinergics, the following structure–activity relationships apply:

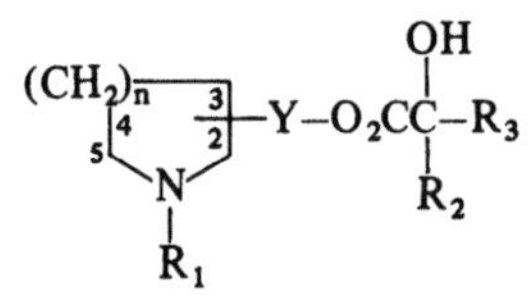

1) As R_1 is increased from methyl to higher alkyls or becomes hydrogen, alkenyl, amino, or aminoalkyl, psychotropic potency diminishes without much effect on peripheral anticholinergic action.

2) R_2 should be an unsubstituted phenyl group, while R_3 must be either a cycloalkyl, alkynyl, thienyl, or unsubstituted phenyl. Alkyl, aryl, halide, or hydroxyl substituents on the phenyl rings abolish central action and diminish anticholinergic potency. R_2 and R_3 can also be replaced by hexahydrofluorenyl (FREITER et al., 1968).

3) As "n" is increased beyond 2 or "Y" beyond zero, psychotropic but not anticholinergic potency decreases. The position of the ester side chain affects central but not peripheral action, with the 4-piperidyl ester being most potent, the 3-ester, second, and the 2-ester, least.

4) R_4 must be an hydroxyl group, while compounds with hydrogen or an isosteric methyl group are devoid of central action and have diminished anticholinergic action. If R_4 is hydrogen and the hydroxyl group is present on phenyl, central potency is retained.

The duration of the psychotropic action of the various anticholinergics is dependent both on the type of heterocyclic amino group as well as R_2 and R_3. The quinuclidinyl and pyrrolidyl derivatives tend to be longer acting than piperidyl, troponyl, or granatonyl, while a cycloalkyl group in R_2 and R_3 prolongs duration. An alkynyl group in R_2 and R_3 decreases duration, while increasing chain length or branching of the alkynyl group correspondingly increases duration.

I. Stereospecifity

The anticholinergic glycolate esters of heterocyclic amino alcohols, including scopolamine and related natural alkaloids, exist as optical isomers, resulting from the asymmetric C of both the amino alcohol and acid moiety. Of the two enantiomers of 3-diphenylacetyl quinuclidine, the (−)-isomer had 25 times the antispasmodic potency of the (+)-isomer; however, the isomers were of equal toxicity, whereas no difference was noted in the antispasmodic potency between the two isomers of the quaternary derivative of 3-quinuclidinyl benzilate (STERNBACH and KAISER, 1952). With respect to their central action, the (+) and (−) enantiomers, which were prepared from the respective quinuclidionols resolved with (+)-camphor-10-sulfonic acid (STERNBACH and KAISER, 1952), differ markedly in their potency (MEYERHOFFER, 1972; LOWY et al., 1976). The (−)-isomer was reported to have about 20 times the potency of the (+)-isomer in producing ataxia in dogs (MEYERHOFFER, 1972); however, with the use of more elaborate behavioral measurements in cats, the potency difference was in excess of 100-fold (LOWY et al., 1976). It is conceivable that the (+)-isomer of 3-quinuclidinyl benzilate is totally devoid of activity on the central nervous system, and the slight activity observed may be attributed to a 1% contamination by the (−)isomer.

II. Nonesteratic Anticholinergics

Although the majority of known centrally active anticholinergics are glycolic acid esters of heterocyclic aminoalcohols, there exist a wide variety of other chemical types. Thioglycolic esters of piperidinol have less antimuscarinic activity both peripherally and centrally, while tending to have a shorter duration of action than the corresponding esters (BUEHLER et al., 1965). Other centrally active anticholinergics include arylether, cycloalkyl ether, and aryl-cycloalkyl derivatives of piperidine and other heterocyclic amino alcohols; however, they are considerably less psychoactive than the esters or ethers (ABOOD, 1968). The phencyclidines, which are widely abused psychotomimetic agents, possess some central antimuscarinic activity (ABOOD, 1968; WEINSTEIN et al., 1973; VINCENT et al., 1978). Phenylcyclohexyl piperidine (PCP) produces behavioral disturbances in man and animals resembling those of other centrally active anticholinergics (ABOOD, 1968). Recently it has been demonstrated that the affinity of PCP for the muscarinic receptors in rat cerebral cortex and brain stem has a K_d of 3×10^{-6} M (ARONSTAM, unpublished), which is 2–3 orders of magnitude less than the glycolate esters.

C. Behavioral and Neurologic Effects

The behavioral and neurologic effects of the more potent anticholinergics in humans have been reviewed elsewhere (Abood and Biel, 1962; Abood, 1968) and will be only briefly summarized. At doses as low as 5 μg/kg (orally or intramuscularly), 3-quinuclidinyl benzilate or *N*-methyl-4-piperidyl benzilate will produce confusion, delirium, hallucinations (visual, auditory, tactile, and gustatory), depersonalization, marked changes in mood, and amnesia. In addition to the spectrum of typical autonomic effects, such as mydriasis, dryness of the mouth, tachycardia, hypertension, and spasmolysis, there occurs a wide variety of neurologic symptoms. Included among these are hyperreflexia, tremors, ataxia, aphasia, apraxia, somnolence, and restlessness. The effects may persist for days following a single dose of 3-quinuclidinyl benzilate or for only 4–8 h with *N*-methyl-4-ethynylphenyl piperidyl glycolate.

In order to evaluate and quantify the behavioral effects of the centrally active anticholinergics, a behavioral technique was developed for the measurement of certain psychophysical parameters (Lowy et al., 1974; Lowy et al., 1976). Cats were trained to respond to a sound signal from either of two speakers by depressing a lever on the same side as the signal in order to receive a food reward. Among the parameters measured were the accuracy in sound localization, sound threshold, preference for left or right lever (laterality), duration of latency to trial onset and response latency, and the number of trials in a 30-min test interval. At 1–5 μg/kg of the more potent glycolate esters (e.g., *N*-quinuclidinyl benzilate or *N*-methyl-4-piperidyl isopentynylphenyl glycolate), number of trials and laterality were markedly affected, while sound threshold and number of errors are unaffected. A good correlation was found between the effect on cats' performance and the psychopharmacologic effectiveness of a group of anticholinergics in humans and other animal experimental paradigms. The results also indicate that the drugs were not producing a loss of sensory acuity in cats, but rather an impairment of the ability of stimuli to act as cues to behavior.

A comparison of the effects of the (+)- and (−)-isomers of 3-quinuclidinyl benzilate on the cat's performance in a sound stimulus learning paradigm (see above) revealed that the (−)-isomer was 100–200 times more effective than the (+)-isomer (Lowy et al., 1976). A single 5 μg/kg dose of the (−)-isomer abolished the ability of the cat to perform for periods lasting up to 7 days.

D. Electrophysiologic Effects

A number of studies have been carried out in man attempting to correlate the encephalographic (EEG) with the behavioral effects following the administration of Ditran (a mixture of *N*-methyl-3-piperidyl and *N*-methyl-2-pyrrolidylmethyl cyclopentylphenylglycolate). A shift in the EEG pattern towards desynchronization was observed with the occurrence of hallucinations, fantasies, illusions, or tremors (Fink, 1960). Such EEG effects were not noted with atropine. Chlorpromazine tended to reverse the EEG and behavioral effects. It was concluded that EEG desynchronization accompanies behavioral disturbances such as anxiety, hallucinations, and confusion, while symptoms such as euphoria, relaxation, and drowsiness are associated with EEG synchronization.

A correlation was found between the degree of the confusional (psychotomimetic) state and the ratio of slow to fast waves concomitant with the dissolution of the alpha rhythm (ITIL, 1966). Alteration of the Ditran-induced confusional and delirious state by a drug, such as chlorpromazine, which eliminated fast activity and potentiated slowing in the EEG, resulted in a comatose state associated with a sleeplike EEG pattern. On the other hand, a partial inhibition in the delirious state was produced by drugs, such as yohimbine and 1,2,3,4-tetrahydroaminoacridine, which decreased the amount of slow EEG activity. Although yohimbine appeared to reverse mainly the Ditran-induced changes in consciousness, tetrahydroaminoacridine also reversed the psychotic symptoms, this latter effect being correlated with the recurrence of alpha activity.

In order to investigate the cholinergic mechanisms involved in the physiologic balance between the corticocaudate and reticular systems, the effects of atropine, Ditran, and physostigmine were compared in cats with electrodes chronically and acutely implanted in the dorsal hippocampus, deep tegmental nucleus of the reticular activating system, head of the caudate nucleus, and right and left sigmoid gyrus (SPRADLIN et al., 1966). Physostigmine was more effective than Ditran in reversing the action of atropine upon the caudate nucleus, while the reversal effects of physostigmine were transient. By simultaneously stimulating the reticular formation the "caudate spindle" phenomenon can be inhibited, and both atropine and Ditran elevated the "inhibition threshold" of reticular inhibition. Despite the slowed cortical rhythms and spontaneous spindles, the cats were hyperactive, disturbed (crying and whining), and displayed defensive movements when approached. In addition, atropine and Ditran had a marked effect upon the hippocampal activity, occasionally producing seizure-like activity. Again, such effects were associated more frequently with Ditran. Since the hippocampal discharge could be interrupted by reticular stimulation, it is not clear whether the discharges seen represent a localized effect or were secondary to the drugs' effect upon the mesodiencephalic activating system. Atropine reverses the inhibitory action of physostigmine on conditioned avoidance responses, operant behavior, and hypothalamic self-stimulation, as well as many of the excitatory (amphetaminelike) actions of physostigmine, such as the shortening of pentobarbital sleeping time, contraversive circus movements, abolition of single shock responses from the midbrain reticular formation, and generalized EEG activation. Both Ditran and scopolamine also block the midbrain reticular activation of the EEG produced by physostigmine.

These observations suggested that there might be some relationship between the reticular depression produced by the anticholinergics and their effect upon the hippocampus. Studies were carried out to demonstrate this relationship by using cats with lesions in the mesencephalic reticular system and measuring the optic evoked response, the recruiting response from stimulation of the anterolateral ventral nucleus and spontaneous hippocampal activity (STERNBERGH and WILSON, 1966). Although atropine decreased the amplitude of the optic evoked response in waking cats but not in cats with reticular lesions, Ditran was without effect in either case. Physostigmine reversed this effect with atropine in waking cats, but had little reversal effect in lesioned animals. The Ditran effect on the evoked response was only reversed by physostigmine in the animals with reticular lesions. In animals with reticular lesions, Ditran facilitated and atropine had no effect on the recruiting response in the anterolateral ventral nucleus. This facilitatory action of Ditran could not be reversed by physostigmine. The unusually high doses for cats (1 mg/kg) of atropine and Ditran produced periodic bursts of beta activity in the hippocampal cortex, an effect which was reversed by physostigmine. Such findings are similar to those observed with LSD and mescaline. It was concluded that alterations of the activity of the visual system are not necessarily produced by drugs with potent hallucinogenic effects; however, such drugs do produce disturbances in the hippocampus which appear not to involve the reticular system.

E. Central Cholinergic Pathways and Systems

Despite the fact that acetylcholine and its associated enzymes are widely distributed in the brain (SHUTE and LEURS, 1963), the clearly defined systems have been restricted to only a few brain areas. Included in this group are the caudate nucleus (BUTCHER and BUTCHER, 1974), hippocampus (LEURS and SHUTE, 1967), interpeduncular nuclei (KAKOTA et al., 1973), and certain subcortical tracts (HEBB et al., 1963). The extent of cholinergic involvement in any region can be determined by the degree of ^{3}H-QNB binding, high-affinity choline uptake, and choline acetylase activity, all parameters appearing to be reasonably well correlated (KUHAR, 1978). Since most neural networks in the brain involve an interaction between two or more different neurotransmitters, it is often difficult to explain the neurologic or behavioral effects on the basis of cholinergic blockade of specific brain regions. The anticholinergics have been used to control tremors associated with Parkinson's disease and use of the major tranquilizers. The tremors apparently result from a deficiency in dopaminergic transmission within the nigrostriatum, a deficiency which is associated with both conditions. Since cholinergic synapses (inhibitory) originating from cells in the caudate nucleus regulate the release of nigrostriatal dopamine, anticholinergics tend to promote dopamine release. Another example is a cholinergically activated noradrenergic inhibitory system in the rat somatosensory cortex, which exhibits marked activation in electric activity when blocked by anticholinergics (MALCOLM et al., 1967).

Another area of the brain with definitive cholinergic mechanisms involves the pyramidal cells of the hippocampus (BISCO and STRAUGHAN, 1966; HERZ and NACIEMENTO, 1965), which appear to contain both muscarinic and nicotinic receptors (KAWAMURA and DOMINO, 1969). Hippocampal theta rhythms, which are cholinergically activated concomitants associated with conditioning, can be suppressed by anticholinergics. Presumably, this action could be responsible for the impairment in learning and memory storage resulting from centrally active anticholinergics.

F. Sites of Anticholinergic Action in Brain

With the use of high affinity radiolabeled anticholinergics, studies have been performed on their regional and cytoplasmic distribution within mammalian brain (ABOOD and RINALDI, 1959; YAMAMURA et al., 1974a). In monkey brain the regional distribution of ^{3}H-3-quinuclidinyl benzilate was found to correlate well with other cholinergic parameters, such as ^{3}H-choline uptake, choline acetyltransferase, and acetylcholinesterase (YAMAMURA et al., 1974b). By far the highest level of all four parameters was in the putamen and caudate nucleus. The cerebral hemispheres, amygdala, and hippocampus contained about half the concentration of the benzilate, but the level of the other cholinergic parameters was a small fraction of that found for the caudate nucleus. Apart from the caudate nucleus, the correlation between the distribution of the anticholinergics and the parameters used to measure cholinergic function was not impressive. By determining the extent to which ^{3}H-3-quinuclidinyl benzilate binding was diminished by pretreatment of rats with atropine, the degree of specific binding for the anticholinergic can be determined in various brain areas (YAMAMURA et al., 1974b). It would appear from such studies that although a correlation was found in some brain areas, e.g., the caudate nucleus, between the distribution of the anticholinergics and other measures of cholinergic action, the binding studies do not permit the conclusion that the drug's distribution is an accurate reflection of the pattern of muscarinic cholinergic receptors in brain.

The utilization of the binding of ^{3}H-anticholinergics to tissue preparations following the lesioning of specific brain areas provides another means of measuring specific receptors for the anticholinergics. If nerve terminals of the cholinergic afferents to the hippocampus contain muscarinic cholinergic receptors, as suggested by pharmacologic studies (MOLENAR and POLAK, 1970; SZERB and SOMOGYI, 1973), then lesioning of the septal–hippocampal cholinergic tract should reduce the drug's binding, a conclusion which was experimentally verified (YAMAMURA and SNYDER, 1974).

I. Competition Between Behavioral Potency and Receptor Affinity

In order to determine whether the centrally active anticholinergics bind to a physiologic receptor, an attempt was made to correlate inhibition binding constants of the various anticholinergic agents to their psychopharmacologic potency (BAUMGOLD et al., 1977). Such a correlation between behavioral and binding data has been attempted with a series of 14 glycolate esters (Fig. 2). A linear relation was observed between the behavioral data and the logarithm of the inhibition constants for binding. The behavioral data were taken from previously published accounts and are expressed quantitatively as BDI (behavioral disturbance index; see GABEL and ABOOD, 1965). From the evidence presented in this study, it can be concluded the ^{3}H-QNB binds to a muscarinic site in brain which is involved in producing the behavioral disturbances elicited by the glycolate esters. This conclusion is based on the low K_d, the saturability and stereospecificity of binding competition studies, and especially on the reasonable correlation observed between behavioral and binding data (Fig. 2). Although the correlation can be useful in predicting the behavioral potency of new glycolate esters, on the basis of their inhibition constants, there are notable exceptions such as atropine, scopolamine, and compound IV. All three drugs had very high affinities for the ^{3}H-QNB binding site, but their behavioral potencies were relatively low. They all contain heterocyclic ring systems other than the piperidine or quinuclidine. In a previous study, where an attempt was made to correlate the behavioral potencies of a series of glycolates with certain physical constants, the correlation tended to be excellent for the quinuclidinyl and piperidyl esters, but not for those having other heterocyclic amino rings such as tropanol and granatonol. On the other hand an excellent correlation was observed between affinity constants and the ability of the anticholinergics to block the acetylcholine-induced contraction of ileum, the correlation being independent of the type of heterocyclic amino ring (BAUMGOLD et al., 1977).

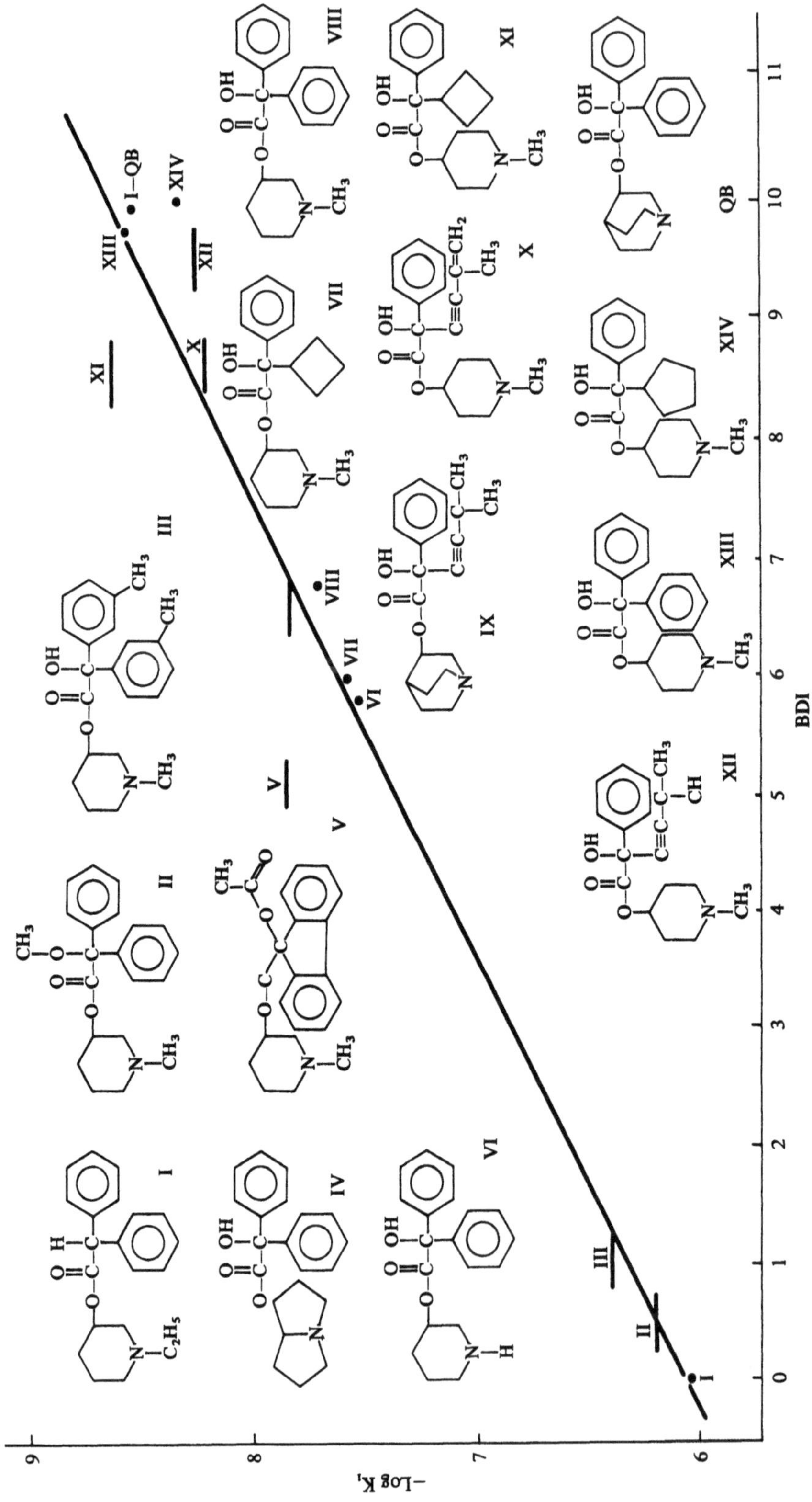

Fig. 2. Correlation of binding affinity of various centrally active anticholinergics to their behavioral disturbance index. Binding affinity is measured by K_I, the drug concentration producing 50% inhibition of ^{3}H-QNB binding to brain membrane preparations. BDI, composite index of behavioral measurements in various animals as a measure of psychotropic potency. Data adapted from BAUMGOLD et al., 1977

A comparison of the receptor binding affinities of the two optical isomers of 3-quinuclidinyl benzilate reveals that the (−)-isomer has about 50 times the affinity of the (+)-isomer for a synaptic membrane preparation from rat caudate nucleus (unpublished). It had been previously reported that the (−)-isomer had only 20 times the affinity of the (+)-isomer to a neural membrane preparation from whole rat brain (BAUMGOLD et al., 1977). The difference may be due to the fact that caudate nucleus contains a greater concentration of cholinergic receptors and that a purified synaptic membrane preparation was used in the later study. The relative binding affinities of the two isomers was, however, still less than the 200:1 potency ratio found in the cat behavioral test (LOWY et al., 1976). A plausible explanation is that the specific neurons associated with the behavioral disturbances of the drugs may possess a greater degree of binding stereospecificity than that exhibited by membrane preparations from either whole brain or caudate nucleus.

G. Conformational Analysis of Glycolate Esters

A conformational analysis has been attempted in order to explain the central action of the glycolate esters (GABEL and ABOOD, 1965). From a consideration of chemical structure–activity relationships and certain physical characteristics of the glycolate esters, it appears that the psychotomimetic effects of the esters may be dependent upon the charge and availability of the lone electron pair of the ring N. It is assumed that the primary site of attachment for the drug molecule is an electrophilic center of the receptor molecule, and that its accessibility is influenced by steric factors affecting the nonbonded electron pair of the heterocyclic N.

An extremely potent psychotomimetic agent of the glycolate series is 3-quinuclidyl benzilate. A unique feature of quinuclidine is its extreme rigidity, which imposes severe restrictions on the rotational and translational movements of the C and N atoms. This rigidity imposes restrictions on the 3-acyl substituent so that it is incapable of intramolecular hydrogen bonding, chelation, and electronic interaction with the N, interactions which would diminish drug efficacy.

Stereochemical considerations may also account for the diminution of pharmacologic activity resulting from alkyl substitution on the carbons adjacent to the ring N, the diminished potency with increasing chain length of the N-alkyl substituent, and the fact that the (β)-isomer of 9-methyl-3-granatanol benzilate is considerably more potent than the α-isomer (ABOOD, 1968).

Verification of the hypothesis that the availability of the nonbonded electron pair on the heterocyclic N is a critical factor in determining psychotropic potency of the anticholinergics requires measurements of such physicochemical parameters as the rate of quaternization of the tertiary N and the charge-transfer stability constants. The rates of quaternization and formation of charge-transfer complexes between chloranil and the drug would be expected to vary directly with the pharmacologic potency, and a reasonably good correlation was found (NOGRADY and ALGIERI, 1968; BAUMGOLD et al., 1975). If the comparisons are limited to the piperidyl, pyrrolizidyl, and quinuclidinyl glycolate esters, the correlation is generally excellent; however, when other heterocyclic amino derivatives, such as tropanyl, granatonyl, or pyrrolizdinyl are included, the correlation is less convincing. It would appear that the nucleophilicity of the heterocyclic N is an essential requirement for pharmacologic activity, but steric-configurational factors optimizing drug-receptor interaction are also important.

H. Theoretical Models of Muscarinic Receptor

It has been suggested that charge-transfer reactions are important in the interaction between a biologic receptor and the anticholinergics (GREEN et al., 1974) as well as other psychotomimetic drugs. The argument that a correlation exists between the ability to form charge-transfer complexes and psychotomimetic potency of the indolealkylamines has been both affirmed (SUNG and PARKER, 1972) and denied (MILLIE et al., 1968). Theoretical models of the cholinergic receptor have been developed by determining the pattern of the molecular electrostatic potential generated by the interaction of acetylcholine with a hypothetical negative site on the receptor (WEINSTEIN et al., 1973). Because of their rigid structure, cholinergic antagonists, although able to generate the characteristic electric potential, are unable to induce the conformational rearrangement of the receptor complex essential for its biologic responsiveness. In an effort to account for the fact that scopolamine has considerably greater central action than atropine, comparative calculations of the protonation affinity of the solvated drugs revealed scopolamine to be more nucleophilic (in the gas phase) and, because of solvation interaction and not intramolecular electronic redistribution, less basic (WEINSTEIN et al., 1977). This observation tends to be in opposition to the experimental pK_as for atropine and scopolamine (9.8 and 7.8 respectively), which suggest that atropine should be more readily protonated than scopolamine. From the molecular electrostatic potential maps for the interaction of the model compounds, tropine and scopine, with the receptor and crystallographic data for scopolamine, the stabilization energy for scopine is calculated to be 2.5 kcal/mol greater than tropine. This difference could account for the fact that scopolamine has a psychotropic action over two orders of magnitude greater than atropine (WEINSTEIN et al., 1977). Insofar as the charge-transfer stability constant is an equilibrium constant, it reflects the stabilization energy of a reactant as well as the nucleophilicity of the drugs.

Quantal mechanical studies were performed on the molecular interaction of phencyclidine derivatives with the cholinergic receptor, utilizing reactivity criteria based on the interaction pharmacophore obtained from the electrostatic potential pattern of the hypothetical drug-receptor complex (WEINSTEIN et al., 1973). A good correlation was found between both the anticholinergic and psychotomimetic properties of the phencyclidines and the structural requirements obtained from the interaction pharmacophore of acetylcholine (WEINSTEIN et al., 1973). Although the study was confined to the phencyclidines, which are weak anticholinergics, it was postulated that the interaction pharmacophore is a useful representation of the electronic structural characteristics required for interaction of the acetylcholine and its antagonists with the receptor. The model accounts for the fact that substituting thienyl or ethynyl for phenyl in phencyclidine does not diminish psychotropic potency, whereas replacement of phenyl by lower alkyl, nitrile, or alkyl or halide-substituted phenyl abolishes psychotropic activity. Such structure–activity relationships are in agreement with those of the substituted glycolic acid derivatives of piperidinol and other cyclic amino alcohols (ABOOD and BIEL, 1962).

I. Multiple Configurational States of the Muscarinic Receptor from Brain

It now appears that several neural receptors, including the muscarinic (Snyder and Bennett, 1976), exist in both agonist and antagonist conformations (Snyder et al., 1975). A more appropriate model considers the receptor to exist in a "high-affinity agonist" and "low-affinity agonist" form, which are interconvertible by modification of sulfhydryl and other functional groups. Reductive alkylation of neural membranes with *N*-ethylmaleimide (NEM) or certain transition metals increases the affinity for muscarinic agonists, such as carbamylcholine, without altering the affinity of anticholinergics (Aronstam et al., 1978). The following scheme has been proposed for the muscarinic receptor which is based on the Katz-Thesleff cyclic model for the nicotinic cholinergic receptor of the motor end plate (Katz and Thesleff, 1951) and attempts to incorporate much of the recent biochemical and physical data on the receptor (Aronstam et al., 1978):

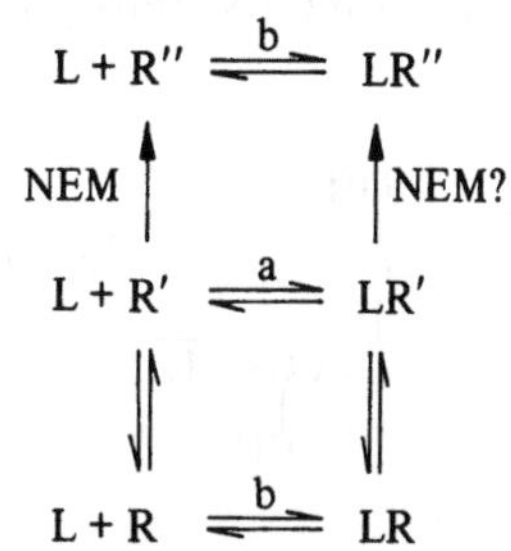

Fig. 3. R and R' represent the low and high agonist-affinity states, respectively. R, receptors that have been converted to the high-affinity form by NEM alkylation and have the same binding properties as R'. L is a ligand, and a and b are the association constants of the ligand with the receptor in the different states

Reductive alkylation of certain sulfhydryl groups appears to stabilize the receptors in the high affinity state, and since the NEM conversion requires elevated temperatures, the NEM-sensitive sulfhydryl groups may be buried within the receptor molecule. The NEM conversion to the high affinity state is more nearly complete in the presence of an agonist than an antagonist or no receptor ligand, although exposure of the receptor to the agonist alone does not alter subsequent agonist binding. Evidently an agonist-induced conformational change within the receptor exposes the buried sulfhydryl groups to NEM, and insofar as the change is not produced by anticholinergics, it may reflect the physiologic response of the receptor to the agonist. In the case of the Katz-Thesleff model the equivalent of R refers to a refractory state of the receptor, so that a pharmacologic response occurs only after the association of the agonist in the active state (R, in the model above). It has been suggested that the high agonist-affinity state of the end organ of the electric eel is correlated with desensitization, insofar as preconditioning of nicotinic receptors increases receptor affinity for agonists (Weber et al., 1975).

The association of the anticholinergic with the muscarinic receptor is distinctly different from that of acetylcholine and other agonists, despite the fact that both contain an esteratic and cationic site. The difference is attributable to the presence of aromatic or other large hydrophobic substituents on the anticholinergics which contribute to their interaction with hydrophobic sites of both phospholipids and proteins. Both the degree of hydrophobicity and steric factors contribute to the interaction of anticholinergics with their receptor, probably eclipsing esteratic-cationic forces. Thermodynamic studies of the brain muscarinic receptor suggest that hydrophobic forces are preponderant over ionic and polar forces; furthermore, chaotropic ions, which weaken hydrophobic interaction by disrupting water structure, reversibly decrease anticholinergic affinity to receptors (ARONSTAM et al., 1977).

II. Use of Affinity-Labeled Sepharose for Purification of Muscarinic Receptor from Brain

In an attempt to isolate the muscarinic receptor from mammalian brain an affinity column was prepared by coupling to AH-sepharose beads a highly potent anticholinergic, 1-methyl-4-piperidyl phenyl (3-methyl-but-lyne-3-enyl) glycolate (BAUMGOLD and ABOOD, unpublished).

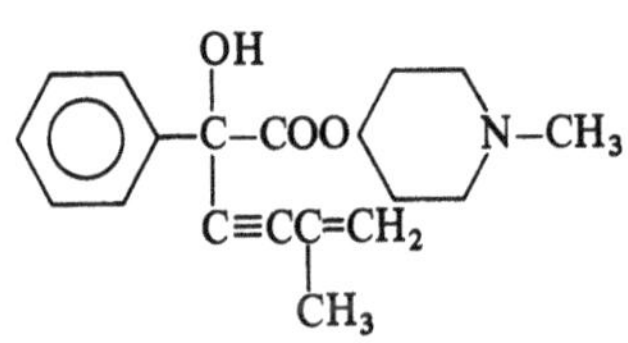

By reacting the alkenyl residue of glycolate with bromine to form the bromide derivative, which is then coupled to AH-sepharose, an affinity gel was obtained having the following structure:

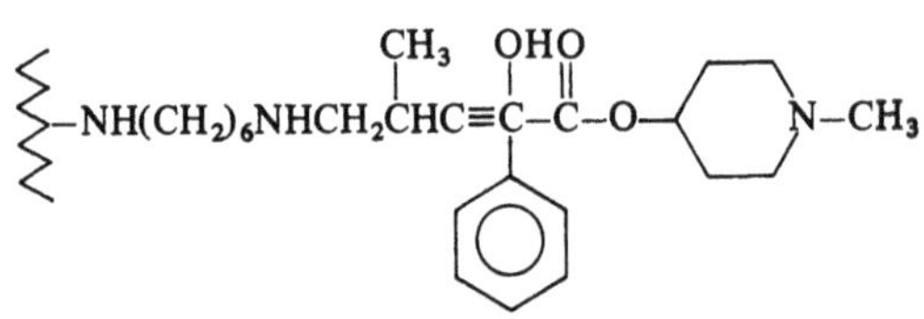

An extract, prepared by homogenization of rat brain membranes in 1% Triton X-100 followed by ultracentrifugation, was passed through the affinity column, and the muscarinic receptor material, which was retained on the column, was eluted with 0.01 M carbamylcholine. The eluted component, which is homogeneous by SDS-acrylamide gel electrophoresis and appears to have a molecular weight in excess of 300,000, exhibits only about five fold enrichment of ^{3}H-QNB binding. Conceivably, the activity was irreversibly diminished by exposure of the receptor to detergent (ARONSTAM et al., 1977).

I. Possible Role of Calcium in Anticholinergic Action

At concentrations of $10^{-5} M$, the centrally active anticholinergics inhibited the spontaneous twitching observed when the frog sartorius muscles were immersed in a Ca-free Ringer's solution (ABOOD et al., 1963). It was shown subsequently that the intracellular resting potential of the muscle after partial depolarization in Ca-deprived media could be restored upon the addition of low concentrations of *N*-methyl-2-pyrrolidylmethyl cyclopentylphenylglycolate (PMCG) to the medium. Evidently the drug was acting in a manner similar to Ca in restoring the resting potential and, thereby, excitability of the muscle. A similar action of Ca and PMCG was observed on the negative after-potential of an excited single muscle fiber. At a concentration of $10^{-5}M$, PMCG produced a marked prolongation of the negative after-potential, usually seen when the Ca concentration of Ringer's solution is increased from 2 to 5 m*M*. Accompanying the prolongation of the negative after-potential in the presence of $10^{-5}M$ PMCG is a significant increase in the degree of isometric contraction of the frog muscle. The stimulation of the muscle anaerobic glycolysis accompanying the depolarization resulting from either Ca removal or high $K+$ is also blocked by the addition of $10^{-5}M$ PMCG (ABOOD, 1962). Evidently the drug's action is at the level of the Ca-linked excitation-coupling system of the muscle. Since the concentration of PMCG used in such studies is considerably greater than that needed to produce central effects in mammals, one might question their relevance to the drug's action on brain. Nevertheless, in view of the general regulatory role of Ca in excitability as well as neurotransmitter storage, release, and action, the possibility should be considered that some of the central actions of the anticholinergics may be attributable to their interference with Ca.

J. Clinical Use of Anticholinergics

A number of centrally active anticholinergics are used clinically in the treatment of various psychiatric disorders as well as Parkinsonism and the extrapyramidal side effects of the major tranquilizers (see Table 1). As early as 1951, large doses of atropine were used in the management of psychotics, the dose (32 mg) being sufficient to produce confusion, delirium, and coma (FORRER, 1951). In the course of investigating the central effects of Ditran in humans, it was observed that some subjects exhibited a marked elevation in mood, characterized by increased euphoria, initiative, and activity (ABOOD and MEDUNA, 1958). Subsequently, it was shown that following an intramuscular dose of 5–15 mg Ditran to depressed patients, which produced hallucinations, delirium, and confusion, there occurred an amelioration of many of the symptoms (ABOOD and MEDUNA, 1958; FINKELSTEIN, 1961).

Benactyzine, a drug which was introduced in the early days of the psychotherapeutic drugs, is probably the only anticholinergic used chronically for the treatment of psychoneuroses (JACOBSEN, 1964). Its peripheral anticholinergic potency is about one-tenth that of atropine, and its central action, one-tenth that of Ditran.

A number of widely used psychotherapeutic drugs are known to produce anticholinergic side effects including central manifestations. Included in this group are the tricyclic antidepressants, phenothiazines, and anti-Parkinsonism drugs (DAVIES et al., 1971; GERSHON et al., 1962; VAN DER KOLK et al., 1978). Among the central effects produced in man are anxiety, delirium, hallucinations, stupor, and coma, all of which are characteristic of the potent anticholinergics. With the use of the QNB-receptor binding assay, it can be shown that the tricyclic antidepressant, amitriptyline and clozapine had about 5% the potency of atropine, while imipramine had about 10%

Table 1. Psychotherapeutic anticholinergics.

Name	Chemical structure	Dose (mg)	Treatment
Atropine	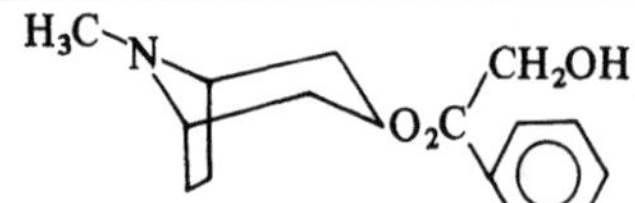	30	Psychosis
Ditran	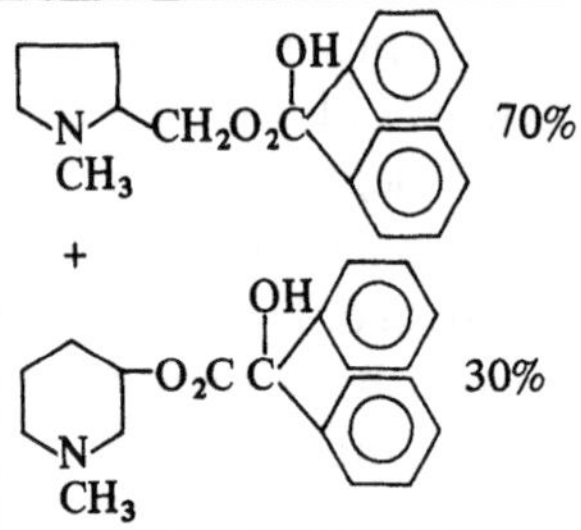	5–15	Depression
Benactyzine	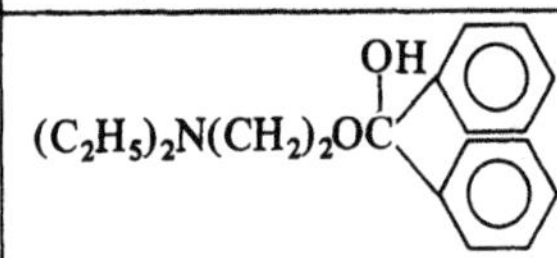	3–10	Depression
Trihexylphenidyl	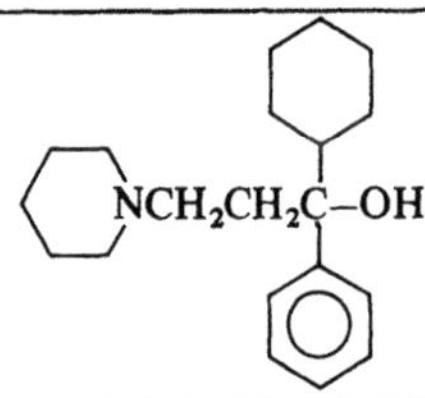	1–2	Parkinsonism
Benztropine	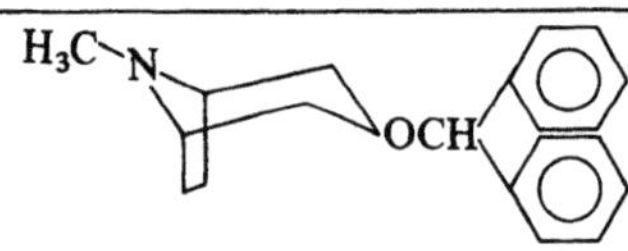	1–2	Extra-pyramidal symptoms Pyrkinsonism
Thiothixene	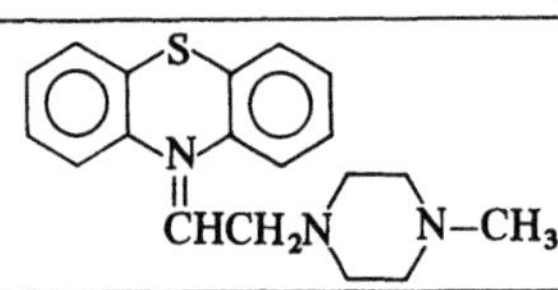	10–20	Psychosis
Thioridazine	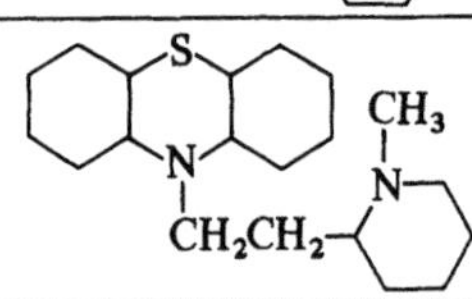	200–800	Psychosis
Amitriptyline	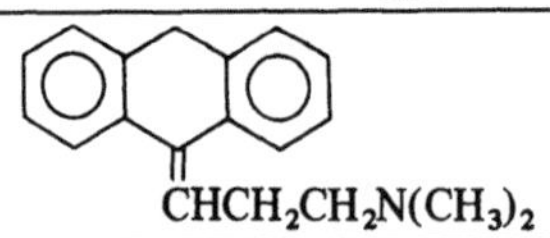	75–150	Depression
1–Cyclohexylpiperidine	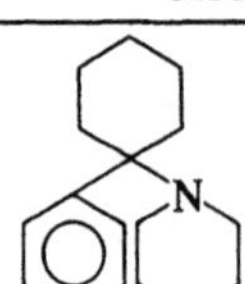		Anesthesia (dissociative)

and chlorpromazine about 1% the binding affinity to brain preparations as did amitriptyline (SNYDER and YAMAMURA, 1977). Such studies prompted the conclusion that the anticholinergic properties may be in part responsible for the antidepressant effects (SNYDER and YAMAMURA, 1977), but in a clinical study little correlation was found (VAILLANT, 1969).

A number of major tranquilizers, such as clozapine and thiroidazine, have a low incidence of extrapyramidal side effects, whereas others, such as the butyrophenones and trifluoperaine, have a high incidence. The difference is explainable on the basis that drugs such as clozapine exert a central anticholinergic effect at dose levels needed for tranquilization. By examining the relative affinity of a variety of antipsychotic drugs for the muscarinic receptor, it was shown that the ability to produce extrapyramidal side effects was inversely related to the affinity to the muscarinic receptor (SNYDER et al., 1974).

References

Abood, L.G.: The psychotomimetic glycolate esters. In: Drugs affecting the central nervous system. Burger, A. (ed.), pp. 127–165. New York: Dekker 1968

Abood, L.G., Biel, J.H.: Anticholinergic psychotomimetic agents. Int. Rev. Neurobiol. *4*, 218–271 (1962)

Abood, L.G., Koyoma, I., Kimizuka, H.: A possible mechanisms of action of calcium and some psychotomimetic agents on membranes. Nature *197*, 367–369 (1963)

Abood, L.G., Meduna, L.J.: Some effects of a new psychotogen in depressive states. J. Nerv. Ment. Dis. *127*, 546–549 (1958)

Abood, L.G., Rinaldi, F.: Studies with a tritium-labeled psychotomimetic agent. Psychopharmacology *1*, 117–123 (1959)

Aronstam, R.S., Abood, L.G., Baumgold, J.: Role of phospholipids in muscarinic binding in neural membranes. Biochem. Pharmacol. *26*, 1689–1695 (1977)

Aronstam, R.S., Abood, L.G., Hoss, W.: Influence of sulfhydryl reagents and heavy metals on the functional state of the muscarinic acetylcholine receptor in rat brain. Mol. Pharmacol. *14*, 575–586 (1978)

Baumgold, J., Abood, L.G., Aronstam, R.: Studies on the relationship of binding affinity to psychoactive and anticholinergic potency of a group of psychotomimetic glycolates. Brain Res. *124*, 331–340 (1977)

Baumgold, J., Abood, L.G., Hoss, W.P.: Chemical factors influencing the psychotomimetic potency of glycolate esters. Life Sci. *17*, 603–612 (1975)

Biel, J.H., Abood, L.G., Hoya, W.K., Leiser, H.A., Nuhfer, P.A., Kluchesky, E.F.: Central Stimulants II Cholinergic Blockade. J. Org. Chem. *26*, 4096–4103 (1961)

Biscoe, T.J., Straughan, D.W.: Microelectrophoretic studies of neurones in the cat hippocampus. J. Physiol. (Lond.) *183*, 341–359 (1966)

Buehler, C.A., Thames, S.F., Abood, L.G., Biel, J.H.: Physiologically active compounds. VI. Cyclic amino thiolesters of substituted chloroacetic, benzilic, and glycolic acids. J. Med. Chem. *8*, 643–647 (1965)

Butcher, S.G., Butcher, L.L.: Origin and modulation of acetylcholine activity in the striatum. Brain Res. *71*, 167–171 (1974)

Davies, R.K., Tucker, G.J., Harrow, M., Detre, T.P.: Confusional episodes and antidepressant medication. Am. J. Psychiatry *128*, 95–99 (1971)

Feldberg, W.: A Pharmacological approach to the brain, pp. 84–88. Boston: Williams & Wilkins 1963

Fink, M.E.: Effect of anticholinergic compounds on post-convulsive electroencephalogram and behavior of psychiatric patients. Electroencephalogr. Clin. Neurophysiol. *12*, 359–369 (1960)

Finkelstein, B.A.: Ditran, a psychotherapeutic advance: A review of one hundred and three cases. J. Neuropsychiatr. *2*, 144–148 (1961)
Forrer, G.R.: Atropine toxicity in the treatment of mental disease. Am. J. Psychiatry *108*, 107 (1951)
Freiter, E.R., Cannon, J.G., Milne, L.D., Abood, L.G.: Synthesis of compounds with potential psychotomimetic activity. J. Med. Chem. *11*, 1041–1045 (1968)
Gabel, N., Abood, L.G.: Stereochemical factors related to the potency of anticholinergic psychotomimetic drugs. J. Med. Chem. *8*, 616–619 (1965)
Gershon, S.: Behavioral effects of anticholinergic psychotomimetics and their antagonism in man and animals. Recent Adv. Biol. Psychiatr. *8*, 141–149 (1966)
Gershon, S., Holmberg, G., Mattson, E., Mattson, N., Marshall, A.: Imipramine hydrochloride. Arch. Gen. Psychiatry *6*, 96–101 (1962)
Green, J.P., Johnson, C.L., Kang, S.: Application of quantum chemistry to drugs and their interaction. Ann. Rev. Pharmacol. *14*, 319–342 (1974)
Hebb, C.O., Krnjevic, K., Silver, A.: Effect of undercutting on the acetylcholine and choline acetyltransferase activity in the cats cerebral cortex. Nature *198*, 692 (1963)
Herz, A., Nacimento, A.C.: Über die Wirkung von Pharmaka auf Neurone des Hippocampus nach mikroelektrophoretischer Verabfolgung. Naunyn Schmiedebergs Arch. Pharmacol. *251*, 295–314 (1965)
Itil, T.M.: Quantitative EEG changes induced by anticholinergic drugs and their behavioral correlates in man. Recent Adv. Biol. Psychiatr. *8*, 151–158 (1966)
Jacobsen, E.: Benactyzine. In: Psychopharmacological agents. Gordon, M. (ed.), Vol. *1*, pp. 287–298. New York: Academic Press 1964
Kakota, K., Nakamura, Y., Hassler, R.: Habenulo-interpeduncular tract: a possible cholinergic neuron in brain. Brain Res. *62*, 264–267 (1973)
Katz, B., Thesleff, S.: A study of desensitization produced by acetylcholine at the motor end plate. J. Physiol. (Lond.) *138*, 63–80 (1957)
Kawamura, H., Domino, E.G.: Differential actions of m and n cholinergic agonists on the brainstem activating system. Int. J. Neuropharmacol. *8*, 105–115 (1969)
Kosman, M.E.: Effects of amphetamine on the learning and performance of mice in a swimming maze. Proc. Soc. Exp. Biol. Med. *115*, 728–731 (1964)
Kuhar, M.J.: Central cholinergic pathways: Physiological and pharmacologic aspects. In: Psychopharmacology. Lipton, M.A., Dimascio, A., Killiam, K.E. (eds.), pp. 199–203. New York: Raven 1978
Leurs, P.K., Shute, C.C.D.: The cholinergic limbic system. Brain *90*, 521–540 (1967)
Lipman, V., Abood, L.G., Shurrager, P.S.: Effect of anticholinergic psychotomimetic agents on motor activity and body temperature. Arch. Int. Pharmacodyn. Therap. *146*, 174–191 (1963)
Lowy, K., Weiss, B., Abood, L.G.: Influence of an anticholinergic psychotomimetic agent on behavior in cats controlled by an auditory stimulus. Neuropharmacology *13*, 707–718 (1974)
Lowy, K., Abood, L.G., Raines, H.: Behavioral effects and binding affinities of two stereoisomeric psychotomimetic glycolates. J. Neurosci. Res. *2*, 157–165 (1976b).
Lowy, K., Abood, M.E., Drexler, M., Abood, L.G.: Antagonism by cholinergic drugs of behavioral effects in cats of an anticholinergic psychotomimetic drug and enhancement by nicotine. Neuropharmacology *16*, 399–403 (1976a)
Malcolm, J.L., Sarawa, P., Spear, P.J.: Cholinergic and adrenergic inhibition in the rat cerebral cortex. Int. J. Neuropharmacol. *6*, 509–527 (1967)
Meyerhoffer, A.: Absolute configuration of 3-quinuclidinyl benzilate and the behavioral effect in dog of the optical isomers. J. Med. Chem. *15*, 994–995 (1972)
Millie, P., Mairieu, J.P., Benoim, J., Lallemand, J.Y., Julia, M.: Researches in the indole series. Quantal mechanical calculations and charge-transfer complexes of substituted indoles. J. Med. Chem. 207–211 (1968)
Molenar, P.C., Polak, P.L.: Stimulation by atropine of acetylcholine release and synthesis in cortical slices from rat brain. Br. J. Pharmacol. *40*, 406–417 (1970)
Nogrady, T., Algieri, A.A.: Charge transfer complexes in medicinal chemistry. I. Correlations with the psychotropic activity of piperidinol esters and related compounds. J. Med. Chem. *11*, 212–213 (1968)

Polidora, V.: A sequential response method for studying complex behavior in animals and its application to the measurement of drug effects. J. Exp. Anal. Behav. *6*, 271–277 (1963)
Shute, C.C.D., Leurs, P.R.: Cholinesterase-containing systems of the brain of the rat. Nature *199*, 1160–1164 (1963)
Snyder, S.H., Bennett, J.P.: Neurochemical receptors in the brain: Biochemical identifiaction. Ann. Rev. Physiol. *38*, 153–175 (1976)
Snyder, S.H., Chang, K.J., Kuhar, M.J., Yamamura, H.I.: Biochemical identification of the muscarinic cholinergic receptor. Fed. Proc. *34*, 1915–1921 (1975)
Snyder, S., Yamamura, H.: Antidepressants and the muscarinic acetylcholine receptor. Arch. Gen. Psychiatry *34*, 236–239 (1977)
Spradlin, W.W., Sternbergh, W.C.A., Wilson, W.P., Hughes, J.L.: Anticholinergic hallucinosis: I. Effects of atropine and JB 329 on caudate spindle phenomena and electrical activity of cat hippocampus. Recent Adv. Biol. Psychiatr. *8*, 175–185 (1966)
Sternbach, L.H., Kaiser, S.: Antispasmodics. II: Esters of basic bicyclic alcohols. J. Am. Chem. Soc. *74*, 2219–2221 (1952)
Sternbergh, W.C.A., Wilson, W.P.: Anticholinergic hallucinosis: II. Effects of atropine and JB 329 on activity of the visual system, nonspecific projection system, and hippocampus in animals without reticular system lesions. Recent Adv. Biol. Psychiatr. *8*, 187–197 (1966)
Sung, M.T., Parker, J.A.: Amphetamine correlation of activity with stability of molecular complexes. Proc. Natl. Acad. Sci. USA *69*, 1346–1347 (1972)
Szerb, J.C., Somogyi, G.T.: Depression of acetylcholine release from cerebral cortical slices by cholinesterase inhibition and oxotremorine. Nature (New Biol.) *241*, 121–122 (1973)
Vaillant, G.E.: Clinical significance of anticholinergic effects of imipramine-like drugs. Am. J. Psychiatry *125*, 1600–1602 (1969)
Van der Kolk, B.A., Shader, R.I., Greenblatt, D.J.: Autonomic effects of psychotropic drugs. In: Psychopharmacology. Lipton, M.A., Dimascio, A., Killiam, K.E. (eds.), pp. 1009–1020. New York: Raven 1978
Vincent, J.P., Cavey, D., Kamenka, J.M., Geneste, P., Lazdunski, M.: Interaction of phencyclidines with the muscarinic and opiate receptors in the central nervous system. Brain Res. *152*, 176–182 (1978)
Weber, M.,David-Pfeutychangeux, J.P.: Regulation of binding properties of the nicotinic receptor protein by cholinergic ugands in membrane fragments of torpedo marmoti. Proc. Natl. Acad. Sci. USA *72*, 3443–3447 (1975)
Weinstein, H., Srebrenik, S., Mayaani, S., Sokolovsky, M.: A theoretical model study of the comparative effectiveness of atropine and scopolamine action in central nervous system. J. Theor. Biol. *64*, 295–309 (1977)
Weinstein, H., Maayani, S., Srebrenik, S., Cohen, S., Sokolovsky, M.: Psychotomimetic drugs as anticholinergic agents. II. Quantum mechanical study of molecular interaction potentials of 1-cyclohexylpiperidine derivatives with cholinergic receptor. Mol. Pharmacol. *9*, 820–834 (1973)
Weiss, B., Heller, A.: Methodological problems in evaluating the role of cholinergic mechanisms in behavior. Fed. Proc. *28*, 135–145 (1969)
Yamamura, H.L., Snyder, S.H.: Postsynaptic localization of muscarinic cholinergic receptor binding in rat hippocampus. Brain Res. *78*, 320–326 (1974)
Yamamura, H.L., Kuhar, M.J., Greenberg, D., Snyder, S.H.: Muscarinic cholinergic receptor binding: regional distribution in monkey brain. Brain Res. *66*, 541–546 (1974a)
Yamamura, H.L., Kuhar, M.J., Snyder, S.H.: In vivo identification of mucarinic cholinergic receptor binding in rat brain. Brain Res. *800*, 170–176 (1974b)

CHAPTER 16

Central Nervous Actions of Beta-Adrenoceptor Antagonists

D. A. BUXTON, D. T. GREENWOOD, and D. N. MIDDLEMISS

A. Introduction

The development during the 1960s of drugs which specifically antagonise β-adrenoceptors has led to the introduction of a new class of therapeutic agents of established value in the treatment of a variety of cardiovascular diseases, including angina, cardiac arrhythmia and hypertension. It has been assumed that these effects are mediated primarily by the antagonism of the effects of noradrenaline at receptor sites within the peripheral autonomic nervous system. In hypertension, however, the mode of action is by no means certain, and evidence has been put forward in support of a centrally mediated component (DAY and ROACH, 1973). Various central nervous system effects have been noted in both animals and man, and these effects may provide a basis for the claimed therapeutic benefits seen in some psychiatric and neurological disorders. The mechanisms underlying these therapeutic claims are poorly understood, since β-adrenoceptor antagonists have pharmacological actions other than at β-adrenoceptors and the role of the latter in the CNS is unknown.

We review the evidence that there are β-adrenoceptors in the CNS, and that β-adrenoceptor antagonists have central biochemical, behavioral, and electrophysiological effects in animals and man as well as the extent to which these may be related to their therapeutic actions in psychiatric and neurological disorders.

The CNS actions of β-adrenoceptor antagonists have been the subject of several previous reviews (GREENBLATT and SHADER, 1972; JEFFERSON, 1974; WHITLOCK and PRICE, 1974; CONWAY et al., 1978).

B. Pharmacological Heterogeneity and Access to the Brain of Beta-Adrenoceptor Antagonists

Of fundamental importance to studies of β-adrenoceptor antagonists in the CNS is the appreciation that these agents form a heterogeneous class of compounds with respect to pharmacological activity. These drugs may have selectivity for different subtypes of β-adrenoceptor; thus, β_1-receptors are largely characteristic of heart tissue and β_2-receptors of lung and blood vessels. They may have intrinsic sympathomimetic (ISA or partial agonist) activity and/or may have membrane stabilising activity (MSA), a property which is related to lipophilicity and therefore to ease of brain penetration of these agents. A summary of the commonly used β-adrenoceptor antagonists and their known properties is given in Table 1.

As well as possessing pharmacological heterogeneity, these drugs also show different abilities to enter the CNS. There have been a number of animal studies designed

Table 1. Pharmacological activities of some β-adrenoceptor antagonists

Generic name	Proprietary name	β-Antagonist activity	Selectivity	ISA[a]	MSA[b]	Brain access
Dichloroisoprenaline (DCI)	—	+	None	+++	+	NA[c]
Propranolol	Inderal (1)	+	None	None	+	+
D-Propranolol	—	Very weak	None	None	+	+
Pronethalol	Alderlin (1)	+	None	++	+	+
INPEA	—	+	None	+	None	Poor
Butoxamine	—	+	β_2	+	NA[c]	NA[c]
Pindolol	Visken (2)	++	None	++	+	+
Alprenolol	Aptin (3)	+	None	None	+	+
Oxprenolol	Trasicor (4)	+	None	+	+	+
Sotalol	Betacardone (5) Sotacor (6)	+	None	None	None	Poor
Practolol	Eraldin (1)	+	β_1	+	None	Poor
Atenolol	Tenormin (7)	+	β_1	None	None	Poor
Metoprolol	Lopressor (8) Betaloc (3)	+	β_1	None	None	Poor/+
Acebutolol	Sectral (9)	+	β_1	+	+	Poor/+

[a] Intrinsic sympathomimetic activity
[b] Membrane-stabilising activity
[c] Data not available
+, ++, +++ Increasing intensity/potency
(1) ICI, (2) Sandoz, (3) Astra, (4) CIBA, (5) Duncan Flockhart, (6) Bristol, (7) Stuart, (8) Geigy, (9) May and Baker

to measure CNS penetration of these agents after both acute and chronic administration (MASUOKA and HANSSON, 1967; SCALES and COSGROVE, 1970; HAYES and COOPER, 1971; BODIN et al., 1974; GARVEY and RAM, 1975; MYERS et al., 1975; JOHNSSON and REGARDH, 1976; LEVY et al., 1976; DAY et al., 1977; SCHNECK et al., 1977; VAN ZWIETEN and TIMMERMANS, 1979; STREET et al., 1979; CRUIKSHANK et al., 1979) which show that all the commonly used β-antagonist drugs do penetrate the CNS to some extent. Radioactivity can be detected in the mouse brain as early as 5 min after systemic administration of radiolabelled β-adrenoceptor antagonists, albeit to varying degrees (STREET et al., 1979). Distribution equilibrium between the brain and plasma is achieved within 30 min for propranolol (HAYES and COOPER, 1971) and alprenolol (BODIN et al., 1974), but takes 12 to 24 h for practolol (SCALES and COSGROVE, 1970). The degree of penetration of the CNS can be explained on the basis of the lipophilicity of individual drugs. Thus propranolol, alprenolol, oxprenolol and pindolol readily penetrate the CNS, acebutolol and metoprolol somewhat less so, and sotalol, atenolol and practolol penetrate very poorly (see previously quoted references in this section). There is a slight initial preferential uptake of the L-isomer of propranolol into brain tissue after intravenous administration in mice (LEVY et al., 1976), which cannot be explained in terms of the lipophilicity of the D- and L-isomers which are identical. This difference may be explicable in terms of a cardiovascular phenomenon since propranolol has been demonstrated to alter cerebral blood flow (MACKENZIE et al., 1976).

The relevance of these animal studies to man may be judged from a post-mortem study in patients who had received a prolonged intravenous infusion of D-propranolol as part of a treatment for paraquat poisoning (MYERS et al., 1975). This study showed that the brain/plasma ratio of propranolol in man under these conditions is similar to that observed in the rabbit ($\sim$15:1), and therefore this β-adrenoceptor antagonist is highly concentrated in brain tissue.

C. Evidence for Beta-Adrenoceptors in the CNS

I. Biochemical Evidence

β-adrenoceptor antagonists principally block sympathetic stimulation, an effect which is thought to occur via adrenoceptors linked to an adenylate cyclase. It is therefore possible that central nervous effects may also be due to the attenuation of central sympathetic stimulation. A necessary condition for this to occur is that β-adrenoceptors should be demonstrable in the CNS.

The first biochemical demonstration of β-adrenoceptors in the CNS was by KAKIUCHI and RALL (1968) who showed that an adenylate cyclase from rabbit cerebellum, when stimulated by isoprenaline, produced an increase in cyclic AMP, which was antagonized by dichloroisoprenaline, a β-adrenoceptor antagonist. Stimulation of adenylate cyclase by isoprenaline has subsequently been demonstrated in rat brain homogenates (HORN and PHILLIPSON, 1976), in the cortex of the primate brain (AHN et al., 1976) and in the cerebellum of the human brain (TSANG and LAL, 1978). Each of these isoprenaline-stimulated adenylate cyclases was blocked by propranolol (for a recent review see KEBABIAN, 1977). WURTMAN et al. (1971) demonstrated that the synthesis of serotonin and melatonin in the pineal body of the rat is mediated through a β-adrenoceptor. These studies all suggest the presence of β-adrenoceptors in the CNS.

Technical difficulties involved in the preparation of catecholamine-responsive adenylate cyclases from brain tissue, however, have hampered further research in this area. More recent work has concentrated on the demonstration of β-adrenoceptors in the CNS, using receptor binding techniques.

A variety of radioligands has been used to demonstrate and quantify β-adrenoceptors in the CNS. These include [^{3}H] propranolol (NAHORSKI, 1976), dihydro [^{3}H] alprenolol (ALEXANDER et al., 1975; BYLUND and SNYDER, 1976), [^{125}I] iodohydroxybenzylpindolol (SPORN and MOLINOFF, 1976) and [^{3}H] adrenaline (U'PRICHARD and SNYDER, 1977). The binding properties of the radioligands to CNS homogenates have the characteristics of receptors in that the binding was in each case rapid, reversible, stereospecific and of high affinity. The order of potency of catecholamine agonists in displacing these ligands was found to be isoprenaline > adrenaline > noradrenaline, which fulfills the criteria for beta-adrenoceptors. Depending on the tissue source, the receptors were found to be predominantly of the β_1 type (ALEXANDER et al., 1975; BYLUND and SNYDER, 1976; DOLPHIN et al., 1979), β_2 type (NAHORSKI, 1976; U'PRICHARD and SNYDER, 1977; COTE and KEBABIAN, 1978) or a mixture of the two subtypes (NAHORSKI, 1978). The ontogeny of both the [^{125}I] iodohydroxybenzylpindolol binding site and isoprenaline-stimulated adenylate cyclase has been studied in the rat, and it is concluded that the development of β-adrenoceptors permits the expression of catecholamine-sensitive adenylate cyclase activity. Normal levels of β-receptors are reached 14 days after birth (HARDEN et al., 1977). There is a good correlation between the potencies of β-agonists and antagonists against dihydro [^{3}H] alprenolol binding and catecholamine-stimulated adenylate cyclase in both the rat cortex (DOLPHIN et al., 1979) and rabbit cerebellum (COTE and KEBABIAN, 1978). It is therefore likely that in the CNS the dihydro [^{3}H] alprenolol binding site and the β-adrenoceptor coupled to an adenylate cyclase are identical. Despite the fact that β-receptors have been detected on glial cells (MAGUIRE et al., 1976), it is probable that the majority of the β-adrenergic radioligand binding sites are of synaptic location and hence may play a role in synaptic transmission (BYLUND and SNYDER, 1976; DAVIS and LEFKOWITZ, 1976; DOLPHIN et al., 1979). Further evidence for a synaptic localisation of β-adrenoceptors has been provided by the use of a fluorescent analogue of propranolol, 9-aminoacridine-propranolol, which has been claimed to selectively label, in vivo, the presynaptic β-receptors in the cerebellum (MELAMED et al., 1976). More recent studies have suggested, however, that the fluorescence seen in this study was a result of autofluorescent granules (HESS, 1979).

II. Electrophysiological Evidence

Evidence that β-adrenoceptors may be functional entities in the CNS comes from micro-iontophoretic studies in which micro-iontophoretic application of adrenergic agonists and antagonists has been shown convincingly to influence the electrical activity of cortical neurons of the cat (STRAUGHAN et al., 1968). The presence of both excitatory and inhibitory β-adrenoceptors in cat cortex has been demonstrated (BEVAN et al., 1974; BEVAN et al., 1977).

D. Neuropharmacological and Behavioral Effects of Beta-Adrenoceptor Antagonists

I. Central Nervous Effects in Animals

Despite the convincing demonstration of the presence of β-adrenoceptors in the CNS, it is not clear what contribution antagonism at these receptors may play in the observed central effects of β-adrenoceptor antagonists.

Much of the work on central actions of β-adrenoceptor antagonists follows administration by systemic routes, and therefore debate exists concerning the relative importance of peripheral and central mechanisms and the possibility of actions other than those at β-adrenergic sites playing a role.

If central β-blockade is of importance during treatment with these drugs, one may anticipate changes in central noradrenaline levels or turnover. Many studies on the effect of both acute and chronic administration of β-adrenoceptor antagonists on brain biogenic amine concentrations have been published, but these are mainly contradictory in their findings. Thus, one or more of the amine levels have been found to be increased (ARO and KLINGE, 1971; MAHON et al., 1977; MILMORE and TAYLOR, 1976), decreased (BRUNNER et al., 1966; HERMAN et al., 1971) or unaffected (LAVERTY and TAYLOR, 1968; GREEN and GRAHAME-SMITH, 1976; MAZURKIEWICZ-KWILECKI and ROMAGNOLI, 1970).

Studies on amine turnover in rats, after acute administration of propranolol, claim to show an enhancement of dopamine turnover in the limbic regions of the brain (FUXE et al., 1976a; WIESEL, 1976) or no change in whole brain (ANDEN and STROMBOM, 1974), but no change in the striatum after chronic dosing (LAVERTY and TAYLOR, 1968). Noradrenaline turnover is apparently reduced and increased by L- and D-propranolol, respectively, in the cortex cerebri (FUXE et al., 1976b) and is increased (WIESEL, 1976) or unchanged (ANDEN and STROMBOM, 1974) in whole brain by DL-propranolol administration. 5-HT turnover is either reduced (MILMORE and TAYLOR, 1976) or unaffected (GREEN and GRAHAME-SMITH, 1976) by acute propranolol administration to rats. It is our opinion that no conclusions can be drawn from such conflicting data, and a definitive study of the effect of a range of β-adrenoceptor antagonists on biogenic amine levels and turnover is required.

Other biochemical effects which have been noted following administration of β-adrenoceptor antagonists include alterations in the activity of tyrosine hydroxylase (SULLIVAN et al., 1972; PETERS and MAZURKIEWICZ-KWILECKI, 1975; RAINE and CHUBB, 1977), dopamine β-hydroxylase (RAINE and CHUBB, 1977) and monoamine oxidase (MAO) (MILMORE and TAYLOR, 1976). The last of these changes, the inhibition of monoamine oxidase by propranolol, is likely to be due to the membrane-stabilising property of propranolol since the effect occurs only at high concentrations (0.26 mM). This membrane-stabilising effect is also likely to account for the activity of β-adrenoceptor antagonists against [^{3}H] haloperidol (BREMNER et al., 1978) and [^{3}H] naloxone receptor binding (CHARALAMPOUS and ASKEW, 1974). Presynaptic β-adrenoceptors are thought to mediate noradrenaline release, and blockade by β-adrenoceptor antagonists has been demonstrated in brain slices (SHENOY and ZIANCE, 1979). Chronic propranolol administration is also claimed to induce β-receptor supersensitivity as measured by adenylate cyclase responsiveness to noradrenaline (DOLPHIN et al., 1977) or dihydro [^{3}H] alprenolol binding (DOLPHIN et al., 1979). This may not be a functional supersensitisation during chronic administration of the drug, since acute administration of propranolol actually reduces the apparent number of β-receptors in rat brain if care is taken not to wash away propranolol bound to the membranes (CONNELL et al., 1980).

Propranolol has been shown to modify both brain oxygen consumption (ANDJELKOVIC, 1974; BERNTMAN et al., 1978) and glycolysis (LEONARD, 1972; BERNTMAN et al., 1978) and, following intraventricular administration, to elevate serum prolactin (GALA et al., 1972) and also to reverse the effect of dopamine on growth hormone release (COLLU et al., 1972).

Other studies following central administration of β-adrenoceptor antagonists have suggested the possible role of β-adrenergic systems in the hypothalamic control of both feeding behavior (LEIBOWITZ, 1970) and blood pressure (PHILIPPU and KITTEL, 1977).

A variety of neuropharmacological and behavioral properties have been attributed to β-adrenoceptor blocking drugs. Many of these relate to central nervous system depression. Thus, LESZKOVSKY and TARDOS (1965), MURMAN et al. (1966), BARAR and MADAN (1973), TRIVEDI and SHARMA (1973) and IZQUIERDO et al. (1974) describe reduced spontaneous locomotor activity in rodents following propranolol, pronethalol and alprenolol, but nifenalol (INPEA) may be unique in possessing CNS stimulant properties (MURMAN et al., 1966; ILYUTCHENOK et al., 1972; BARAR and MAdan, 1973). Ksiazek and Kleinrok (1974) have examined effects on locomotor behavior following intraventricular administration, and although very small doses of propranolol caused increased activity, higher doses of propranolol and all doses of alprenolol and sotalol tested decreased activity. Reports of potentiation of barbiturate and ethanol hypnosis by β-adrenoceptor antagonists support these general findings (Shah et al., 1974; Barar and Madan, 1973, and Iyer et al., 1975). Sedative effects of a more subtle nature are evident from observations reported of the effects of β-adrenoceptor antagonists on hyperarousal or aggression following septal lesions in rats (Bainbridge and Greenwood, 1971), the behavior of isolated mice (Weinstock and Speiser, 1973), mouse shock-induced fighting (Murman et al., 1966) and both amphetamine and LSD-induced behaviors (Weinstock and Speiser, 1974; Kocur et al., 1977). There is a report that propranolol reverses the aberrant behavior induced in dogs by the anticholinergic drug Ditran, an effect considered by the experimenters to be predictive of antidepressant activity (Korol and Brown, 1967), but there have been no clinical reports of such activity. Muscle relaxation and inhibition of tremor induced by oxotremorine have been reported for several antagonists of this class (Agarwal and Bose, 1967; Sharma et al., 1971; Leslie et al., 1972; Singh et al., 1973; Ganguly, 1976). Various effects on conditioned behavior have been reported, including effects of propranolol on rat conflict behavior (Sepinwall et al., 1973; Robichaud et al., 1973), timing behavior (Richardson et al., 1972) and conditioned avoidance (Merlo and Izquierdo, 1971; Izquierdo et al., 1974) and by oxprenolol on conditioned hyperthermia (Noble and Delini-Stula, 1976). It is unlikely that the bulk of these generally CNS depressant effects are related to β-blockade. Not only are they seen at doses many times higher than those required for β-blockade, but they are also commonly produced by similar doses of the drugs' stereo-isomers where these are available, e.g. propranolol and oxprenolol, which differ markedly in β-adrenoceptor antagonist potency. Also, not all β-adrenoceptor blockers which reach the CNS show depressant activity. Nifenalol, as seen previously, appears to be a CNS stimulant. It may be noted in this context that INPEA is structurally an ethanolamine whilst most antagonists discussed here are propanolamine in structure. The mechanism common to many of these drugs of membrane stabilising activity, shared equally by the isomers of propranolol, has frequently been invoked as a likely mechanism for non-specific CNS depressant effects of which sedation may be one.

Anticonvulsant properties of β-adrenoceptor antagonists have been repeatedly described. These include inhibition of audiogenic seizures and those induced by maximal electroshock and strychnine in rodents (Leszkovsky and Tardos, 1965; Murman et al., 1966; Trivedi and Sharma, 1973; Shah et al., 1974; Madan and Barar, 1974; Iyer et al., 1975; Saelens et al., 1973, 1974, 1977; Jaeger et al., 1978). Propranolol is a potent inhibitor of maximal electroshock seizures in the rat ($ED_{50}=4.5$ mg/kg) (Jaeger et al., 1978), but there is little doubt that this property is also independent of β-blockade since the D-isomer of propranolol is also a potent anticonvulsant (Jaeger et al., 1978). Work by Saelens et al. (1973, 1974, 1977) strongly suggests that a major metabolite of propranolol, propranolol glycol, contributes to this anticonvulsant effect.

Examples of neuropharmacological and behavioral effects which may arise from blockade of β-adrenoceptors in the CNS are rare and perhaps not surprisingly since little is understood of central β-receptor function. Ethanol-induced behavior in rodents is believed to be catecholamine dependent (CARLSSON et al., 1972) and has a stimulant phase believed to be mediated by α-adrenoceptors but also a depressant phase which is inhibited by propranolol (MATCHETT and ERICKSON, 1977; ENGEL and LILJEQUIST, 1976).

More extensive, however, is the evidence that some β-adrenergic antagonists have effects at central serotonin receptors.

The recent demonstration using receptor binding techniques of a stereospecific interaction of propranolol and other β-adrenoceptor antagonists with the 5-HT receptor on rat brain synaptic preparations indicates an activity of β-antagonists which may be of importance in interpreting some of the central effects of these drugs seen in animals and man (MIDDLEMISS et al., 1977). The blockade of the [^{3}H] 5-HT binding site may explain the antagonism of a 5-HT-sensitive adenylate cyclase noted by KOCUR et al. (1975) and the blockade of LSD-induced biochemical and behavioral changes in the mouse (KOCUR et al., 1977) since propranolol and other β-adrenoceptor antagonists also displace [^{3}H] LSD from its receptor (CONNEL et al., 1979).

The study of several β-adrenoceptor antagonists in isolated tissue and ganglion preparations (SCHECHTER and WEINSTOCK, 1974; WEINSTOCK and SCHECHTER, 1975), and in several behavioral syndromes related to raised functional brain 5-HT activity, are consistent with these drugs having 5-HT antagonist activity. Thus, propranolol and several other β-adrenoceptor antagonists inhibit the development in rats of a hyperactivity syndrome produced by the administration of the 5-HT precursor L-tryptophan and a monoamine oxidase (MAO) inhibitor (GREEN and GRAHAME-SMITH, 1976; COSTAIN and GREEN, 1978 and DEAKIN and GREEN, 1978; BUXTON et al., 1979) and a probably related syndrome induced by MAO inhibition and reserpine (DELINI-STULA and MEIER, 1976). Where stereo-isomers exist, as in the case of propranolol, the L-isomer shows the more potent effect in these experiments. This observation is also true of propranolol's inhibitory effect on another syndrome resulting from 5-HT precursor loading, namely head twitches in mice following 5-HTP (WEINSTOCK et al., 1977). There is a report that sleep induced by 5-HT in young chicks, which lack a blood brain barrier, is also inhibited stereospecifically by propranolol (WEINSTOCK et al., 1977), but this does not appear to be a consistent finding (BUXTON and FRIEND, 1979, in preparation). YEROUKALIS et al. (1978) have shown convincingly that propranolol applied iontophoretically to Purkinje fibres of the cerebellum inhibits 5-HT induced excitation. The balance of evidence from these studies suggests that it is likely that some β-adrenoceptor blocking drugs may act in vivo as 5-HT antagonists.

II. Central Nervous Effects in Man

In contrast to findings in animals, there is relatively little unequivocal evidence indicative of direct effects of β-adrenoceptor antagonists on the human CNS.

Conflicting results have been obtained from studies of the effects of β-adrenoceptor antagonists on the human EEG. Several investigators have recorded no changes in response to single or repeated low oral or intravenous doses of propranolol and acebutolol (DUNLEAVY et al., 1971; LADER and TYRER, 1972; STRAUMANIS and SHAGASS, 1976; KAYED and GODTLIBSEN, 1977a), whereas others have observed minimal or transient effects following propranolol, metoprolol and acebutolol (RUSER, 1976; KAYED and GODTLIBSEN, 1977b; ORZACK et al., 1973). The latter investigators showed that at a dose of 330 mg/day, propranolol selectively increased fast β-wave activity. This effect was not, however, apparent at the higher dose level of 675 mg/day. In contrast, other studies have shown more pronounced EEG changes attributable to propranolol (Comparato and Montuori, 1973; Moglia et al., 1976; Roubicek, 1976 and 1977) and pindolol (Roubicek, 1977). These effects are reportedly characterised by increased amplitude and frequency of both α- and fast β-wave activity somewhat similar to changes observed following the administration of benzodiazepine anxiolytics and tricyclic antidepressant drugs. Impaired performance in several psychomotor function tests, e.g. pursuit rotor and reaction time, has been demonstrated after administration of single oral doses of oxprenolol, atenolol, and propranolol (Glaister et al., 1973; Bryan et al., 1974; Landauer et al., 1979). Other similar studies, including critical flicker frequency tests (CFF), have yielded conflicting results (Tyrer and Lader, 1974a, b; Ogle and Turner, 1974). In addition, neither atenolol nor propranolol exerted any significant effects on the performances of either the Stroop colour-word test or on car driving skills (Harvey et al., 1977; Clayton et al., 1977). It may be significant that performance of those tests which are primarily dependent on cerebral function, i.e. CFF and serial subtraction, invariably remain unaffected by β-adrenoceptor blocking drugs. The decrement in performance noted by some authors may thus be a consequence of an action on skeletal muscle rather than a direct depressant effect on the CNS.

Several clinical investigators have sought corroborative biochemical evidence for an action of β-adrenoceptor antagonists at central sites by measuring neurotransmitter metabolites and neuro-endocrine levels. Belmaker et al. (1978) failed to detect any effects of propranolol on cerebrospinal fluid (CSF) cyclic nucleotide concentration. In contrast, propranolol has been found to modify human growth hormone secretion (Imura et al., 1968; Massara and Camanni, 1972) and to attenuate by 80% the nocturnal rise in serum melatonin secretion (Hanssen et al., 1977).

Studies of changes in the level of prolactin following the administration of β-adrenoceptor antagonists are of particular interest because of the reported beneficial actions of these drugs in the treatment of psychosis. Ridges et al. (1977) reported a transient elevation in serum prolactin levels after propranolol, whereas later investigators reported either no effect (Elizure et al., 1978) or a small decrease (Hanssen et al., 1978; Wilson et al., 1979) following administration of this drug to schizophrenic patients. Elevated prolactin levels, either in response to metoclopramide infusion (Wilson et al., 1979) or in women with hyperprolactinaemia (Board et al., 1977) do not appear to be reduced by propranolol administration, suggesting that the slight decrease observed in some schizophrenic patients is unlikely to be due to changes in dopaminergic receptor function.

The therapeutic administration of β-adrenoceptor blocking drugs has been associated with a range of side effects which, though of a low overall incidence, collectively suggest that these drugs do exert central effects in man. These side effects include vivid dreams, insomnia, visual and tactile hallucinations, disorientation and "acute brain syndrome" (Stephen, 1966; Prichard and Gillam, 1964; Hinshelwood, 1969; Tyrer and Lader, 1973; Shopsin et al., 1975; Topliss and Bond, 1977; Helson and Duque, 1978). Paradoxical, in view of the reported benefit in some schizophrenic patients, are isolated reports of "propranolol psychosis" with auditory hallucinations (Frazer and Carr, 1976; Steinert and Pugh, 1979) and disorientation and paranoid delusions (Peters et al., 1978).

E. Therapeutic Effects in Psychiatric and Neurological Disorders

Irrespective of the significance of the various biochemical, neuropharmacological and behavioral properties of β-adrenoceptor antagonists which have been demonstrated in animals, there is an increasing interest in the use of these drugs in the treatment of several psychiatric and neurological disorders in which a direct action on the CNS may be implicated.

I. Anxiety

The use of β-adrenoceptor antagonists in the control of anxiety was reported by GRANVILLE-GROSSMAN and TURNER (1966), who showed that propranolol was more effective than a placebo in relieving the autonomically mediated symptoms of clinical anxiety. Many subsequent clinical trials have demonstrated the value of propranolol (GOTTSCHALK et al., 1974; BECKER, 1976), oxprenolol (GAIND et al., 1975; JAMES et al., 1977; NUM, 1977), sotalol (TYRER and LADER, 1972) and metoprolol (HEIDBREDER et al., 1978) in alleviating the somatic manifestations of anxiety. These symptoms, e.g. tachycardia, palpitations and gastro-intestinal disturbances, arise as a consequence of excessive stimulation of peripheral β-adrenoceptors and commonly occur during states of acute emotional arousal.

Although the "psychic" elements of anxiety may also respond to β-adrenoceptor antagonists, the balance of evidence favours a predominantly peripheral site of action (GOTTSCHALK et al., 1974; GRANVILLE-GROSSMAN, 1974). The observation that the D-isomer of propranolol, which is virtually devoid of β-adrenoceptor antagonist activity, is ineffective in treating anxiety is of particular relevance in this context (BONN and TURNER, 1971). Furthermore, practolol, a drug which enters the brain poorly, is clinically effective (BONN et al., 1972).

II. Drug Dependence and Abuse

Excessive stimulation of the sympathetic nervous system is also a common finding in alcoholism and drug dependence, suggesting a logical application of β-adrenoceptor antagonists in the management of these conditions. Conflicting reports have appeared concerning the effects of propranolol in the treatment of alcoholics (CARLSSON and JOHANSSON, 1971; NOBLE et al., 1973; GALLANT et al., 1973; CARLSSON and FASTH, 1976; SELLERS et al., 1977) and opiate addicts (GROSZ, 1972; LOWENSTEIN, 1973) and in alleviating adverse reaction to LSD and marijuana (LINKEN, 1971; DREW et al., 1972). The behavioral interactions observed in animals between β-adrenoceptor antagonists and alcohol or certain stimulant drugs may indicate that central actions are involved in addition to effects at peripheral β-adrenoceptors.

III. Tremor

Numerous reports have appeared during the past decade of the value of several β-adrenoceptor antagonists in treating various forms of tremor. Beneficial effects have been reported in tremor associated with anxiety (GRANVILLE-GROSSMAN and TURNER, 1966; SUZMAN, 1976), thyrotoxicosis (MARSDEN et al., 1968), lithium therapy for mania (KIRK et al., 1973; FLORU et al., 1974) and in benign essential tremor (GILLIGAN et al., 1972; DUPONT et al., 1973; WINKLER and YOUNG, 1974; TERAVAINEN et al., 1977), also in Parkinson's disease when given alone or in combination with other anti-tremor drugs (HERRING, 1964; OWEN and MARSDEN, 1965; BHASKAR et al., 1977; KISSEL et al., 1974).

Although a central component in the action of propranolol in benign essential tremor has been implicated (YOUNG et al., 1975), it is probable that a major component in the therapeutic action of β-adrenoceptor antagonists resides in their ability to block peripheral β-adrenoceptors located in the region of the intrafusal fibres of muscle spindles (MARSDEN et al., 1967; BOWMAN and NOTT, 1970). Evidence exists for the sympathetic innervation of at least some muscle spindle poles (BALLARD, 1978), and intravenous infusion of adrenaline and other sympathomimetic amines enhances both physiological and pathological tremor (MARSHALL and SCHNEIDEN, 1966), presumably by an exclusively peripheral mechanism.

Beneficial effects of propranolol in clonus (MAI and PEDERSEN, 1976) and in Ekbom's syndrome have been claimed (STRANG, 1967), but pindolol may precipitate this condition (MORGAN, 1975).

IV. Migraine

Propranolol and certain other β-adrenoceptor antagonists have been shown to be effective as a prophylactic treatment for migraine (WEBER and REINMUTH, 1972; MALVEA et al., 1973; ANTHONY, 1977). However, the aetiology of this condition and, therefore, the mode of action of β-adrenoceptor blocking drugs in alleviating it remains uncertain. The relative contribution of central and peripheral neuronal components is unclear, and both noradrenergic and serotonergic factors have been implicated. Thus, although the blockade of peripheral β-receptors may be an important feature in the action of these drugs (JOHNSON, 1978), possible effects at central noradrenergic and tryptaminergic sites may yet be demonstrated.

V. Schizophrenia and Other Behavioral Disorders

Of great potential interest and possible theoretical importance are the claims for beneficial effects of high doses of propranolol in various psychotic states. Interest was initially aroused following the observation of improved mental state during treatment of acute porphyria with propranolol (ATSMON and BLUM, 1970). Improvements in florid symptomatology have subsequently been claimed in both acute and chronic schizophrenics and in manic patients after propranolol (ATSMON et al., 1972; ATSMON, 1973; YORKSTON et al., 1974; VON ZERSSEN, 1976; YORKSTON et al., 1977; SHEPPARD, 1979) and oxprenolol (VOLK et al., 1972) administration. Patients who improved on propranolol appeared to be those who exhibited a high urinary excretion of catecholamines and 3-methoxy-4-hydroxy-phenylglycol (MHPG) while taking the drug (ATSMON et al., 1972).

Where beneficial effects have been observed, doses have been high in relation to those normally required to effect peripheral β-adrenoceptor blockade, suggesting that other actions of these drugs or their metabolites might be involved. In contrast, other investigators (ORZACK et al., 1973; GARDOS et al., 1973; RACKENSPERGER et al., 1974) have observed no benefit. It is hoped that further controlled studies now in progress will allow a definitive conclusion to be drawn as to whether propranolol is useful in the treatment of schizophrenia. If β-adrenoceptor antagonists prove to be useful in the treatment of certain forms of psychosis, important theoretical issues will be raised since these drugs are devoid of classic neuroleptic, i.e. dopamine antagonist, activity possessed by the phenothiazine and butyrophenone drugs. As previously pointed out, they also do not cause the marked elevation in plasma prolactin concentration which is characteristic of neuroleptic medication. There are also anecdotal reports that propranolol may alleviate certain aspects of belligerent behavior and "explosive rage" following head injury (ELLIOT, 1976, 1977).

F. Summary and Conclusions

Neuropharmacological and biochemical studies have provided convincing evidence that certain β-adrenoceptor antagonists have central effects in animals, and these studies also suggest several possible mechanisms by which these effects may be brought about. First, there is good evidence that central β-adrenoceptors exist and that they may be widely distributed in brain tissue. There is also good evidence that β-adrenoceptor antagonists are effective at central β-receptors in vitro. Since many drugs of this class are also known to pass into the brain easily it may be assumed, therefore, that they may also act in vivo as central β-adrenoceptor antagonists. A second possible mechanism of action is membrane stabilisation which is possessed by many β-adrenoceptor antagonists. Antagonists such as propranolol and oxprenolol, which possess stereo-isomers, show a separation between the isomers for β-blocking effects but not for membrane stabilisation. Since several effects in animals, including sedative, antitremor and anticonvulsant effects, are common to both isomers, it is possible that such a non-specific effect is responsible. A third central mechanism of potential importance comes from evidence that certain adrenoceptor antagonists may also act centrally as 5-HT antagonists.

With this information, and considering the range of effects reported in animals, it is perhaps surprising that clinical pharmacology has demonstrated relatively few CNS effects in man, with the exception of some EEG changes and minor performance deficits. However, some of the reported side effects in man, e.g. hallucinations and vivid dreams, are probably better evidence for central action of some of these drugs. Although there have been numerous claims for therapeutic uses of β-adrenoceptor antagonists, it is difficult in most cases to distinguish the relative effects of peripheral and central contributions to the therapeutic effect. Whilst therapeutic efficacy seems certain in some anxiety states, in control of tremor and migraine it may not be necessary to invoke a central mechanism of action by adrenoceptor antagonists although the possibility of a central mechanism cannot be ruled out. The evidence for efficacy in the management of major psychosis by β-adrenoceptor antagonists is less strong, and the results of more controlled studies are required. If this effect is confirmed, a major new role for drugs of this type may emerge and, in this instance, it would presumably be necessary to assume a central mechanism of action.

References

Agarwal, S.L., Bose, D.: A study of the role of brain catecholamines in drug induced tremor. Br. J. Pharmacol. Chemother. *30*, 349–353 (1967)

Ahn, H.S., Mishra, R.K., Demirjia, C., Makinan, M.H.: Catecholamine-sensitive adenylate cyclase in frontal cortex of primate brain. Brain Res. *116*, 437–454 (1976)

Alexander, R.W., Davis, J.N., Lefkowitz, R.J.: Direct identification and characterisation of β-adrenergic receptors in rat brain. Nature *258*, 437–440 (1975)

Anden, N.E., Strombom, U.: Adrenergic receptor blocking agents: Effects on central noradrenaline and dopamine receptors and on motor activity. Psychopharmacology *38*, 91–103 (1974)

Andjelkovic, D.: Effect of adrenergic substances on oxygen consumption of rat brain tissue. J. Pharm. Pharmacol. *26*, 138–139 (1974)

Anthony, M.: Beta blockers in migraine prophylaxis. Curr. Ther. *18*, 17–18 (1977)

Aro, S., Klinge, E.: Influence of β-adrenergic blockade on the catecholamine content of some tissues of the rat. Scand. J. Clin. Lab. Invest. *27*, Suppl. 116, 72 (1971)

Atsmon, A.I.: Propranolol therapy helps some patients with mental disorders. J. Am. Med. Assoc. *224*, 173–174 (1973)

Atsmon, A.I., Blum, M.: Treatment of acute porphyria variegata with propranolol. Lancet *1970 I*, 196–197

Atsmon, A.I., Blum, M., Steiner, M., Latz, A., Wijsenbeek, K.: Further studies with propranolol in psychotic patients. Relation to initial psychiatric state, urinary catecholamines and 3-methoxy-4-hydroxy-phenyl-glycol excretion. Psychopharmacology *27*, 249 (1972)

Bainbridge, J.G., Greenwood, D.T.: Tranquillising effects of propranolol demonstrated in rats. Neuropharmacology *10*, 453–458 (1971)

Ballard, K.J.: Typical sympathetic noradrenergic endings in a muscle spindle of the cat. J. Physiol. (Lond.) *285*, 61 P (1978)

Barar, F.S.K., Madan, B.R.: Effects of ten beta-adrenoceptor blocking agents on spontaneous motility and pentobarbital-induced anaesthesia in mice. Indian J. Physiol. Pharmacol. *17*, 235–240 (1973)

Becker, A.L.: Oxprenolol and propranolol in anxiety states. A double blind comparative study. S. Afr. Med. J. *50*, 627–629 (1976)

Belmaker, R.H., Ebstein, R.P., Biederman, J., Stern, R., Berman, M., Van Praag, H.M.: The effect of L-DOPA and propranolol on human CSF cyclic nucleotides. Psychopharmacology *58*, 307–310 (1978)

Berntman, L., Carlsson, C., Siesjo, B.K.: Influence of propranolol on cerebral metabolism and blood flow in the rat brain. Brain Res. *151*, 220–224 (1978)

Bevan, P., Bradshaw, C.M., Szabadi, E.: Potentiation and antagonism of neuronal responses to monoamines by methysergide and sotalol. Br. J. Pharmacol. *50*, 445 P (1974)

Bevan, P., Bradshaw, C.M., Szabadi, E.: The pharmacology of adrenergic neuronal responses in the cerebral cortex: Evidence for excitatory α- and inhibitory β-receptors. Br. J. Pharmacol. *59*, 635–641 (1977)

Bhaskar, P.A., Bhaskar, E.A., Jagannathan, K.: Clinical observations on the tremorolytic action of propranolol (a beta-adrenergic blocker). Antiseptic *74*, 30–34 (1977)

Board, J.A., Fierro, R.J., Wasserman, A.J., Bhatnagar, A.S.: Effects of α and β adrenergic blocking agents on serum prolactin levels in women with hyperprolactinaemia and galactorrhoea. Am. J. Obstet. Gynecol. *127*, 285–287 (1977)

Bodin, N.O., Borg, K.O., Johansson, R., Obianwu, H., Svensson, R.: Absorption, distribution and excretion of alprenolol in man, dog and rat. Acta Pharmacol. Toxicol. (Kbh) *35*, 261–269 (1974)

Bonn, J.A., Turner, P.: D-propranolol and anxiety. Lancet *1971 I*, 1355–1356

Bonn, J.A., Turner, P., Hicks, D.: Beta-adrenergic blockade with practolol in treatment of anxiety. Lancet *1972 I*, 814–815

Bowman, W.C., Nott, M.W.: Actions of some sympathomimetic bronchodilator and beta-adrenoceptor blocking drugs on contractions of the cat soleus muscle. Br. J. Pharmacol. *38*, 37–49 (1970)

Bremner, R.M., Greengrass, P.M., Morville, M., Blackburn, K.J.: Effect of tolamolol and other beta-adrenoceptor blocking drugs on [^{3}H] haloperidol binding to rat striatal membrane preparations. J. Pharm. Pharmacol. *30*, 388–389 (1978)

Brunner, H., Hedwall, P., Maitre, L., Meier, M.: Beeinflussung des pressorischen Eserin-Effekts durch Propranolol. Naunyn Schmiedebergs Arch. Pharmacol. *254*, 45–55 (1966)
Bryan, P.C., Efiong, D.O., Stewart-Jones, J., Turner, P.: Propranolol on tests of visual function and central nervous activity. Br. J. Clin. Pharmacol. *1*, 82–84 (1974)
Buxton, D.A., Friend, J., Kent, A.P.: β-adrenoreceptor antagonists in L-tryptophan and L-DOPA induced behavioural syndromes. Br. J. Pharmacol. 68, 176P (1980)
Bylund, D.B., Snyder, S.H.: β-adrenergic receptor binding in membrane preparations from mammalian brain. Mol. Pharmacol. *12*, 568–580 (1976)
Carlsson, A., Engel, J., Svensson, T.H.: Inhibition of ethanolol induced excitation in mice and rats by α-methyl-p-tyrosine. Psychopharmacology *26*, 207–312 (1972)
Carlsson, C., Fasth, B.G.: A comparison of the effects of propranolol and diazepam in alcoholics. Br. J. Addict. *71*, 321–326 (1976)
Carlsson, C., Johansson, T.: The psychological effects of propranolol in the abstinence phase of chronic alcoholics. Br. J. Psychiatry *119*, 605–606 (1971)
Charalampous, K.O., Askew, W.E.: Effect of non-opiate antagonists on stereospecific opiate receptor binding of tritiated naloxone. Res. Commun. Chem. Pathol. Pharmacol. *8*, 615–622 (1974)
Clayton, A.B., Harvey, P.G., Betts, T.A.: The psychomotor effects of atenolol and other antihypertensive agents. Postgrad. Med. J. *53*, Suppl. 3, 157–161 (1977)
Collu, R., Fraschini, F., Visconti, P., Martini, L.: Adrenergic and serotonergic control of growth hormone secretion in adult male rats. Endocrinology *90*, 1231–2137 (1972)
Comparato, M.R., Montuori, E.: Accion del propranolol sobre el comportamiento sexual. Obstet. Ginecol. Lat.-Am. *31*, 320–329 (1973)
Connell, D.J., Middlemiss, D.N., Stone, M.A.: Further evidence for an interaction of propranolol with the central 5-hydroxytryptamine (5-HT) receptor. Br. J. Pharmacol. *68*, 173P (1980)
Conway, J., Greenwood, D.T., Middlemiss, D.N.: Central nervous actions of beta-adrenoreceptor antagonists. Clin. Sci. Mol. Med. *54*, 119–124 (1978)
Costain, D.W., Green, A.R.: β-adrenoceptor antagonists inhibit the behavioural responses of rats to increased brain 5-hydroxytryptamine. Br. J. Pharmacol. *64*, 193–200 (1978)
Cote, T.E., Kebabian, J.W.: β-adrenergic receptor in the brain: Comparison of [^{3}H] DHA binding sites and a β-adrenergic receptor regulating adenylyl cyclase activity in cell free homogenates. Life Sci. *23*, 1703–1714 (1978)
Cruikshank, J.M., Neil-Dwyer, G., Cameron, M., McAinsh, J.: β-blockers and the central nervous system. 6th Scientific Meeting of Int. Soc. Hypertension, Goteborg, June 1979 (Abstr.)
Davis, J.W., Lefkowitz, R.J.: β-adrenergic receptor binding: Synaptic localisation in rat brain. Brain Res. *113*, 214–218 (1976)
Day, M.D., Roach, A.G.: β-adrenergic receptors in the central nervous system of the cat concerned with control of arterial blood pressure and heartrate. Nature (New Biol.) *242*, 30–31 (1973)
Day, M.D., Hemsworth, B.A., Street, J.A.: The central uptake of beta-adrenoceptor antagonists. J. Pharm. Pharmacol. *29*, S 52P (1977)
Deakin, J.F.W., Green, A.R.: The effects of putative 5-hydroxytryptamine antagonists on the behaviour produced by administration of tranylcypromine and L-tryptophan or tranylcypromine and L-DOPA to rats. Br. J. Pharmacol. *64*, 201–209 (1978)
Delini-Stula, A., Meier, M.: Inhibitory effects of propranolol and oxprenolol on excitation induced by a MAO inhibitor and reserpine in the mouse. Neuropharmacology *15*, 383–388 (1976)
Dolphin, A., Sawaya, M.C.B., Jenner, P., Marsden, C.D.: Behavioural and biochemical effects of chronic reduction of cerebral noradrenaline receptor stimulation. Naunyn Schmiedebergs Arch. Pharmacol. *299*, 167–173 (1977)
Dolphin, A., Adrien, J., Hamon, M., Bockaert, J.: Identity of [^{3}H]-dihydroalprenolol binding sites and β-adrenergic receptors coupled with adenylate cyclase in the central nervous system: Pharmacological properties, distribution and adaptive responsiveness. Mol. Pharmacol. *15*, 1–15 (1979)
Drew, W.G., Kiplinger, G.F., Miller, L.L., Marx, M.: Effects of propranolol on marihuana-induced cognitive dysfunctioning. Clin. Pharmacol. Ther. *13*, 526–533 (1972)
Dunleavy, D.L.F., Maclean, A.W., Oswald, I.: Debrisoquine, guanethidine, propranolol and human sleep. Psychopharmacology *21*, 101–110 (1971)

Dupont, E., Hanssen, H.J., Dalby, M.A.: The treatment of benign essential tremor with propranolol. Acta Neurol. Scand. *49*, 75–84 (1973)
Elizure, A., Segal, Z., Yeret, A., Davidson, S., Ben-David, M.: Antipsychotic activity and mode of action of propranolol vs. neuroleptic drugs. Isr. J. Med. Sci. *14*, 493–494 (1978)
Elliot, F.A.: The neurology of explosive rage. The dyscontrol syndrome. Practioner *217*, 51–60 (1976)
Elliot, F.A.: Propranolol for the control of belligerent behaviour following acute brain damage. Ann. Neurol. *1*, 489–491 (1977)
Engel, J., Liljequist, S.: Behavioural effects of β-receptor blocking agents in experimental animals. Adv. Clin. Pharmacol. *12*, Suppl., 45–50 (1976)
Floru, von L., Floru, L., Tegeler, J.: Wirkung von Rezeptorenblockern (Pindolol und Practolol) auf den Lithium bedingten tremor-klinischen Versuch und theoretische Erwägungen. Arzneim. Forsch. *24*, 1122–1125 (1974)
Frazer, H.S., Carr, A.C.: Propranolol psychosis. Br. J. Psychiatry *129*, 508–512 (1976)
Fuxe, K., Bolme, P., Agnati, L., Everitt, B.J.: The effect of DL-, L- and D-propranolol on central monoamine neurones. I. Studies on dopamine mechanisms. Neurosci. Lett. *3*, 45–52 (1976a)
Fuxe, K., Bolme, P., Agnati, L., Everitt, B.J.: The effect of DL-, L- and D-propranolol on central monoamine neurones. II. Studies on noradrenaline mechanisms. Neurosci. Lett. *3*, 53–60 (1976b)
Gaind, R., Suri, A.M., Thomson, J.: Use of beta blockers as an adjunct in behavioural techniques. Scott. Med. J. *20*, 284–286 (1975)
Gala, R.R., Janson, P.A., Kuo, E.Y.: The influence of neural blocking agents injected into the third ventricle of the rat brain and hypothalamic electrical stimulation on serum prolactin. Proc. Soc. Exptl. Med. *140*, 569–572 (1972)
Gallant, D.M., Swanson, W.C., Guerrero-Figueroa, R.: A controlled evaluation of propranolol in chronic alcoholic patients. J. Clin. Pharmacol. *13*, 41–43 (1973)
Ganguly, D.K.: Antioxotremorine action of propranolol. Br. J. Pharmacol. *56*, 21–24 (1976)
Gardos, G., Cole, J.O., Volicer, L., Orzack, M.H., Oliff, A.C.: A dose response study of propranolol in chronic schizophrenics. Curr. Ther. Res. *15*, 314–323 (1973)
Garvey, H.L., Ram, N.: Comparative antihypotensive effects and tissue distribution of β-adrenergic blocking drugs. J. Pharmacol. Exp. Ther. *194*, 220–233 (1975)
Gilligan, B.S., Veale, J.L., Wodak, J.: Propranolol in the treatment of tremor. Med. J. Aust. *1*, 320–322 (1972)
Glaister, D.H., Harrison, M.H., Allnutt, M.F.: Environmental influences on cardiac activity. In: New perspectives in β-blockade. Burley, D.M., Frier, J.H., Rondel, R.K., Taylor, S.H. (eds.), pp. 241–267. Horsham, England: CIBA 1973
Gottschalk, L.A., Stone, W.N., Gleser, G.C.: Peripheral versus central mechanisms accounting for antianxiety effects of propranolol. Psychosom. Med. *36*, 47–56 (1974)
Granville-Grossman, K.L., Turner, P.: The effect of propranolol on anxiety. Lancet *1966 I*, 788–790
Granville-Grossman, K.: Propranolol, anxiety and the CNS. Br. J. Clin. Pharmacol. *1*, 361–363 (1974)
Green, A.R., Grahame-Smith, D.G.: (−)-propranolol inhibits the behavioural responses of rats to increased 5-hydroxytryptamine in the central nervous system. Nature *262*, 594–596 (1976)
Greenblatt, D.J., Shader, R.I.: On the psychopharmacology of β-adrenergic blockade. Curr. Ther. Res. *14*, 615–625 (1972)
Grosz, H.J.: Successful treatment of heroin addict with propranolol: Implications for opiate addiction treatment and research. J. Indiana State Med. Assoc. *65*, 505–509 (1972)
Hanssen, T., Heyden, T., Sundberg, I., Wetterberg, L.: Effect of propranolol on serum melatonin. Lancet *1977 II*, 309–310
Hanssen, T., Heyden, T., Sundberg, I., Wetterberg, L., Eneroth, P.: Decrease in serum prolactin after propranolol in schizophrenia. Lancet *1978 I*, 101–102
Harden, T.K., Wolfe, B.B., Sporn, J.R., Perkins, J.P., Molinoff, P.B.: Ontogeny of β-adrenergic receptors in rat cerebral cortex. Brain Res. *125*, 99–108 (1977)
Harvey, P.G., Clayton, A.B., Betts, T.A.: The effects of four antihypertensive agents on the Stroop colour-work test in normal male subjects. Psychopharmacology *54*, 133–138 (1977)

Hayes, A., Cooper, R.G.: Studies on the absorption, distribution and excretion of propranolol in rat, dog and monkey. J. Pharmacol. Exp. Ther. *176*, 302–311 (1971)

Heidbreder, E., Pagel, G., Rockel, A., Heidland, A.: Beta-adrenergic blockade in stress protection. Limited effect of metoprolol in psychological stress reaction. Eur. J. Clin. Pharmacol. *14*, 391–398 (1978)

Helson, L., Duque, L.: Acute brain syndrome after propranolol. Lancet *1978 I*, 8055 (1978)

Herman, Z.S., Kmieciek-Kolada, K., Drybanski, A., Sokola, A., Trzeciak, H., Chrusciel, T.L.: The influence of alprenolol on the central nervous system of the rat. Psychopharmacology *21*, 66–73 (1971)

Herring, A.B.: Action of pronethalol on parkinsonian tremor. Lancet *1964 II*, 892

Hess, A.: Visualization of β-adrenergic receptor sites with fluorescent β-adrenergic blocker probes – or autofluorescent granules? Brain Res. *160*, 533–538 (1979)

Hinshelwood, R.D.: Hallucinations and propranolol. Br. Med. J. *1969 II*, 445

Horn, A.H., Phillipson, O.T.: A noradrenaline sensitive adenylate cyclase in the rat limbic forebrain: Preparation properties and the effects of agonists, adrenolytics and neuroleptic drugs. Eur. J. Pharmacol. *37*, 1–11 (1976)

Ilyutchenok, R.Yu., Gilinsky, M.A., Yeliseyeva, A.G., Jivotikoff, B.P., Loskutova, L.V., Pastoukhoff, Y.F.: The central effects of the beta-adrenergic blocking agent INPEA. Neuropharmacology *11*, 609–614 (1972)

Imura, H., Kato, Y., Ikeda, M.: Effects of adrenergic blocking or stimulating drugs on growth hormone (HGH) secretion in man. In: 3rd International Congress of Endocrinology. Gual, G. (ed.), pp 17. Amsterdam: Excerpta Medica 1968

Iyer, K.S., Govindankutty, A., Radha, M.: Central nervous system pharmacology of propranolol. Indian J. Physiol. Pharmacol. *19*, 152–156 (1975)

Izquierdo, J.A., Fabian, H.E.M., Chemerinski, E.: Effects of d- and l-propranolol on spontaneous motility and retention in male mice. Acta Physiol. Lat.-Am. *24*, 669–670 (1974)

Jaeger, V., Esplin, B., Capek, R.: The anticonvulsant effects of propranolol and β-adrenergic blockade. Experientia *35*, 80–81 (1978)

James, I.M., Pearson, R.M., Griffith, D.N.M., Newbury, P.: Effect of oxprenolol on stage-fright in musicians. Lancet *1977 II*, 952–954

Jefferson, J.W.: Beta-adrenergic receptor blocking drugs in psychiatry. Arch. Gen. Psychiatry *31*, 681–691 (1974)

Johnson, E.S.: A basis for migraine therapy – the autonomic theory reappraised. Postgrad. Med. J. *54*, 231–242 (1978)

Johnsson, G., Regardh, C.G.: Clinical pharmacokinetics of Beta-adrenoreceptor blocking drugs. Clin. Pharmacokinet. *1*, 233–263 (1976)

Kakiuchi, S., Rall, T.W.: The influences of chemical agents on the accumulation of adenosine 3′,5′-phosphate in slices of rabbit cerebellum. Mol. Pharmacol. *4*, 367–378 (1968)

Kayed, K., Godtlibsen, O.B.: Central effects of the beta-adrenergic blocking agent acebutolol – a quantitative EEG study using normalised slope descriptors. Eur. J. Clin. Pharmacol. *12*, 327–331 (1977a)

Kayed, K., Godtlibsen, O.B.: Effects of the beta-adrenoceptor antagonists acebutol and metoprolol on sleep pattern in normal subjects. Eur. J. Clin. Pharmacol. *12*, 323–326 (1977b)

Kebabian, J.W.: Biochemical regulation and physiological significance of cyclic nucleotides in the nervous system. Adv. Cyclic Neucleotide Res. *8*, 421–508 (1977)

Kirk, L., Baastrup, P.C., Schou, M.: Propranolol treatment of lithium-induced tremor. Lancet *1973 II*, 1086–1087

Kissel, P., Tridon, P., Andre, J.M.: Levodopa-propranolol therapy in parkinsonian tremor. Lancet *1974 I*, 403–404

Kocur, J., Jurkowski, A., Kedziora, J., Czernicki, J.: The influence of 5-hydroxytryptamine and some β-adrenolytic compounds on adenylate cyclase in rabbit brain in vivo. Pol. J. Pharmacol. Pharm. *27*, Suppl., 113–117 (1975)

Kocur, J., Jurkowski, A., Kedziora, J.: The influence of haloperidol and propranolol on behaviour and biochemical changes in the brain of mice treated with LSD. Pol. J. Pharmacol. Pharm. *29*, 281–288 (1977)

Korol, B., Brown, M.L.: The role of the beta-adrenergic system in behaviour: Antidepressant effects of propranolol. Curr. Ther. Res. *9*, 269–279 (1967)

Ksiazek, A., Kleinrok, Z.: Central action of drugs affecting beta-adrenergic receptor. II. The central action of intraventricularly applicated propranolol in rats. Pol. J. Pharmacol. Pharm. *26*, 297–304 (1974)
Lader, M.H., Tyrer, P.J.: Central and peripheral effects of propranolol and sotalol in normal human subjects. Br. J. Pharmacol. *45*, 556–560 (1972)
Landauer, A.A., Pocock, D.A., Prott, F.W.: Effects of atenolol and propranolol on human performance and subjective feelings. Psychopharmacology *60*, 211–215 (1979)
Laverty, R., Taylor, K.M.: Propranolol uptake into the central nervous system and the effect on rat behaviour and amine metabolism. J. Pharm. Pharmacol. *20*, 605–609 (1968)
Leibowitz, S.F.: Hypothalamic β-adrenergic "satiety" system antagonises an α-adrenergic "hunger" system in the rat. Nature *226*, 963–964 (1970)
Leonard, B.E.: A comparison between the effects of phenoxybenzamine, phentolamine and propranolol on mouse brain glycolysis. Biochem. Pharmacol. *21*, 109–113 (1972)
Leslie, G.B., Hayman, D.G., Ireson, J.D., Smith, S.: The effects of some beta-adrenergic blocking agents on the central and peripheral actions of tremorine and oxotremorine. Arch. Int. Pharmacodyn. Ther. *197*, 108–111 (1972)
Leszkovsky, G., Tardos, L.: Some effects of propranolol on the central nervous system. J. Pharm. Pharmacol. *17*, 518–519 (1965)
Levy, A., Ngai, S.H., Finck, A.D., Kawashima, K., Spector, S.: Disposition of propranolol isomers in mice. Eur. J. Pharmacol. *40*, 93–100 (1976)
Linken, A.: Propranolol for LSD-induced anxiety states. Lancet *1971 II*, 1039–1040
Lowenstein, H.: Propranolol as a psychotropic agent. Lancet *1973 I*, 559–560
MacKenzie, E.T., McCulloch, J., Harper, A.M.: Influence of endogenous norepinephrine on cerebral blood flow and metabolism. Am. J. Physiol. *231*, 489–494 (1976)
Madan, B.R., Barar, F.S.K.: Anticonvulsant activity of some beta-adrenoceptor blocking agents in mice. Eur. J. Pharmacol. *29*, 1–4 (1974)
Maguire, M.E., Wicklund, R.A., Anderson, H.J., Gilman, A.G.: Binding of (^{125}I) Iodohydroxybenzyl pindolol to putative β-adrenergic receptors of rat glioma cells and other cell clones. J. Biol. Chem. *251*, 1221–1231 (1976)
Mahon, B., O'Donnell, J., Leonard, B.E.: Effect of acute and chronic administration of dl-propranolol on brain catecholamine concentrations in the rat. J. Med. Sci. *5*, 44 (1977)
Mai, J., Pedersen, E.: Clonus depression by propranolol. Acta Neurol. Scand. *53*, 395–398 (1976)
Malvea, B.P., Gwon, N., Graham, J.R.: Propranolol prophylaxis of migraine. Headache *12*, 163–167 (1973)
Marsden, C.D., Foley, T.H., Owen, D.A.L., McAllister, R.G.: Peripheral β-adrenergic receptors concerned with tremor. Clin. Sci. Mol. Med. *33*, 53–65 (1967)
Marsden, C.D., Gimlette, T.M.D., McAllister, R.G., Owen, D.A.L., Miller, T.N.: The effects of β-adrenergic blockade on finger tremor and achilles reflex time in anxious and thyrotoxic patients. Acta Endocrinol. *57*, 353–362 (1968)
Marshall, M., Schneiden, H.: Effect of adrenaline, noradrenaline, atropine and nicotine on some types of human tremor. J. Neurology Neurosurg. Psychiatry *29*, 214–218 (1966)
Massara, F., Camanni, F.: Effect of various adrenergic receptor stimulating and blocking agents on human growth hormone secretion. J. Endocrinol. *54*, 195–206 (1972)
Masuoka, D., Hansson, E.: Autoradiographic distribution studies of adrenergic blocking agents II ^{14}C-propranolol a β-receptor-type blocker. Acta Pharmacol. Toxicol. *25*, 447–455 (1967)
Matchett, J.A., Erickson, C.K.: Alteration of ethanol-induced changes in locomotor activity by adrenergic blockers in mice. Psychopharmacology *52*, 201–206 (1977)
Mazurkiewicz-Kwilecki, I.M., Romagnoli, A.: Cardiac catecholamine levels and blood pressure after chronic treatment with β-adrenergic blocking agents. J. Pharm. Pharmacol. *22*, 235–237 (1970)
Melamed, E., Lahav, M., Atlas, D.: Direct localisation of β-adrenoceptor sites in rat cerebellum by a new fluorescent analogue of propranolol. Nature *261*, 420–421 (1976)
Merlo, A., Izquierdo, J.: The effect of post-trial injection of β-adrenergic blocking agents on a conditioned reflex in rats. Psychopharmacology *22*, 181–186 (1971)
Middlemiss, D.N., Blakeborough, L., Leather, S.R.: Direct evidence for an interaction of beta-adrenergic blockers with the 5-HT receptor. Nature *267*, 289–290 (1977)

Milmore, J.E., Taylor, K.M.: Propranolol inhibits rat brain monoamine oxidase. Life Sci. *17*, 1843–1848 (1976)
Moglia, A., Arrigo, A., Tatara, A., Savoldi, F., Bo, P.: Studio eegraphico preliminare sugli effetti del propranolol nell'uomo. Farmaco (Prat.) *31*, 568–573 (1976)
Morgan, L.K.: Restless legs precipitated by β-blocker, relieved by orphenadrine. Med. J. Aust. *2*, 753 (1975)
Murman, W., Almirante, L., Saccani-Guelfi, M.: Central nervous system effects of four β-adrenergic receptor blocking agents. J. Pharm. Pharmacol. *18*, 317–318 (1966)
Myers, M.G., Lewis, P.J., Reid, J.L., Dollery, C.T.: Brain concentration of propranolol in relation to hypotensive effects in the rabbit with observations on brain propranolol levels in man. J. Pharmacol. Exp. Ther. *192*, 327–335 (1975)
Nahorski, S.: Association of high affinity stereospecific binding of [^{3}H] propranolol to cerebral membranes with β-adrenoceptors. Nature *259*, 488–489 (1976)
Nahorski, S.: Heterogenecity of cerebral β-adrenoreceptor binding sites in various vertebrate species. Eur. J. Pharmacol. *51*, 199–209 (1978)
Noble, E.P., Parker, E., Alkana, R., Cohen, H., Birch, H.: Propranolol-ethanol interaction in man. Fed. Proc. *32*, 724 (1973)
Noble, W., Delini-Stula, A.: Effect of oxprenolol on some fear induced behavioural responses and hyperthermia in rats subjected to inescapable shocks. Psychopharmacology *49*, 17–22 (1976)
Num, R.G.: Blocking exam nerves. Lancet *1977 II*, 1133
Ogle, C.W., Turner, P.: The effects of oral doses of oxprenolol and of propranolol on CNS function in man. J. Pharmacol. Clin. *1*, 256–261 (1974)
Ogle, C.W., Turner, P., Markomihelakis, H.: The effects of high doses of oxprenolol and of propranolol on pursuit rotor performance, reaction time and critical flicker frequency. Psychopharmacology *46*, 295–299 (1976)
Orzack, M.H., Branconnier, R., Gardos, G.: CNS effects of propranolol in man. Psychopharmacology *29*, 299–306 (1973)
Owen, D.A.L., Marsden, C.D.: Effect of adrenergic β-blockade on parkinsonian tremor. Lancet *1965 II*, 1259
Peters, D.A.V., Mazurkiewicz-Kwilecki, I.M.: Tyrosine hydroxylase activity in rat brain regions after chronic treatment with propranolol. J. Pharm. Pharmacol. *27*, 671–676 (1975)
Peters, N.L., Anderson, K.C., Reid, P.R., Taylor, G.J.: Acute mental status changes caused by propranolol. Johns Hopkins Med. J. *143*, 163–164 (1978)
Phillipu, A., Kittel, E.: Presence of β-adrenoreceptors in the hypothalamus; their importance for the pressor response to hypothalamic stimulation. Naunyn Schmiedebergs Arch. Pharmacol. *297*, 219–225 (1977)
Prichard, B.N.C., Gillam, P.M.S.: Use of propranolol ("Inderal") in the treatment of hypertension. Br. Med. J. *1964 II*, 725–727
Rackensperger, W., Gaupp, R., Mattke, D.J., Schwartz, D., Stutte, K.H.: Behandlung von akuten schizophrenen Psychosen mit Beta-Receptoren Blockern. Arch. Psychiatr. Nervenkr. *219*, 29–36 (1974)
Raine, A.E.G., Chubb, I.W.: Long term β-adrenergic blockade reduces tyrosine hydroxylase and dopamine hydroxylase activities in sympathetic ganglia. Nature *267*, 265–267 (1977)
Richardson, J.S., Stacey, P.D., Russo, N.J., Musty, R.E.: Effects of systemic administration of propranolol on the timing behaviour (DRL) of rats. Arch. Int. Pharmacodyn. Ther. *197*, 66–71 (1972)
Ridges, A.P., Lawton, K., Harper, P., Ghosh, C., Hindson, N.: Propranolol in schizophrenia. Lancet *1977 II*, 986
Robichaud, R.C., Sledge, K.L., Hefner, M.A., Goldberg, M.E.: Propranolol and chlordiazepoxide on experimentally induced conflict and shuttle-box performance in rats. Psychopharmacology *32*, 157–160 (1973)
Roubicek, J.: Effect of β-adrenoceptor blocking drugs on EEG. Br. J. Clin. Pharmacol. *3*, 661–665 (1976)
Roubicek, J.: The EEG profile of beta adrenoceptor blockers. Electroencephalogr. Clin. Neurophysiol. *42*, 438–439 Abst. 26 (1977)
Ruser, I.: Die Wirkung von Propranolol auf den Verlauf der Hirnstromkurve. Deut. Gesundh.-Wes. *31*, 1987–1989 (1976)

Saelens, D.A., Walle, T., Privitera, P.J., Knapp, D.R., Gaffney, T.: The psychopharmacological effects of a new metabolite of propranolol. Adv. Biochem. Psychopharmacol. *7*, 107–112 (1973)
Saelens, D.A., Walle, T., Privitera, P.J., Knapp, D.R., Gaffney, T.: Central nervous system effects and metabolic disposition of a glycol metabolite of propranolol. J. Pharmacol. Exp. Ther. *188*, 86–92 (1974)
Saelens, D.A., Walle, T., Gaffney, T.E., Privitera, P.J.: Studies on the contribution of active metabolites to the anticonvulsant effects of propranolol. Eur. J. Pharmacol. *42*, 39–46 (1977)
Scales, B., Cosgrove, M.B.: The metabolism and distribution of the selective adrenergic blocking agent, practolol. J. Pharmacol. Exp. Ther. *175*, 338–347 (1970)
Schechter, Y., Weinstock, M.: β-adrenoceptor blocking agents and response to adrenaline and 5-hydroxytryptamine in rat isolated stomach and uterus. Br. J. Pharmacol. *52*, 283–287 (1974)
Schneck, D.W., Pritchard, J.F., Hayes, A.H.: Studies on the uptake and binding propranolol by rat tissues. J. Pharmacol. Exp. Ther. *203*, 621–629 (1977)
Sellers, E.M., Zilm, D.H., Degani, N.C.: Comparative efficacy of propranolol and chlordiazepoxide in alcohol withdrawal. J. Stud. Alcohol *38*, 2096–2108 (1977)
Sepinwall, J., Grodsky, F.S., Sullivan, J.W., Cook, L.: Effects of propranolol and chlordiazepoxide on conflict behaviour in rats. Psychopharmacology *31*, 375–382 (1973)
Shah, U.H., Jindal, M.N., Patel, V.K., Kelkar, V.V.: Central actions of some beta-adrenoceptor blocking agents. Arzneim. Forsch. *24*, 1581–1581 (1974)
Sharma, J.N., Singh, G.B., Dhawan, B.N.: Effect of beta-adrenergic blockade on tremorine tremors in mice. Jpn. J. Pharmacol. *21*, 675–677 (1971)
Shenoy, A.K., Ziance, R.J.: Comparative regulation of potassium and amphetamine induced release of [^{3}H] norepinephrine from rat brain via presynaptic mechanisms. Life Sci. *24*, 255–264 (1979)
Sheppard, G.P.: High-dose propranolol in Schizophrenia. Br. J. Psychiatry *134*, 470–476 (1979)
Shopsin, B., Hirsch, J., Gershon, S.: Visual hallucinations and propranolol. Biol. Psychiatry *10*, 105–107 (1975)
Singh, K.P., Bhandari, D.S., Mahawar, M.M.: Effects of some beta-adrenergic blocking agents on tremorine induced tremor, hypothermia and cholinergic effects in rats. Indian J. Med. Res. *61*, 1544–1549 (1973)
Sporn, J.R., Molinoff, P.B.: β-adrenergic receptors in rat brain. J. Cyclic Nucleotide Res. *2*, 149–161 (1976)
Steinert, J., Pugh, C.R.: Two patients with schizophrenic-like psychosis after treatment with beta-adrenergic blockers. Br. Med. J. *1979 I*, 790
Stephen, S.A.: Unwanted effects of propranolol. Am. J. Cardiol. *18*, 463–472 (1966)
Strang, R.R.: The symptom of restless legs. Med. J. Aust. *1*, 1211–1213 (1967)
Straughan, D.W., Roberts, M.H.T., Sobiezek, A.: The effect of noradrenaline on single neurones in the cat cerebral cortex. Yugoslav Physiol. Pharmacol. Acta *4*, 145–147 (1968)
Straumanis, J.J., Shagas, C.: Electrophysiologic effects of triiodothyronine and propranolol. Psychopharmacology *46*, 283–288 (1976)
Street, J.A., Hemsworth, B.A., Roach, A.G., Day, M.D.: Tissue levels of several radiolabelled β-adrenoceptor antagonists after intravenous administration to rats. Arch. Int. Pharmacodyn. Ther. *237*, 180–190 (1979)
Sullivan, J.L., Segal, D.S., Kuczenski, R.T., Mandell, A.J.: Propranolol-induced rapid activation of rat striatal tyrosine hydroxylase concomitant with behavioural depression. Biol. Psychiatry *4*, 193–204 (1972)
Suzman, M.M.: Propranolol in the treatment of anxiety. Postgrad. Med. J. *52*, Suppl. 4, 168–174 (1976)
Teravainen, H., Larsen, A., Fogelholm, R.: Comparison between the effects of pindolol and propranolol on essential tremor. Neurology *27*, 439–442 (1977)
Topliss, D., Bond, R.: Acute brain syndrome after propranolol treatment. Lancet *1977 II*, 1133–1134
Trivedi, C.P., Sharma, R.D.: Neuropharmacological studies on propranolol – a beta-adrenergic blocking agent. Indian J. Med. Sci. *27*, 753–758 (1973)

Tsang, D., Lal, S.: Accumulation of cyclic adenosine 3′,5′ monophosphate in human cerebellar cortex slices: effect of monoamine receptor agonists and antagonists. Brain Res. *140*, 307–313 (1978)

Tyrer, P.J., Lader, M.H.: Some clinical and physiological effects of sotalol in chronic anxiety. Psychopharmacology *26*, Suppl., 50 (1972)

Tyrer, P.J., Lader, M.H.: Effects of β-adrenergic blockade with sotalol in chronic anxiety. Clin. Pharmacol. Ther. *14*, 418–426 (1973)

Tyrer, P.J., Lader, M.H.: Physiological and psychological effects of propranolol, + propranolol and diazepam in induced anxiety. Br. J. Clin. Pharmacol. *1*, 379–385 (1974a)

Tyrer, P.J., Lader, M.H.: Physiological response to propranolol and diazepam in chronic anxiety. Br. J. Clin. Pharmacol. *1*, 387–390 (1974b)

U'Prichard, D.C. Snyder, S.H.: Differential labelling of and noradrenergic receptors in calf cerebellum membranes with [^{3}H]-adrenaline. Nature *270*, 261–263 (1977)

Volk, W., Bier, W., Braun, J.P., Gruter, W., Spiegelberg, U.: Behandlung von erregten Psychosen mit einem Beta-Rezeptoren-Blocker (Oxprenolol) in hoher Dosierung. Nervenarzt *43*, 491–492 (1972)

Weber, R.B., Reinmuth, O.M.: The treatment of migraine with propranolol. Neurology *22*, 366–369 (1972)

Weinstock, M., Schechter, Y.: Antagonism by propranolol of the ganglion stimulant action of 5-hydroxytryptamine. Eur. J. Pharmacol. *32*, 293–301 (1975)

Weinstock, M., Speiser, Z.: The effect of DL-propranolol, D-propranolol and practolol on the hyperactivity induced in rats by prolonged isolation. Psychopharmacology *30*, 241–250 (1973)

Weinstock, M., Speiser, Z.: Modification by propranolol and related compounds of motor activity and stereotype behaviour induced in the rat by amphetamine. Eur. J. Pharmacol. *25*, 29–35 (1974)

Weinstock, M., Weiss, C., Gitter, S.: Blockade of 5-hydroxytryptamine receptors in the central nervous system by β-adrenoceptor antagonists. Neuropharmacology *16*, 273–276 (1977)

Wiesel, F.A.: The effect of propranolol on central monoamine metabolism. Acta Physiol. Scand. [Suppl.] *440*, 143 (1976)

Wilson, J.D., King, D.J., Sheriden, B.: Plasma prolactin levels before and during propranolol in chronic schizophrenia. Br. J. Clin. Pharmacol. *7*, 313–314 (1979)

Winkler, G.F., Young, R.R.: Efficacy of chronic propranolol therapy in action tremors of the familial, senile or essential varieties. N. Engl. J. Med. *290*, 984–988 (1974)

Whitlock, F.A., Price, J.: Use of β-adrenergic receptor blocking drugs in psychiatry. Drugs *8*, 109–124 (1974)

Wurtman, R.J., Shein, H.M., Larin, F.: Mediation of β-adrenergic receptors of norepinephrine on pineal synthesis of [^{14}C] serotonin and [^{14}C] melatonin. J. Neurochem. *18*, 1683–1687 (1971)

Yeroukalis, D., Gatzonis, S., Alevizos, B., Stefanis, C.: Effect of propranolol isomers on monoamine neurons in rat cerebellum. 11th CINP Congress, Vienna, July 1978. Abstr., p. 221, 1978

Yorkston, N.J., Zaki, S.A., Malik, M.K.U., Morrison, R.C., Havard, C.W.H.: Propranolol in the control of schizophrenic symptoms. Br. Med. J. *1974 IV*, 633–635

Yorkston, N.J., Gruzelier, J.H., Zaki, S.A., Hollander, D., Pitcher, D.R., Sergeant, H.G.: Propranolol as an adjunct to the treatment of schizophrenia. Lancet *1977 II*, 575–578

Young, R.R., Growdon, J.H., Shahani, B.T.: Beta-adrenergic mechanisms in action tremor. N. Engl. J. Med. *293*, 950–953 (1975)

Von Zerssen, D.: Beta-adrenergic blocking agents in the treatment of psychoses. A report of 17 cases. In: Neuropsychiatric effects of adrenergic beta-blocking agents. Adv. Clin. Pharmacol. *12*, 105–114 (1976)

Van Zwieten, P.A., Timmermans, P.B.M.W.M.: Comparison between the acute haemodynamic effects and brain penetration of atenolol and metoprolol. J. Cardiovasc. Pharmacol. *1*, 85–95 (1979)

CHAPTER 17

Caffeine

C.-J. ESTLER

A. Introduction

Caffeine in the form of caffeine-containing beverages is probably one of the most widely used psychostimulatory agents. The use of coffee beans is first reported in the fifteenth century in Ethiopia and Arabia. The habit of coffee drinking soon became popular, first in the Near East and about 100 years later in Europe. From there it spread over the western hemisphere. Today the per capita consumption of coffee in various countries is in the range of several kilograms per annum (Table 1).

The use of tea stems from the Far East. It was indroduced to China in the fourth century and to Japan in the ninth century. In the sixteenth century the first tea-leaves were brought to Europe, where in some countries tea soon became a favourite drink (Table 1).

Maté is a popular drink in South America. Its caffeine content is slightly lower than that of tea. Cocoa-like drinks made from the seeds of the cocoa tree, which contain 1.5%–3% theobromine and 0.05%–0.15% caffeine, have been in use in Mexico and Peru since old ages and were introduced to Europe in 1520, but only in the nineteenth century did the production of cocoa powder became really important. In recent

Table 1. Per capita consumption of coffee beans and tea-leaves in various countries (1972). (According to GILBERT, 1976)

	Coffee beans[a] (kg)	Tea-leaves[b] (kg)
Canada	4.1	0.9
Denmark	12.6	0.4
Finland	12.0	—
France	5.1	0.1
Germany (Federal Republic)	4.9	0.2
Japan	0.5	1.0
Italy	3.4	0.1
Netherlands	9.3	0.6
Norway	10.3	—
Sweden	13.5	0.2
Switzerland	6.2	0.2
United Kingdom	2.2	3.8
United States	6.3	0.3

[a] Coffee beans contain 0.8%–2.5%
[b] Tea-leaves contain ca. 2% caffeine

Table 2. Caffeine content of various beverages. (According to GOODMAN and GILMAN, 1975; GILBERT, 1976, LEVENSON and BICK, 1977)

	Range (mg/cup)	Average (mg/cup)
Coffee		
Ground	60–150	85
Instant	40–100	60
Decaffeinated[a]	1– 8	3
Tea	25–100	40
Cocoa (depending on type of preparation)	7– 50	—
Cola drinks	20– 50 mg/10 oz	—

[a] Decaffeinated coffee contains a maximum of 0.08% caffeine according to regulations valid in the Federal Republic of Germany; in the United States at least 97% of the caffeine must be removed (VITZTHUM, 1976)

Table 3. Caffeine content of various kinds of coffee. (According to VITZTHUM, 1976)

	Amount of coffee used[a] (g/l)	Percent of caffeine extracted
Regular coffee as used in central European countries	50	90
Mocca	100	75
Espresso	150	60

[a] Roasted coffee beans contain 0.8%–2.5% (normal range, 0.9%–1.3%) caffeine

decades the so-called cola drinks named after the kola nut, which contains about 2% caffeine, have become very popular.

Surely the above-mentioned beverages are consumed not only because of their pleasant taste, but also because of their stimulating properties, which correlate fairly closely to their caffeine content. However, the caffeine content may vary widely depending on the mode of preparation of the drink (Tables 2 and 3). Furthermore, these beverages contain a host of other ingredients (Table 4) that may influence the absorption of caffeine from the gastro-intestinal tract or modify its action. Chlorogenic acid, for instance, which is present in coffee in greater amounts than caffeine, possesses central stimulatory properties and is held responsible for stimulatory effects produced by decaffeinated coffee (CZOK, 1966). These facts must be considered when the results of studies with coffee, tea or caffeine are compared.

The beneficial effects of caffeine on psychomotor performance seem to be well-known. In textbooks of pharmacology (e.g. GOODMAN and GILMAN, 1975) they are described with phrases such as the following: "Caffeine is a powerful CNS stimulant... Its main action is to produce a more rapid and clearer flow of thought, and to allay drowsiness and fatigue. After taking caffeine one is capable of a greater sustained intellectual effort and a more perfect association of ideas. There is also keener appreciation of sensory stimuli, and reaction time to them is appreciably

Table 4. Main constituents of coffee beans and tea-leaves. (According to LEVENSON and BICK, 1977; VITZTHUM, 1976)

Coffee beans roasted		Tea-leaves	
Carbohydrates	~24%–30%	Carbohydrates	>25%
Proteins	~ 9%–13%	Cellulose	
Lipids	~13%	Amino acids	
Minerals	~ 4%	Lignin	
Caffeine	~ 0.9%–2.5%	Tannins or polyphenols	
Chlorogenic acid	~ 3.5%	Caffeine	1.5%–5%
		Theobromine	0.2%
		Theophyllin	0.1%

diminished... In addition, motor activity is increased...." Of course, adverse effects can be also observed, especially when larger quantities of caffeine have been ingested, and there is a limited number of individuals who do not tolerate caffeine very well.

But in spite of the fact that the favourable effects of caffeine on psychomotor functions appear to be beyond any doubt, trials to substantiate the empirically well-known psychomotor effects by way of sophisticated psychological methods yield equivocal results. There are a number of reasons for the discrepancies, which are to be mentioned briefly: A large part of the original experiments on the psychological effects of coffee and caffeine were carried out in the first decades of this century. These studies were often poorly devised and in many cases uncontrolled and performed on only a few subjects who, moreover, had not been properly selected. Sometimes subjective ratings substitute for objective measurements and statistical evaluations are missing. Such studies that do not fulfill the criteria of modern experimental design must be judged with proper reserve. But even more recent investigations are sometimes defective with regard to standardization and control. This is especially true for studies with coffee. In most studies only one dose of caffeine or coffee has been tested. Despite the fact that different investigators have used different doses of caffeine, dose–response relations cannot be easily established, since the ways in which the drinks were prepared or the drugs administered vary widely. Furthermore, only a few investigators gave attention to their subjects' habits in caffeine consumption, and very few were aware of the possibility that the outcome of the experiments might be influenced or falsified by tolerance to caffeine in caffeine-treated subjects or by withdrawal symptoms in untreated controls.

B. Experiments in Humans

I. Effects on Various Psychological Parameters

The effect of caffeine on psychomotor performance has been surveyed in earlier papers. The reader is referred also to the earlier reviews by EICHLER (1938, 1976), CALHOUN (1971), CZOK (1966), GILBERT (1976), LANDIS (1958), SELBACH (1969), and WEISS and LATIES (1962).

1. Mood

Effects of caffeine on mood have been mostly tested by self-rating of the subjects studied. Such ratings show a great variation. In experiments by FLORY and GILBERT (1943) 30 of 43 subjects receiving ~160 mg caffeine did not feel that they had received a stimulant. According to BACHRACH (1966) there was no difference on the rating of interest, attentiveness and wakefulness between caffeine- (~130 mg) and placebo-treated subjects. In experiments by NASH (1972) the alleviation of feeling of fatigue brought about by 100 mg caffeine/m^2 body surface was only at the borderline of significance, and in experiments by LADER (1969) only small increases in alertness and "quickness" have been observed with 300 mg caffeine, 150 mg being ineffective. Subjective arousal was little influenced by a very high dose of 750 mg caffeine (FRÖBERG et al., 1969). MITCHELL et al. (1974), who treated their subjects with 150–300 mg caffeine, placebo, disguised drugs or no drug, judged caffeine to be an active placebo which was effective only when the subjects knew they received the drug. On the other hand, persons receiving ~240 mg caffeine felt talkative, excited, exhilarated and less sleepy than placebo-treated controls (SEASHORE and IVY, 1953). Persons doing exhausting work rated their effort as being significantly less strenuous, though total work output was increased (COSTILL et al., 1978). Similarly, students treated with 150–200 mg caffeine rated themselves more alert and more active physically and noted an increased nervousness. The latter effect was dose related (GOLDSTEIN et al., 1965b).

In more detailed studies on young women the same authors showed that the response to coffee experienced by the subjects was correlated with the amount of coffee used. Persons accustomed to heavy amounts of coffee reported more of the desirable stimulant and euphoric effects and less nervousness and irritability than light users or abstainers from coffee, who often reacted negatively to caffeine, complaining of nervousness and jitteriness (GOLDSTEIN et al., 1969a). Based on studies on different types of individuals, VON KLEBELSBERG and MOSTBECK (1963) stated that trophotropic persons treated with coffee believed their performance to be more positively influenced than ergotropic subjects. In studies by ADLER et al. (1950) caffeine reduced negative symptoms, especially at a simulated altitude (18,000 ft). These studies show that the effect of caffeine and caffeine-containing beverages is not only dose and time dependent but also depends to a considerable extent on the initial value, which may be influenced by the caffeine consumption habits of the individuals tested. Anticipation of caffeine effects may also play an important role. Moreover, the experiments by GOLDSTEIN et al. (1969a, b) on coffee users and abstainers provide evidence of tolerance or habituation (see this Chap., Sect. B.IV).

2. Attention, Concentration and Vigilance

Attention and concentration are prerequisites for carrying out complicated tasks. Changes in these parameters will, therefore, influence the results of complex psychomotor tests. There are some studies in which an objective estimation of attention and vigilance, apart from other psychomotor parameters, has been aimed at. They yielded equivocal results.

HAWK (1929) found that overdosage of caffeine (two to six cups) impaired the ability of subjects to concentrate, (HAWK, 1929) while STANLEY and SCHLOSSBERG (1953) found that tea had only a detrimental (if any) effect on sustained attention. VON KLE-

BELSBERG and MOSTBECK (1963) observed only an insignificant improvement of the *Konzentrationsleistungstest* (test of ability to concentrate) in non-fatigued subjects. LIENERT and HUBER (1966) reported better results when the *Konzentrationsleistungstest* was performed as a speed test. Similarly, caffeine diminished lapses of attention in a prolonged complex test under boring conditions (BAKER and THEOLOGUS, 1972). In a vigilance test caffeine exhibited a positive effect only on those subjects who showed a decrement in performance under placebo (extroverts) but not on those who showed no such decrement (introverts) (KEISTER and MCLAUGHLIN, 1972).

Similar equivocal results have been obtained in studies in which the galvanic skin reaction, which is considered to reflect the affective arousal of the CNS (AMBROZI and BIRKMAYER, 1970), was measured. AMBROZI and BIRKMAYER (1970) noted a decrease of the reaction. SWITZER (1935a, b) reported an increase in amplitude, a decrease of latency and a retardation of extinction.

3. Fatigue and Sleep

As mentioned in Sect. B.I, caffeine may dose dependently induce the feeling of alertness and stimulate attitude to work. When applied in sufficient amounts it reduces fatigue. Fatigue as a subjective feeling cannot be estimated quantitatively. Therefore flicker fusion frequency, which is considered an indicator of neural fatigue, has often been measured. It was found to be unaffected by caffeine at doses ranging from 200 to 900 mg (ADLER et al., 1950; AMBROZI and BIRKMAYER, 1970; LEHMANN and CSANK, 1957). A positive result is reported by MÜCHER and WENDT (1951). However, these experiments were not performed on exhausted persons. In fatigued persons an improvement was noted by SEASHORE and IVY (1953). According to results by LANDGREBE (1960), healthy persons habituated to coffee showed an increase of the flicker fusion frequency, while persons with autonomic instability and unaccustomed to caffeine showed a decrease.

The effect of tea on fatigue rating was only small (STANLEY and SCHLOSSBERG, 1953). Caffeine (~250 mg) reduced the feeling of fatigue effectively in persons doing exhaustive work (FOLTZ et al., 1942). Under the same amount of caffeine truck drivers judged themselves able to do their work for a longer time (SEASHORE and IVY, 1953); they even had trouble falling asleep. Students receiving coffee containing 150–200 mg caffeine 1 h before retiring also complained of delayed onset of sleep (GOLDSTEIN et al., 1964, 1965a). In addition, those subjects who habitually drank coffee tended to report having slept less soundly after caffeine-containing than after decaffeinated coffee. Similar effects have been reported earlier by HAWK (1929); HOLLINGWORTH (1912) and MULLIN et al. (1933 cit. according to LANDIS, 1958).

More objective determinations (electroencephalogram, electro-oculogram, electromyelogram etc.) of sleeping behaviour have been performed in recent experiments. BŘEZINOVA (1974), KARACAN et al. (1976) and NICHOLSON and STONE (1977), but not MÜLLER-LIMMROTH (1972), found a dose-dependent decrease of total sleeping time. The onset of sleep was significantly delayed in young men by one to four cups of coffee or an equivalent amount of caffeine (KARACAN et al., 1976), and in middle-aged people by 300 mg caffeine (BŘEZINOVA, 1974). In contrast using 100–300 mg caffeine NICHOLSON and STONE (1977) found no change of sleep latency in their subjects. An increased number of awakenings have been reported by BŘEZINOVA (1974), KARACAN

Table 5. Changes of sleep parameters after coffee. (According to MÜLLER-LIMMROTH, 1972)

	Duration of sleep (min) Stages				Motor activity Stage	
	1	2	3	4	1	REM
Placebo	56	166	92	134	4.5	3.6
Decaffeinated coffee	61	183	83	132	17.9	6.0
Coffee	70	191	75	116	28.0	6.0

et al. (1976) and MÜLLER-LIMMROTH (1972). Interestingly, there is also objective evidence that a reduction of sleep quality is caused by caffeine. In MÜLLER-LIMMROTH's (1972) experiments, regular coffee reduced the duration of stages 3 and 4 sleep and enhanced stages 1 and 2. This effect was less pronounced with decaffeinated coffee. In the studies by KARACAN et al. (1976) decaffeinated coffee was without detrimental effect, but regular coffee and caffeine shifted stages 3 and 4 to the later portions of the night; it also increased stages 1 and 2 during the earlier phase. REM sleep was shifted from the third to the first portion of the night. The percentage of REM sleep was not decreased. This is in good argreement with earlier observations by BŘEZINOVA (1974) and NICHOLSON and STONE (1977). A disturbed soundness of sleep due to coffee also becomes apparent from an increasing motor activity (number and amplitude of movements) of sleeping persons (MÜLLER-LIMMROTH, 1972; SCHWERTZ and MARBACH, 1965). Insomnia has also been found to occur after cola drinks (SILVER, 1971). COLTON et al. (1968) reported that there is some indication that tolerance will develop: Only non-coffee drinkers reported disturbances in sleep patterns.

As will be discussed later, the caffeine-induced diminution of boredom and the delay of fatigue and sleepiness undoubtedly play a central role in many of the beneficial effects of caffeine (i.e. attentiveness, accuracy and psychomotor performance).

II. Effects on Motor Performance

1. Total Work Output

A broad discussion of the effects of caffeine on human physical performance is beyond the scope of this review, since working capacity is not solely dependent on psychological functions but to a large degree also on metabolic conditions and other factors (e.g. mobilization and availability of substrates for skeletal muscle, cardiovascular function etc.) that may be greatly influenced by caffeine (for review see EICHLER, 1976).

Several authors have reported that working periods on ergometers were prolonged in subjects treated with coffee or caffeine (COSTILL et al., 1978; FOLTZ et al., 1942; KOLEY et al., 1973; SCHIRLITZ, 1930) and that even if working became less economical (SCHIRLITZ, 1929) the total work done was increased (KOLEY et al., 1973; SCHIRLITZ, 1929). In addition, caffeine shortened the recovery from exhaustive work (KOLEY et al., 1973) and significantly enhanced the working capacity in a second period of work that had to be done following a short rest after a first period of exhausting work (FOLTZ et al., 1942). For more extensive discussion of this type of studies see EICHLER (1976) and WEISS and LATIES (1962).

2. Tapping

The maximum frequency of tapping a key with one finger is often determined in order to estimate the maximum speed of voluntary motor discharge. Among others this test is sensitive to emotional tension and, if performed over a prolonged period, also to muscular fatigue. The results range from 5%–10% decrease after coffee (GILLILAND and NELSON, 1939), through no effect (ADLER et al., 1950; DAHME et al., 1972; FLORY and GILBERT, 1943; VON KLEBELSBERG and MOSTBECK, 1963) to increase (CLUBLEY et al., 1977; LEHMANN and CSANK, 1957; THORNTON et al., 1939; WENZEL and RUTLEDGE, 1962). A correlation of the effect to the drug dose applied or the state of the individual tested is not apparent from these studies.

3. Hand Steadiness, Motor Skill and Accuracy

Special types of motor performance requiring motor skill and accuracy, such as needle threading (DUREMAN, 1962), hitting a small target with a stylus (HORST et al., 1934a) or handwriting (SEYFFERT, 1954), may be impaired by caffeine under some conditions. In a more complicated test requiring acquired greater skill the rapidity of movements was facilitated, but precision was impaired (HORST et al., 1934b). Unexpectedly the deteriorating effects on writing and threading became manifest only 5–6 h after the ingestion of caffeine, while shortly after the coffee ingestion writing was improved (more clear and energetic). This is in line with the observations by HORST et al. (1934b) that impaired performance in the target test was preceded by a transient improvement. Accordingly, GOLDSTEIN et al. (1965b) did not observe a negative effect on co-ordination in a simple task (following lines with a pencil) within 3 h after ingestion of coffee.

The detrimental effects on motor performance can easily be ascribed to tremor and decreased hand steadiness and dexterity, which have been observed repeatedly in caffeine-treated persons (FOLTZ et al., 1942; FRANKS et al., 1975; GILLILAND and NELSON, 1939; HULL, 1935; LEHMANN and CSANK, 1957; SWITZER, 1935a; THORNTON et al., 1939; for review see CALHOUN, 1971). The negative effects on motor performance, especially those an hand steadiness, though strictly speaking not psychotropic in nature, may affect in various ways the results of psychomotor tests in which motor responses are involved (e.g. tapping, typewriting etc.) and may mask positive effects and speed of reaction of similar parameters.

III. Effects on Psychomotor Parameters

1. Reaction Time

Because of its simplicity reaction time is frequently tested despite a number of drawbacks that make definite assessment of the results difficult. Being a function of the sense modality stimulated reaction time varies widely with the complexity of the experimental conditions. Good performance in such tests requires not only reaction speed but also attention, and under some conditions, discrimination of stimuli and motor accuracy. It is highly influenced by boredom and fatigue.

Accordingly, the results of studies on the action of caffeine on reaction time vary greatly. No effect or only slight improvements were observed by DAHME et al. (1972), GILLILAND and NELSON (1939), VON KLEBELSBERG and MOSTBECK (1963), SEASHORE and Ivy (1953) and Thornton et al. (1939), who used low or medium amounts of coffee or caffeine, but also by Lehmann and Csank (1957) with high doses (600–900 mg). On the other hand, in experiments by Clubley et al. (1977) as little as 75–100 mg caffeine reduced auditory reaction time. Cheney (1935) found the effect to be dose dependent: less than 3 mg/kg were ineffective, more than 5 mg/kg caused a reduction of visual reaction time lasting for more than 2 h. The same author obtained better effects on reaction time and accuracy of response with caffeine than with coffee, except during the first half hour when coffee was more effective (Cheney, 1936). A very rapid onset of an improvement of auditory and visual reaction times in persons who had drunk tea or coffee was also noticed by Knowles (1963) and by Stanley and Schlossberg (1953). This led to the suggestion that conditioning to tea or coffee may be involved in this effect. This view is supported by the facts that decaffeinated coffee acted like regular coffee and that the effect of coffee faded away within 60 min (Knowles, 1963). The drug effect may also be dependent on the initial value. Data from Carpenter (1959) suggest that caffeine is effective when the potential for improvement is great, e.g. when the reaction time was lengthened by ethanol (Carpenter, 1959; Franks et al., 1975). Accordingly, Adler et al. (1950) found caffeine to prevent deterioration of choice reaction time at simulated altitude, and Reichard and Elder (1977) detected an enhanced number of correct responses in a choice reaction test in hyperkinetic, but not in normal, children.

Habituation and tolerance towards caffeine also modifies the results. In persons habituated to caffeine, reaction and discrimination times were found to be enhanced. They decreased when the ingestion of coffee or tea was discontinued. In subjects tolerant to caffeine, caffeine shortened their reaction time, while in persons abstaining from caffeine for more than 2 months, reaction time was increased by small doses of caffeine (Eddy and Downs, 1928). In the light of this the prolongation of reaction time after caffeine observed by Hawk (1929) or Schilling (1921) is not inexplicable. Unexplained are, however, the results of Wenzel and Rutledge (1962). In this study the visual reaction time was shortened and complex reaction time was lengthened in a manner inversely related to the dose of caffeine applied (100–300 mg).

2. Simple Tasks (Cancellations, Calculations, Reading etc.)

Simple additions have long been used for estimating the effects of psychotropic drugs. The results obtained with caffeine by Wedemeyer (1919) were inconsistent. Maier (1922) observed an increase of the number of additions performed and a decrease of the errors made. Caffeine-containing and decaffeinated coffee were equally effective; thus the results are dubious. Conversely, a loss of accuracy was reported by Hawk (1929). Bachrach (1966) found no effect of ~130 mg caffeine on adding, whereas Gilliland and Nelson (1939) and Nash (1962a) reported that additions were facilitated by coffee or caffeine. Tea had the same effect, the optimum amount corresponding to 300 mg caffeine (Pauli, 1927). Prüll (1965) (cit. Luff, 1965) found that caffeine increases the amount of calculations but also enhances the fluctuation of the performance. Graf (1961) noted the positive effect to be dose dependent and to be maximal at 0.2 g. In a very remarkable study Barmack (1940) showed that ~130 mg caffeine had no effect during the initial 15-min period of adding, but that it increased the rate of adding towards the latter part of a 2-h session, when given 1–3 h before the trial. Based on these results he put forward the hypothesis that caffeine acts in the first place by adjusting alertness if boredom develops and, thus, its effect becomes manifest mainly when conditions for the maintenance of alertness are not favourable. Up to now this hypothesis has not been refuted.

In another simple task (crossing out certain letters from a given text, i.e. a cancellation test) the performance was improved by ~200 mg (ADLER et al., 1950) and impaired by 600–900 mg caffeine (LEHMANN and CSANK, 1957).

Simple verbal tests such as reading speed, reading comprehension or verbal fluency were not significantly affected by up to 300 mg caffeine (BACHRACH, 1966; FLORY and GILBERT, 1943; FRANKS et al., 1975).

3. Complex Psychomotor Tests (Typewriting, Pursuit Motor Tasks etc.)

The first investigator using a complex psychomotor test for studying the effects of caffeine was HOLLINGWORTH (1912). In experiments on typewriting he showed that writing speed was enhanced by low doses (~65–200 mg) and diminished by high doses (~260–390 mg) of caffeine. The number of errors was slightly reduced. HOLCK (1933), testing the effect of caffeine on playing chess, noticed that problems were solved faster and more accurately by persons treated with 100 mg caffeine.

More recently, various pursuit motor tasks in which alertness, attention, reaction speed, motor skill and accuracy are simultaneously involved have been used. In experiments by DUREMAN (1962) simple code tracking was not affected by caffeine after 3 and 6 h. On the other hand, STRASSER and MÜLLER-LIMMROTH (1971) noted that in a somewhat more complex task caffeine prevented the decrease of performance seen under placebo. Decaffeinated coffee was also effective, but less so than regular coffee. Investigators using different types of airplane simulators generally noticed an improvement of performance by caffeine (ADLER et al., 1950; HAUTY and PAYNE, 1955; SEASHORE and IVY, 1953). An improvement was also seen in simulated car driving: 200–400 mg caffeine enhanced the response to signals, increased attention, inhibited response blocking and reduced the numbers of signals missed, especially when a monotonous situation was simulated (BAKER and THEOLOGUS, 1972; REGINA and SMITH, 1974). Caffeine also partially restored the performance impaired by ethanol (RUTENFRANZ and JANSEN, 1959). On the other hand, non-fatigued subjects treated with 200 mg caffeine drove faster and made more errors (GRAF, 1957, 1961). In a similar test a tendency to drive faster was noticed in ergotropic individuals, while trophotropic persons were slower but better co-ordinated (VON KLEBELSBERG and MOSTBECK, 1963). Using the *Kieler Determinationsgerät* and the *Kugeltest*, both of which measure visual motoric skill, DAHME et al. (1972) and SULC and PORADKOVA (1975) obtained positive results with 200 mg caffeine, while VON KLEBELSBERG and MOSTBECK (1963) found no effect with 100 mg caffeine. According to LUFF et al. (1964) the effect is biphasic, first increasing then decreasing performance.

4. Learning, Memory and Other Intellectual Functions

Learning, memory and intelligence are complex psychological functions that defy qualitative assessment. To circumvent this difficulty a variety of test batteries have been developed and employed in studies with caffeine. Due to the different methodological approaches a comparison of the results is hardly possible. Studying verbal associations, Allers and Freund (1925) had the impression that learning was facilitated but that reproduction was impaired by strong coffee. Catell (1930) likewise found the power of recall and associative performance to be reduced by a medium dose of caffeine (400 mg), whereas a lower dose (200 mg) enhanced the power of recall. Young persons proved to be more susceptible to caffeine than older ones; men were more susceptible than women. Moderate amounts of coffee increased memory span (Gilliland and Nelson, 1939), whereas very high doses of caffeine (600–900 mg) did not show this effect (Lehmann and Csank, 1957). These doses, however, facilitated digit-symbol substitution, which reflects learning and visual motor efficiency (Lehmann and Csank, 1957).

Hull (1935) noticed that persons treated with ~160 mg caffeine and learning series of nonsense syllables showed an excess of anticipatory displacements. Their subjects required longer to memorize. Forming of associative bonds and writing down of verbal combinations was found to be facilitated by one cup of coffee (Reiman, 1934). However, tactile and acoustic associations were impaired by 200 mg caffeine (Hrbeck et al., 1971, 1973). Nash (1962a, b) reported that caffeine (100 mg/m^2 body surface) increased the spontaneity of associations, quickened the formation of thought and enhanced numerical speed, visual thinking and the recall of auditory information. An increase of numerical reasoning together with inductive and spatial reasoning was also reported by Lienert and Huber (1966), while at the same time other sub-tests of the *Intelligenzstrukturtest* (i.e. general information, verbal comprehension) were impaired by 300 mg caffeine. In other experiments the same dose of caffeine was without effect on numerical reasoning (Franks et al., 1975). Using a multiple choice vocabulary test that measured speed of thinking, Flory and Gilbert (1943) even noticed a possible loss of thinking ability in students given ~160 mg caffeine. The discrepancy may be due to the state of the persons tested. In experiments by Revelle et al. (1976) extroverts solved more problems of a verbal ability test under time pressure than did introverts.

IV. Habituation, Tolerance and Dependence

Whether caffeine has to be considered a drug of abuse causing tolerance and dependence is not yet settled. This matter has been extensively discussed by Gilbert (1976). There is no doubt that many people throughout the world habitually consume caffeine-containing beverages in moderate amounts. Excessive use of caffeine seems rare (Czok, 1966, Eichler, 1976). There are few reports on tolerance to caffeine; they deal mostly with somatic functions. For instance sleep disturbance by caffeine was reported less often in coffee drinkers than in abstainers (Colton et al., 1968). Wedemeyer (1919) first reported a decline of enhanced psychomotor performance during the course of 4–5 weeks treatment with caffeine. According to Eddy and Downs (1928) habituation to caffeine-containing beverages appeared to lengthen reaction and discrimination times. At least discontinuance of coffee consumption shortened these parameters. Primavera et al. (1975) did not find significant differences in the personality structure of users and non-users of coffee, although the first group rated themselves more self-confident.

Withdrawal of caffeine may impair the performance of persons habituated to caffeine and may or may not cause mild withdrawal symptoms (DREISBACH and PFEIFFER, 1943; GREDEN, 1974; REIMANN, 1967). FURLONG (1974 cit. according to GILBERT, 1976) had difficulties in encouraging caffeine abstention among persons drinking more than five cups of caffeine-containing beverages a day. The withdrawal symptoms have been investigated by GOLDSTEIN et al. (1964, 1969 a, b), giving coffee with or without added caffeine to heavy users of coffee and to non-users. While abstainers felt normal when given placebo, the users reported dysphoria, uneasiness, irritability, restlessness, nervousness and jitteriness; some felt less alert, lethargic or sleepy. These symptoms appeared 12–16 h after the last ingestion of coffee and were revealed and displaced by pleasant stimulation and contentedness when 150–300 mg caffeine were given.

V. Conclusion

The psychotropic effects of caffeine have been experienced by innumerable individuals, and their existence is unanimously accepted by writers of textbooks and reviews. A great part of these effects can only be evaluated by self-rating of persons treated with caffeine. The number of well-controlled and excellently designed studies is in sharp contrast to the importance of caffeine as a commonly used psychostimulatory drug. Their results are by no means unequivocal or clear-cut. Nevertheless, they substantiate the stimulatory effect on certain psychomotor functions, which becomes especially apparent when these functions are impaired by fatigue. In this way the observations made by KRAEPELIN in 1892 have essentially been confirmed. There is some evidence that caffeine, like other euphoretics, causes a mild degree of habituation and tolerance, but this must still be proven in specially designed experiments.

C. Animal Studies

Parallel to human studies reviewed in Sect. B, experiments on animals have been performed in order to elucidate the psychopharmacological action of caffeine. Such studies have the advantage that the experimental conditions can be better standardized and more clearly defined, but on the other hand the behavioural expressions of the most commonly used animals are very limited. Thus, findings cannot be easily transferred to humans. The animal experiments centre on four items: motor activity, response rates, learning and memory and a few kinds of social behaviour.

I. Motor Activity

The motor activity of animals is determined using simple measures of sedation or excitation. There is general agreement that caffeine enhances running and exploratory activity of various animal species (BOISSIER and SIMON, 1967; DEWS, 1953; ESTLER, 1973, 1979; HEIM et al., 1955, 1971; KNOLL, 1961; MENGE, 1961; NIESCHULTZ, 1967; WALDECK, 1975; for review see CALHOUN, 1971; EICHLER, 1976). Obviously this effect is dose dependent and biphasic: an increase of the activity is only observed within a certain dose range, higher doses are ineffective or even reduce the activity. However, the doses yielding maximum response differ widely from investigation to investigation. KNOLL (1961) noted a linear increase of activity with caffeine doses ranging from 25 to 150 mg/kg in mice, whereas in experiments by DEWS (1953) or MENGE (1961) in the same species the activity was reduced by doses of 50 mg/kg or higher. The effect is also dependent on the state of the animals. According to GREENBLATT and OSTERBERG (1961 a, b), caffeine increased activity only in grouped mice and reduced the motility of isolated animals. This is in line with similar results of VALZELLI and BERNASCONI (1973) who, moreover, showed that the effect also depends on the state of aggressiveness of the animals. KEHRHAHN (1973) demonstrated caffeine to be most effective during daytime.

Furthermore, different types of motor performance were differently affected. Ambulation was increased by doses of caffeine (5–10 mg/kg) that did not affect rearing and slightly decreased novelty preference (HUGHES and GREIG, 1976). MARRIOTT (1968) showed that caffeine (12–50 mg/kg) increased the activity of rats in a treadmill but not within a maze. Spontaneous alterations in a Y-maze were found to be enhanced in experiments by COX (1970) and HUGHES and GREIG (1976). Running speed was measured and found to be increased by BARRY and MILLER (1965), MILLER and MILES (1935) and WANNER and BÄTTIG (1965). The effect was also dependent on the motivation state of the animals and especially pronounced in animals performing poorly because of low drive (MILLER and MILES, 1935; WANNER and BÄTTIG, 1965).

It may well be that immobilization of animals treated with high doses of caffeine is due to impaired motor co-ordination. Experiments in which co-ordination was measured yielded no conclusive results: low doses of caffeine had no effect in an acute experiment (PLOTNIKOFF et al., 1962), and an improvement was seen in a prolonged study (ESTLER et al., 1978). A systematic investigation seems to be required to clarify this matter.

There have been only a few experiments on long-term effects of caffeine. ESTLER et al. (1978) and NEUMANN (1965) reported that the swimming endurance of mice was reduced by caffeine. TAINTER (1943) assumed that tolerance may develop to the hyperkinetic effect of caffeine. According to BOYD et al. (1965) the activity of rats is depressed during withdrawal of caffeine.

II. Response Rates

As noted in Sect. C.I, running performance of rats is enhanced by caffeine when they are motivated by a rewarding stimulus (BARRY and MILLER, 1965; MILLER and MILES, 1935; WANNER and BÄTTIG, 1965). An increased response rate after caffeine was also observed in other experimental situations. SKINNER and HERON (1937) observed increased bar pressing for food in rats treated with 10 mg/kg caffeine. MEDEK et al. (1971) found conditioned alimentary motor reactions to be improved by very low doses of caffeine (0.02–0.6 mg/kg). Increased response rates were also observed in rats by SOLYOM et al. (1968) and in pigeons by BLOUGH (1957). MECHNER and LATRANYI (1963) studied the dose–response relations of caffeine. Similar to motor activity (see this Chap., Sect. C.I), operant behavior was improved by medium doses and impaired by high doses of caffeine. Similarly WAYNER et al. (1976) demonstrated that schedule-dependent reactions (lever pressing, licking, water consumption) were inversely influenced by low (3 mg/kg) and high (100 mg/kg) doses of caffeine. The positive effect of the low dose was absent in undernourished animals. A tolerance to caffeine was also noted. STINNETTE and ISAAC (1975) showed that light and dark may also affect the operant behaviour.

In experiments with a differential reinforcement of low rates schedule, the frequency of short inter-response times was greatly enhanced by caffeine doses ranging from 6 to 24 mg/kg; 48 mg/kg was uneffective (WEBB and LEVINE, 1978). A similar effect was observed by ANDO (1973). Shortened reaction times were reported by NIESCHULZ (1963) and by MATTHIES and ERDMANN (1957). In an unusual test NIESCHULZ (1963) found the distractibility of rats to be greatly increased by caffeine, and training effects were markedly reduced.

An important observation is that caffeine increased the rate of self-stimulation in monkeys with electrodes implanted in the medium forebrain bundle (MALIS et al., 1960). This effect was noted even with a rather high dose (200 mg/kg) of caffeine that in other experiments usually depresses activity.

III. Learning

1. Discrimination

A short review on the effects of caffeine on learning has been given by ESSMAN (1971).

Learning of animals has often been studied by way of various types of mazes. Early experiments by LASHLEY (1917) and MACHT (1932) were not very conclusive. COOPER et al. (1969) and CASTELLANO (1976) reported that learning of a discrimination task in a maze was facilitated by 1 mg/kg caffeine; higher doses were inhibitory. In similar experiments RAHMANN (1963) found 0.5 mg/kg to be the dose most effective in regard to learning, relearning and retention. Doses of 1–10 mg/kg impaired both parameters. In CASTELLANO's (1976) experiments memory stabilization was improved when 1 mg/kg caffeine was given during the training period. The long-term store of memory was unaffected by 5 mg/kg caffeine citrate in mice (CRABBE and ALPERN, 1973). Doses of 10 and more mg/kg caffeine disrupted the performance due to excitation and inco-ordination of the animals (CASTELLANO, 1976; STRIPLING and ALPERN, 1974). On the other hand, 20–25 mg/kg caffeine was able to block the amnesia produced by inhibitors of protein synthesis (FLEXNER and FLEXNER, 1975; FLOOD et al., 1978). Relearning of reinforced conditioned behaviour disrupted by throwing the animals into confusion and frustration was facilitated by caffeine (MATTHIES and ERDMANN, 1957).

Visual discrimination was not affected by 2.5 mg/kg, facilitated by 5 mg/kg and impaired by 10 mg/kg caffeine (CASTELLANO, 1977). An acoustic discrimination task was affected in neither direction by 1–60 mg/kg caffeine (GELLER et al., 1971). PARÉ (1961) studied the retention in rats trained on visual discrimination. The number of errors in the retention trials was reduced by 30 mg/kg caffeine, but only when the drug was given 5 s after the criterion was reached. When given after 2 min or later, caffeine was without effect. There is no reasonable explanation for this unique observation. Another kind of discrimination experiment was made by KULKARNI (1972). Rats had to discriminate two levers to avoid shock. In these experiments 25 mg/kg caffeine increased the correct and decreased the wrong lever response. Wrong responses increased with 100 mg/kg caffeine. The same inverse effects were observed with signal association.

2. Avoidance

Conditioned avoidance or escape responses are other often studied parameters for learning and memory. BARRY and MILLER (1965) observed an increased running performance of rats in order to avoid electroshock. HEARST (1964) demonstrated that caffeine (20 and 80 mg/kg) clearly increased the frequency of lever pressing on a given light signal to avoid shock. In addition, the animals learned better to discriminate light of different intensity. An increased responding in various shock avoidance schedules was also observed by CARPI et al. (1974), DAVIS and KENSLER (1973), HUGHES and FORNEY, (1961), MORPURGO (1965), PLOTNIKOFF (1962), PLOTNIKOFF and FITZLOFF (1963) and TONINI and BABBINI (1961). On the other hand, OLIVERIO (1967) observed only very small effects. IZQUIERDO (1974), MARINO and CUOMO (1974) and SANSONE (1975) found no effects of various doses of caffeine on conditioning, deconditioning by reserpine and reconditioning after reserpine. Part of these discrepancies may be due to the fact that caffeine seems to act biphasically: increase or no effect with lower doses, decrease of performance with higher doses (BÄTTIG and GRANDJEAN, 1955; CASTELLANO et al., 1973; NIESCHULZ, 1969). It is conceivable that doses impairing motor performance also interfere with escape reactions. Species and strain differences also seem to be involved (SATINDER, 1971; CASTELLANO, 1977). As in discriminative behaviour caffeine not only facilitates learning, but also improves retention, when given shortly before or immediately after training (ROUSSINOV and YONKOV, 1974, 1976).

When rats were confronted with a conflict situation (motivation either to drink or to avoid shock), caffeine caused the animals to drink and accept shocks (HOROVITZ et al., 1972). The authors' ascribe this effect to an antianxiety action of caffeine, but this explanation appears disputable.

IV. Social Behaviour

In an open field test caffeine increased the gregariousness of rats (CAPPELL and LATANÉ, 1969). However, the contacts between the animals were short lasting. On the other hand, caffeine in the same dose range reduced the huddling behaviour (i.e., lying piled up into a heap) (GIURGEA and VAN KEMEULEN, 1974). Sexual activity was enhanced; latencies for mounting and copulation were decreased (ZIMBARDO and BARRY, 1958). Very high doses inhibited copulation and blocked the growth of population in rats (BOVET-NITTI and MESSERI, 1975). The reason may be an increased aggressiveness of caffeine-treated animals (CAPPELL and LATANÉ, 1969; BOVET-NITTI and MESSERI, 1975). PETERS (1967) and PETERS and BOYD (1967) also observed an increased auto-aggression and automutilation in rats.

Some investigators found that caffeine or coffee reduced the uptake of food and water (ESTLER et al., 1978, TAINTER, 1943) or weight gain (ESTLER et al., 1978; STRUBELT et al., 1973). Increased water consumption occurred in rats chronically treated with caffeine (BOYD et al., 1965).

V. Conclusion

The animal experiments essentially confirm the experiments on humans, but in general they do not allow conclusions that exceed those made from human studies. The special advantages of animal experiments lie in the greater simplicity of the methodology, the greater ease of standardization and control and the possibility to perform simultaneous investigations on concomitant changes in cerebral metabolism or neuronal function in order to gain insight into the basic mechanism of the psychotropic effects. Unfortunately, at present such studies, though numerous, have not yet reached a point, where well-founded conclusions can be drawn (for review see ESTLER, 1976).

References

Adler, H.F., Burkhardt, W.L., Ivy, A.C., Atkinson, A.J.: Effect of various drugs on psychomotor performance at ground level and at simulated altitudes of 18,000 feet in a low pressure chamber. J. Aviat. Space Environ. Med. *21*, 221–236 (1950)

Allers, R., Freund, E.: Zur Kenntnis der psychischen Wirkung von Arzneimitteln und anderen Stoffen; I. Die Wirkung des Kaffees. Z. Gesamte Neurol. Psychiatrie *97*, 749–769 (1925)

Ambrozi, L., Birkmayer, W.: Über die Objektivierbarkeit von psychopharmakologischen Drogen am Beispiel von Coffein und coffeinfreiem Kaffee. Int. Z. Klin. Pharmacol. Ther. Toxicol. *3*, 167–173 (1970)

Ando, K.: Profile of drug effects on temporally spaced responding rats. Pharmacol. Biochem. Behav. *3*, 833–841 (1973)

Bachrach, H.: Note on the psychological effects of caffeine. Psychol. Rep. *18*, 86 (1966)

Baker, W.J., Theologus, G.C.: Effects of caffeine on visual monitoring. J. Appl. Psychol. *56*, 422–427 (1972)

Barmack, J.E.: The time of administration and some effects of 2 grs. of alkaloid caffeine. J. Exp. Psychol. *27*, 690–698 (1940)

Barry, H., Miller, N.E.: Comparison of drug effects on approach, avoidance, and escape motivation. J. Comp. Physiol. Psychol. *59*, 18–24 (1965)

Bättig, K., Grandjean, E.: Die Wirkung von Barbitalum solubile und von Coffeinum Na-benz. auf einen bedingten Reflex bei der Ratte. Helv. Physiol. Pharmacol. Acta *13*, C 54-C 55 (1955)

Blough, D.S.: Some effects of drugs on visual discrimination in the pigeon. Ann. NY Acad. Sci. *66*, 733–739 (1957)

Boissier, J.R., Simon, P.: Influence de la caféine sur le comportement en situation libre de la souris. Arch. Int. Pharmacodyn. Ther. *166*, 362–369 (1967)

Bovet-Nitti, F., Messeri, P.: Central stimulating agents and population growth in mice. Life Sci. *16*, 1393–1402 (1975)

Boyd, E.M., Dolman, M., Knight, L.M., Sheppard, E.P.: The chronic oral toxicity of caffeine. Can. J. Physiol. Pharmacol. *43*, 995–1007 (1965)

Březinová, V.: Effect of caffeine on sleep: EEG study in late middle age people. Br. J. Clin. Pharmacol. *1*, 203–208 (1974)

Calhoun, W.H.: Central nervous system stimulants. In: Pharmacological and biophysical agents and behaviour. Furchtgott, E. (ed.), pp. 181–268. New York, London: Academic Press 1971

Cappell, H., Latané, B.: Effects of alcohol and caffeine on the social and emotional behavior of the rat. Q. J. Stud. Alcohol *30*, 345–356 (1969)

Carpenter, J.A.: The effect of caffeine and alcohol on simple visual reaction time. J. Comp. Physiol. Psychol. *52*, 491–496 (1959)

Carpi, C., Banfi, S., Cornelli, U.: A proposal of a screening method for substances active on learning and memory. J. Pharmacol. [Suppl. 2] *5*, 16 (1974)

Castellano, C.: Effects of caffeine on discrimination learning, consolidation, and learned behaviour in mice. Psychopharmacology *48*, 255–260 (1976)

Castellano, C.: Effects of pre- and post-trial caffeine administrations on simultaneous visual discrimination in three inbred strains of mice. Psychopharmacology *51*, 255–258 (1977)

Castellano, C., Sansone, M., Renzi, P., Annecker, L.: Central stimulant drugs on avoidance behaviour in hamsters. Pharmacol. Res. Commun. *5*, 287–293 (1973)

Cattell, R.B.: The effects of alcohol and caffeine on intelligent and associative performance. Br. J. Med. Psychol. *10*, 20–33 (1930)
Cheney, R.H.: Comparative effect of caffeine per se and a caffeine beverage (coffee) upon the reaction time in normal young adults. J. Pharmacol. Exp. Ther. *53*, 304–313 (1935)
Cheney, R.H.: Reaction time behavior after caffeine and coffee consumption. J. Pharmacol. Exp. Ther. *19*, 357–369 (1936)
Clubley, M., Henson, T., Peck, A.W., Riddington, C.: Effects of caffeine and cyclizine alone and in combination on human performance and subjective ratings. Br. J. Clin. Pharmacol. *4*, 652 (1977)
Colton, T., Gosselin, R.E., Smith, R.P.: The tolerance of coffee drinkers to caffeine. Clin. Pharmacol. Ther. *9*, 31–39 (1968)
Cooper, B.R., Potts, W.J., Morse, D.L., Black, W.C.: The effects of magnesium pemoline, caffeine and picrotoxin on a food reinforced discrimination task. Psychon. Sci. *14*, 225–226 (1969)
Costill, D.L., Dalsky, G.P., Fink, W.J.: Effects of caffeine ingestion on metabolism and exercise performance. Med. Sci. Sports *10*, 155–158 (1978)
Cox, T.: The effects of caffeine, alcohol, and previous exposure to the test situation on spontaneous alternation. Psychopharmacologia *17*, 83–88 (1970)
Crabbe, J.C., Alpern, H.P.: Facilitation and disruption of the long-term store of memory with neural excitants. Pharmacol. Biochem. Behav. *1*, 197–202 (1973)
Czok, G.: Untersuchungen über die Wirkung von Kaffee. Darmstadt: Steinkopff 1966
Dahme, G., Lienert, G., Malorny, G.: Einflüsse von Alkohol und Kaffee auf die Psychomotorik sowie auf die subjektive Einschätzung des eigenen Befindens. Z. Ernährungswiss. [Suppl.] *14*, 36–46 (1972)
Davis, T.R.A., Kensler, C.J.: Comparison of behavioral effects of nicotine, d-amphetamine, caffeine and dimethylheptyl-tetra-hydrocannabinol in squirrel monkeys. Psychopharmacology *32*, 51–65 (1973)
Dews, P.B.: The measurement of the influence of drugs on voluntary activity in mice. Br. J. Pharmacol. *8*, 46–48 (1953)
Dreisbach, R.H., Pfeiffer, C.: Caffeine-withdrawal headache. J. Lab. Clin. Med. *28*, 1212–1219 (1943)
Dureman, E.I.: Differential patterning of behavioral effects from three types of stimulant drugs. Clin. Phrmacol. Ther. *3*, 29–33 (1962)
Eddy, N.B., Downs, A.W.: Tolerance and cross-tolerance in the human subject to the diuretic effect of caffeine, theobromine and theophylline. J. Pharmacol. Exp. Ther. *33*, 167–174 (1928)
Eichler, O.: Kaffee und Coffein, 1st ed. Berlin: Springer 1938
Eichler, O.: Kaffee und Coffein, 2nd ed. Berlin, Heidelberg, New York: Springer 1976
Essmann, W.B.: Drug effects and learning and memory processes. Adv. Pharmacol. Chemother. *9*, 241–330 (1971)
Estler, C.-J.: Effect of α- and β-adrenergic blocking agents and parachlorophenylalanine on morphine- and caffeine-stimulated locomotor activity of mice. Psychopharmacology *28*, 261–268 (1973)
Estler, C.-J.: Stoffwechsel einzelner Organe. In: Kaffee und Coffein. Eichler, O. (ed.), 2nd Ed., pp. 183–214. Berlin, Heidelberg, New York: Springer 1976
Estler, C.-J.: Influence of pimozide on the locomotor hyperactivity produced by caffeine. J. Pharm. Pharmacol. *31*, 126–127 (1979)
Estler, C.-J., Ammon, H.P.T., Herzog, C.: Swimming capacity of mice after prolonged treatment with psychostimulants. I. Effect of caffeine on swimming performance and cold stress. Psychopharmacology *58*, 161–166 (1978)
Flexner, J.B., Flexner, L.B.: Puromycin's suppression of memory in mice as affected by caffeine. Pharmacol. Biochem. Behav. *3*, 13–17 (1975)
Flood, J.F., Rosenzweig, M.R., Jarvik, M.E.: Memory: Modification of anisomycin-induced amnesia by stimulants and depressants. Science *199*, 324–326 (1978)
Flory, C.D., Gilbert, J.: The effects of benzedrine sulphate and caffeine citrate on the efficiency of college students. J. Appl. Psychol. *27*, 121–134 (1943)
Foltz, E., Ivy, A.C., Barborka, C.J.: The use of double work periods in the study of fatigue and the influence of caffeine on recovery. Am. J. Physiol. *136*, 79–87 (1942)

Franks, H.M., Hagedorn, H., Hensley, V.R., Hensley, W.J., Starmer, G.A.: The effect of caffeine on human performance, alone and in combination with ethanol. Psychopharmacology *45*, 177–181 (1975)

Fröberg, J., Karlsson, C.-G., Levi, L., Linde, L., Seeman, K.: Test performance and subjective feelings as modified by caffeine-containing and caffeine-free coffee. In: Coffein und andere Methylxanthine. Heim, F., Ammon, H.P.T. (eds.), pp. 15–20. Stuttgart, New York: Schattauer 1969

Furlong, cit. accord. Gilbert

Geller, I., Hartmann, R., Blum, K.: Effects of nicotine, nicotine monomethiodide, lobeline, chlordiazepoxide, meprobamate and caffeine on a discrimination task in laboratory rats. Psychopharmacology *20*, 355–365 (1971)

Gilbert, R.M.: Caffeine as a drug of abuse. In: Research advances in alcohol and drug problems. Gibbins, R.J., Israel, Y., Kalant, H., Popham, R.E., Schmidt, W., Smart, R.G. (eds.), Vol. 3, pp. 49–176. New York: Wiley & Sons 1976

Gilliland, A.R., Nelson, D.: The effects of coffee on certain mental and physiological functions. J. Gen. Psychol. *21*, 339–348 (1939)

Giurgea, M., van Kemeulen, R.: Social behavior and central nervous system stimulants. Proc. Eur. Soc. Stud. Drug Toxicol. *15*, 25–32 (1974)

Goldstein, A.: Wakefulness caused by caffeine. Arch. Exp. Pathol. Pharmacol. *248*, 269–278 (1964)

Goldstein, A., Warren, R., Kaizer, S.: Psychotropic effects of caffeine in man. I. Individual differences in sensitivity to caffeine-induced wakefulness. J. Pharmacol. Exp. Ther. *140*, 156–159 (1965a)

Goldstein, A., Kaizer, S., Warren, R.: Psychotropic effects of caffeine in man. II. Alertness, psychomotor coordination, and mood. J. Pharmacol. Exp. Ther. *150*, 146–151 (1965b)

Goldstein, A., Kaizer, S.: Psychotropic effects of caffeine in man. III. A questionnaire survey of coffee drinking and its effects in a group of housewives. Clin. Pharmacol. Ther. *10*, 477–488 (1969a)

Goldstein, A., Kaizer, S., Whitby, O.: Psychotropic effects of caffeine in man. IV. Quantitative and qualitative differences associated with habituation to coffee. Clin. Pharmacol. Ther. *10*, 489–497 (1969b)

Goodman, L.S., Gilman, A.: The pharmacological basis of therapeutics, 5th ed. New York: MacMillan 1975

Graf, O.: Genußmittel, Genußgifte und Leistungsfähigkeit. Sportmedizin *8*, 17–22 (1957)

Graf, O.: Arbeit und Pharmaka. Handb. Gesamt. Arbeitsmed., vol. 1, pp. 512–553. Berlin, München, Wien: Urban & Schwarzenberg 1961

Greden, J.F.: Anxiety or caffeinism: A diagnostic dilemma. Am. J. Psychiatry *131*, 1089–1092 (1974)

Greenblatt, E.N., Osterberg, A.C.: Effect of drugs on maintenance of exploratory behavior in mice. Fed. Proc. *20*, 397 (1961)

Greenblatt, E.N., Osterberg, A.C.: Correlations of activating and lethal effects of excitatory drugs in grouped and isolated mice. J. Pharmacol. Exp. Ther. *131*, 115–119 (1961)

Hauty, G.T., Payne, R.B.: Mitigation of work decrement. J. Exp. Psychol. *49*, 60–67 (1955)

Hawk, Ph.B.: A study of the physiological and psychological reactions of the human organism to coffee drinking. Am. J. Physiol. *90*, 380–381 (1929)

Hearst, E.: Drug effects on stimulus generalization gradients in the monkey. Psychopharmacology *6*, 57–70 (1964)

Heim, F., Haas, B.: Der Einfluß von Megaphen auf Motilität und Sauerstoffverbrauch weißer Mäuse in Ruhe und Erregung. Arch. Exp. Pathol. Pharmakol. *226*, 395–402 (1955)

Heim, F., Hach, B., Mitznegg, P., Ammon, H.P.T., Estler, C.-J.: Coffein-antagonistische Wirkungen des Theobromins und coffeinartige Eigenschaften von Theobromin-Metaboliten. Arzneim. Forsch. *21*, 1039–1043 (1971)

Holck, H.G.O.: Effect of caffeine upon chess problem solving. J. Comp. Physiol. Psychol. *15*, 301–311 (1933)

Hollingworth, H.L.: The influence of caffeine on the speed and quality of performance on typewriting. Psychol. Rev. *19*, 66–73 (1912)

Horovitz, Z.P., Beer, B., Clody, E., Vogel, J.R., Chasin, M.: Cyclic AMP and anxiety. Psychosomatics *13*, 85–92 (1972)

Horst, K., Buxton, R.E., Robinson, W.D.: The effect of the habitual use of coffee or decaffeinated coffee upon blood pressure and certain motor reactions of normal young men. J. Pharmacol. Exp. Ther. *52*, 322–337 (1934a)

Horst, K., Robinson, W.D., Jenkins, W.L., Bao, D.L.: The effect of caffeine, coffee and decaffeinated coffee upon blood pressure, pulse rate and certain motor reactions of normal young men. J. Pharmacol. Exp. Ther. *52*, 307–321 (1934b)

Hrbek, J., Komenda, S., Mačáková, J., Široká, A.: Acute effect of chlorprothixen (5 mg), caffeine (200 mg), and the combination of both drugs on verbal associations. Act. Nerv. Super. *13*, 207–208 (1971)

Hughes, R.N., Greig, A.M.: Effects of caffeine, methamphetamine and methylphenidate on reactions to novelty and activity in rats. Neuropharmacology *15*, 673–676 (1976)

Hughes, F.W., Forney, R.B.: Alcohol and caffeine in choice-discrimination tests in rats. Proc. Soc. Exp. Biol. Med. *108*, 157–159 (1961)

Hull, C.L.: The influence of caffeine and other factors on certain phenomena of rote learning. J. Gen. Psychol. *13*, 249–274 (1935)

Izquierdo, I.: Effect on pseudoconditioning of drugs with known central nervous activity. Psychopharmacology *38*, 259–266 (1974)

Karacan, I., Thornby, J.I., Anch, A.M., Booth, G.H., Williams, R.L., Salis, P.J.: Dose-related sleep disturbances induced by coffee and caffeine. Clin. Pharmacol. Ther. *20*, 682–689 (1976)

Kehrhahn, O.H.: Das Verhalten männlicher Albinomäuse im Laufrad-Versuch. Arzneim. Forsch. *23*, 981–991 (1973)

Keister, M.E., McLaughlin, R.J.: Vigilance performance related to extroversion-introversion and caffeine. J. Exp. Res. Pers. *6*, 5–11 (1972)

Klebelsberg, D. v., Mostbeck, A.: Wirken sich mittlere Dosen von Kaffee und Koffein auf psychische Funktionen der Fahrtüchtigkeit aus? Psychol. Prax. *7*, 23–35 (1963)

Knoll, J.: Motimeter, a new sensitive apparatus for the quantitative measurement of hypermotility caused by psychostimulants. Arch. Int. Pharmacodyn. Ther. *130*, 141–154 (1961)

Knowles, J.B.: Conditioning and the placebo effect: The effects of decaffeinated coffee on simple reaction time in habitual coffee drinkers. Behav. Res. Ther. *1*, 151–157 (1963)

Koley, J., Koley, B.N., Maitra, S.R.: Effect of drinking tea, coffee and caffeine on work performance. Indian J. Physiol. Allied Sci. *27*, 96–106 (1973)

Kraepelin, E.: Über die Beeinflussung einfacher psychischer Vorgänge durch einige Arzneimittel. Jena: Fischer 1892

Kulkarni, A.S.: Avoidance acquisition and CNS stimulants. Arch. Pharmacol. *273*, 394–400 (1972)

Lader, M.: Comparison of amphetamine sulphate and caffeine citrate in man. Psychopharmacology *14*, 83–94 (1969)

Landgrebe, B.: Vergleichende Untersuchungen mit dem Flimmertest nach coffeinhaltigem und coffeinfreiem Kaffee. Med. Welt *2*, 1486–1490 (1960)

Landis, C.: Physiological and psychological effects of the use of coffee. In: Problems of addiction and habituation. Hoch, P., Zubin, H. (eds.), pp. 37–48. New York: Grune & Stratton 1958

Lashley, K.S.: The effects of strychnine and caffeine upon the rate of learning. Psychobiol. *1*, 141–169 (1917)

Lehmann, H.E., Csank, J.: Differential screening of phrenotropic agents in man: Psychophysiologic test data. J. Clin. Psychopathol. *18*, 222–235 (1957)

Levenson, H.S., Bick, E.C.: Psychopharmacology of caffeine. In: Psychopharmacology in the practice of medicine. Jarvik, M.E. (ed.), pp. 451–463. New York: Appleton-Century-Croft 1977

Lienert, G.A., Huber, H.P.: Differential effects of coffee on speed and power tests. J. Psychol. *63*, 269–274 (1966)

Luff, K.: Die Kaffeewirkung auf das zentrale Nervensystem. Ärztl. Praxis *17*, 5–7 (1965)

Luff, K., Vogler, Th., Bardong, H.: Uber den Einfluß des Coffeins auf das Leistungsverhalten am Kugeltestgerät. Zentralbl. Verkehrsmed. Verkehrspsychol. Luft-Raumfahrtmed. *10*, 74–83 (1964)

Macht, D.I.: Effect of adenine and caffeine injections on behavior of rats in a circular maze. Proc. Soc. Exp. Med. *29*, 953–954 (1932)

Maier, H.W.: Untersuchungen über die Wirkungen des Koffeins und des Kaffees auf den Menschen. An Hand von Experimenten mit gewöhnlichem Kaffee und Kaffee „HAG“. II. Teil. Untersuchungen über die Beeinflussung der geistigen Leistungsfähigkeit. Schweiz. Arch. Neurol. Neurochir. Psychiatr. *10. 11.*, 80–99 (1922)
Malis, J.L., Brodie, D.A., Moreno, O.M.: Drug effects on the behavior of self-stimulation monkeys. Fed. Proc. *19*, 23 (1960)
Marino, A., Cuomo, V.: Fattori psicologici e azioni farmacologiche della caffeina. Arch. Sci. Med. (Torino) *131*, 29–37 (1974)
Marriott, A.S.: The effects of amphetamine, caffeine and methylphenidate on the locomotor activity of rats in an unfamiliar environment. Int. J. Neuropharmacol. *7*, 487–491 (1968)
Matthies, H., Erdmann, D.: Die Wirkung von Coffein auf bedingtreflektorische Reaktionen der Ratte und auf eine experimentelle Zerrüttung des Nervensystem. Pharmazie *12*, 561–567 (1957)
Mechner, F., Latranyi, M.: Behavioral effects of caffeine, methamphetamine, and methylphenidate in the rat. J. Exp. Anal. Behav. *6*, 331–342 (1963)
Medek, A., Hrbek, J., Navratil, J., Komenda, S.: The effect of chlorprothixene and caffeine on the conditioned alimentary motor reflexes in cats. Act. Nerv. Super. *13*, 210–211 (1971)
Menge, G.: Tierexperimentelle Untersuchungen zur zentral stimulierenden Wirkung eines neuen Theophyllin-Derivates. Arzneim. Forsch. *11*, 271–273 (1961)
Miller, N.E., Miles, W.R.: Effect of caffeine on the running speed of hungry, satiated, and frustrated rats. J. Comp. Physiol. Psychol. *20*, 397–412 (1935)
Mitchell, V.E., Ross, S., Hurst, P.M.: Drugs and placebos: Effects of caffeine on cognitive performance. Psychol. Rev. *35*, 875–883 (1974)
Morpurgo, C.: Drug-induced modifications of discriminated avoidance behavior in rats. Psychopharmacology *8*, 91–99 (1965)
Mücher, H., Wendt, H.-W.: Gruppenversuch zur Bestimmung der kritischen Verschmelzungsfrequenz beim binokularen Sehen: Änderungen unter Koffein und nach normaler Tagesarbeit. Arch. Exp. Pathol. Pharmakol. *214*, 29–37 (1951)
Müller-Limmroth, W.: Der Einfluß von coffeinhaltigem und coffeinfreiem Kaffee auf den Schlaf des Menschen. Z. Ernährungswiss. [Suppl.] *14*, 46–53 (1972)
Mullin, cit. accord. Landis
Nash, H.: Alcohol and caffeine: A study of their psychological effects. Springfield: Thomas 1962a
Nash,H.: The double-blind procedure: rational and empirical evaluation. J. Nerv. Ment. Dis. *134*, 34–47 (1962b)
Neumann, K.-H.: Tierversuche zur Frage körperlichen Leistungsvermögens nach Aufnahme von Koffein. Med. Klin. *60*, 1354–1356 (1965)
Nicholson, A.N., Stone, B.M.: Studies on the sleep of the young adult after caffeine. Br. J. Clin. Pharmacol. *4*, 717P (1977)
Nieschulz, O.: Über Aussagemöglichkeiten psychopharmakologischer Tierversuche. Med. Monatsschr. *17*, 566–571 (1963)
Nieschulz, O.: Über Nachweismöglichkeiten zentraler Wirkungen des Coffeins in Tierversuchen. 3me Colloqu. Int. sur le Chimie des Cafés, pp. 277–285. Paris: ASIC 1967
Nieschulz, O.: Lernverhalten von Mäusen nach experimentellen Hirnschäden. Arzneim. Forsch. *19*, 357–360 (1969)
Oliverio, A.: Effetto antifatica dell'amfetamina e di farmaci stimolanti centrali sulle prestazioni di topi durante sedute di condizionamento prolungate. Il Farmaco *22*, 159–171 (1967)
Paré, W.: The effect of caffeine and seconal on a visual discrimination task. J. Comp. Physiol. Psychol. *54*, 506–509 (1961)
Pauli, R.: Der Einfluß von Tee auf geistige Arbeit. Arch. Ges. Psychol. *59*, 391–416 (1927)
Peters, M.: Caffeine-induced hemorrhagic automutilation. Arch. Int. Pharmacodyn. Ther. *169*, 139–145 (1967)
Peters, J.M., Boyd, E.M.: The influence of sex and age in albino rats given a daily oral dose of caffeine at a high dose level. Can. J. Physiol. Pharmacol. *45*, 305–311 (1967)
Plotnikoff, N.: Bioassay of psychoactive agents on escape from auditory stress. Fed. Proc. *21*, 420 (1962)
Plotnikoff, N., Fitzloff, J.: Effects of stimulants on isolated rats. Arch. Int. Pharmacodyn. Ther. *145*, 421–429 (1963)

Plotnikoff, N., Reinke, D., Fitzloff, J.: Effects of stimulants on rotarod performance. J. Pharm. Sci. *51*, 1007–1008 (1962)
Primavera, L.H., Simon, W.E., Camisa, J.M.: An investigation of personality and caffeine use. Br. J. Addict. *70*, 213–215 (1975)
Prüll, G.: Über die Wirkung von Weckmitteln (Coffein und Pervitin) auf die psychophysische Leistungsfähigkeit nach Alkoholgenuß. Med. Dissertation, Frankfurt/Main 1965
Rahmann, H.: Einfluß von Coffein auf das Gedächtnis und das Verhalten von Goldhamstern. Pflügers Arch. *276*, 384–397 (1963)
Regina, E.G., Smith, G.M.: Effects of caffeine on alertness in simulated automobile driving. J. Appl. Psychol. *59*, 483–489 (1974)
Reichard, C.C., Elder, Th.: The effects of caffeine on reaction time in hyperkinetic and normal children. Am. J. Psychiatry *134*, 144–148 (1977)
Reiman, G.: The influence of coffee on the association constant. J. Exp. Psychol. *17*, 93–104 (1934)
Reimann, H.A.: Caffeinism: A cause of long-continued, low-grade fever. J. Am. Med. Wom. Assoc. *202*, 131–132 (1967)
Revelle, W., Amaral, Ph., Turriff, S.: Introversion/extroversion, time stress, and caffeine: effect on verbal performance. Science *192*, 149–150 (1976)
Roussinov, K.S., Yonkov, D.I.: Comparative study of the influence of caffeine and theophylline on the learning and memory of albino rats. Dokl. Bolgarsk. Acad. Nauk. *27*, 1605–1608 (1974)
Roussinov, K., Yonkov, D.: Comparative study of the effect of caffeine, strychnine and echinopsin on learning and memory in albino rats. Acta Physiol. Pharmacol. Bulg. *2*, 66–71 (1976)
Rutenfranz, J., Jansen, G.: Über die Kompensation von Alkoholwirkungen durch Coffein und Pervitin bei einer psychomotorischen Leistung. Z. Physiol. Arbeitsphysiol. *18*, 62–81 (1959)
Sansone, M.: Effects of chlordiazepoxide, CNS-stimulants and their combinations on avoidance behaviour in mice. Arch. Int. Pharmacodyn. Ther. *215*, 190–196 (1975)
Satinder, K.P.: Genotype-dependent effects of D-amphetamine sulphate and caffeine on escape-avoidance behavior of rats. J. Comp. Physiol. Psychol. *76*, 359–364 (1971)
Schilling, W.: The effect of caffeine and acetanilid on simple reaction time. Psychol. Rev. *28*, 72–79 (1921)
Schirlitz, K.: Über Coffein bei ermüdender Muskelarbeit. Arbeitsphysiol. *2*, 273–297 (1930)
Schwertz, M.-Th., Marbach, G.: Effects physiologiques de la caféine et du meprobamate au cours du somneil chez l'homme. Arch. Sci. Physiol. *19*, 425–479 (1965)
Seashore, R.H., Ivy, A.C.: The effects of analeptic drugs in relieving fatigue. Psychol. Monographs *67*, 1–13 (1953)
Selbach, H.: Coffein, vegetative Regulationen und Zentralnervensystem. In: Coffein und andere Methylxanthine. Heim, F., Ammon, H.P.T. (eds.), pp. 21–43. Stuttgart, New York: Schattauer 1969
Seyffert, H.-M.: Physiologische und psychologische Wirkungen von Kaffee und Coffein. Arzneim. Forsch. *4*, 207–209 (1954)
Silver, W.: Insomia, tachycardia, and cola drinks. Pediatrics *47*, 635 (1971)
Skinner, B.F., Heron, W.T.: Effects of caffeine and benzedrine upon conditioning and extinction. Psychol. Record *1*, 340–346 (1937)
Solyom, L., Enesco, H.E., Beaulieu, C.: The effect of RNA, uric acid and caffeine on conditioning and activity in rats. J. Psychiatr. Res. *6*, 175–183 (1968)
Stanley, W.C., Schlossberg, H.: The psychophysiological effects of tea. J. Psychol. *36*, 435–448 (1953)
Stinnette, M.J., Isaac, W.: Behavioral effects of d-amphetamine and caffeine in the squirrel monkey. Eur. J. Pharmacol. *30*, 268–271 (1975)
Strasser, H., Müller-Limmroth, W.: Vergleichende Untersuchungen über die Wirkung von Koffein und Chlorogensäure auf die Psychomotorik des Menschen. Ärztl. Forsch. *25*, 209–217 (1971)
Stripling, J.S., Alpern, H.P.: Nicotine and caffeine: disruption of the long-term store of memory and proactive facilitation of learning in mice. Psychopharmacology *38*, 187–200 (1974)

Strubelt, O., Siegers, C.-P., Breining, H., Steffen, J.: Tierexperimentelle Untersuchungen zur chronischen Toxizität von Kaffee und Coffein. Z. Ernährungswiss. [Suppl.] *12*, 252–260 (1973)
Sulc, J., Poradkova, M.: The effect of low doses of analgesics and caffeine on psychomotor function. Act. Nerv. Super. *17*, 285–286 (1975)
Switzer, St.C.A.: The effect of caffeine on experimental extinction of conditioned reactions. J. Gen. Psychol. *12*, 78–94 (1935a)
Switzer, St.C.A.: The influence of caffeine upon "inhibition of delay". J. Comp. Physiol. Psychol. *19*, 155–175 (1935b)
Tainter, M.L.: Effects of certain analeptic drugs on spontaneous running activity of the white rat. J. Comp. Physiol. Psychol. *36*, 143–155 (1943)
Thornton, G.R., Holck, H.G.O., Smith, E.L.: The effect of benzedrine and caffeine upon performance in certain psychomotor tasks. J. Abnorm. Soc. Psychol. *34*, 96–113 (1939)
Tonini, G., Babbini, M.: Individual variations of pharmacological central reactions. Biochem. Pharmacol. *8*, 59 (1961)
Valzelli, L., Bernasconi, S.: Behavioral and neurochemical effects of caffeine in normal and aggressive mice. Pharmacol. Biochem. Behav. *1*, 251–254 (1973)
Vitzthum, O.G.: Chemie und Bearbeitung des Kaffees. In: Kaffee und Coffein. Eichler, O. (ed.), 2nd. ed. pp. 3–64. Berlin, Heidelberg, New York: Springer 1976
Waldeck, B.: Effect of caffeine on locomotor activity and central catecholamine mechanisms: a study with special reference to drug interaction. Acta Pharmacol. Toxicol. [Suppl. 4] *36*, 1–23 (1975)
Wanner, H.U., Bättig, K.: Pharmakologische Wirkungen auf die Laufleistung der Ratte bei verschiedener Leistungsbelohnung und verschiedener Leistungsanforderung. Psychopharmacology *7*, 182–202 (1965)
Wayner, M.J., Jolicoeur, F.B., Rondeau, D.B., Barone, F.C.: Effects of actue and chronic administration of caffeine on schedule dependent and schedule induced behavior. Pharmacol. Biochem. Behav. *5*, 343–348 (1976)
Webb, D., Levine, T.E.: Effects of caffeine on DRL performance in the mouse. Pharmacol. Biochem. Behav. *9*, 7–10 (1978)
Wedemeyer, Th.: Über die Gewöhnung psychischer Funktionen an das Coffein. Arch. Exp. Pathol. Pharmakol. *85*, 339–358 (1919)
Weiss, B., Laties, V.G.: Enhancement of human performance by caffeine and the amphetamines. Pharmacol. Rev. *14*, 1–36 (1962)
Wenzel, D.G., Rutledge, Ch.O.: Effects of centrally-acting drugs on human motor and psychomotor performance. J. Pharm. Sci. *51*, 631–644 (1962)
Zimbardo, Ph.G., Barry, H.: Effects of caffeine and chlorpromazine on the sexual behavior of male rats. Science *127*, 84–85 (1958)

CHAPTER 18

Research Methodology in Clinical Trials of Psychotropic Drugs

H. HEIMANN and H. J. GAERTNER

A. General Principles for the Clinical Investigation of Psychotropic Drugs

I. Introduction

Compared to the assessment of pharmacological effects on body functions, clinical testing of psychotropic drugs presents us with particular problems. The *treatment objective*, namely to influence psychiatric syndromes, is on a higher level of complexity than the goals of other pharmacotherapy, e.g., reduction of blood pressure or regulation of blood sugar level. Psychiatric syndromes can only be defined descriptively and can be distinguished from the personality of the patient, who must be treated as a whole, only by means of rough schematization. Therefore, the first step in the clinical investigation of psychotropic drugs is to bring to mind the different levels on which psychiatric syndromes can be quantified and the corresponding methods which can be used for this purpose.

The *treatment targets*, namely structures of the central nervous system and their conditions of functioning, are highly complex. Functional drug effects which have been experimentally demonstrated on certain animal brain structures cannot simply be transposed to human circumstances when the effect of the preparations is to be judged *on the level of behavior and experience*, i.e., the desired effects on man. Recent studies of the direct behavioral and experiential effects of psychotropic drugs on healthy volunteers using precise psychological methods show that these effects depend not only on the substance administered and on its dosage, but also on other factors which must be considered in the evaluation of a preparation. It is in this connection that the differences between the initial psychophysiological condition of healthy subjects and that of psychiatric patients must receive special consideration. Only under this aspect can the problem of the *specificity of a psychotropic effect* and its *generalizability* be discussed. For example, can psychiatric syndromes be reliably distinguished at the symptom level? Does a certain psychotropic substance affect a particular symptom or a certain group of symptoms, so that we can precisely delineate the specificity of this psychotropic effect? Or can the psychotropic effect of a drug only be vaguely differentiated from a nonspecific placebo effect? In contrast to other fields of pharmacology, the main and side effects of psychotropic agents cannot always be clearly discriminated.

After a thorough consideration of the special problems posed by the testing of psychiatric drugs on patients, we discuss the currently accepted *strategy of clinical testing*.

In a third section, we give critical attention to a number of factors responsible for the fact that precise differences in effect between various psychotropic drugs can only be reliably proven on a very gross level. Certain factors, whose investigation must remain the subject of further research, prevent the precise determination and reliable, differentiated proof of these differences.

II. Methods for the Assessment of Psychiatric Disorders

At present, psychiatric syndromes can in principle be measured at five different levels.
1. Level of diagnosis (diagnostic entities)
2. Syndrome level (nosological nonspecificity)
3. Level of single symptoms or characteristics (nosological and syndrome nonspecificity)
4. Level of psychophysiological reactivity
5. Level of clinical-biochemical methods of investigation.

These different levels of measurement must be considered in clinical trials, although their specific meaning for the effects of psychotropic substances is presently unclear. They play a particular role in the discussion of *homogeneity of sample populations*. For example, it is not sufficient to characterize the subjects of a test on the diagnostic level alone. It has been shown that the effects of psychotropic medication do not restrict themselves to nosological categories. Nevertheless, it is necessary to specify the patients in a testing sample diagnostically. For this purpose, it has become customary to use the WHO classification (ICD) (DEGKWITZ et al., 1980). For particular research purposes, the diagnostic criteria of FEIGHNER et al. (1972) have proved useful.

Of particular importance for the characterization of a test sample is the *syndrome level*. Psychiatric syndromes can be defined in various ways. One can employ the classical clinical-descriptive method and specify a syndrome diagnosis in addition to the nosological diagnosis. For example: endogenous depression, agitated or inhibited syndrome. More often, syndromes are determined by *factor analysis* as a means of secondary quantification of behavior characteristics. Pathological behavior is described and quantified for single characteristics using rating scales. Syndromes are then validated on large samples of psychiatric patients by means of factor analysis. Examples of such rating scales are those of LORR (1963), OVERALL and GORHAM (1962), or WITTENBORN (1955). For the description of depressive syndromes, HAMILTON's (1960) scale is most often used. A summary of the most frequently used scales for the description of samples on the syndrome or symptom level can be found in CIPS (1977).

Symptom measurement in the classical clinical sense is the basis of the AMP system (ANGST et al., 1969). In contrast to the rating scales already mentioned, this system is based on the precise definition of traditional psychiatric symptoms and arranges them according to clinical aspects. Factor analysis has also been used to define syndromes in the AMP system. These essentially correspond to the well-known psychiatric-clinical syndromes (compare BAUMANN, 1974; PIETZCKER et al., 1977; SULZ-BLUME et al., 1979).

These first three levels in the clinical assessment of psychiatric syndromes make it clear that any quantification necessary for the analysis of a therapeutic effect is *based on an abstraction*. At the root of the measurement lies the relationship of the observer to the patient and the description of the patient's observed behavior or mood within this context. Only secondarily, by means of consensual definition, can units of description, characteristics, or symptoms be delineated and tabulated as items on predetermined scales. The numerical values in these scales, which are essentially quantitative statements about psychiatric phenomena, have at most a nominal or ordinal scale niveau. However, a particular position on such a scale always signifies a complex measure and can refer to very different things. For instance, the same score on the Hamilton scale can represent predominantly somatic complaints in one depressive patient, while for another patient it can signify more psychic symptoms of depression. For this reason, quantitative values on these three clinical-descriptive levels of assessment are complex entities based on a myriad of interdependent circumstances.

The fourth level of measurement for psychiatric syndromes, *psychophysiological reactivity*, has gained importance in recent years. Technical developments have made it possible to monitor physiological parameters in psychiatric patients as a matter of routine. In particular, the quantification of the electorencephalogramm has led to progress in discriminating between the effects of psychotropic medication on patients and on healthy volunteers (see BENTE, et al. 1976, BENTE, 1977; ITIL, 1974; SALETU, 1976). Not only the electroencephalogram at rest, but especially the investigation of electric brain potentials produced in response to certain sensory events make the psychophysiological differentiation between psychiatric syndromes possible today. Measures of psychophysiological reactivity include evoked potentials, in particular their latter segments (see SUTTON and TUETING, 1978), the expectancy wave or CNV (see TIMSIT-BERTHIER, 1973; HEIMAN, 1979; GIEDKE et al., 1980), and numerous aspects of peripheral autonomic variables (heart rate, blood pressure, pulse amplitude, etc.) under certain conditions of stimulation (see review by LADER, 1975). On this psychophysiological level, the results of very complex processes are measured. However, the measurements yield clear quantitative values with interval scale niveau. For certain psychiatric syndromes, e.g., depression, schizophrenia, or neurosis, differences in psychophysiological reactivity can be specified.

These same characteristics apply to the *level of clinical-biochemical assessment*, which has attained particular importance in recent decades. Of primary significance is the exact determination of monoamine metabolites in liquor, plasma and urine. This allows identification of subgroups of psychiatric syndromes, for instance in depressive patients. An example of this methodology can be found in the studies by VAN PRAAG (1974, 1977) on serotonin metabolism in the brain. He assayed 5-HIAA (5-Hydroxyindolacetic acid) in the liquor of depressive patients before and after probenizid administration. Other examples are studies by SCHILDKRAUT et al. (1978), MAAS (1975), and GOODWIN and POTTER (1979) on the noradrenaline metabolite MHPG (3-Methoxy-4-hydroxyphenylglycol) in urine and cerebrospinal fluid. Recently, studies on the stimulation of hypothalamic system using neurohormones have allowed analysis of the reactivity of such structures (MATUSSEK, 1978; SACHAR et al., 1971; LANGER et al., 1976; LAAKMANN, 1979).

Studies on the metabolism of the neurotransmitters noradrenaline and serotonin have yielded some clues to the classification of depressive disorders and the prediction of drug response. Concerning the clinical significance of blunted growth hormone response, blunted thyroid-stimulating hormone response, altered dexamethasone suppression test, increased cortisone exrection, etc., a lively dispute is still in progress. This is also the case for findings pertinent to those enzymes involved in neurotransmitter metabolism (monoamino oxidase, catechol-*O*-methyltransferase, dopamine-β-

hydroxylase). The diagnostic and therapeutic significance of increased endorphin concentrations in the liquor of schizophrenic patients is also currently unclarified (TERENIUS and WAHLSTRÖM, 1979). The frequently inadequate psychopathological monitoring of patients under investigation has certainly contributed to the difficulties of interpreting these biochemical findings. The best understanding of biochemical parameters has been achieved for patients with bipolar depression, a disorder which also exhibits as well-defined course.

Recent studies (COURSEY et al., 1979; KNORRING et al., 1980) indicate that the simultaneous monitoring of biochemical and psychophysiological parameters is more likely to produce clinically relevant results than are isolated measurements on either level.

Notwithstanding the importance of progress on both biological levels, the psychophysiological and the biochemical, it must not be forgotten that the *decisive criterion for the therapeutic efficacy* of a psychotropic substance is *clinical judgment*, with all its imperfections and problems of satisfactory quantification. This short review of the assessment of psychiatric syndromes using currently available scientific methods makes it clear that we cannot expect to find simple 1:1 correspondence between the different levels of measurement, particularly in the comparison of the clinical-descriptive and the biological levels.

III. Factors Influencing the Effect of Psychotropic Substances

As behavior and experience are always the results of very different factors, and as psychopathological behavior patterns as discussed in Section 2 must be regarded as the common end stretch in the course of complex conditional relationships, the psychotropic effect of a drug is not determined by *chemical structure* and *dosage* alone. Additional factors can also modify this effect. Of these, the *influence of personality structure* and of *situation*, or of certain attitudes of expectancy, have been best investigated to date. A third factor to be considered is the *general initial state of the central nervous system* in psychiatric patients, who exhibit increased or decreased levels of activation.

Questionnaires allow *personality types* to be objectified, e.g., extroverted or introverted personalities, high (unstable) or low (stable) neuroticism scores. Instruments for the diagnosis of these four personality types within the normal range are the FPI (FAHRENBERG et al., 1973), the 16 PF by CATTELL (1956), or the EPI by Eysenck (EGGERT, 1973).

Studies proving the *differential influence of personality* on the effect of psychotropic drugs deal primarily with sedatives, anxiolytics, and minor tranquilizers (see JANKE et al., 1979; HEIMANN, 1976). For example, minor tranquilizers improve performance in subjects with high neuroticism scores, whereas stable subjects exhibit a performance impairment on psychometric tests. Similarly, the condition of unstable subjects is improved by these drugs, whereas stable subjects experience the minor tranquilizers as unpleasant. Sedatives shift introverted subjects in the direction of extroversion, whereas stimulants cause extroverted subjects to move in the direction of introversion (EYSENCK, 1960). We have shown that this drug postulate cannot always be replicated (HEIMANN and STRAUBE, 1979).

Situational influences can also be demonstrated by employing suitable methods. JANKE and GLATHE (1964), for instance, have investigated the influence of *perfor-*

mance demands on the effects of minor tranquilizers and neuroleptics. They found that these preparations atypically do not produce emotionally stabilizing effects under conditions in which great demands are placed on the subjects. On the contrary, they sometimes even have an activating and mood-worsening effect. *Emotionally stressful conditions of investigation*, e.g., *noise*, influence the psychotropic effect, according to JANKE, W. and JANKE, A. (1961, unpublished work), in the following manner: under noise-free conditions, the sensibility of test subjects is shifted in the direction of anhedonia; under noise conditions, however, these negative displacements occur only infrequently and sometimes even displacements in the direction of positive mood are found.

Of particular significance are the *situational effects* of the communicative relationship, e.g., the attitude of the physician toward the medication he prescribes, as shown by SARWER-FONER and KERENYI (1961), MAY (1976), DANCKWARDT (1978), and RÜGER (1979). Minor tranquilizers had a more definite anxiolytic effect on patients with anxiety syndromes when the physician had a positive attitude toward the prescription of such medications. The effect was weaker when he held the drug to be ineffective. In the context of an experiment on sensory physiology, REED and WITT (1968) were even able to induce or suppress the effects of LSD in two subjects under placebo conditions.

It is characteristic for all of these studies that *replication* often yields contradictory results. In our opinion, this is caused by the subject's *initial state*. Most of these investigations were conducted on *healthy volunteers* who were at most on the border to pathology. The observed effects were relatively weak. For strongly effective substances such as neuroleptics in larger doses or narcotics, a differential effect could not be proved. Therefore, in a differential study both the strength of the psychotropic action and the initial condition of the subject's central nervous system must be taken into consideration (HEIMANN, 1976).

The clinical observation that healthy subjects only tolerate hallucinogens, neuroleptics, antidepressants, and tranquilizers in relatively small doses, whereas the psychiatric patient can tolerate doses many times as large, characterizes the altered initial psychophysiological reactivity of patients' central nervous systems. For example, a single dose of 75 mg imipramine leads to strong autonomic distress or even vomiting in healthy subjects , whereas depressives tolerate three times the amount without the appearance of considerable autonomic side effects. Even more marked is the difference in tolerable dosage of neuroleptics. Our healthy subjects, for instance, exhibit considerable performance decrements in all psychomotoric tests and strong dysphoric sedation effects after administration of 10 mg of clozapine. The average dose of clozapine for the treatment of schizophrenics is ca. 400 mg. Even for minor tranquilizers a similar relation can be observed. As little as 5 mg of diazepam leads to unpleasant sedative effects in healthy subjects, whereas anxious patients need many times that amount for the alleviation of distress.

We have attempted to explain the differences in initial state between healthy subjects and psychiatric patients within the framework of the *general theory of arousal* (see LEGEWIE, 1968; HEIMANN, 1975). In this connection, it must be remembered, however, that from a psychophysiological point of view psychiatric patients (schizophrenics and depressives) are not merely displaced in a certain direction, i.e., overaroused or underaroused. These patients suffer from a restriction in their adaptive ability to modulate psychophysiological systems. We were able to verify this hypothesis by showing that stronger intercorrelations exist between different psychophysiological systems in depressives than in healthy controls (HEIMANN, 1979; GIEDKE et al., 1980; GILLIN et al., 1979). This also applies to the orienting response in schizophrenics with respect to skin resistance amplitude and the pupillary light reaction (STRAUBE, 1980). Thus, it appears that the condition of psychiatric patients before treatment can be characterized not only by a shift in tonic arousal but also by a *reduction in degrees of freedom in the various psychophysiological systems* (autonomic variables on the periphery, evoked potentials, expectancy wave, etc.) under stimulation conditions. These systems exhibit greater cohesion in psychiatric patients than in healthy subjects under comparable conditions.

IV. Specificity of Psychotropic Effects

The preceding discussion makes it clear that hardly any general statements can be made about pharmacological effects on psychic disturbances. The clinical classification of psychotropic drugs is therefore merely a coarse schematization, although it has proved ot be relatively useful in practice. There is extensive overlapping between the different groups of psychotropic substances with regard to indication. Furthermore, under certain external circumstances we invariably find numerous deviations from the intended effect. The naive notion that psychic disorders can be nosologically or pathophysiologically discriminated in a manner similar to somatic diseases or that the psychophysiological basis of a syndrome with relatively constant overt appearance is always the same must be rejected. This also applies to the idea that a substance which affects a certain neurotransmitter system must produce the same effects in every case and at all times on the level of behavior and experience.

It is quite probable that a drug's *direct* effect on cerebral structures and functions merely sets certain processes in motion which in turn combine with *the reactions of the organism* to these external influences. This combination is then responsible for observed effects in the area of behavior and experience. That means that what we can observe in the patient is the *result of a directly pharmacologically induced psychic syndrome which enters into interaction with psychophysiological conditions of the psychiatric syndrome and, in the most propitious case, leads to alleviation or to disappearance of the latter*. This conveys the complexity of psychotropic action and must be considered when one regards the numerous, partially contradictory, partially very unsatisfactory results of clinical trials with psychotropic substances.

For the sake of simplicity it has become customary to neglect these complex relationships involved in the psychotropic effect. One speaks of "*antipsychotic action*" or of "*antidepressive*" and "*anxiolytic action*," although these simple terms conceal great complexity. Thus, a strategy for the clinical investigation of psychotropic drugs can only be understood *in analogy to other clinical-pharmacological investigations with patients*, and must not neglect the special conditions of psychic syndromes, their assessment and influence, as well as the complexity of the psychotropic effects of medication.

Nothing demonstrates the consequences of inadmissable simplification more clearly than *placebo research*. The idea that so-called placebo reactors, i.e., subjects with certain personality characteristics who regularly react to placebos with psychic effects, could be identified by employing psychometric methods has proved to be false. According to FISHER (1967) and SHAPIRO (1968), anyone can exhibit reactions to placebos under certain external or internal situational conditions, either with psychic symptoms or with abatement of existing disturbances. The placebo rate for depressive syndromes is ca. 30%. For anxiety neurosis it is certainly higher, whereas for acute schizophrenia, obsessive neurosis, and serious psychic disorders in connection with organic brain defects it is considerably lower. The *placebo effect* is therefore *dependent* on the *severity of the general psychic disorder*. For instance, a psychotic disintegration of personality can hardly be influenced by placebo in the way that light anxiety neurotic complaints can. On the other hand, as we have seen, the magnitude of a compound's psychic action is inversely proportional to the significance of the nonspecific factors of personality and situation. A highly effective neuroleptic at a high dosage, for instance, leads to similar effects in different personality types, whereas a minor tranquilizer with mild, sedative effect produces differing results.

For this reason, in the field of psychotropic drugs no *unambiguous* definition for the specificity of effect can be given. Only the general direction relative to other types of effects can be determined. Thus, for psychiatric syndromes of modest to intermediate severity, the placebo control is indispensable in order to objectify a psychotropic, therapeutically relevant effect. Only nonspecific, but nonetheless generalizable effects are exhibited by placebo; the effects of psychotropic substances can be more clearly speciefied, always in comparison to placebo, only when the psychic syndromes to be influenced can be reliably discriminated. The *specificity of a psychotropic effect* is therefore a *relative term* and exists as it were *in contradiction to generalizability*. Specificity can only be determined in comparison to the placebo effect and with reference to clearly defined test populations. This must be kept in mind for the strategy of clinical investigation.

B. Strategy of Clinical Investigation

I. Introduction

The problem of preclinical screening on animals as a means of arriving at hypotheses on clinical psychiatric effects or side effects cannot be treated here (see ZBINDEN, 1976). The *responsibility* for the treatment of psychiatric patients with an investigational drug resides with the physician conducting the investigation. He must be provided with the complete results of all pharmacological and toxicological studies on the drug being evaluated. In his role as partner to the clinical investigation, a competent pharmacologist must summarize the obtained results and discuss them with the investigator, who must provide reasons and assume responsibility for a therapeutic experiment with patients or a pharmacological investigation involving normal volunteers.

It has become customary that this rationale must also be presented to an ethics committee. Furthermore, there are legal provisions to be adhered to in different countries before proceeding from animal pharmacology to clinical pharmacology with humans.

Clinical investigations are executed in three phases. These are not always uniformly defined, but in principle they begin with the study of pharmacokinetics and pharmacodynamics (as a rule on healthy subjects and perhaps on patients) and proceed to the actual clinical trials on patient samples in open and in controlled form. Extensive instructions for clinical investigations can be found in WITTENBORN (1977) and in LEVINE (1979).

II. Phase I

1. Pharmacokinetics

Using clinical-pharmacological methods, absorption, distribution, half-life, metabolism, and excretion of a drug must be studied in human subjects (usually volunteers, more seldom patients). Currently the emphasis in these investigations lies on the technical-pharmacological side. It is of great importance, however, that even during the earliest clinical-pharmacological studies, the psychic effects observed in subjects or patients be carefully registered and documented. They may possibly contain clues to subsequent clinical indication.

The effective dosage can be determined by means of increasing single doses or multiple doses. Especially in the case of repeated administration, careful laboratory controls of the hemopoietic system and liver functions are indispensible. Today it is generally necessary to develop sensitive assay techniques for a new compound in order to make blood level controls possible.

2. Pharmacodynamics

The investigation in Phase I concerns psychotropic drugs whose effects at the level of objectively observable and subjective behavior of humans can only be predicted within limits based on preclinical screening. For this reason, the exact observation and documentation of subjects on the behavior and the subjective level is essential.

Whereas relatively small subject samples are sufficient for pharmacokinetic studies and the investigation of the metabolism of new drug, it is problematic to test such small numbers of subjects repeatedly with different substances in order to determine psychic effects. Expectations can lead to observable effects despite placebo controls; earlier experiences with a certain class of drugs can distort results. For precise details on the psychic effects of a psychotropic substance, for example in the areas of subjective condition, psychomotor performance, cognitive disturbance, memory functions, or vigilance, larger samples of healthy volunteers are necessary (20–30 subjects). The psychotropic effects as compared to placebo are verified and measured quantitatively on these subjects using differentiated psychometric techniques. The study design can call for a single dose or multiple doses in a group comparison with placebo. If the sequence of administration of medication at different dosage levels and of placebo is suitably balanced, an intraindividual comparison of effects is also possible. The advantage of an intraindividual comparison is based on lower interindividual variance. Such a crossover design with a balanced time factor treatment sequence is only adequate in this very early phase involving healthy subjects, but does offer differentiated effect profiles for different substance categories (see HEIMANN, 1974; JANKE, 1965). For certain questions it is even useful to resort to a very small group of subjects (i.e., 10–20) and to select tests which can be repeated frequently in order to reduce the effect of the situational factor (i.e., inner motivation; see HEIMANN and STRAUBE, 1979).

III. Phase II

In this phase, a new drug is to be tested with reference to its possible indications, clinically effective dosage and dosage range, the latency of onset, duration of effect, and side effects. Early in Phase II, these goals dictate that a substance must be tested in an *open experiment* with *increasing doses* and under careful control of effects and side effects as well as laboratory controls on a nonhomogenous patient population. For ethical reasons, children, aged patients, women who may become pregnant, and patients with other organic illnesses are excluded here. This early stage of Phase II is of decisive importance for the discovery of new types of psychotropic effects. It requires particularly broad clinical experience in association with and treatment of psychiatric patients as well as extensive experience in the investigation of psychotropic drugs. In this phase, important observations were made by experienced clinicians during the period of explosive development in psychopharmacology.

Today, investigation is aimed at determining *finer differences* in effect and especially at discovering drugs with less disturbing side effects, as the field of treatment is already populated by numerous effective but not always satisfactory preparations. In this context, the investigator's clincial experience assumes an even more important role. His observations of the first patients tested yield *hypotheses on the psychotropic effect* of a substance. These are subsequently the targets of critical testing. Therefore, it is essential that a new agent be tested by *several very experienced investigators* in this early part of Phase II, and that their observations be painstakingly recorded. In addition to rating scales for the evaluation of psychic effects by the physician, it is also always necessary, in our opinion, to include the *observation of personnel* (free description and/or, for example, the NOSIE scale; HONIGFELD et al., 1976).

For the patient, the primary risk lies in the possibility that the investigational drug could be ineffective or less effective than standard medication. After receiving a full explanation of the investigation he must give his informed consent in written from. In this early planning stage, it is important to keep in mind that a *maximum amount of information* should be extracted from each treatment trial. This means that in addition to clinical observation and documentation, suitable measures should be recorded at all three clinical levels and, if possible, on both biological levels of assessment for psychic syndromes.

If first observations involving psychiatric patients concerning the effectiveness of a drug have yielded hypotheses pointing to a certain type of indication, appropriate methods must be selected to test them. Whereas nonhomogenous samples of psychiatric syndromes were advantageous for the discovery of new treatment hypotheses early in Phase II, at this point the focus must be shifted to *homogenization of sample populations for double-blind tests*. In general, it is necessary for the investigator to begin with open tests in order to convince himself of the efficacy of a drug and of its appropriate dosage range.

In double-blind tests the diagnoses, syndromes, and symptoms of the hospitalized patients must be documented with particular care. *Random assignment of the test preparation and placebo or reference drug is indispensable*. The key to this assignment may only be provided after completion of the clinical trial. This is particularly important, as such information, when accessible during an investigation, can influence subsequent judgment. The appropriate size of experimental groups for antidepressants and anxiolytics is at least 30–50 patients; for neuroleptics 60–80. An exact description of the sample must be recorded before starting the experiment in order to facilitate the reliable interpretation of results. This documentation cannot be restricted to the momentary psychiatric diagnosis at commencement of treatment alone, but rather must include the previous case histories and treatment. A washout period of at least 8–10 days, according to the pharmacokinetics of previous medication, must be provided. Unfortunately, this washout period cannot always be observed under the conditions of practice in psychiatric clinics. If it is included, however, it often shows that a number of hospitalized patients, especially those with depressive syndromes, improve spontaneously to such an extent that they should not be included in the controlled double-blind experiment.

Group comparison has proved superior to a cross over design within one patient group for investigations of psychotropic drugs, especially because of the spontaneous course of psychic syndromes and because of possible carry-over effects.

Important is the *control of serum levels*, although experience regarding the relationship of serum concentration to therapeutic efficacy is ambiguous. According to KRAG-SØRENSEN et al. (1976), the serum levels found after *identical* doses are so varied that unintended underdosage or possibly even overdosage may distort the results of a clinical trial (see also SJÖQVIST, 1979). This is especially true when a fixed dose is administered, and for a double-blind test a fixed dose is more expedient than varying dosage within a prescribed range. As a compromise, a double-blind study can begin with a fixed dose and, if the resulting effect is insufficient, follow up with a predetermined dosage increase. The control of serum levels is also useful for the judgment of *compliance*. COPPEN (1976) estimates that one-fifth of all psychiatric patients do not take the prescribed medications as instructed. This naturally depends on individual circumstances, particularly on the motivation and instruction of the staff.

The principle elaborated above for the early stages of Phase II also apply to double-blind studies. Namely, *side effect* and *laboratory controls* must be executed with particular care. For the study of anxiolytics and minor tranquilizers a test duration of 2–4 weeks, for antidepressants 3–4 weeks, and for neuroleptics at least 4 weeks and preferably 6–8 weeks should be observed.

A special problem is that of dropouts. They must be conscientiously documented. Records must include reasons for termination, which can be very rapid and complete recovery (possibly an effect independent of medication) or ineffectiveness of or intolerance to a substance.

The question of a placebo control in double-blind studies with psychiatric patients is particularly controversial. From a methodological point of view this control is necessary, as the comparison with a standard drug *does not allow the conclusion of equal effectiveness* when investigational substance and standard medication produce the same success rate. This point is illustrated in the following example. Depending on the size of the sample, when the placebo rate for depressive patients is 30%, the success rate of a reference drug 70%, and that of the study drug 50%, the difference between standard drug and new drug can be statistically nonsignificant, while the standard drug and the placebo can exhibit a significant difference in effect. Because of factors (discussed in the first section) complicating the clinical investigation of psychotropic effects, such a type II error is particularly likely. Unfortunately, the ability to discriminate between the effect of the drug and that of the placebo as well as between the two effective substances at the clinical level remains restricted. Especially in the case of antidepressants, however, a placebo comparison is at present practically unfeasible.

For reasons of medical ethics at least those depressive patients in clinical treatment, i.e., with marked depression and high suicide risk, cannot be assigned to the less effective placebo group.

The *evaluation of treatment effect* takes place using rating scales. As a baseline, two ratings should be made during the washout period. Thereafter, ratings should be carried out at least weekly. The intervals between ratings must be determined beforehand and strictly observed. In the course of the experiment, the same raters should always judge the patients condition.

We cannot treat details of *statistical analysis* here. The precise quantitative description of the cases, for which various calculation procedures have been proposed (cf. WITTENBORN, 1977; LEVINE, 1979; FERNER, 1977), is not sufficient. A global rating and rank ordering of treatment success in each case should also occur. This is important because significant differences at the item or syndrome level do not always correspond to an improvement with relevance for the patient (compare Sect. C).

IV. Phase III

Guided by the hypotheses obtained up to this point, Phase III of the investigation is primarily concerned with comparative studies involving a larger patient sample and aiming at confirmation of the indication. Furthermore, the safety of long-term medication (3–6 months) and finally the clarification of particular effect mechanisms and implications must be established.

As the results of Phase II allow a fairly reliable estimation of the efficacy of the investigational drug, the sample population can now be broadened in Phase III to include women of child-bearing potential, patients with organic diseases and perhaps also with concurrent medication, children, and aged patients. These groups must be evaluated separately as to age, socioeconomic status, special treatment situations, etc. The various treatment groups should be as homogenous as possible. Group size should roughly equal that in the latter stage of Phase II.

As a rule, the experimental design selected for this stage should be *double-blind*, as in late Phase II. If possible, interactions with other substances should be controlled for, and special treatment conditions as well as out-patient treatment should be studied. In Phase III, *multicenter studies* are preferable. The planning must be just as conscientious as in Phase II. However, psychiatric institutions whose staffing does not allow the investment of the methodological effort necessary in the previous phases can also collaborate here. During interpretation, not only global results but also results in the individual treatment groups should receive consideration, as such comparisons often uncover interesting differences. When possible, the double-blind test should include a placebo condition.

The experiments in this phase involving long-term treatment with a study drug should allow the evaluation of administration under in-patient and out-patient conditions. The documentation of cases, including diagnosis, syndrome, symptoms, and assessment devices, can now be substantially simplified. However, sufficient laboratory controls are necessary in all cases, particularly when treatment continues over several months, as the administration of the test preparation to a larger population allows the discovery of rare treatment complications.

C. Special Problems

I. Introduction

In the first section we discussed *general* difficulties encountered in trials with psychotropic substances. We shall now try to provide at least a few insights into some questions left open for future research. For example, from the standpoint of pharmacological effect alone, numerous circumstances actually present in the treatment of psychiatric patients appear as *interfering factors*. Also, the *quantification* of descriptive methodology for the evaluation of psychic effects is not satisfactory and demands improvement. Here, various parameters involved in the formation of an evaluation must be considered. Finally, the *conditions* of a *double-blind comparison* with a placebo or with a reference substance also raise critical questions. In particular, the investigational strategy now widely adopted is suitable for delivering proof of effectiveness and for judging the safety of a medication. This strategy is based on a therapeutic experiment with a large sample under double-blind conditions. However, because a large number of patients with relatively uniform overt symptomatology are included in the sample, a new problem is created. As we know, very different pathogenetic of pathophysiological states can underlie one and the same psychic manifestation. For this reason, therapy failures achieve particular importance, as long as the patients concerned have received sufficient doses. Their comparison with successful cases is extremely valuable. In other words, the extreme cases in a treatment experiment are of particular interest to the researcher. The question arises as to whether careful single case studies in these extreme groups should not be carried out in addition to the necessary investigation based on group statistics. These single case studies would have to be conducted in great detail over extended periods of time, demanding the investment of considerable additional effort.

II. Interfering Factors

Interfering factors are factors which cannot be attributed directly to the medication. They can be classified into four groups (compare SCHMOCKER, 1977; BUSCH, 1977) according to their sources: a) those that concern the *patient and his illness directly*, e.g., the spontaneous course of the illness, personality traits, or special previous experiences with medication; b) those concerning the *attending physician*, e.g., his attitude towards pharmacotherapy, his therapeutic ability, and training; c) those relating to the *treatment milieu*, e.g., various conditions of stationary treatment, concurrent psycho- or sociotherapy; and d) those concerning the *private milieu of the patient*, e.g., family situation, existence or nonexistence of a significant other who may influence therapeutic progress. For the evaluation of neuroleptics in acute psychosis, the spontaneous course of the disorder is of primary importance. This also applies to the testing of antidepressants on phasic depressives. Also, the patient's private milieu and socioeconomic circumstances must be considered in the evaluation of these drugs. Particularly in the area of neurotic disorders, these two last-mentioned factors play an important role in the evaluation of anxiolytics and minor tranquilizers. When possible, interfering factors should be recorded and considered in interpretation.

III. Criticism of Quantification

Available rating scales and assessment devices are rough simplifications and schemas of what occurs between the patient and the investigator in a context of social interaction. It is very easy to demonstrate that those behavior patterns of psychiatric patients which are recorded as identical items on such scales often have different meanings for different patients. If one applies several quantitative evaluation instruments to one patient, for instance, and correlates the scores obtained before and after treatment, it can be shown that different rating scales tap varying aspects of information at different points in time. The intercorrelation between scores is generally lower before than after treatment (compare *Heimann* and *Schmocker*, 1974; HEIMANN, 1977). These differences are not caused by variations in distribution, but rather by qualitatively different information components entering into the quantitative description.

The necessary repeated assessment with the same instrument before, during, and at the end of treatment also poses special problems when psychic syndromes are concerned. There exists a *time series effect* in the sense that for the observer, "improvement" can be induced, especially when his contact with the patient improves. On the other hand, schizophrenic patients incapable of communicating certain pathological experiences at the onset of treatment may become able to do so as neuroleptics take effect or as their contact with the investigator improves.

These questions can be summarized under the concept of the *observer parameter*, referring primarily to the problems of rating scales and time series effects. In the first area, systematic training can reduce error, as reliability studies using video recordings of patient interviews have shown. In order to enable the investigator to adhere strictly to the conventions of description, examples illustrating the symptoms and items on a rating scale must be presented during training. Even so, the limit of training is soon reached. This limit is rooted in the second parameter: in *the symptom or the item itself as it refers to a patient sample*. The time series effect can be reduced, as RENFORDT and BUSCH (1976) and BOBON (1978) have demonstrated, by making video recordings of interviews showing the patient's current condition. These recordings are subsequently presented to the raters in *random order*.

Every descriptive symptom contains a certain *semantic ambiguity*, not only for the observer but above all for the patient himself. This can most easily be proved by analyzing the *self-report inventories* which have been developed to measure anxiety and depression. We were able to demonstrate that depressed patients are *not capable of reliably discriminating between subjective anxiety and depression in their own experience*. The correlation between the results of a self-report anxiety scale and a depression inventory is greater than $r = 0.9$ (HEIMANN and GIEDKE, to be published). A trained observer, however, was able to discriminate between the anxiety and the depression items on the Hamilton scale with reasonable accuracy, as confirmed by comparison with the patients' psychophysiological arousal niveau (spontaneous fluctuations in skin resistance). It should also be noted that the *frequency distributions of symptoms or items* in a patient sample can vary considerably. Some items are relatively scarce, but have the reputation of being quite specific to certain states of illness. On the other hand, there are items which exhibit a fairly nonspecific distribution over all diagnostic groups. Furthermore, there are items or symptoms which show marked quantitative increments corresponding to the severity of the disorder, whereas others remain relatively constant in degree. One must consider all of these aspects in order to understand that psychiatric scales using single items or symptoms *as units* which can be utilized in factor analysis or other statistical procedures are really nothing more than rough schemas.

Finally, too little research has been devoted to the question of whether or not the *psychopathological manifestations* of a patient as reflected in rating scores are really relevant to *practical use*, i.e., to the evaluation of therapeutic effect. In any case it is necessary to investigate this question for the various psychiatric syndromes. It is possible that in chronic schizophrenia, for instance, a certain measure of psychotic behavior is a better basis for eventual reintegration in society than the neuroleptic suppression of all psychotic phenomena, especially when lethargy and apathy are the price which must be paid.

IV. Double-Blind Conditions

There currently exists a general consensus that the effectiveness and safety of a psychoactive drug as compared to a placebo or a referent drug can only be assessed in a double-blind design. Furthermore, this is only possible when a strictly random assignment of subjects to experimental groups takes place. Besides the fact that various ethical objections can be made to this procedure, one must also consider the problem of testing whether or not this condition has actually been met. On the one hand this is not always feasible because of possible side effects (e.g., extrapyramidal symptoms in the case of neuroleptics). On the other hand there are also prejudices among physicians, as some believe that double-blind conditions are impossible with certain drugs. In a comparison between amitriptyline and maprotiline on depressive patients, for instance, it was contested that the double-blind conditions could not be met because amitriptyline sedates more heavily. Nevertheless, the double-blind study was conducted and observers were unable to identify the different substances during the experiment.

Finally, double-blind comparisons involving larger patient samples deliver only relatively global results for a particular indication. The success rate is generally about 70%. Replications of double-blind studies yield similar results at best, i.e., they can confirm the effectiveness, but if samples were selected only on the basis of clinical criteria, they cannot answer the question of which drug is the right one for a certain patient. For example, the failure of an antidepressive therapy cannot be predicted on the basis of the momentary symptomatic manifestations at the onset of treatment (compare ANGST et al., 1974). For this reason it is necessary to conduct double-blind studies on subgroups selected on the basis of such biological aspects as psychophysiological reactivity or special clinical-biochemical measures. To illustrate this point, it has been shown that depressive patients whose 5-HIAA liquor values indicate normal serotonin brain metabolism cannot be distinguished at the clinical level from those whose serotonin turnover is diminished. This also applies to depressive patients with normal or diminished urinary MHPG levels. Only the group of bipolar depressives exhibits distinct behavior with reference to this biochemical parameter. Therefore, intensive investigations of the extreme groups of so-called therapy responders and non-responders assume special significance. It is the results of such studies which will finally enable us to find criteria for answering the decisive question of which drug is suitable for which patient.

References

Angst, J., Battegay, R., Bente, D., Berner, P., Broesen, W., Cornu, F., Dick, P., Engelmeier, M.P., Heimann, H., Heinrich, K., Helmchen, H., Hippius, H., Pöldinger, W., Schmidlin, P., Schmitt, W., Weis, P.: Das Dokumentations-System der Arbeitsgemeinschaft für Methodik und Dokumentation in der Psychiatrie (AMP). Arzneim. Forsch. (Drug Res.) *19*, 399 (1969)

Angst, J., Baumann, U., Hippius, H., Rothweiler, R.: Clinical aspects of resistance to Imipramin therapy. Pharmacopsychiatry *7*, 211–216 (1974)

Baumann, U.: Diagnostische Differenzierungsfähigkeit von Psychopathologie-Skalen. Arch. Psychiat. Nervenkr. *219*, 89–103 (1974)

Bente, D.: Vigilanz: Psychophysiologische Aspekte. Verh. Deut. Ges. Inn. Med. *83*, 945–952 (1977)

Bente, D., Frick, K., Lewinsky, M., Penning, J., Scheuler, W.: Signalanalytische Untersuchungen zur Wirkung des Andidepressivums Nomifensin auf das EEG gesunder Probanden. Arzneim. Forsch. *26*, 1120–1125 (1976)

Bobon, D.P.: Time-blind evaluation of psychopathology in drug research. Acta. Psychiat. Belg. *78*, 635–645 (1978)

Busch, H.: Kontrolle von Störfaktoren. Zur Kontrolle untersucherabhängiger Störfaktoren bei der klinischen Prüfung. Pharmakopsychiatry *10*, 152–162 (1977)

Cattell, R.B.: Validation and intensification of the sixteen personality factor questionnaire. J. Clin. Psychol. *12*, 205–214 (1956)

CIPS (Collegium Internationale Psychiatriae Scalarum) (Hrsg.): Internationale Skalen für Psychiatrie. Berlin: Sekretariat E., Grethlein 1977

Coppen, A.: Assessment of drugs in schizophrenia. Discussion on basic trial design. Brit. J. Clin. Pharmacol. *3*, 381–383 (1976)

Coursey, R.D., Buchsbaum, M.S., Murphy, D.L.: Platelet MAO activity and evoked potentials in the identification of subjects biologically at risk for psychiatric disorders. Br. J. Psychiatry *134*, 372–381 (1979)

Danckwardt, J.F.: Zur Interaktion von Psychotherapie und Psychopharmakotherapie. Psyche *32*, 111–154 (1978)

Degkwitz, R., Helmchen, H., Kockott, G., Mombour, W. (Hrsg.): Diagnosenschlüssel und Glossar psychiatrischer Krankheiten. Berlin, Heidelberg, New York: Springer 1980

Eggert, D.: Eysenck-Persönlichkeits-Inventar E-P-I. Göttingen: Verlag für Psychologie Dr. C.J. Hogrefe 1973

Eysenck, H.J.: Drug postulates, theoretical deductions, and methodological considerations. In: Drugs and behaviour. Uhr, L., Miller, J.G. (eds.), pp. 352–359. New York, London: Wiley 1960

Fahrenberg, J., Selg, H., Hampel, R.: Das Freiburger Persönlichkeitsinventar (FPI). Göttingen: Verlag für Psychologie Dr. C.J. Hogrefe 1973

Feighner, J.P., Robbings, E., Guze, S.B., Woodruff, R.A., jr., Winokur, G., Murray, R.: Diagnostic criteria for use in psychiatric research. Arch. Gen. Psychiatry *26*, 57–63 (1972)

Ferner, U.: Planung von Psychopharmakaprüfungen. Statistische Aspekte zur Planung von Psychopharmakaprüfungen. Pharmakopsychiatry *10*, 132–139 (1977)

Fisher, S.: The placebo reactor: thesis, antithesis, synthesis and hypothesis. Dis. Nerv. Syst. *28*, 510–515 (1967)

Giedke, H., Bolz, J., Heimann, H.: Evoked potentials, expectancy wave, and skin resistance in depressed patients and healthy controls. Pharmakopsychiatry *13*, 91–101 (1980)

Gillin, J.C., Duncan, W., Pettigsew, K.D., Frankel, B.L., Snyder, F.: Successful separation of depressed, normal, and insomniac subjects by EEG sleep data. Arch. Gen. Psychiatry *36*, 85–90 (1979)

Goodwin, F.K., Potter, W.Z.: Noradrenergic function in affective illness. In: Proceedings of the 11th Congress of the Collegium Internationale Neuro-Psychopharmacologicum, Vienna 1978. Saletu, B., Berner, P., Hollister, L. (eds.), pp. 127–137. Oxford: Pergamon Press 1979
Hamilton, M.: A rating scale for depression. J. Neurol. Neurosurg. Psychiatry *23*, 56–62 (1960)
Heimann, H.: Prüfung psychotroper Substanzen am Menschen. Arzneim. Forsch. (Drug Res.) *24*, 1341–1346 (1974)
Heimann, H.: Pharmakogen induzierte Verhaltensänderungen beim Menschen. In: Anfall – Verhalten – Schmerz. Int. Symp. St. Moritz 1975. Birkmayer, W. (Hrsg.), pp. 217–226. Bern, Stuttgart, Wien: Huber 1976
Heimann, H.: Wirkung von Psychopharmaka und zugrundeliegende theoretische Vorstellungen. Pharmakopsychiatry *10*, 119–129 (1977)
Heimann, H.: Psychophysiologie endogener Psychosen. Schweiz. Arch. Neurol. Neurochir. Psychiatry *125*, 231–252 (1979)
Heimann, H., Giedke, H.: Psychophysiology of anxiety, fear and phobia. 11th C.I.N.P. Congress, Vienna July 9–14 (1978). Progress in Neuro-Psychopharmacology (to be published)
Heimann, H., Schmocker, A.M.: Zur Problematik der Beurteilung des Schweregrades psychiatrischer Zustandsbilder. Arzneim. Forsch. (Drug Res.) *24*, 1004–1006 (1974)
Heimann, H., Straube, E.: Personality and arousal. Systematic modification with d-Amphetamine and Phenobarbital. In: Pharmacology of the states of alertness. Passouant, P. (ed.), pp. 179–188. Oxford, New York: Pergamon Press 1979
Honigfeld, G., Gillis, R.D., Klett, C.J.: NOSIE. Nurses' observation scale for in-patient evaluation. In: ECDEU assessment manual for psychopharmacology. Guy, W. (ed.), pp. 265–273. Maryland: Rev. Ed. Rockville 1976
Itil, T.M.: Quantitative pharmaco-electroencephalography. In: Psychotropic drugs and the human EEG. Modern problems in pharmacopsychiatry. Itil, T. (ed.), vol. 8, pp. 43–75. New York: Karger 1974
Janke, W.: Über einige methodische Probleme bei pharmako-psychologischen Untersuchungen mit Tranquilantien, Neuroleptika und Sedativa. Arch. Ges. Psychol. *117*, 107–117 (1965)
Janke, W., Glathe, H.: Experimentelle Untersuchungen zur psychischen Wirkung von Sedativa unter Normal- und Belastungsbedingungen. Psychol. Forsch. *27*, 377–402 (1964)
Janke, W., Debus, G., Longer, N.: Differential psychopharmacology of tranquilizing and sedating drugs. In: Differential psychopharmacology of anxiolytics and sedatives. Boissier, J.-R. (ed.), vol. 14, pp. 13–98. Basel: Karger 1979
Knorring, L. von, Perris, C., Ross, S.B.: Serum Dopamine-β-hydroxylase and the augmenting-reducing response. Biol. Psychiatry *3*, 397–405 (1980)
Kragh-Sørensen, P., Hansen, C.E., Baastrup, P.C., Hvidberg, E.F.: Self-inhibiting action of Nortriptylin's antidepressive effect at high plasma levels: a randomized double-blind study controlled by plasma concentrations in patients with endogenous depression. Psychopharmacology *45*, 305–312 (1976)
Laakmann, G.: Neuroendocrine differences between endogenous and neurotic depression as seen in stimulation of growth hormone secretion. In: Neuroendocrine correlates in neurology and psychiatry. Müller, E.E., Agnoli, A. (eds.), pp. 263–271. Amsterdam, New York, Oxford: Elsevier/North Holland Biomedical Press 1979
Lader, M.: The psychophysiology of mental illness. London, Boston: Routledge & Kegan Paul 1975
Langer, G., Heinze, G., Reim, B., Matussek, N.: Reduced growth hormone responses to Amphetamine in endogenous depressive patients. Arch. Gen. Psychiatry *33*, 1471–1475 (1976)
Legewie, H.: Persönlichkeitstheorie und Psychopharmaka. Kritische Untersuchungen zu Eysencks Drogenpostulat. Meisenheim (Glan): A. Hain 1968
Levine, J.: Coordinating clinical trials in psychopharmacology: planning, documentation, and analysis. DHEW Publication No. (ADM) 79–803. Washington D.C.: U.S. Government Printing Office 1979
Lorr, M.: In-patient multidimensional psychiatric scale. Palo Alto, Calif.: Consulting Psychologists Press 1963
Maas, J.W.: Biogenic amines and depression. Biochemical and pharmacological separation of two types of depression. Arch. Gen. Psychiatry *32*, 1357–1361 (1975)

Matussek, N.: Neuroendokrinologische Untersuchungen bei depressiven Syndromen. Nervenarzt *49*, 569–575 (1978)

May, P.R.A.: When, What and Why? Psychopharmacotherapie and other treatments in schizophrenia. Comprehens. Psychiatry *17*, 683–693 (1976)

Overall, J.E., Gorham, D.R.: The brief psychiatric rating scale. Psychol. Rep. *10*, 799–812 (1962)

Pietzcker, A., Gebhardt, R., Freudenthal, K.: Ein Vergleich nosologisch-diagnostischer mit cluster-analytisch gefundenen Gruppen anhand AMP-dokumentierter psychopathologischer Befunde. Nervenarzt *48*, 276–282 (1977)

Praag, H.M. van: Towards a biochemical typology of depression. Pharmakopsychiatry *7*, 281–292 (1974)

Praag, H.M. van: Significance of biochemical parameters in the diagnosis, treatment, and prevention of depressive disorders. Biol. Psychiatry *12*, 101–131 (1977)

Reed, C.F., Witt, P.N.: Factors contributing to unexpected reactions in two human drug placebo experiments. Confin. Psychiatry (Basel) *8*, 57–68 (1968)

Renfordt, E., Busch, H.: Time-blind analysis of TV-stored interviews. An objective method to study antidepressive drug-effects. Int. Psychopharmacopsychiatry *11*, 129–134 (1976)

Rüger, M.: Kombinationen von psychiatrischer Pharmakotherapie und Psychotherapie. Nervenarzt *50*, 491–500 (1979)

Sachar, E.G., Finkelstein, J., Hellmann, L.: Growth hormone responses in depressive illness. I. Response to insuline tolerance test. Arch. Gen. Psychiatry *25*, 263–269 (1971)

Saletu, B.: Psychopharmaka, Gehirntätigkeit und Schlaf. Basel, München, Paris, London, New York, Sydney: S. Karger, 1976

Sarwer-Foner, G.J., Kerenyi, A.B.: Accumulated experience with transference and countertransference aspects of the psychotropic drugs 1953–1960. In: Neuropsychopharmacology. Rothlin, E. (Hrsg.), pp. 385–391. Amsterdam: Elsevier 1961

Schildkraut, J.J., Orsulak, P.J., LaBrie, R.A., Schatzberg, A.F., Gudeman, J.E., Cole, J.O, Rohde, W.A.: Toward a biochemical classification of depressive disorders. II. Application of multivariate discriminant function analysis to data on urinary catecholamines and metabolites. Arch. Gen. Psychiatry *35*, 1436–1439 (1978)

Schmocker, A.M.: Kontrolle von Störfaktoren. Pharmakopsychiatry *10*, 149–151 (1977)

Shapiro, A.K.: Semantics of the placebo. The psychiatric quarterly. State Hospitals Press, Utica, N.Y., October 1968

Sjöqvist, F.: Monitoring of antidepressant drug plasma levels: the next ten years. Progr. Neuro-Psychopharmacol. *3*, 201–210 (1979)

Straube, E.: Reduced reactivity and psychopathology. Examples for research on schizophrenia. In: Functional states of the brain: Their determinants. Koukkou, M., Lehmann, D., Angst, J. (eds.), pp. 291–307. Amsterdam: Elsevier 1980

Sulz-Blume, B., Sulz, K.D., von Cranach, M.: Zur Stabilität der Faktoren-Struktur der AMDP-Skala. Arch. Psychiat. Nervenkr. *227*, 353–366 (1979)

Sutton, S., Tueting, P.: Evoked potentials and diagnosis. In: Critical issues in psychiatric diagnosis. Spitzer, R.L., Klein, D.F. (eds.), pp 265–279. New York: Raven Press 1978

Terenius, L., Wahlström, A.: Endorphins in psychotropic drug action. In: Biochemical clinical pharmacology. J.P. Tillement (ed.), pp. 59–67. Oxford: Pergamon Press 1979

Timsit-Berthier, M., Delannoy, J., Komincky, N., Rousseau, J.C.: Slow potential changes in psychiatry. I. Contingent negative variation. Electroenceph. Clin. Neurophysiol. *35*, 355–361 (1973)

Wittenborn, J.R.: Mannual: Wittenborn psychiatric rating scales. New York: Psychological Corporation 1955

Wittenborn, J.R.: Guidelines for clinical trials of psychotropic drugs. Pharmakopsychiat. Neuro-Psychopharmakol. *10*, 205–231 (1977)

Zbinden, G.: Progress in toxikology, vol. 2. Berlin, Heidelberg, New York: Springer 1976

CHAPTER 19

An International Convention on the Control of Psychotropic Substances

H. HALBACH

The "Convention on Psychotropic Substances, 1971" (in the following designated as "the Convention") was initiated by the United Nations' Commission on Narcotic Drugs, a functional commission of the Economic and Social Council, and the Expert Committee on Drug Dependence of the World Health Organization (WHO) because of the legal difficulty in controlling drugs other than those of the morphine, cocaine or cannabis type under the existing international conventions on narcotics control.

According to its preamble, the intent of the Convention is to prevent and combat the adverse effect on public health and the social problems resulting from the abuse of psychotropic substances, and the illicit traffic connected with such abuse, through rigorous measures designed to restrict their use to legitimate medical purposes. At the same time the Convention recognizes that the availability of the drugs so controlled for medical and scientific purposes should not be unduly restricted.

The public health and social problems arising from drug dependence and abuse which the Covention purports to combat must be delineated. In its attempt to do so the WHO Expert Committee [1] stated:

"If such a drug abuse or dependence is likely to be, or is known to be, only sporadic or infrequent in the population, if there is little danger of its spread to others, and if its adverse effects are likely to be, or are known to be, limited to the individual user, there is no public health problem. ... On the other hand, if the drug dependence is associated with behavioural or other responses that adversely affect the user's interpersonal relations or cause adverse physical, social, or economic consequences to others as well as to himself, and if the problem is actually widespread in the population or has a significant potential for becoming widespread, then a public health problem does exist."

The Convention does not qualify nor quantify the public health and social problems except by stating that "there is sufficient evidence that the substance is being or is likely to be, abused so as to constitute a public health and social problem warranting the placing of the substance under international control."

To the extent that social problems and those of public health are often linked and in view of the definition of health in the WHO Constitution as "a state of complete physical, mental, and social well being" it is understood that the WHO must make an appraisal of the overall consequences of drug taking before it recommends to the Commission on Narcotic Drugs to control the drug in question by adding it to one of four lists (so-called schedules) providing for graded measures of control. The ulti-

1 WHO Technical Report Series, No. 407, 1969, pp. 6–7

mate decision is left to the Narcotics Commission. Changes in the control status of a drug or its removal from control are handled in the same way.

The objective of the Convention is not to control any psychotropic substance likely to lead to adverse effects on public health and to social problems through abuse, but only those which are capable of producing "(1) a state of dependence and (2) central nervous system stimulation or depression resulting in hallucinations or disturbances in motor function or thinking or behavior or perception or mood." This and some other formulations in the Convention are the result of diplomatic rather than scientific disputes between the states signatories of the Convention.

Evidence of the capacity to produce the effects enumerated under clauses (1) and (2) above is, however, not required if the incriminated substance can produce "similar abuse and similar ill effects" as a substance already controlled by the Convention. A finding regarding similarity will normally require a detailed investigation of the dependence-producing and psychic or behavioral effects. The reason for including the alternative criterion of similarity was the desire to cover substances which might not produce a clear state of dependence (such as certain hallucinogens), but are nevertheless abused.

The recognition by the Convention of the production of dependence as a major criterion will preclude the control of psychotoxic substances without dependence-producing properties.

The criteria regarding dependence and certain psychic and behavioral effects as well as the criterion of similarity provide for the possibility of covering new types of substances different from those envisaged by the Convention at its inception. This distinguishes the Convention from the earlier international treaties on narcotics control which are applicable to three categories of drugs only, i.e., those of the morphine, cocaine, and cannabis type. Candidates for possible future coverage by the Convention would be alcohol (ethanol) and khat (catha edulis), since they fulfill the criteria for control. Whether such control is warranted would depend on its appropriateness and practicability.

The Convention requires evidence of the dependence-producing properties of a drug and of its abuse "already occurring" or "likely to occur."

The state of dependence, whether physical (physiological) or psychic (psychological) in origin and outcome, is the result of an interaction between a chemical and an organism (human or animal). Dependence is thus a biological phenomenon amenable to scientific experimental investigation and describable in adequate biological terms. Hence, the dependence-producing potential of a drug can be tested.

In contrast, the actual abuse of a dependence-producing drug occurs in response to an interplay of a wide range of personal and environmental factors of, inter alia, a psychological, anthropological, sociological, cultural, and economic nature. The resultant abusive behavior and the consequences of such abuse for the individual and society must be the subjects of an evaluation that takes into account the pharmacological and above all the dependence-producing properties of the substance in question. In the absence of reproducibility, evaluation is a less precise, less reliable, and less conclusive procedure than pharmacologic testing. Confronted with this situation and the desirable preventive function of the Convention, a decision regarding control, especially of a new substance, will have to rely heavily on estimates inferred from data obtainable through the testing of its psychopharmacologic properties.

Finally, the control status of a drug will depend on the balance between the risks of its abuse and its therapeutic benefits, in order not to limit unduly its availability for legitimate medical purposes by way of too stringent control measures.

Current pharmacologic approaches towards establishing, as required by the Convention, the dependence potential and therapeutic usefulness of a psychotropic substance have been outlined by the WHO Expert Committee on Drug Dependence in its 21st report: WHO Technical Report Series, No. 618, 1978, pp. 10–25; 30–32. In the following the relevant parts of this report are reproduced with the gratefully acknowledged permission of the World Health Organization.

3. ANIMAL STUDIES ON PSYCHOTROPIC AND DEPENDENCE-PRODUCING DRUGS

3.1. General pharmacology and toxicology

To be relevant to the problem of abuse the study of a psychotropic substance in animals must be designed to demonstrate a specific profile of effects, including the overall side-effects and toxic effects. The specific effects that are to be searched for correspond, at least in part, to the drug's potential psychic toxicity and potential therapeutic properties; the balance between these two is one of the major bases for the evaluation of the drug. As some relevant effects of known psychotropic drugs are not present or not pronounced in all laboratory animals, it is essential to use the appropriate animal species and strain for studying these effects. Several routes of administration may be used.

3.1.1. Single-dose studies

Numerous techniques are available in single-dose studies, ranging from the simple observation of locomotor disturbances and abnormal movements and postures to examinations of specific sensory or motor systems. Changes in sexual function, appetite, vigilance, arousal, and the performance of learnt activities should be observed and physiological effects should be studied by means of electrocardiography, electroencephalography, and the measurement of heart rate, blood pressure, temperature, respiration, and pupillary changes. Further information might be obtained from biochemical investigations – in particular, the determination of the levels and turnover of biogenic amines and other brain components and the affinity of some psychotropic drug, such as lysergide, for specific receptors.

The profile determined in the acute studies might permit the drug in question to be assigned to an already well characterized class of drugs. The psychotropic drugs scheduled in the 1971 Convention belong to the following classes:

(1) hallucinogens of the lysergide, STP, or tetrahydrocannabinol type,

(2) central nervous system (CNS) stimulants of the amphetamine type, and

(3) CNS depressants of the barbiturate and other types.

Phencyclidine, which is also scheduled, displays a mixed profile. Of course, numerous types of psychoactive drugs are not represented in the four schedules of the Convention, e.g., hallucinogens of the belladonna alkaloid type, stimulants of the

MAO-inhibitor type, and depressants of the benzodiazepine type. Furthermore, in the future there will be drugs with differently combined or absolutely new profiles.

The profiles include not only psychotoxic activity but also therapeutically useful activity such as anorexigenic, sleep-inducing, or tranquilizing effects.

The study of general side-effects with conventional methods is also necessary because abuse-liability is affected by their presence or absence. Abuse is less likely to occur, for instance, when the drug in question is irritating or produces diarrhoea.

3.1.2. Multiple-dose studies

Many important characteristics of drugs will be disclosed only in studies with repeated administrations. Some of these studies are conventional, such as the short- and long-term toxicity tests that disclose perturbations in food intake, growth, blood cells, clinical chemistry, histology, etc. Other studies are less conventional, referring more specifically to behavioural disturbances that appear only after repeated administration and are subject to factors such as tolerance or sensitization. For instance, it has been shown that repeated administration of amphetamines can lead to profound behavioural alterations in animals accompanied by irreversible neurochemical and neurophysiological manifestations.

Similarly, conventional teratological and fertility studies are prerequisites for a thorough evaluation of any drug to be used in humans, and particular emphasis should be placed on possible disturbances in the behaviour of the offspring.

Although "rebound" phenomena (e.g., depression following stimulation or vice versa) might sometimes be observed after a single administration, they are much more likely to occur after repeated doses.

3.1.3. Antagonism, cross-tolerance, and interactions

The use of antagonists is often very helpful in determining the profile of a compound. However, the interpretation must be made with caution because there is no antagonist as yet that can be considered specific to one single class of substances scheduled in the Convention (i.e., that will antagonize a given effect only of these substances and not of any other drug). There is also no antagonist that will suppress all the effects of a single psychotropic substance.

When a class of psychotropic drugs displays the phenomenon of tolerance, evidence of cross-tolerance with a new substance under study may be considered one of the most valid criteria for the existence of a close resemblance between the new product and the prototype. It may be difficult, however, to establish the specificity of a particular instance of cross-tolerance. Nevertheless, the use of antagonism and cross-tolerance may be helpful in characterizing mechanisms of action.

Besides drug antagonism and cross-tolerance, other interactions might be worth studying for both scientific and practical reasons. These include the interactions between psychotropic drugs and ethanol, between barbiturates and amphetamines, and between reserpine and amphetamines.

3.1.4. Pharmacokinetics

The determination of the pharmacokinetics of a psychotropic substance given by one or several routes is essential for the design of experiments involving repeated administrations and for predicting the dependence potential. Naturally, the time course of absorption, distribution, and excretion depends not only on the chemical constitution of a given drug but also on its physical characteristics (solubility, polarity, etc.) and the kind of formulation. Drugs that remain in the body for long periods of time might present special hazards. The drugs most likely to produce dependence are those whose effects have a rapid onset. The choice of the appropriate animal species for dependence studies on particular drugs can be based on such factors as pharmacokinetic and pharmacodynamic similarity to man, susceptibility to the substance, and availability of valid methods. However, when these factors are not well known the use of a variety of animal species is of great importance.

A report by a WHO scientific group on the bioavailability of drugs provides further information on this subject.

3.1.5. Environmental factors

The effects of psychotropic drugs may be influenced by environmental and even social factors. For instance, temperature, temporal rhythm, and the size and nature of the cage have been shown to modify the intensity and duration of various stimulatory or depressant phenomena. The effects of psychotropic drugs on learnt behaviour is, to a great extent, determined by the reward contingencies maintaining the behaviour. Typically, crowding increases the toxicity of amphetamine-like drugs in suitable strains of mice. The administration of a psychotropic drug to one member of a monkey colony may profoundly modify the behaviour of the other animals.

3.2. Physical dependence studies

On the basis of many years of study with the opiates, well defined methods have been developed for the assessment of physical dependence in animals. In general the drug under investigation must satisfy two requirements: first, it must have the ability to substitute for a known dependence-producing agent in animals physically dependent on that agent; secondly, it must be capable of inducing primary dependence when administered at the appropriate doses and time intervals for an appropriate period of time. Methods utilizing these principles have been developed for drugs of the sedative-hypnotic class, and these will be discussed in more detail below. A recent symposium[1] has summed up much of the present state of the art. Physical dependence has been definitely established only for central nervous system depressants. The question of physical dependence on drugs of the amphetamine type and on some hallucinogenic substances has still not been completely resolved. The relationship of physical dependence to drug-seeking behaviour has been established for only a few drugs.

3.2.1. Direct induction studies

The production of primary dependence on sedative-hypnotic drugs depends on the proper choice of dose, dosing interval, duration of treatment, and route of admin-

1 Thompson, T., Unna, K.R. (ed.): Predicting the abuse dependence of stimulant and depressant drugs. Baltimore: University Park Press 1977

istration. On termination of drug treatment, withdrawal signs are seen the severity of which depends on the degree of physical dependence. Withdrawal signs for the sedative hypnotics are characterized by hyperirritability, tremor, "delirium", and convulsions. A variety of rating scales have been used in attempts to quantitate the degree and severity of the dependence. The method of Jones and co-workers[1] is probably the most sophisticated and best validated system. On the other hand, the monkey may offer some advantage in the clarity of withdrawal signs.[2] Extensive work in this regard has also been carried out in the cat.[3]

Rodents have not proved to be as useful, although they have the advantage of lower cost. Mention should be made of some newer rodent techniques which, although promising, have not yet been validated. These include schedule-induced polydypsia[4] and continuous intraperitoneal infusion.[5,6]

3.2.2. Substitution studies

For several decades attempts have been made to develop methods for determining whether new drugs would substitute for barbiturates in animals. The first practical method was probably that of Deneau & Weiss,[7] which involved dogs maintained on barbital sodium. Signs and symptoms of withdrawal were semiquantitated, and the ability of the test drug to substitude for barbital was determined. Similar methods have been developed for the monkey,[8] and recently quantitative procedures have been developed for the dog.[9] Procedures using rodents have not been as well validated, although mention should be made of the methods of GOLDSTEIN.[10]

3.3. Self-administration studies

3.3.1. Reinforcing property of drugs

A reinforcing effect on drug-seeking and drug-taking behaviour is an essential property of drugs common to all types of psychotropic substances that produce and/or perpetuate the repeated use of drugs in man. Physical dependence may be regarded as of secondary importance because it does not necessarily develop with all types of dependence-producing psychotropic substances. Laboratory methods of assessing the reinforcing effect of drugs in animals have been developed over the past 15 years and are now being used for the prediction of the dependence potential in man.[11]

1 Jones, B.E., et al.: Psychopharmacologia *47*, 7 (1976)
2 Yanagita, T.: J. Pharmacol. Exp. Ther. *172*, 163 (1970)
3 Okimoto, M., et al.: J. Pharmacol. Exp. Ther. *192*, 555 (1975)
4 Falk, J.L.: Personal communication
5 Teiger, D.G.: J. Pharmacol. Exp. Ther. *190*, 408 (1974)
6 Patrick, G.A., et al.: Proceedings of the Committee on Problems of Drug Dependence. Washington DC: National Research Council, National Academy of Sciences 1976
7 Deneau, G.A., Weiss, S.: Pharmakopsychiatry, Neuro-psychopharmakol. *1*, 270 (1968)
8 Yanagita, T.: J. Pharmacol. Exp. Ther. *185*, 307 (1973)
9 Jones, B.E. et al.: Psychopharmacologia *47*, 7 (1976)
10 Goldstein, D.B.: J. Pharmacol. Exp. Ther. *183*, 14 (1972)
11 Johanson, C.E., Schuster, C.R.: In: Predicting the abuse dependence of stimulant and depressant drugs. Thompson, T., Unna, K.R. (eds.). Baltimore: University Park Press 1977

In these tests conditions are arranged so that a selected behavioural response is followed by the administration of the drug. If the response increases in frequency, the reinforcing effect is said to be positive and the behaviour can be called drug-seeking and/or drug-taking behaviour.

Self-administration techniques have been developed using rats,[1] cats,[2] dogs,[3] and monkeys.[4,5] In most cases the pressing of a lever by the animal activates an infusion pump, and a preset amount of drug solution is delivered to the animal through a permanently implanted catheter. The most widely used route of self-administration is the intravenous route, but other routes such as intragastric[6] and intranasal[7] are also in use for water-insoluble and inhalant forms of drugs.

The use of these techniques has shown that substances abused by man – such as opiates, some synthetic analgesics, cocaine, sedative-hypnotics, alcohol, stimulants, nicotine, and organic solvents – have a reinforcing effect in animals.[7,8,9] No animal studies have demonstrated reinforcing effects with lysergide,[10] and problems exist for Δ^9-tetrahydrocannabinol[11] and methaqualone.[12]

Thus, within the above limitation, the assessment of the reinforcing effect in laboratory animals is believed to be a useful approach for predicting the dependence potential of psychotropic substances in man.

3.3.2. Cross self-administration – "substitution"

Animals are trained to self-administer a prototypic drug intravenously at a dose previously determined to be effective in producing lever-pressing at a significantly higher rate than that for the vehicle. Typically, daily experimental sessions last for several hours, during which the drug is delivered once for every fixed number of responses (e.g., 1, 5, or 10). After establishment of a stable rate and pattern of drug-reinforced responding, a test drug may be substituted for the standard drug. The rate and pattern of response maintained by the test drug are compared with the rate and pattern observed with the standard drug and the vehicle. If the response rate for the test drug is higher than that for the vehicle, the test drug is considered to have a positive reinforcing effect. Tests must be made of a broad range of unit doses (i.e., the dose contained in each infusion) in order to determine whether a drug has positive reinforcing properties.

---

1 Weeks, J.R.: Science *138*, 143 (1962)
2 Balster, R.L. et al.: Psychopharmacologia *46*, 229 (1976)
3 Jones, B.E., Prada, J.: Psychopharmacologia *30*, 1 (1973)
4 Yanagita, T. et al.: Excerpta Med. Int. Congr. Ser. *87*, 453 (1965)
5 Thompson, T., Schuster, C.R.: Psychopharmacologia *5*, 87 (1964)
6 Yanagita, T., Takahashi, S.: J. Pharm. Exp. Ther. *185*, 307 (1973)
7 Yanagita, T.: Jpn. J. Clin. Pharmacol. *1*, 13 (1973)
8 Thompson, T., Unna, K.R. (eds.): Predicting the abuse dependence of stimulant and depressant drugs. Baltimore: University Park Press 1977
9 Deneau, G.A., Inoki, R.: Ann. N. Y. Acad. Sci. *142*, 277 (1967)
10 Yanagita, T.: Bull. Narc. *25* (4), 57 (1973)
11 Kaymakçalan, S.: Bull. Narc. *25* (4), 39 (1973)
12 Yanagita, T.: Personal communication

3.3.3. Continuous self-administration

In this procedure animals are allowed to self-administer drugs, intravenously or by some other route, without dose or time limitation. The experiment is usually started with self-administration of the vehicle for 1–2 weeks to observe the baseline response rate for each animal. The test drug is then substituted. The initial unit dose used is based on results obtained in preliminary tests or in the above-mentioned cross self-administration experiment.

If a significant increase in response rate is generated by the test drug, the experiment is continued for several weeks and the daily dose levels, the drug-taking patterns, and the overt physical and behavioural manifestations of the effects of the drug are observed.[1] If no increase in response rate is seen with the test drug, shifts of unit dose and/or forced programmed administration of the drug for a certain period (e.g., 2 weeks) should be attempted to determine whether the animal will then initiate and maintain self-administration. Withdrawal signs and changes of the response rate may be observed by depriving the animal of the drug for 24–48 h or longer. The use of experimentally naive animals is regarded as an essential part of this experiment for demonstration of the primary reinforcing property of drugs. This procedure permits assessment not only of the reinforcing effect but also of some other properties of drugs, such as behavioural effects and toxicity at the self-regulated dose regimen.

3.3.4. Procedures designed to assess reinforcing efficacy

The mere fact that a drug has a reinforcing effect is not sufficient evidence to predict its abuse liability in man. For that purpose the reinforcing efficacy of the drug must be determined. Several attempts have been made to establish procedures to quantitate the reinforcing effects.

Progressive-ratio procedure. Responding is first established with a standard drug, then the test drug is substituted and the number of responses required for drug reinforcement is systematically increased. The response requirement that the animal fails to meet is called the breaking-point. Results obtained from this procedure have a good predictive value for certain classes of psychotropic drugs.[2, 3]

Choice procedure. This procedure permits the experimental animal to choose between two drug solutions. Animals are trained to choose between a prototypic drug and saline. After initial training, the test drug may be substituted at various doses. Two measures can be derived – the percentage choice of one solution compared with the other and rate of response maintained by the two solutions. This procedure appears to have considerable promise in the rank-ordering of drugs for reinforcement efficacy.[4, 5]

---

1 Johanson, C.E. et al.: Pharmacol. Biochem. Behav. *4*, 45 (1976)
2 Griffiths, J.D. et al.: Psychopharmacologia *43*, 81 (1975)
3 Yanagita, T.: Bull. Narc. *25* (4), 57 (1973)
4 Johanson, C.E., Schuster, C.R.: J. Pharmacol. Exp. Ther. *193*, 676 (1975)
5 Balster, R.L., Schuster, C.R.: Cocaine and other stimulants, p. 571. New York: Plenum 1977

Second-order schedule procedure. Animals are trained to respond on a simple reinforcement schedule in which a brief stimulus (e.g., a light or tone) is presented concurrently with a drug. It is found that the stimulus is able to sustain behaviour even when only intermittently coupled with drug delivery. This procedure has not been applied to the prediction of relative abuse liability of drugs although it has the advantage that extended samples of behaviour leading to drug reinforcement can be maintained with little or no confounding effect of previous drug administration (e.g., earlier the same day).[1]

3.3.5. Importance of other observations during self-administration studies

The possible information obtainable in continuous self-administration experiments concerns the animals' drug-taking patterns, the self-regulated dose levels that are specific to each drug, and the ability of the drug to produce physical and behavioural effects and toxicities at the self-regulated dose regimen. The development of tolerance and physical dependence to a drug can also be observed in continuous self-administration procedures.[2,3]

Although physical dependence is of only secondary importance for prediction of the abuse liability of psychotropic substances, its development is relevant to the prediction of abuse liability when some aversive withdrawal signs (due to physical dependence) intensify drug-seeking behaviour. This has been shown by comparing the reinforcing efficacy in physically dependent and non-dependent monkeys.[4,5]

3.4. Other procedures

3.4.1. Discriminative stimulus techniques

The dependence potential of psychotropic drugs is largely related to their subjective effects, which are qualitative. Drug discrimination studies are based on the hypothesis that the property of psychoactive drugs that enables them to function as discriminative stimuli in animals is analogous to the property responsible for producing subjective effects in man. For the evaluation of the discriminative stimulus properties of drugs, rats or monkeys are trained to make one response following the administration of a prototypic drug in order to obtain a reinforcement (presentation of food or water or termination of shock) and to make a different response following the administration of the drug vehicle. A test drug is judged to produce discriminative stimuli similar to those produced by the training drug if the animals emit the drug-appropriate response following administration of appropriate doses of the test compound.[6] The procedure has been validated for narcotic analgesics as well as analgesics with mixed agonist and narcotic antagonist properties.[1-6]

1 Goldberg, S.R. et al.: Fed. Proc. *34*, 1771 (1975)
2 Deneau, G.A. et al.: Psychopharmacologia *16*, 30 (1969)
3 Johanson, C.E. et al.: Pharmacol. Biochem. Behav. *4*, 45 (1976)
4 Yanagita, T.: Pharmacol. Rev. *27* (4), 503 (1976)
5 Schuster, C.R.: Fed. Proc. *29*, 2 (1970)
6 Schuster, C.R., Balster, R.L.: Adv. Behav. Pharmacol. *1*, 85 (1977)

Discrimination procedures for evaluating psychomotor stimulants have also been developed.[7,8] They permit differentiation between dexamphetamine and levamfetamine as well as between amphetamine-like and other stimulants.

These procedures may be of particular importance when considering hallucinogenic drugs that are not self-administered by animals. Unfortunately, the evaluation of discriminative properties is not as complete for the hallucinogenic drugs as it is for the opiate and stimulant classes of drugs.[9,10,11]

3.4.2. Techniques for evaluating lysergide-like hallucinogens

No positive reinforcing properties have been demonstrated for lysergide-like hallucinogens, but these drugs can nevertheless be identified through the analysis of pharmacological syndromes. For instance, these agents produce head twitching in mice, bizarre behavior in several animal species, and hyperthermia in rabbits.[12] Furthermore, in monkeys they act as negative reinforcers. The "chronic spinal dog" has also proved to be of value for the study of lysergide-like hallucinogens.[13] As in man, lysergide produces in the "chronic spinal dog" pupillary dilation, tachycardia, increased respiratory rate, increased body temperature, facilitation of the hind limb flexor reflex, and evocation of the stepping reflex. When lysergide is administered repeatedly, tolerance develops to some of these effects, and cross-tolerance has been shown to other lysergide-like hallucinogens. Conversely other lysergide-like hallucinogens can induce tolerance as well as cross-tolerance to lysergide. Serotonin and tryptamine antagonists selectively antagonize certain actions of lysergide-like agents.[14] Thus serotonin and tryptamine antagonism may be of value in identifying lysergide-like activity. By means of these procedures, the actions of lysergide and amphetamine can be separated.[1] Validation of some of these procedures for hallucinogens has been made by testing mescaline, psilocin, and

---

1 Shannon, H.E., Holtzman, S.G.: J. Pharmacol. Exp. Ther. *198*, 54 (1976)
2 Kuhn, D.M. et al.: J. Pharmacol. Exp. Ther. *196*, 121 (1976)
3 Colpaert, F.C. et al.: J. Pharmacol. Exp. Ther. *197*, 180 (1976)
4 Holtzman, S.G. et al.: Discriminative properties of narcotic antagonists. In: Discriminative stimulus properties of drugs. Lal, H. (ed.), p. 47. New York: Plenum Press 1977
5 Colpaert, F.C. et al.: Life Sci. *16*, 705 (1975)
6 Hirschhorn, I.D., Rosecrans, J.A.: Psychopharmacologia *47*, 65 (1975)
7 Silverman, P.B., Ho, B.T.: Characterization of discriminative response control by psychomotor stimulants. In: Discriminative stimulus properties of drugs. Lal, H. (ed.), p. 107. New York: Plenum Press 1977
8 Schechter, M.D., Rosecrans, J.A.: Eur. J. Pharmacol. *21*, 212 (1972)
9 Schechter, M.D., Rosecrans, J.A.: Psychopharmacologia *26*, 313 (1972)
10 Winter, J.C.: Fed. Proc. *33*, 1825 (1974)
11 Kuhn, D.M. et al.: Discriminative stimulus properties of hallucinogens: behavioural assay of drug action. In: Discriminative stimulus properties of drugs. Lal, H. (ed.), p. 137. New York: Plenum Press
12 Jacob, J.: Proc. Eur. Soc. Study Drug Toxicity *8*, 59 (1967)
13 Martin, W.R. et al.: Drug Alcohol Depend. *3*, 113 (1978)
14 Jacob, J., Girault, J.M.: Serotonin. In: Body temperature: regulation, drug effects and therapeutic indication. Lomax, P., Schönbaum, E. (eds.). New York: Dekker

STP. These psychotomimetic drugs produce pharmacological profiles predominantly similar to those of lysergide. In addition, several other substituted amphetamine derivatives have been evaluated.[2,3] The problem of classifying these compounds is complex since some have mixed lysergide- and amphetamine-like effects, some have predominantly amphetamine-like effects, and some have effects that resemble neither those of lysergide nor those of dexamphetamine. Despite these problems, the evaluation techniques (including the use of antagonists) show promise of being able to differentiate the various hallucinogenic substances.

4. HUMAN PHARMACOLOGY

4.1. General pharmacology

Prior to any specific evaluation, a careful study to determine the possible range of drug doses – from minimally effective doses to those producing undesirable side-effects – must be carried out in man. Such a study should include complete monitoring of both physiological characteristics (e.g., blood pressure readings, ECG, neurological examination) and behavioural characteristics (e.g., overt signs and symptoms, assessment according to behavioural rating scales). The study must include clinical chemistry and haematology examinations and urinalysis. When possible, both single-dose and multiple-dose studies should be carried out, and both a placebo and a positively acting substance should be included. In the ideal situation, pharmacokinetic data (e.g., half life) may also be obtained.

Information from such studies is invaluable in planning the more complex abuse liability studies described below. In addition, real and potential drug toxicity might be discovered in such studies.

As with all human studies, such experiments should be subject to peer review and the customary constraints and safeguards, based both on common sense and on ethical considerations. Initiation and continuation of subject participation in a study should be voluntary. All subjects should be informed of the purpose of the study and the associated risks and that they are free to withdraw from the study at any time.

4.2. Physical dependence

Long-term administration studies show that certain sedative-hypnotics in large doses produce physical dependence with abstinence syndromes characterized by convulsions and toxic psychosis. The morbidity and possible mortality associated with drug withdrawal preclude the use of this method for the testing of new drugs;

1 Vaupel, D.B. et al.: Pharmacologist *18*, 128 (1976)
2 Vaupel, D.B. et al.: Drug Alcohol Depend. *2*, 45 (1977)
3 Nozaki, M. et al.: Eur. J. Pharmacol. (in press)

however, there is a possibility that some manifestations of withdrawal could be detected after the experimental long-term administration of therapeutic doses.

It was demonstrated many years ago that secobarbital could prevent the toxic psychosis and convulsions associated with the pentobarbital withdrawal syndrome. These results demonstrate that substitution studies with sedative hypnotics can be conducted under experimental conditions. Again the ethical issues associated with high-dose dependence on sedative-hypnotics preclude the use of this method.

In general, the amphetamine-like stimulants and hallucinogens do not produce a significant degree of physical dependence. There is, however, evidence that abrupt withdrawal after long-term administration of a high dose of amphetamine [1] and Δ^9-tetrahydrocannabinol [2] leads to the production of withdrawal signs and symptoms.

4.3. Subjective effects

In doses that may be used therapeutically, dexamphetamine sulfate produces in nontolerant drug abusers a characteristic set of alterations in mood, feeling states, perception, physiological characteristics, and behaviour. One evaluated effect is "euphoria" or feelings of elation, well-being and contentment that are considered by many to be indicative of the ability of dexamphetamine to induce drug-seeking behaviour. A series of experimental studies indicate that a number of other agents produce this characteristic profile of subjective behavioural and physiological effects – e.g., methamphetamine, phenmetrazine, methylphenidate, ephedrine, diethylpropion and phentermine. On the other hand, fenfluramine and chlorphentermine are clearly distinguishable from dexamphetamine. This methodology allows the early identification of agents with amphetamine-like activity.[3]

In near therapeutic doses, pentobarbital also produces a characteristic profile of alterations in mood, perception, feeling states and behaviour in nontolerant drug abusers, as well as a type of euphoria. In addition, pentobarbital facilitates postrotatory nystagmus, a physiological effect useful for bioassay of sedative hypnotics. Limited experimental studies indicate that other agents can produce these pentobarbital-like effects (secobarbital, phenobarbital, and methaqualone) and suggest that this methodology will allow the early identification of agents with pentobarbital-like activity.[4]

Among the hallucinogens, lysergide produces a characteristic syndrome of subjective and physiological effects, to which tolerance develops. Other agents pro-

1 Jaffee, J.H.: In: The pharmacological basis of therapeutics. Goodman, L.S., Gilman, A. (eds.). New York: Macmillan 1975
2 Jones, R.T., Benowitz, N.: In: Pharmacology of marihuana. Braude, M.C., Szara, S. (eds.), vol. 2. New York: Raven Press 1976
3 Martin, W.R. et al.: Clin. Pharmacol. Exp. Ther. *12*, 245 (1971)
4 Jasinski, D.R. et al.: Progress report on studies from the clinical pharmacological section of the Addiction Research Center. Presented at the meeting of the Committee on Problems of Drug Dependence, Cambridge, Massachusetts, July 1977

duce a similar syndrome of lysergide-like subjective and physiological effects and show cross-tolerance in lysergide-tolerant individuals. These agents may also produce a type of euphoria. Other hallucinogens probably produce other distinct syndromes in man. However, there are no experimental studies to demonstrate the utility of the method in classifying these agents for abuse potential. With perhaps the exception of nonpsychotogenic doses of the tetrahydrocannabinols, it is likely that ethical considerations will prevent the experimental study of hallucinogenic drugs in man.

4.4. Behavioural techniques

There have been several investigations of the reinforcing effects of psychotropic drugs in human volunteers allowed to engage in an operant procedure that is reinforced with the delivery of a drug. Alcohol,[1] cannabis,[2] heroin, and pentobarbital[3] function as positive reinforcers. In addition, the behavioural toxicity produced by these self-administered drugs may be evaluated.[2] These operant procedures could assist also in estimating the dependence potential of psychotropic drugs in man.

More recently an attempt has been made to measure the relative reinforcing efficacy of stimulant drugs using a choice procedure.[4] Subjects experience two different drugs; later, they each choose the one they prefer. This procedure shows promise for estimating the relative dependence potential of stimulant drugs. It may be applicable to other classes of psychotropic drugs and may serve as a means of validating prediction based on studies of the reinforcing properties of drugs in animals.

4.5. Relevance of pharmacological and behavioural data to abuse liability

Prediction of the likelihood of abuse and the risks attendant on abuse of psychotropic substances involves four steps. The first step is the accumulation of pharmacological and toxicological data, mostly obtained from animals but some from man. The extent of the studies in man might vary considerably, depending on the properties of the drug in question. The second step is the use of these data to form a judgement on the dependence potential in man. The third step is the prediction of the likelihood that the substances will be abused by certain individuals within a society or culture. This prediction is based not only on the dependence potential of the substances but also on other factors such as the socioeconomic conditions, the availability of the substances, their therapeutic use, and the record of previous drug abuse in the society concerned. However, it is obvious that the pharmacological properties of the substances play a primary role in initiating and/or maintaining drug abuse. In this regard the relative efficacy of the reinforcing effects and the

1 Bigelow, G. et al.: Fed. Proc. *34*, 1785 (1975)
2 Mendelson, J. et al.: J. Pharmacol. Exp. Ther. *198*, 42 (1976)
3 Griffiths, R.R. et al.: J. Pharmacol. Exp. Ther. *197*, 488 (1976)
4 Johanson, C.E., Uhlenuth, E.: Presented at the meeting of the American Psychological Association, 1977

identification of the substances with a particular class of drugs may be of special importance. The fourth step is the prediction of the risk to both the individual and society when the substances are abused. Again this involves factors other than drug properties, but consideration of the following drug properties may be the most logical approach to prediction of the risk of abuse.

(1) A possible reinforcing effect, which would lead to compulsive drug-seeking behavior.

(2) Possible pharmacological effects, which would produce behavioral disorders at a dose level consistent with a self-administered regimen.

(3) Possible toxic effects, which would produce pathological changes at a dose level consistent with a self-administered regimen.

(4) Severity of the withdrawal manifestations including risk to life.

4.6. Decision-making

It is important to recognize that pharmacological techniques necessarily play a predominant role in the scheduling of new psychotropic substances that are being introduced into therapeutics. In the case of an agent that has a pharmacological profile similar to that of a prototypic drug of abuse (e.g., pentobarbital, dexamphetamine, lysergide), a decision to control it can be made with a relative certainty that it has the capacity to be abused. Two provisos must be emphasized, however. First, there is evidence of inherent species differences in reactivity to individual drugs within given classes. Thus some knowledge of the human pharmacology of the drug must be available to validate the techniques used in animals. Secondly, the actual incidence of abuse of an agent is influenced by factors other than its pharmacological properties. Many of these factors are unknown, but it is generally felt that the customs and passing fashions of the particular culture, the availability of the drug, the physicochemical properties of the drug, the type of pharmaceutical preparation, and the abuser's knowledge of the effects of the drug all contribute to the actual incidence of abuse. Thus, certain drugs may have the pharmacological profile of a prototypic drug of high abuse potential, but at any given time or in a particular society their incidence of abuse may be low or nil.

New psychotropic agents developed for their unique therapeutic value will not usually produce pharmacological profiles similar to those of prototypic drugs. This fact constitutes a major problem for the prediction of a new drug's dependence-producing potential. Complications already arise with agents that only partially resemble the prototypic agent or have a mixed profile of effects.

6. ASSESSMENT OF THERAPEUTIC USEFULNESS

In contrast to earlier treaties on the international control of drugs, the Convention on Psychotropic Substances requires from WHO an assessment of the therapeutic usefulness of a substance or preparation notified for control. This requirement responds to the view expressed in the sixteenth report of the WHO Expert Committee on Drug Dependence[1] that "the need, type and degree of international control must be based on two considerations: (*a*) the degree of risk to public health and (*b*) the usefulness of the drug in medical therapy." The drug's usefulness must be weighed against the potential or established risks from its abuse, and the resulting ratio determines both the need for control and the degree of control.

Because of the established therapeutic usefulness and the necessary and legitimate use of many of the drugs included in the schedules of the Convention (and of other drugs that may become candidates for inclusion), the impact of the Convention on medical practice may be greater than that of other international Conventions concerned with drug control. The responsibility of WHO in implementing the Convention is amplified by considerations concerning individual and public health. Thus WHO must make every effort to ensure that the inclusion of drugs in the schedules is justified by the appropriate assessment of the balance between risk and benefit.

In the absence of precise evidence on the criterion for therapeutic usefulness, recourse must be had to reputed usefulness, which reflects the general opinion of practitioners or expert panels. This opinion may change with time or even vary between countries.

With the passage of time therapeutic usefulness itself may be subject to change. For instance, new effects (desired or undesired) may be discovered, and the need for a drug may increase or the drug may become obsolete.

6.1. Therapeutic efficacy and safety

The proof of efficacy and the demonstration of safety should be basic conditions for obtaining permission to launch a drug on to the market. The scientific approach to the evaluation of both efficacy and safety is of recent date. It involves many disciplines, including toxicology, pathology, pharmacology, clinical pharmacology, behavioural science, biopharmacy, biochemistry, and biometrics. General principles for the evaluation of the efficacy and safety of drugs have been formulated by a number of WHO expert groups.[2]

Many governments have accepted the responsibility of ensuring that the drugs made available to doctors and patients comply with established standards of efficacy and safety. To the extent that these responsibilities are discharged appropriately, the basic requirements for the determination of the usefulness of a drug can be presumed to have been fulfilled. In these circumstances WHO would not have to scrutinize the relevant preclinical and clinical data.

The situation is quite different with substances, like some of those in Schedule I of the Convention, which have not been introduced into medical practice (or which have been introduced only in a limited way). In such cases WHO would itself have to engage in studying or possibly generating the documentation needed for the assessment of efficacy and safety and the resultant therapeutic value.

1 WHO Technical Report Series, No. 407, 1969, p. 18
2 WHO Technical Report Series, No. 341, 1966; No. 364, 1967; No. 403, 1968; No. 425, 1969; No. 426, 1969; No 482, 1971; No. 536, 1974; No. 563, 1975.

The consideration of efficacy and safety should not be limited to the study of information available at the time of official approval (registration) and marketing of the drug but should extend to postregistration information such as that resulting from long-term application.

As required by the Convention, a comparison must be made with existing drugs. Differences must be expected in the pharmacological profiles of drugs of similar chemical structure – except those with very minor modifications known not to entail differences in respect of pharmacokinetics or mechanism of action. Even slight structural changes might lead to differences in effects, which again would make it difficult to equate substances of similar chemical structure with regard to their usefulness.

Cases are known where new therapeutic properties and uses were detected in a drug after it had been used in medical practice for some time. For example, methaqualone was developed as an antimalarial drug; later on its value in relieving arthritic pain was discovered. Today methaqualone is used as a hypnotic only. It is conceivable that events might occur in the reverse order – i.e., the initial use of a psychoactive substance might be followed by the discovery of other possibly more valuable therapeutic properties. Such discoveries might be forestalled by too rigid control at an early stage of drug development.

Author Index

Page numbers in *italics* refer to bibliography

Subject Index

Handbook of Experimental Pharmacology

Continuation of "Handbuch der experimentellen Pharmakologie"

Volume 11
Lobelin und Lobeliaalkaloide

Volume 12
Morphin und morphinähnlich wirkende Verbindungen

Volume 14: Part 1
The Adrenocortical Hormones I

Part 2
The Adrenocortical Hormones II

Part 3
The Adrenocortical Hormones III

Volume 16
Erzeugung von Krankheitszuständen durch das Experiment/Experimental Production of Diseases

Part 1
Blut (In Vorbereitung)

Part 2
Atemwege

Part 3
Heart and Circulation

Part 4
Niere, Nierenbecken, Blase

Part 5
Liver

Part 6
Schilddrüse
(In Vorbereitung)

Part 7
Zentralnervensystem

Part 8
Stütz- und Hartgewebe

Part 9
Infektionen I

Part 10
Infektionen II

Part 11A
Infektionen III

Part 11B
Infektionen IV

Part 12
Tumoren I

Part 13
Tumoren II

Part 14
Tumoren III
(In Vorbereitung)

Part 15
Kohlenhydratstoffwechsel, Fieber/ Carbohydrate Metabolism, Fever

Volume 17
Ions alcalino-terreux

Part 1
Systèmes isolés

Part 2
Organismes entiers

Volume 18
Histamine and Anti-Histaminics

Part 1
Histamine. Its Chemistry, Metabolism and Physiological and Pharmacological Actions

Part 2
Histamine II and Anti-Histaminics

Volume 19
5-Hydroxytryptamine and Related Indolealkylamines

Volume 20: Part 1
Pharmacology of Fluorides I

Part 2
Pharmacology of Fluorides II

Volume 21
Beryllium

Volume 22: Part 1
Die Gestagene I

Part 2
Die Gestagene II

Volume 23
Neurohypophysical Hormones and Similar Polypeptides

Volume 24
Diuretica

Springer-Verlag
Berlin
Heidelberg
New York

Handbook of Experimental Pharmacology

Continuation of "Handbuch der experimentellen Pharmakologie"

Springer-Verlag
Berlin
Heidelberg
New York

Volume 25
Bradykinin, Kallidin and Kallikrein

Volume 26
H. Fischer: **Vergleichende Pharmakologie von Überträgersubstanzen in tiersystematischer Darstellung**

Volume 27
Anticoagulantien

Volume 28: Part 1
Concepts in Biochemical Pharmacology I

Part 3
Concepts in Biochemical Pharmacology III

Volume 29
Oral wirksame Antidiabetika

Volume 30
Modern Inhalation Anesthetics

Volume 32: Part 1
Insulin I

Part 2
Insulin II

Volume 34
Secretin, Cholecystokinin, Pancreozymin and Gastrin

Volume 35: Part 1
Androgene I

Part 2
Androgens II and Antiandrogens/ Androgene II und Antiandrogene

Volume 36
Uranium – Plutonium – Transplutonic Elements

Volume 37
Angiotensin

Volume 38: Part 1
Antineoplastic and Immunosuppressive Agents I

Part 2
Antineoplastic and Immunosuppressive Agents II

Volume 39
Antihypertensive Agents

Volume 40
Organic Nitrates

Volume 41
Hypolipidemic Agents

Volume 42
Neuromuscular Junction

Volume 43
Anabolic-Androgenic Steroids

Volume 44
Heme and Hemoproteins

Volume 45: Part 1
Drug Addiction I

Part 2
Drug Addiction II

Volume 46
Fibrinolytics and Antifibrinolytics

Volume 47
Kinetics of Drug Action

Volume 48
Arthropod Venoms

Volume 49
Ergot Alkaloids and Related Compounds

Volume 50: Part 1
Inflammation

Part 2
Anti-Inflammatory Drugs

Volume 51
Uric Acid

Volume 52
Snake Venoms

Volume 53
Pharmacology of Ganglionic Transmission

Volume 54: Part 1
Adrenergic Activators and Inhibitors I

Part 2
Adrenergic Activators and Inhibitors II

Volume 55: Part 1
Antipsychoticcs and Antidepressants I

Part 2
Antipsychotics and Antidepressants II